"This matchless volume offers a defining culturally based neuropsychology resource. We owe deep appreciation to the Editor for assembling an exceptional group of scholars using evidence-based scholarly inquiry and case exemplars from around the world. The experienced authors share their insights and personal reflections in a manner no other text provides. This well-organized text offers practical skills and is a must have for my shelf and yours."

Marc A. Norman, PhD, ABPP-CN
University of California, San Diego, USA

"Not just that we *should* have broader knowledge and awareness, but a place to begin the dive into the impossibly beautiful, complicated intersection of brain and behavior in the context of culture."

Karen Postal, PhD, ABPP-CN
Clinical Instructor in Psychology, Harvard Medical School, Massachusetts, USA

"With elaborate and consistently well-crafted detail, this book addresses the complex and multi-layered topic of cultural diversity, the most timely and important issue confronting clinical neuropsychologists in all parts of the world. International experts deliver impressive and authoritative guidance, including compelling applications of original and widely-used normative data."

Jerry J. Sweet, PhD, ABPP-CN
Emeritus, NorthShore University HealthSystem, Evanston, Illinois, USA

T0386156

Cultural Diversity in Neuropsychological Assessment

Cultural Diversity in Neuropsychological Assessment provides a platform for clinical neuropsychologists, psychologists, and trainees to bridge cultures and speak to each other about the ethnically diverse communities they serve throughout the world. It allows readers to peek into their clinical filing cabinets and examine how they worked with diverse individuals from indigenous and migrant communities of Arab, Asian, European, Israeli, Latin American and Caribbean, Persian, Russian, Sub-Saharan African, and North American origin.

The book first reviews important foundations for working with diverse communities that include key knowledge, awareness, skills, and action orientation. It then provides a collection of cases for each cultural geographic region. Each section begins with an introductory chapter to provide a bird's eye view of the historical and current state of clinical and research practice of neuropsychology in that region. Then, each chapter focuses on a specific community by providing surface and deep-level cultural background knowledge from the authors' unique perspectives. A case study is then covered in depth to practically showcase an evaluation with someone from that community. This is followed by a summary of key strategic points, lessons learned, references, further readings, and a glossary of culture specific terminology used throughout the chapter. In the end, the appendix provides a list of culturally relevant tests and norms for some communities.

This ground-breaking peer-reviewed handbook provides an invaluable clinical resource for neuropsychologists, psychologists, and trainees. It increases self-reflection about multicultural awareness and knowledge, highlights practical ways to increase cultural understanding in neuropsychological and psychological assessments, and sparks further discussion for professional and personal growth in this area.

Dr. Farzin Irani's background includes a PhD from Drexel University, an internship at Brown University, a post-doctoral fellowship at the University of Pennsylvania, and board certification by the American Board of Professional Psychology. She is actively involved in clinical practice, teaching, mentorship, scholarship, service, and advocacy in neuropsychology. She currently serves in leadership positions in several local and national professional organizations including the Asian Neuropsychological Association, Society for Clinical Neuropsychology, American Academy/ Board of Clinical Neuropsychology and the Philadelphia Neuropsychology Society.

Cultural Diversity in Neuropsychological Assessment

Developing Understanding through Global Case Studies

Edited by Farzin Irani
Foreword by Desiree Byrd

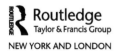
Routledge
Taylor & Francis Group

NEW YORK AND LONDON

Cover image: © Getty Images

First published 2022
by Routledge
605 Third Avenue, New York, NY 10158

and by Routledge
4 Park Square, Milton Park, Abingdon, Oxon, OX14 4RN

*Routledge is an imprint of the Taylor & Francis Group,
an informa business*

Library of Congress Cataloging-in-Publication Data
A catalog record for this title has been requested

ISBN: 9780367509293 (hbk)
ISBN: 9780367509262 (pbk)
ISBN: 9781003051862 (ebk)

DOI: 10.4324/9781003051862

Typeset in Times New Roman
by KnowledgeWorks Global Ltd.

Contents

E. Action

PART II
Case Studies

Black American

Coast Salish Native American

Indigenous Canadian

Overview

Lebanese

Overview

F. Latin America and the Caribbean

List of Contributors

Kristina A. Agbayani, PhD, ABPP-CN
Polytrauma Network Site
VA Palo Alto Health Care System
Palo Alto, CA, USA

Mohammed Alsubaie, MS
Department of Clinical Psychology
Seattle Pacific University
Seattle, WA, USA

Seyed Reza Alvani, PhD
Kashan University of Medical Sciences
    (KAUMS)
Kashan, Iran

Kendra M. Anderson, PhD
Louis A. Faillace, MD, Department of
    Psychiatry and Behavioral Sciences
McGovern Medical School at UTHealth
Houston, Texas 77021, USA

Joseph Arboleda-Velasquez, MD, PhD
Schepens Eye Research Institute,
    Massachusetts Eye and Ear
Harvard Medical School
Boston, MA, USA

Caroline Ba, PsyD
Department of Psychiatry
Virginia Hospital Center, Washington
    School of Psychiatry
Arlington, VA, USA

Eagle Runs Around Bear
Lummi Nation

Katrina E. Belen, PsyD
Licensed Psychologist
Rehabilitation Neuropsychology
Plano, TX 75075, USA

Jacob A. Bentley, PhD, ABPP
Department of Clinical Psychology
Seattle Pacific University
Seattle, WA, USA

Shaquanna Brown, PhD
Postdoctoral Fellow
Department of Psychiatry and Human
    Behavior
Warren Alpert Medical School
    of Brown University, Providence,
    Rhode Island

Carrie Bourassa, PhD
Community Health and Epidemiology,
    Medicine
University of Saskatchewan
Saskatoon, SK, Canada

Lisa Bourke-Bearskin, RN, PhD
School of Nursing
Thompson Rivers University
Kamloops, BC, Canada

Claudia García de la Cadena, PhD
Postgrados y Maestría en Neuropsicología
Departamento de Psicología
Universidad del Valle de Guatemala
Guatemala, Guatemala, Guatemala

(Lic.) Adriana Puente Calzada
Ciudad de Mexico, Mexico

Esther Chin, PhD
Neuropsychology Services
AMITA Health Neurosciences
    Institute/Women and Children's
    Hospital
Elk Grove Village/Hoffman Estates,
    IL, USA

(Lcda) Isis Yahaira Marroquin Jerez de Cifuentes
Maestría en Neuropsicología Clínica
Departamento de Psicología
Universidad del Valle de Guatemala
Guatemala, Guatemala

Kate Cockcroft, PhD
School of Human and Community
Development
Department of Psychology
University of the Witwatersrand
Johannesburg, Gauteng, South Africa

Julia C. Daugherty, PhD
Center for Research on the Mind,
Brain and Behavior
University of Granada
Granada, Andalucía, Spain

Paula Karina Pérez Delgadillo, PsyD
New York University Langone Health
Rusk Rehabilitation, New York, NY, USA

Mirella Díaz-Santos, PhD
Adjunct Assistant Professor
Center for Cognitive Neuroscience
Director of Research
Hispanic Neuropsychiatric Center of
Excellence
Department of Psychiatry and
Biobehavioral Sciences
David Geffen School of Medicine
University of California
Los Angeles, CA, USA

Artemisa R. Dores, PhD
Degree, master, PhD, post PhD, Specialist
in Clinical and Health Psychology,
and Specialist in Neuropsychology
by the Portuguese Psychologists
Association
Center for Rehabilitation Research (CIR),
School of Health, Polytechnic Institute
of Porto (P. Porto), 4200-072
Porto, Portugal
Laboratory of Neuropsychophysiology
Faculty of Psychology and Educational
Sciences of University of Porto, 4200-135
Porto, Portugal

Vonetta M. Dotson, PhD
Department of Psychology and
Gerontology Institute
Georgia State University
Atlanta, GA, USA

Mario F. Dulay Jr., PhD
Department of Neurological Surgery
Houston Methodist Neurological
Institute
Houston, TX, USA

Ahmed F. Fasfous, PhD
Department of Social Sciences
Bethlehem University
Bethlehem, Palestine

Aline Ferreira-Correia, PhD
HPCSA Registered Clinical Psychologist/
Neuropsychologist
Psychology Department
University of the Witwatersrand
Johannesburg, Gauteng, South Africa

Sanne Franzen, MSc
Department of Neurology
Erasmus MC University Medical Center
Rotterdam, the Netherlands

Daryl Fujii, PhD, ABPP-CN
Veterans Affairs Pacific Island Health
Care Services
Honolulu, Hawaii, USA

Andreia Geraldo, PhD candidate
Degree, master, PhD candidate,
Specialist in Clinical and Health
Psychology by the Portuguese
Psychologists Association
Laboratory of Neuropsychophysiology
Faculty of Psychology and Educational
Sciences of University of Porto, 4200-135
Porto, Portugal

Bruno Joseph Giordani, PhD
Department of Psychiatry
The University of Michigan
Ann Arbor, MI, USA

Dov Gold, PsyD
William James College
Newton, MA, USA

Miriam Goudsmit, Clinical psychologist
Department of Psychiatry and Medical
  Psychology
OLVG Hospital
Amsterdam, the Netherlands

Sandra Guerreiro, PhD
Specialist in Clinical and Health Psychology,
  and specialist in Neuropsychology by the
  Portuguese Psychologists Association
CRPG—Centro de Reabilitação Profissional
  de Gaia (CRPG—Gaia Vocational
  Rehabilitation Centre) & Institute of Health
  Sciences
Universidade Católica Portuguesa
Porto, Portugal

Farah Hameed, MD
Department of Rehabilitation and
  Regenerative Medicine
Columbia University Irving Medical
  Center
New York, NY, USA

Anita Herrera Hamilton, PhD, ABPP-CN
Pediatric Neuropsychologist
Department of Pediatrics
Children's Hospital Los Angeles
Assistant Professor
University of Southern California
Keck School of Medicine, Los Angeles,
  CA, USA

Kimi Hashimoto, MS
Department of Clinical Psychology
Seattle Pacific University
Seattle, WA, USA

Yue Hong, PsyD
Neuropsychological Assessment
  Center
Salem Hospital
Salem, MA, USA

Dan Hoofien, PhD
Department of Psychology
The Israeli Academic College at Ramat
  Gan and The Tel Aviv-Jaffa Academic
  College
The Hebrew University of Jerusalem,
  Jerusalem, Israel

Jean N. Ikanga, PhD
Staff Scientist
Department of Rehabilitation Medicine
Division of Neuropsychology
Emory University School of Medicine,
  Atlanta, GA, USA

Farzin Irani, PhD, ABPP-CN
Private Practice (AAA Neuropsychology)
Malvern, PA, USA
West Chester University of Pennsylvania
Department of Psychology (Retired Faculty)
West Chester, PA, USA

Mi-Yeoung Jo, PsyD, ABPP-CN
Independent Practice
Sherman Oaks, CA 91403, USA

Velissa M. Johnson, PhD, ABPP-CN
Pediatric Neuropsychologist
Helen DeVos Children's Hospital—Division of
  Neurosciences
Grand Rapids, Michigan, USA

Tedd Judd, PhD, ABPP-CN
Maestría en Neuropsicología Aplicada
Universidad del Valle de Guatemala
Guatemala, Guatemala
School of Psychology, Family, and Community
Seattle Pacific University
Seattle, WA, USA
Neuropsychological and Psychoeducational
  Services
Bellingham, WA, USA

Sagar S. Lad, PsyD, CSP
Board Certified Specialist in Psychometry
Advanced Psychology Fellow-
  Neuropsychology Specialty
W.G. (Bill) Hefner Veteran Affairs
  Healthcare System
Adjunct Faculty (Neurology)—Wake Forest
  School of Medicine, Winston-Salem, NC,
  USA

Sumaya Laher, PhD
School of Human and Community
  Development
Department of Psychology
University of the Witwatersrand
Johannesburg, Gauteng, South Africa

Sanam J. Lalani, PhD
Department of Psychiatry
Lab of Cognitive Imaging
University of California
San Diego, CA, USA
Lalani Neuropsychology Services
3245 Geary Blvd. #591252
San Francisco, CA, USA

Laiene Olabarrieta Landa, PhD
Departamento de Ciencias de la Salud
Universidad Pública de Navarra
Pamplona, Spain

Juan Carlos Arango Lasprilla, PhD
Biocruces Bizkaia Health Research Institute
Cruces University Hospital
Barakaldo, Spain
Ikerbasque, Basque Foundation for Science
Bilbao, Spain
Department of Cell Biology and Histology
University of the Basque Country
    (UPV/EHU)
Leioa, Spain

Dongwook D. Lee, PhD, ABPP
WCG MedAvante-ProPhase
Hamilton, NJ 08619, USA

David Lerner, PhD, ABN
Independent Practice
Dallas, TX, USA

Jorge J Llibre-Guerra, MD
Department of Neurology
National Institute of Neurology and
    Neurosurgery
La Habana, Cuba
Department of Neurology
Washington University
St Louis, MO, USA

María Jesús Gómez López, PhD
Clínica Uner
Alicante, Spain

Francisco Lopera, MD
Grupo de Neurociencias de Antioquia
Universidad de Antioquia, Medellin,
    Colombia

Beatriz MacDonald, PhD
Department of Pediatrics, Section of
    Psychology
Baylor College of Medicine & Texas
    Children's Hospital
Houston, TX, USA

Lingani Mbakile-Mahlanza, DPsyc
Department of Psychology
Faculty of Social Sciences
University of Botswana
Gaborone, Botswana

Michelle Miranda, PhD, MPH
Department of Neurology
University of Utah
Salt Lake City, Utah, USA

Mansha Mirza, PhD
Department of Occupational
    Therapy
University of Illinois at Chicago
Chicago, IL, USA

Farhiya Mohamed, M.S.W.
Somali Family Safety Task
    Force
Seattle, WA, USA

Maria Soledad Montero, PsyD
University of California,
    Davis
Sacramento, CA, USA

Diana Múnera, BS
Massachusetts General
    Hospital
Harvard Medical School
Boston, MA, USA

Ann T. Nguyễn, MA
Department of Psychology
Loma Linda University
Loma Linda, CA, USA

Christopher Minh Nguyễn, PhD
Department of Psychiatry and
    Behavioral Health
The Ohio State University Wexner
    Medical Center
Columbus, OH, USA

T. Rune Nielsen, PhD
Authorized Psychologist
Danish Dementia Research Center
Copenhagen University Hospital,
    Rigshospitalet
Copenhagen, Denmark

Megan E. O'Connell, PhD, RD Psych
Department of Psychology
University of Saskatchewan
Saskatoon, SK, Canada

Carlos Oliveira, MA
Alliant International University
Sacramento, CA, USA

Rafael E. Oliveras-Rentas, PsyD
School of Behavioral and Brain Sciences
Ponce Health Sciences University
Ponce, Puerto Rico

Cherry Ordoñez, MA
California School of Professional Psychology
Alliant International University
San Francisco Bay Area, CA, USA

June Yu Paltzer, PhD, ABPP-CN
Department of Neurology
UC Davis School of Medicine
Sacramento, CA, USA

Ivan Panyavin, PhD
Department of Psychology
University of Saskatchewan
Saskatoon, SK, Canada

Ana I Peñalver-Guía, MSc
Department of Neurology
National Institute of Neurology and
    Neurosurgery
La Habana, Cuba

Ana Paula Almeida de Pereira, MS, PhD
Department of Psychology
Federal University of Paraná
Curitiba, Paraná, Brazil

Irene Piryatinsky, PhD, ABPP-CN
Board Certified Neuropsychologist Assistant
    Professor of Neurology Tufts University
    School of Medicine
Neuropsychological Assessment
    Clinic at the Brighton Marine
Brighton, MA 02135

Maiko Sakamoto Pomeroy, PhD
Associate Professor, Clinical
    Psychologist/Neuropsychologist
Faculty of Medicine
Saga University, Saga, Japan

Yakeel T. Quiroz, PhD
Grupo de Neurociencias
    de Antioquia
Universidad de Antioquia
Medellin, Colombia
Massachusetts General
    Hospital
Harvard Medical School
Boston, MA, USA

Amir Ramezani, PhD
Private Practice: Center for Cognition
    & Compassion
University of California,
    Davis
VA Whole Health
Pleasanton, CA, USA

Arash Ramezani, BA
Fair Oaks, CA, USA

Diego Rivera, MPH, PhD
Departamento de Ciencias
    de la Salud
Universidad Pública de Navarra
Pamplona, Spain

Walter Rodríguez-Irizarry, PsyD
Department of Social Sciences and
    Humanities, Interamerican University
    of Puerto Rico, San Germán
    Campus
San German, Puerto Rico
School of Behavioral & Brain
    Sciences, Ponce Health Sciences
    University
Ponce, Puerto Rico

Ana M Rodriguez-Salgado, MSc
Department of Neurology, National
    Institute of Neurology and
    Neurosurgery, 29 y D Vedado
La Habana, Cuba
Global Brain Health Institute, University of
    California
San Francisco, CA, USA

Regilda Anne A. Romero, PhD
Division of Psychology
Department of Psychiatry
University of Florida
Gainesville, FL, USA

Orlando Sánchez, PhD
Mental Health Service Line,
    Veterans Affairs Puget Sound
    Health Care System—American
    Lake Division
Tacoma, WA, USA
Department of Psychiatry and Behavioral
    Sciences
University of Washington
Seattle, WA, USA
Maestría en Neuropsicología
    Aplicada
Universidad del Valle de
    Guatemala
Guatemala, Guatemala

Ana Linda Diaz Santos, PsyD
Neuropsychology Postdoctoral
    Fellow, Spanish/Cross-Cultural
    Track
Department of Neurology
Baylor College of Medicine
Houston, TX, USA

Dorothee Schoemaker, PhD
Massachusetts General Hospital
Harvard Medical School
Boston, MA, USA
Schepens Eye Research Institute,
    Massachusetts Eye and Ear
Harvard Medical School
Boston, MA, USA

**Mathew Staios, Master of Clinical
    Neuropsychology**
PhD Candidate
Turner Institute for Brain and Mental Health
School of Psychological Sciences
Monash University, Melbourne, Australia

Anthony Y. Stringer, PhD, ABPP-CN
Department of Rehabilitation Medicine
Emory University
Atlanta, GA, USA

Adriana M. Strutt, PhD, ABPP-CN
Department of Neurology
Baylor College of Medicine
Houston, TX, USA
Maestria en Neuropsicología Aplicada
Universidad del Valle de Guatemala
Guatemala, Guatemala

Rex M. Swanda, PhD, ABPP-CN
Private Practice
Albuquerque, New Mexico

Nicholas S. Thaler, PhD, ABPP-CN
Assistant Clinical Professor
UCLA Semel Institute for Neuroscience
    & Human Behavior
Los Angeles, CA, USA

Shushan Tigranyan, PsyD
Kaiser Permanente
South Sacramento, CA, USA

BaoChan Tran, PsyD
Department of Neurology
University of Pennsylvania
Philadelphia, PA, USA

Valentine Afamefuna Ucheagwu, PhD
Department of Psychology
Nnamdi Azikiwe University
Awka, Anambra, Nigeria

Daniela Ramos Usuga, MSc
Biomedical Research Doctorate Program
University of the Basque Country (UPV/EHU)
Leioa, Spain
BioCruces Bizkaia Health Research Institute
Barakaldo, Spain

Özgül Uysal-Bozkir, PhD
Department of Psychology, Education and
    Child Studies
Erasmus University Rotterdam
Rotterdam, the Netherlands

Eli Vakil, PhD
Department of Psychology and Leslie
    and Susan Gonda (Goldschmied)
    Multidisciplinary Brain Research Center
Bar-Ilan University
Ramat-Gan, Israel

Gloria M. Morel Valdés, PsyD
Department of Neurology
University of Wisconsin School of Medicine
    and Public Health
Madison, WI, USA

Mairim Vega-Carrero, PsyD
Clinical Psychology (PsyD) Program
Albizu University, Mayagüez University
    Center
Mayagüez, Puerto Rico

Lina Velilla-Jiménez, MS
Grupo de Neurociencias de Antioquia
Universidad de Antioquia
Medellín, Colombia
Senior Atlantic fellow for equity in brain
    Health
Global Brain Health Institute/University of
    California
San Francisco, CA, USA

Jennifer Walker, PhD
School of Rural and Northern Health
Laurentian University
Sudbury, ON, Canada

Louise F. Wheeler, PhD
Department of Counseling Psychology and
    Special Education
Counseling and Psychological Services
Brigham Young University
Provo, UT, USA

Christina G. Wong, PhD
Cleveland Clinic Lou Ruvo Center for Brain
    Health
Las Vegas, NV, USA

Mimi K.W. Wong, PhD
ZSFG Neuropsychology Service
UCSF Department of Psychiatry
Zuckerberg San Francisco General Hospital
    and Trauma Center
San Francisco, CA, USA

Isabel González Wongvalle, PsyD
Private Practice
Miami, Florida, USA

Karim Z. Yamout, PsyD, ABPP-CN
Private Practice
Bradenton, FL, USA

Janet J. Yañez, MA
Clinical Psychology, Doctoral Candidate
Jackson Health System in affiliation with the
    University of Miami (UM) Miller School of
    Medicine
Christine E. Lynn Rehabilitation Center for
    The Miami Project to Cure Paralysis at
    UHealth/Jackson Memorial, Miami, FL

Emmanuel A. Zamora, PsyD
Private Practice
University of California, Davis
Sacramento, CA, USA

List of Reviewers

Maleeha Abbas, PhD
Evidence Based Treatment Centers of Seattle
(EBTCS), PLLC
Seattle, WA, USA

Lynette Abrams-Silva, PhD, ABPP-CN
Department of Psychology
University of New Mexico
Albuquerque, New Mexico, USA

Anna V. Agranovich, PhD, ABPP
Department of Physical Medicine and
Rehabilitation
Johns Hopkins University School
of Medicine
Baltimore, MD, USA

Franchesca Arias, PhD
Assistant Scientist I, Aging Brain Center
Marcus Institute for Aging Research,
Hebrew SeniorLife
Instructor of Neurology, Harvard Medical
School, Boston, MA
Staff Neuropsychologists
Beth Israel Deaconess Medical Center
Boston, MA 02131, USA

Carol L. Armstrong, PhD, ABN
Adjunct Associate Professor
Perelman School of Medicine
University of Pennsylvania
Philadelphia, PA, USA

Majid Azzedine, PhD
Federal Way Psychology Clinic
Federal Way, WA 98003
Child Study and Treatment Center
Lakewood, Washington

Michelle Braun, PhD, ABPP-CN
Clinical Neuropsychologist
Department of Neurology and
Neurosurgery
Ascension Healthcare System—All Saints
Hospital
Racine, WI 53405, USA

Ayca Coskunpinar Byerley, PhD, HSPP
Clinical Neuropsychologist, Co-Owner
Neuropsychology Associates
Carmel, IN, USA

Stefano F. Cappa, MD
University School for Advanced Studies
(IUSS-Pavia) and IRCCS Mondino
Foundation
Pavia, Italy

Melissa Castro, PsyD, ABPP-CN
Minneapolis Clinic of Neurology
Minneapolis, MN, USA

Freeman M. Chakara, PsyD, ABPP-CN
Clinical Director
Providence Behavioral Health
600H Eden Rd
Lancaster, PA 17601, USA

Angeles M. Cheung, PhD, ABPP
Board Certified in Clinical
Neuropsychology
American Board of Professional
Psychology
Clinical Instructor of Rehabilitation and
Human Performance
Icahn School of Medicine at Mount Sinai
New York, NY, USA

Jennifer L. Gallo, PhD
Clinical Neuropsychologist, Global
  Neurosciences Institute
Associate Professor of Neurology,
  Drexel University College of
  Medicine
Upland, PA | Philadelphia, PA, USA

Vidyulata Kamath, PhD, ABPP-CN
Department of Psychiatry and Behavioral
  Sciences
The Johns Hopkins University School of
  Medicine
Baltimore, MD, USA

Kelly Kollias, PsyD
AAA Neuropsychology, LLC
Malvern, PA, USA

Mary H. Kosmidis, PhD
School of Psychology
Aristotle University of Thessaloniki
Thessaloniki, Greece

Margaret Lanca, PhD
Department of Psychiatry
Harvard Medical School/Cambridge Health
  Alliance
Cambridge, MA 02139, USA

Sophie H. Longwill PsyD, MBA
Private Practice
18 W. King St
Malvern, PA 19355, USA

Maria Raquel Lopa-Ramos, PhD
Ledesma Group for Neuropsychological
  Services
Neurodevelopmental Center—St. Luke's
  Medical Center, Quezon City
Metro Manila, Philippines

Dawn Mechanic-Hamilton, PhD, ABPP-CN
Department of Neurology
University of Pennsylvania
Philadelphia, PA, USA

Michelle Miranda, PhD, MPH
Department of Neurology
University of Utah
Salt Lake City, Utah, USA

Tanya T. Nguyen, PhD
Department of Psychiatry
University of California
  San Diego
VA San Diego Healthcare System
La Jolla, CA, USA

Marc Norman, PhD, ABPP-CN
Department of Psychiatry
University of California,
  San Diego
San Diego, CA, USA

Shelley Peery, PhD
San Francisco Neuropsychology PC
San Francisco, CA, USA

Karen Postal, PhD, ABPP-CN
Department of Psychiatry
Harvard Medical School
Cambridge, MA, USA

Courtney Ray, MDiv, PhD
Department of Psychology
City University of New York Brooklyn
  College
New York, NY, USA

Johanna Rengifo, PhD
Clinical Neuropsychologist
  (Spanish bilingual)
Department of Neurology
UC Davis School of Medicine
Alzheimer's Disease Center
Walnut Creek, CA, USA
San Francisco Neuropsychology PC
San Francisco, CA, USA

Diomaris Eliana Safi, PsyD
Department of Psychiatry and Behavioral
  Sciences
UCLA Hispanic Neuropsychiatric
  Center of Excellence
University of California
  Los Angeles
Los Angeles, CA 90095, USA

Shalom Shapiro, PsyD
Department of Neuropsychology
Kennedy Krieger Institute
Baltimore, MD, USA

Anita Sim, PhD, ABPP
Department of Physical Medicine &
  Rehabilitation
Minneapolis VA Health Care System
Minneapolis, MN 55417, USA

Paola Suarez, PhD
Department of Psychiatry and Biobehavioral
  Sciences
University of California, Los Angeles
Westwood, CA 90095, USA

Preeti Sunderaraman, PhD
K99/R00 Associate Research Scientist
  (Affiliation at the time of review)
Columbia University Medical Center
The Taub Institute and The Gertrude H.
  Sergievsky Center
Department of Neurology
630 West 168th Street
New York, NY 10032, USA
Assistant Professor of Neurology
  (Current Affiliation)
Department of Neurology
Boston University School of Medicine
Medical Campus
72 East Concord Street
MA 02118, USA
Assistant Professor of Neurology
The Framingham Heart Study—Brain Aging
  Program
73 Mount Wayte Avenue
Framingham, MA 01702, USA

Sharon Truter, D. Litt, Et Phil
HPCSA-registered Neuropsychologist and
  Counselling Psychologist
Honorary Research Associate, Psychology
  Department
Rhodes University
Grahamstown, South Africa

David Tsai, PhD, ABPP-CN
Coatesville VA Medical Center
Coatesville, PA, USA

Clemente Vega, PsyD, ABPP-CN
Department of Psychiatry
Harvard Medical School
Boston, MA, USA

Karen E. Wills, PhD, ABPP-CN
Private Practice & Affiliated Professional Staff
Children's Hospitals and Clinics
Minneapolis, MN, USA

Acknowledgments

Like many of us, my grandmothers loved to tell us meaningful stories. One of those stories was about a little bird who emerged in a world with a beloved family who didn't have a big nest or a lot of food but had the wisdom to teach her life lessons. They taught her that different birds get different lotteries of birth. Some can fly, and some can't. Those birds that can fly see the world from the sky. Those birds that can't fly see the world from the ground. All these beautiful birds take care of each other. They help each other learn to fly and land safely. That's the way the flocks thrive. "Know your flocks," said my grandmother.

My first multicolored flock is one that looks, loves, achieves, believes, and thrives differently. They are my children, parents, spouse, brother, nieces/nephews, aunts/uncles, cousins, and extended family of in-laws, friends, and sisters/brothers-from-other-mothers. Some of my first flock watch over us from high in the sky and will always stay in our memories. This first flock provides core strength and safety.

A second flock gave this project flight. They said, "Okay, so you want to write a book. Let us give you the wings to help you fly." This flock included dearest mentors, Drs. Karen Postal, Paul Moberg and Doug Chute, who provided unfaltering support that gave confidence to try and flutter my wings. Then came an AACN conference where I gathered the guts to go to a publishers' booth and share an idea about using a novel, storytelling, case study approach to help our neuropsychology community learn more about culturally diverse communities globally. Taylor & Francis/Routledge's, Senior Publisher Lucy Kennedy's eagerness and support was instrumental in propelling the project forward. The anonymous reviewers who also expressed enthusiasm about the idea then allowed take-off in 2019.

A third powerful flock then stepped up and said, "This is a needed project. Let us help. We know other birds that we can connect you with." This flock started with Drs. Daryl Fujii and Tedd Judd who have been instrumental in helping build the flock and providing key wisdom and insights along the way. The project would not have been possible without your support, responsiveness, and eagerness to help. Other key influencers included Drs. T. Rune Nielson, Marc Norman, Preeti Sunderaraman, Anita Herrera Hamilton, Tony Stringer, Vidya Kamath, Juan Carlos Arango Lasprilla, June Paltzer, Rex Swanda, Orlando Sanchez, Michelle Miranda, Mirella Diaz-Santos, Kendra Anderson, Christina Wong, Adriana Strutt, Christine Salinas, Julie Bobholz, Ann Shuttleworth-Edwards, Sharon Truter, Freeman Chakara, Kira Armstrong, Monica Rosselli, and Carol Armstrong. You all know how to help others strengthen their flocks.

We also need to especially honor a late giant in our field, Dr. Alfredo Ardilla. Despite health struggles, he supported this project with great kindness and warmth. One of his last words to me were "I hope to see your interesting book published very soon" and I feel badly that wasn't realized. But we did focus on his last encouragement to "Go ahead with this excellent project." Thank you for helping many flocks soar, Dr. Ardilla. Your legacy lives on in our work.

Next came a key fourth flock of contributors who said, "Yes! We want to share our stories about our flocks." This group of authors delivered their chapters with passion, hard work, and commitment. This was despite a double pandemic superimposed on top of existing daily work demands and ongoing personal, structural, and systemic barriers. Some authors were experienced contributors and some first-time authors in English. Please accept deep gratitude for your tireless efforts, responses to "nudges," and openness to consider editorial and reviewer suggestions. You each honor this project with your wisdom. You will help many see different perspectives from both the ground and the sky.

The fifth expert flock then came through and said, "We will help everyone land safely." Thank you to the external reviewers and advisors who offered their time, cultural or neuropsychological content expertise, as well as careful and constructive comments to enhance the work of others and build cultural bridges. You helped improve our work.

A special shout-out goes to my student editorial assistant, Sana Arastu, who volunteered her time to provide referencing and editorial support in the midst of managing her own dissertation and school demands. Saloni Singhania has also been a welcome support through the publisher. Just as important are my local sustenance crew of Michele Grasso, Dr. Kelly Kollias, Dr. Samantha Foreman, and our students, all of whom keep us grounded and provided essential support for clinical and training activities throughout this project. A safe landing was also not possible without the various local and national equity forum group members, especially the invaluable nest provided by the Asian Neuropsychology Association through challenging times. Dr. Desiree Byrd's beautiful words and enthusiastic support have empowered beyond what words can express. Amazing people who send good vibes—you too are part of the flock and valued.

Our final flocks are perhaps the most important of all. You are the individuals and families who we work with. You share your stories with us and present views from the sky and the ground. This book would not exist without you. You are also the readers who want to appreciate different perspectives. You serve many different types of birds and help them soar and land safely. You are not alone on these journeys, and we hope that you "know your flocks" too.

Thank you, dear flocks. We grow and thrive together.

Farzin Irani

Preface

A lot of different flowers make a bouquet.

Anonymous

Our ability to reach unity in diversity will be the beauty and the test of our civilization.

Mahatma Gandhi

This peer-reviewed clinical handbook builds on ongoing efforts to keep neuropsychology relevant in an increasingly diverse and global world. It provides a platform for clinical neuropsychologists/psychologists/trainees to bridge cultures and speak to each other about the ethnically diverse communities we represent and serve internationally. It allows readers to peek into our clinical filing cabinets and learn how we have understood and assessed diverse people from indigenous and migrant communities of Arab, Asian, European, Israeli, Latin American and Caribbean, Persian, Russian, Sub-Saharan African, and North American origin.

Before delving into learning more about specific communities and case studies, readers are invited to consider some foundational supports for their journeys. Dr. Fujii offers his ECLECTIC framework to gain **Knowledge** about cultural neuropsychology within the context of current and future directions for the field. Drs. Sanchez and Judd share their training model to obtain **Skills** in multicultural education and training in neuropsychology. Dr. Swanda highlights the importance of **Awareness of Self** through a reflective local practice model. Dr. Hamilton's group highlights **Awareness of Others** by drawing attention to microaggressions experienced by BIPOC neuropsychologists and trainees. Finally, Dr. Diaz-Santos's group highlights that **Action** is more important than affirmation and reviews the role of neuropsychologists in social justice advocacy.

After these introductory chapters, we invite you to join us for a tour around the world to experience the beauty of its people. We offer a collection of neuropsychology case study chapters that showcase brain-behavior assessments in communities which are organized alphabetically by cultural geographic region. When there is a large enough group of communities within a region, there is also an overview chapter that provides a bird's eye view of the *historical and current state of research and clinical practice of neuropsychology within the region.*

Understanding the context of each case requires background knowledge about the community being served. In each chapter, Section I presents *surface and deep level **Background Information*** about a community from the authors' perspective. This includes aspects of terminology, authors' perspectives, geography, history, immigration/relocation, languages, communication, education, literacy, socio-economic status, values and customs, gender and sexuality, spirituality and religion, acculturation and systemic barriers, mental health views, and approaches to neuropsychological assessment in the country of origin and country of practice. The below figure highlights the framework used throughout this book to increase cultural understanding.

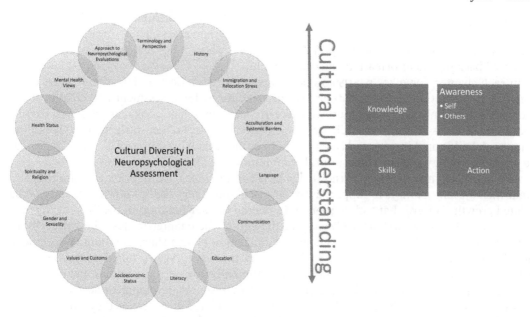

Framework for increasing cultural understanding in neuropsychology

This knowledge is presented from the *authors' worldview*. The tone of these case study chapters is intended to be personalized and reflect the voice of authors who may be culturally matched or not to the community of focus. Author perspectives are sometimes from the country of origin, sometimes from the country where they practice, and sometimes reflect a collaboration between both. When comfortable, some authors have chosen to use a story-telling writing style or share personal anecdotes and professional experiences to increase practical understanding and applicability of the content to bring it to life. Writing styles are as diverse as the people served.

It is worth noting that when presenting this background information, the authors do not claim to speak for all members of a community. This section is also not meant to be an encyclopedic coverage of all that is known about a community. Readers are instead encouraged to consider this background knowledge as one source of information to spark further curiosity. The individuality of those we work with deserves equal attention, and we need to have the humility to know that we will always be limited in our understanding of another person.

This background review then sets the stage in Section II to introduce an interesting, deidentified neurological/psychiatric/psychological **Case Study**. These case studies showcase a neuropsychological assessment conducted with a member of the community based on the neuropsychologists' practicing framework. Neuropsychology and the authors are at various stages of development in clinical and research practice internationally with different training backgrounds and practicing frameworks. Authors include eminent international neuropsychologists/psychologists who have spent their careers doing cross-cultural work, as well as newer ethnically diverse authors who have rich clinical experiences and cultural expertise working within their communities. All these voices are centered and equally important.

The book has tried to capture *a snapshot of cultures of neuropsychology* across the globe at this moment without judgment. The focus of the case studies is, therefore, less on educating about neuropsychology syndromes and instead on highlighting *contextual considerations in neuropsychological assessment and rehabilitation practices*. The intended clinical tone is meant to be based on empirical foundations and sound clinical practice while also introducing new ideas and challenges in conducting culturally and linguistically appropriate assessments throughout the world. Cultural and neuropsychological expert peer reviewers who are familiar with a community have reviewed background information and case content.

In each chapter, some key pearls and perils are captured in Section III, which covers **Lessons Learned**. This section provides authors' recommendations for assessment and treatment when working with members of a community. There are many excellent books, articles, and resources that focus on cross-cultural research in the science and practice of neuropsychology. This clinical handbook builds on this work and is not meant to be an exhaustive source of all knowledge related to neuropsychology and the multicultural communities we serve.

As contexts change, so will our knowledge base and practices. Readers are encouraged to continue their *life long journeys* to support awareness (self and other), skills, knowledge, and advocacy related growth. Toward that end, authors have offered further readings in the form of **References** within each chapter as well as a **Glossary** at the end of the chapter to describe culturally relevant terms (indicated by **bold** in the chapter). Some authors also share community specific **Test and Norm Resources in the Appendix** at the back of the book. Again, this does not serve as an exhaustive review of all tests/norms available for ethnically diverse communities, but does capture some current tools while underscoring gaps and future resource development needs. Readers are encouraged to keep up with the evolving literature for updated measures as they emerge.

We hope that the current sampling highlights that there is much more to learn and the *scope for ongoing growth in appreciating the importance of culture in neuropsychology is immense.* There are *many more cultures and subcultures* that could have been featured in this handbook. The focus on some ethnically diverse communities here does not exclude the crucial limelight that many other culturally diverse groups deserve. Perhaps future editions will allow systematic coverage of other groups and brain-behavior functions within their cultural contexts. For now, we also recognize the interconnected nature of other social categorizations beyond race and ethnicity and interweave aspects of intersectionality throughout the chapters. This includes considerations for gender, LGBTQ+ identities, socioeconomic status, age, developmental and acquired disability, religion/spirituality, indigenous heritage, and national origin.

Overall, we hope that your ongoing journey will be as personally and professionally rewarding as it has been for us. This handbook reflects hard work and collaboration among authors and reviewers to continue to provide resources that *increase self-reflection about multicultural awareness and knowledge, highlight practical ways to provide culturally aware neuropsychological and psychological assessment and treatment services, and spark further discussions for professional and personal growth in this area.*

Farzin Irani

Foreword

This is the book that we have been waiting for. In an age when there is a thirst for new disciplinary knowledge and practices that are grounded in equity, this text answers the call. **Cultural Diversity in Neuropsychological Assessment: Developing Understanding through Global Case Studies** brings us back to the center of our discipline, the assessment process, and frames it through a cultural lens that traverses oceans, languages, religions, and borders. In this handbook, assessments with people from all corners of the world receive dignified and respectful attention and none are relegated to the margins as anomalies or spectacles. Variety is the point, not the exception and in this text, the contours of diversity are beautifully normalized and honored. This orientation is a welcomed relief because for far too long North America and Europe, with rare exception, have dominated the neuropsychological print narrative and centered the assessment process within the narrow confines of its people, who are primarily monolingual, with relatively high levels of education and enjoy the privilege of health care and stable political structures. In these traditional orientations, assessment with people who were diverse was contextualized as special, exotic, etc. In this Global Case Studies text, that trope is abandoned, and uniqueness is the standard. Often, direct client quotes open case studies, centering the experience and perspective of the person, as it should be. In this, the book reminds us of our shared humanity and the global common interests of the practice of neuropsychology.

Though this book has been in the making for years, its publication in 2021 coincides with a time of international reckoning with racial injustices and other systemic inequities. A time when neuropsychology, like most other disciplines, is being forced to take a critical look at its own track record in the treatment of diversity. As is well known, the record is tainted and fraught with harm, abuse, and abject disregard. The addition of the Global Cases book to our canon shifts the arc toward inclusiveness. Books like these and their forerunners are invaluable cornerstones that ground us and offer inspiration and direction when we need it the most.

The text holds special relevance for practitioners who work with people who have migrated from their home countries and resettled in others. Chapter authors provide vivid descriptions of cultural contexts and customs that accompany immigrants to assessment appointments but cannot be summarized in data tables or easily communicated from client to practitioner. Yet, as the authors beautifully demonstrate, these factors are as influential in the assessment dynamics as the neurological insult prompting the referral. These contextual factors arise in response to forces such as power hierarchies, cultural norms of obedience to authority figures, social desirability, and varying comfort levels with self-disclosure. This book shines a caring light onto these soft spots, sensitizing us to what we might otherwise miss or so that we can elevate the humanity in our profession. By expanding our awareness of the client experience during assessment, we become more responsive clinicians.

While many chapters articulate the challenges associated with practicing neuropsychological assessment in regions where resources are low, this is not the book's focus. Refreshingly, the authors share their cases in a solution-focused frame, showcasing their resourcefulness and creativity. Those of us with the privilege of practicing in resource-rich settings have much to learn from our global colleagues.

Another standout design aspect of this collection is the range of nationalities of the authors. Of the 36 case study chapters, half are written by non-US-based neuropsychologists and psychologists who practice in their native countries. Many of the other authors share ancestral origins with the regions they write about and/or co-write with persons who are native to those lands. Gaining access to first-hand accounts from such a worldly roster is a welcomed and rare gem. Such an author list does not happen by chance; the editor was clearly intentional in her commitment to be inclusive and to identify practitioners from countries not typically included in American-based neuropsychological texts on diversity. In doing so, the editor shows us what is possible when commitment aligns with intent. This global sampling is a gift in many ways. The cultural congruence between the authors and the places that they write about free the readers from the breath holding that we are accustomed to doing when reading what is written about us, wondering whether colonial themes will skew the narrative and disappoint us in the end. On the contrary, these authors offer authentic accounts and holistic case presentations. I appreciated that the authors were candid and transparent about their process in the larger disciplinary context. Some authors shared personal stories that provided glimpses into their individual struggles with identity and experiences with testing, their feelings about language competencies, and their navigation of difficult cultural territories within the scope of their practice. Such examples of vulnerability will resonate with all of us who are honest about how our personal and professional identities often intersect in the assessments that we conduct.

Overall, the contents of this book are like a gumbo mix of treats offering up innumerable gifts to all who are ready to learn. Readers who are history buffs will enjoy the tracing of the history of neuropsychology in various corners of the world and learning about the educational requirements for neuropsychologists in various countries. The book provides exposure to this variability while leveling the contribution from each author, helping us expand our perception of what a neuropsychologist is. We learn that they are not all doctoral level trained, but they are all doing the critical work of assessing and treating persons suffering brain-based behavioral disturbance. For those of us hungry for practical examples of how to complete assessments with people from cultures that we know little about, we get plenty in this handbook: richly conceptualized and presented immediately after the background regional informational. The pairing of the case studies with the regional information is another genius design benefit that makes this handbook particularly valuable. We are reminded that after the national statistics, prevalence rates, and regional profiles, we are all individual humans who need help sometimes and deserve to get it in settings where our uniqueness is respected and honored. This handbook helps us all feel seen.

The open and accepting tone of the handbook make it a valuable educational tool for all of us: student and elder professional alike. Such an editorial tone helps us negotiate our own shortcomings and provide starting points for self-improvement. In reading this text, you will be humbled by learning so much of what you do not know. You will be inspired by colleagues who do more with less. You will grow from the expanded exposure to variable models of practice and constructs. Most of all, you will be filled with gratitude to the editor and authors and gift this book to your colleagues and trainees.

Desiree Byrd, PhD, ABPP-CN

Part I

Introductory Foundations

A. Knowledge

1 Cultural Neuropsychology

Current State and Future Directions

Daryl Fujii

International population trends portend an increased need for neuropsychological services around the world. The first trend is the aging of the world population. According to World Health Organization,[1] the number of people over age 60 will reach 2 billion by 2050, which is almost double the current population (12%–22%). Moreover, persons aged 80 or older will be more than triple from 125 to 434 million. The greatest growth will occur in low- and middle-income countries where 80% of the world's older people live. Unfortunately, these countries have a relatively short time (20–30 years) to adapt to such drastic increases in the elderly and their risks for significantly more health problems and cognitive decline than younger populations. Morbidities not only impact the quality of life but also have significant economic implications. To address issues associated with the aging population, one of the current goals of the WHO dementia plan is to develop the capacity to diagnose 50% of persons with dementia in 50% of countries by 2025.[2]

A second major trend is the increase in international migration. There were an estimated 272 million migrants in 2019, which represented an increase of 51 million since 2010. Migration is motivated by work opportunities, family reunification, and seeking asylum. International migrants comprise 3.5% of the global population with roughly half residing in the following countries: United States (US) (51 million), Germany and Saudi Arabia (13 million each), Russia (12 million), United Kingdom (10 million), United Arab Emirates (9 million), France, Canada, and Australia (around 8 million each), and Italy (6 million). The leading countries of origin for migrants are India (18 million), Mexico (12 million), China (11 million), Russia (10 million), and the Syrian Arab Republic (8 million).[3] A significant challenge for migrant hosting countries is providing access to healthcare, including psychological and neuropsychological services. As many migrants do not speak or are not fluent in the language of the host country, a major barrier to healthcare is the lack of interpreters and appropriate language services.[4]

As these migration data indicate, there is a great need for neuropsychological services for diverse populations. In addition to many immigrants in the Hispanic (18.5%) and Asian (5.9%) communities, other US minority groups include African American (13.5%) and Native American/Hawaiians (1.5%), who together account for almost 40% of the US population.[5] Indeed, it is projected that ethnic minorities will outnumber European Americans by the year 2044.[6]

A third and most recent occurrence is the sheer number of persons infected with COVID-19 around the world. As of January 2021, over 100 million persons were infected with the virus resulting in over 2.2 million deaths.[7] Preliminary data indicate that COVID-19 is associated with cerebral vascular events, encephalopathy, and acute respiratory distress, often requiring a respirator for breathing support. Although results significantly vary as to how many experience long-term cognitive problems, early findings suggest enduring cognitive deficits for persons who suffered severe COVID-19 illness.[8] In addition, patients of past pandemics have demonstrated diverse

DOI: 10.4324/9781003051862-2

neuropsychiatric symptoms, such as encephalopathy, psychosis, or demyelinating processes that can follow infections months or longer in recovered patients.[9]

This chapter describes in broad strokes how the world and the United States are dealing with the increased need for neuropsychological services for diverse populations. First, the state of current services around the world will be described. Next, initiatives in the United States for addressing cultural issues in neuropsychological training and assessment will be covered with a summary of current shortcomings and needs. The chapter closes with a discussion of future trends and recommendations to meet the increased need for neuropsychological services around the world.

Neuropsychology around the World

Neuropsychological practices around the world are highly variable and largely dependent on cultural, economic, and political factors, with most development occurring within the past 25 years.[10] Growth is reflected in the increase in international contributors to the major clinical neuropsychology journals over the past 20 years: Journal of International Neuropsychology (2000–8 articles; 2020–46 articles), Archives of Clinical Neuropsychology (2000–9 articles; 2020–19 articles), The Clinical Neuropsychologist (2000–3 articles; 2020–18 articles). The globalization of neuropsychology and the development of infrastructure is also illustrated by the recent addition of mid-year International Neuropsychological Society (INS) conferences around the world, including Israel (2014), Australia (2015, 2021), the United Kingdom (2016), South Africa (2017), Czech Republic (2018), Brazil (2019), and the upcoming conference in Taiwan (2023).

The development of neuropsychology has taken variable paths across the world. For example, in Japan, neuropsychology developed from the country's neurology and psychiatry disciplines.[11] In Singapore, Hong Kong, Taiwan, or the Philippines, neuropsychology was developed by nationals who studied abroad in the United States or Australia and brought knowledge and technology back to their countries, whereas in countries, such as Israel, Brazil, and New Zealand, neuropsychology developed within the context of rehabilitation.[10] In some low-resource countries such as many African nations, the driver of neuropsychology has been internationally funded research on neurological disorders such as HIV or malaria.[12]

Educational requirements and training for practicing neuropsychology are also highly variable and range from doctoral degrees (United States, Canada), to master's level (Hong Kong, Finland, and South Korea), and bachelor's degrees (Argentina, Mexico, and Spain).[13] By contrast, in some countries such as those in Central and South America, Israel, and India, the practice of neuropsychology is often undertaken by other disciplines, including speech pathologists, occupational therapists, neurologists, and psychiatrists.[10] For example, in Japan, neuropsychologists are psychometrists and only physicians can perform the assessments.[11] Training requirements also differ. The United States uniquely requires a two-year postdoctoral residency for board certification in neuropsychology, while only 5 out of 14 countries surveyed reported processes for board certification.[13]

The most common neurological disorders seen by neuropsychologists around the world include vascular disorders, dementia, and traumatic brain injury (TBI) in adults, and Attention Deficit Hyperactivity Disorder (ADHD), and learning disorders in children. Each region also has disorders which are more prevalent in that region, for example, HIV-related neurocognitive impairment in some African countries.[10] Neuropsychologists in many countries also manage diversity within their country's population, including education, ethnicity, and language.[13]

Despite growth in the discipline, in actuality, neuropsychological services are available to a small minority of people, and generally in countries and for individuals who are economically advantaged. In Canada and Finland, the ratio of neuropsychologists to the population is about

1 per 20,000, whereas in India, China, and South Africa, there is less than one neuropsychologist per 500,000 citizens.[13] By contrast, in many Southeast Asian countries, such as Vietnam, Laos, or Brunei, or much of Central Africa, there are no practicing neuropsychologists.[10]

Even when neuropsychologists are available, barriers exist for competent services, as there is an overreliance on Western tests, for persons who do not speak the country's national language.[10] In addition, there is often a lack of neuropsychologists or trained interpreters who speak the language of diverse regional populations.[4,14]

State of Cultural Neuropsychology in the United States

In 2010, Rivera-Mindt et al.[15] described challenges that the discipline of neuropsychology faces for providing competent services to ethnic minority populations. First is the relatively small number of ethnic minority neuropsychologists in relation to the general population (6% of neuropsychologists, 34% of US Population).[16] This issue is salient for diverse populations due to health and diagnostic disparities, mistrust of providers, naiveté of cultural issues, and linguistic barriers to access services. Numbers in neuropsychology are also low in comparison to other clinical specialties, such as school, counseling, and clinical psychology. There are multiple reasons for the low numbers in graduate school pipelines, including economic issues such as direct costs of undergraduate and graduate school education and the increased need to work during school and after completion of the undergraduate degree. Working during school, which reduces the time for studying, can, in turn, contribute to academic issues such as failure to meet undergraduate requirements to graduate study in neuropsychology and lower Graduate Records Examination (GRE) scores that do not meet program standards, while lack of minority faculty role models and research opportunities for ethnic minorities may also make graduate education in neuropsychology less appealing.[17,18] Second, despite encouragement toward multicultural competence from neuropsychology leadership[19,20] and the American Psychological Association (APA),[21] there is a paucity of details on the knowledge base or skills needed to develop competence or guidelines for training. Third is the low capacity to address linguistic diversity in the US population. Specifically, there is a paucity of neuropsychologists who are fluent in the languages spoken by numerous ethnic minorities, as well as a lack of adequately translated and normed tests. Fourth, ethnic minorities are under-represented in neuropsychological clinical research, which has implications for assessment. This includes questionable validity of neurocognitive models of brain functioning, lack of norms or validation for most neuropsychological tests, and an inability to account for performance differences between ethnic groups.

Results from a 2014 survey of the US and Canadian neuropsychologists examining issues with providing services for diverse patients identified similar concerns.[22] The greatest challenges identified were the lack of appropriate norms, tests, and referral sources, the lack of multicultural training, and the underrepresentation of ethnic minorities in the field of neuropsychology.

Next, the current state of the identified challenges for cultural neuropsychology will be described, including concerns about the development of a pipeline of ethnic minority neuropsychologists, multicultural education and training, capacity to assess linguistic minorities, availability of translated, normed, and validated tests, and research on ethnic minority populations.

Ethnic Minority Pipeline Issues

There have been a number of initiatives by major neuropsychological societies to support ethnic minority students, trainees, and professionals. The National Academy of Neuropsychology's (NAN) Culture and Diversity Committee established the Tony Wong Diversity Award for graduate students or postdoctoral fellows, mentors, and early career professionals in 2013 to recognize excellent ethnic minorities at different career stages. The American Academy of Clinical Neuropsychology (AACN) Relevance 2050 initiative includes travel grants to the annual conference, diversity focused research awards and develops webinars to assist underrepresented minority students and early career professionals into the board certification process. APA's Division 40 Ethnic Minority Affairs Subcommittee has a mentorship program for trainees, travel grants for the annual APA Conference, and diversity focused awards for research and practice. The INS established a student-run committee to address student and trainee needs and facilitate student involvement and contributions to neuropsychological science. The INS Science Committee has offered student awards for students in developing countries. Recently two ethnic minority organizations, the Asian Neuropsychological Association (ANA), and Society for Black Neuropsychology (SBN) have joined the established Hispanic Neuropsychological Society (HNS) to provide additional community-based support for trainees and neuropsychologists.

Current demographic data on neuropsychologists indicate a promising trend for increased numbers of ethnic minorities in neuropsychology training programs, although they remain underrepresented (see Table 1.1). Per 2017 APA Division 40/Society for Clinical Neuropsychology membership data,[16] there are still large gaps between the number of ethnic minority neuropsychologists (5.1%) and the percentage of ethnic minorities in the psychology workforce (15%)[23] and US population (42.1%).[6] In comparison to overall percentages of minority neuropsychologists, there are higher percentages of ethnic minorities who are board certified in clinical neuropsychology (8.4%) which would suggest many achieve high levels of clinical competency. There is no specific demographic data collected by APA or the Association of Postdoctoral Programs in Clinical Neuropsychology (APPCN); however, two recent surveys[24,25] indicate that ethnic minorities make up slightly more than a fourth of current graduate students or trainees in neuropsychology (27%–28.2%). Although these numbers are still significantly lower than the percentages in the US Census (42.2%) or psychology graduates in general (38%),[26] the numbers portend a strong influx of ethnic minority neuropsychologists in the near future. Of note, increases are particularly pronounced for Asian Americans, where percentages in neuropsychology training programs are higher than the overall percentage of Asian Americans in the US Census, while African Americans and Latinx are still underrepresented. It should be mentioned that despite the relatively high numbers of Asian American neuropsychology trainees, because of the heterogeneity within this group, which is comprised of 19 specific ethnicities,[5] many Asian Americans, particularly in the smaller ethnic groups, will still lack services from providers who speak their native language.

Education and Training

Progress has been made in education and training as there are more resources to assist graduate schools and training programs in developing training curriculums. For example, the revised AERA Standards for Psychological Testing[27] describe specific conditions that must be met for psychological tests to be fair to diverse examinees,[28] including examinee comfort with the testing situation, minimalization of testing biases, accessibility in responding, and validity of testing for its intended purposes. The ECLECTIC framework further assists neuropsychologists in developing a context for conceptualizing culturally diverse examinees to guide assessment approaches for collecting accurate data, interpreting data, and making useful recommendations.[29,30] Both tools emphasize that test scores should be conceptualized as performances on Western tests, and in combination, provide concrete strategies for meeting neuropsychological training standards.

Table 1.1 Percent of ethnic minority neuropsychology/psychology students and workforce across time

Ethnicity	2017 Society for Clinical Neuropsychology[a]	2019 American Board of Professional Psychology-Clinical Neuropsychology[b]	2016 Psychology workforce[c]	2020 AACN Survey[d]	2020 Association of Postdoctoral Programs in Clinical Neuropsychology Survey[e]	2018 Psychology Graduate Students[f]	2019 US Census[g]
African American	0.8%	0.9%	4%	5.3%	5.4%	12%	13.4%
Asian American	1.5%	3.4%	4%	9.0%	10.8%	7%	5.9%
Latinx	2.4%	3.4%	5%	7.8%	10.8%	14%	18.5%
Native American	0.4%	0.3%	—	6.1%	—	1%	1.3%
Other	—	0.4%	2%		—	4%	3%
Total	5.1%	8.4%	15%	28.2%	27%	38%	42.1%

Notes:

a APA (2017).[16]
b Personal communication, Rob Davis September 1, 2020.
c Lin et al. (2018).[23]
d Guidotti-Breting et al. (2020).[24]
e Domen et al. (2020).[25]
f Michalski et al. (2019).[26]
g US Census Bureau (2019).[6]

There has also been an increase in cultural neuropsychological educational resources. A number of cultural neuropsychology books have been published on various topics, including Asian Americans,[31,32] diverse populations,[33,34] bilingualism,[35] rehabilitation,[36] assessment of African children,[12] culturally informed neuropsychological assessment,[29] and cultural neuroscience.[37] Testing and cultural resources have been posted on the NAN website. The new edition of the study guide for board certification in clinical neuropsychology includes a chapter describing issues when working with ethnic minorities and persons with disabilities.[38] The Baylor College of Medicine sponsors a weekly continuing education webinar, "Taquitos de Sesos" that is open to all neuropsychologists. Finally, the AACN Relevance 2050 Committee sponsors a cultural CE presentation at every AACN Conference and recently instituted mandatory requirements for including cultural issues in all continuing education presentations.

Despite the progress that has been made, training is still lacking as cultural guidelines for practicum training remain broad and lacking in specifics.[39,40] In addition, a survey of APPCN training directors reported that although ethnic minorities comprise 52% of clinical cases, only 27% of directors rate themselves as having advanced skills in cultural neuropsychology and 33% are not satisfied with the diversity training that they offer.[41]

Linguistic Capacity

Competent neuropsychological assessment of linguistic minorities requires conducting the evaluation in the examinees best language and administering tests that are translated into this language. There have been several developments in these areas. As indicated in the previous section, increasing the numbers of ethnic minority neuropsychologists, particularly from immigrant populations, will be key for providing services to patients whose primary language is not English. Although increasing, the ratio of minority neuropsychologists to the population for many ethnic minority groups is still inadequate.

If a neuropsychologist who speaks the examinee's language is not available, the neuropsychologist performing the evaluation is ethically obligated to use an interpreter. There have been several advancements in promoting the availability, knowledge, and skill base of this discipline. National certification of health care interpreters in the United States began in 2009.[42] Since then, there has been a 42.2% growth of health care interpreter jobs between 2010 and 2020.[43] In addition, there have been increasingly specific discipline guidelines for interpreters for psychology[44,45] and neuropsychology.[46]

A third requirement is the availability of adequately translated tests. To facilitate this goal, the International Test Commission[47] recently revised their guidelines for translating and adapting tests in order to maximize equivalency and minimize biases. Tests such as the Montreal Cognitive Assessment has been translated in over 80 languages,[48] and the Bilingual Aphasia Test has been translated into 74 languages.[49] Although progress has been made, there is still a paucity of translated tests to provide services to the population of linguistic minority examinees, particular for those from low resource countries.[10,22,50]

Test Norms

Related to the lack of translated tests is the paucity of test norms for minority populations. Similar to test translations, there has been a growth in internationally normed and validated tests.[51–54] However, despite this increase in normed tests, there are many ethnic groups, particularly those that come from low resource countries and smaller communities, where no test norms exist. This problem is more pronounced than the availability of test translations, as translation into a language such as Spanish could be used in many countries; however, norms may not be applicable. In addition, in low-resource countries, there may be a translation of a test, but no norms available since collecting normative data is more resource intensive. The lack of normed tests for the different populations that neuropsychologists serve has been identified as the biggest concern for neuropsychologists who provide services to examinees from different cultures.[10,22,50]

As the resource intensive, necessary process of developing norms is underway, an interim alternative to relying on equivalent sample norms is the individual comparison approach, which uses estimates of an examinees' premorbid functioning as a benchmark to interpret test scores using standard norms.[55] However, to use this technique with ethnic minority examinees, there needs to be a manner of estimating premorbid functioning. Fujii[29] developed a strategy to address this issue which entails finding an estimate of average cognitive test performance for people from the examinees country and then titrating the score based upon an estimate of the examinee's functioning within that country. Country test performance estimates on Western tests can be made based upon scores on Western IQ tests.[56] In addition, performance on international academic tests such as the Trends in International Mathematics and Science Study (TIMSS), Progress in International Reading Literacy Study (PIRLS), and Program for International Student Assessment (PISA) can also provide IQ benchmarks, as these tests demonstrate strong correlations with performances on Western IQ tests (0.81–0.88).[57] Another recent development that supports this strategy is new test interpretation guidance which stresses that test performances are "scores" that must be interpreted by a neuropsychologist to determine its significance.[58]

Research

Cultural neuropsychological research has also been increasing as evidenced by increases in the foreign publication in neuropsychological journals. Much of this research provides norms and adaptation of Western style tests for different countries. However, are tests developed in Western countries appropriate for measuring the impact of neurological disorders on populations with different linguistic backgrounds, educational opportunities, or exposure to Western concepts?[10] For example, the growing literature on bilingualism has demonstrated early bilinguals have smaller vocabularies in each language but a composite vocabulary that is equal to monolinguals.[59] Thus, evaluating vocabulary in one language may not accurately measure verbal skills in bilinguals. Understanding bilingualism is particularly important for cultural neuropsychological assessment as most of the world speaks more than one language: 43% are bilingual, 13% are trilingual, and 3% speak more than four languages.[60]

Another growing research area that has significant implications for neuropsychological assessment is clinical cultural neuroscience which examines the cultural impact on brain functioning through functioning imaging data. For example, studies comparing visual perceptual skills of East Asians compared to Westerners report that Westerners perform better on tasks requiring focus on a focal object, while East Asians perform better when the task entails integrating both focal object and background information.[61] This bias was illustrated in a study where European Americans demonstrated increased brain activation in the frontal-parietal areas when asked to attend to both object and context when judging line sizes, while East Asians demonstrated a similar activation pattern when asked to ignore the context and attended solely to the object. In each case, using processing strategies incongruent with cultural preferences resulted in more effortful processing.[62] Perceptual differences are consistent with the differences in cognitive styles and values. Westerners tend to be individualistic, with cognition that is more analytic and emphasizes taxonomic object categorization. By contrast, East Asian cultures are more interdependent, with cognition that emphasizes holistic perception. These differences are believed to fundamentally reflect Greek, and Confucian and Taoist values, which are highly influential in Western and East Asian cultures, respectively.[63]

Future Directions

The COVID-19 pandemic and Black Lives Matter Movement (BLMM) of 2020 have left an indelible mark on the world, American society, as well as on the discipline of psychology. COVID-19 has disproportionally impacted African American, Latinx, and Native American populations, uncovering health disparities for many ethnic minority populations. It has also changed the practice of clinical psychologists with a new reliance on telepsychology for treatment sessions, virtual meetings, and major conferences in order to reduce the risk for spreading infection during face-to-face sessions and large public gatherings. The BLMM increased White majority awareness of institutional racism and demanded support for implementing changes to increase equity in systems. The dual comfort and intrigue with technology and mobilized support of majority populations, in combination with the emerging growth and voice of ethnic minority neuropsychologists appear to have energized the discipline's momentum in achieving the 2010 "Call to Action."

This next section will describe current and proposed initiatives and projects to advance cultural neuropsychology that have been influenced by the confluence of ethnic minority and majority leadership, energized institutional support, and the impact of technology for increasing access to services to underserved populations and educational and training opportunities to neuropsychologists to develop cultural competency within the discipline.

The past few years have seen a significant increase in ethnic minority involvement in shaping the direction of neuropsychology. Ethnic minority neuropsychologists are increasingly holding leadership positions in major neuropsychological associations: Tony Puente served as President of the APA (2018–2019), Anita Sim (2016–2021) served on the AACN Board of Directors and chaired the Relevance 2020 Committee, Marc Norman served on the ABCN Board of Directors (2016–2021), and is currently the Executive Director of INS (2020–20__), Laura Renteria (2017–2022), Veronica Edgars (2019–2024), and Clemente Vega (2020–2025) serve on the ABCN Board of Directors, Anthony Stringer served on the ABCN Board of Directors (2008–2015), was President of ABCN (2015–2017), and is serving on the AACN Board and the new Relevance 2050 Chair (2021–2026), Ozioma Okonkwo serves as the treasurer for INS (2020–2025), and Desiree Byrd is an INS Member at Large (2020–2023). In parallel, the HNS has been a leader in advancing cultural neuropsychology. The organization has sponsored educational opportunities open to all neuropsychologists, including two Neuropsychological Conferences (2015, 2019). Research leaders have been instrumental in publishing Latinx norms for numerous neuropsychological tests.[64,65] HNS leadership has also developed cultural training guidelines from their Houston to Austin Conference summit (Monica Rivera-Mindt, personal communication, 9/13/2020). Future plans include co-hosting conferences with the ANA and SBN.

In addition to increased awareness of institutional racism and support for systemic change, there has been increased movement for increasing the representation of ethnic minority neuropsychologists in decision-making. Perhaps the most significant initiative is the Inter-Organizational Practice Committee (IOPC) approval for the creation of an Inter-Organizational Diversity Committee (IODC), modeled on the IOPC. This new entity gives ethnic minority stakeholders decision-making power for influencing how clinical psychological services are provided to our diverse population. Currently, David Lechuga, Christine Salinas, and Anna Reyes are organizing the development of a Cultural Neuropsychological Council (CNC) comprised of representatives from major neuropsychological organizations to determine practice issues pertaining to culture and diversity that delegates/representatives can bring to the IODC. Issues may include increasing the ethnic minority pipeline, providing guidance for education and training curricula from undergraduate to postgraduate levels, research, legislative and professional practice advocacy, mentorship, fundraising, and liaising with other major neuropsychology (Lechuga, personal communication, 8/24/20).

The major US neuropsychological associations have also introduced new initiatives to address diversity issues. INS is establishing the Black, Indigenous, or Persons of Color (BIPOC) Justice and Equity Task Force to explore the lived experience of being an ethnic minority neuropsychologist to guide institutional reforms for reducing marginalization and microaggressions (Anthony Stringer personal communication, 9/10/20). Similarly, the AACN listserv has initiated Equity Forums to facilitate an exchange of diverse perspectives with the goal of promoting professional development (Anita Herrera-Hamilton, personal communication, 8/8/20). A multiorganizational effort is underway to revise the Houston Conference Training Guidelines (HCTG) with a focus on updating guidelines for cultural neuropsychology training curriculums (Anthony Stringer, personal communication 9/5/20). The APPCN Committee on Diversity and Inclusion is developing projects for recruiting and onboarding international students and updating recruitment procedures for ensure equitable opportunities for students from diverse backgrounds (Amy Heffelfinger, personal communications 9/21/20).

Another ramification of the COVID-19 pandemic is the implementation and acceptance of teleneuropsychology as a viable alternative to traditional face-to-face assessments. Although the technology has received support from validation studies,[66] it was not until the restrictions of the pandemic has the practice become widespread. Concomitant has been the addition of tele-mental health codes and loosening of state licensure requirements for clinical practice across state lines. These two developments have the potential for revolutionizing how cultural neuropsychology is taught and practiced on a global level.

Teleneuropsychology can significantly increase ethnic minority patients' access to treatment from culturally and linguistically competent neuropsychologists, as many bilingual ethnic minority neuropsychologists live in different locations. Teleneuropsychology allows these patients to receive neuropsychological services directly by these distant providers, or local neuropsychologists can use technology for consultation and collaboration with out-of-state cultural experts.

Technology also has far-reaching implications for education and training. Most major neuropsychological conferences in 2020 were virtual conferences. New virtual platforms allow for increased accessibility to continuing education, including cultural neuropsychology, to many ethnic minority students, trainees, and clinicians who would not normally attend due to costs. It could also increase the opportunity for presenting research at conferences and meetings, which are important factors for acceptance into competitive neuropsychology training programs for trainees and tenure/promotion for academic faculty. Training programs that provide services to a diverse population, but lack a diverse faculty, can also benefit from virtual platforms by recruiting ethnic minority neuropsychologists living in other states to assist in providing education, supervision, and mentoring to trainees. Diverse neuropsychologists could be attracted to join training programs through offers of adjunct professorships, stipends, or research collaborations with programs that have access to specific ethnic minority populations.

The aforementioned initiatives can help address ethnic minority pipeline issues, as the lack of minority faculty role models and research opportunities with ethnic minority issues are factors that prevent minorities from specializing in neuropsychology.[17,18] Technology can increase the ability to provide such opportunities and facilitate the recruitment of ethnic minorities at the undergraduate and graduate level by providing virtual talks with university psychology organizations such as Psi Chi or the American Psychological Association of Graduate Students (APAGS).

Finally, technology has significant implications for developing neuropsychology internationally. For many countries, the educational requirement for practicing psychology is a master's or bachelor's degree and many practicing international neuropsychologists have little formal training in the specialization.[10] Moreover, international professionals may not have the resources to attend conferences such as INS for continuing education. With virtual platforms, educational opportunities are accessible to more of the world's neuropsychological providers. Technology also has the potential for facilitating a cross-fertilization of information and ideas. Linguistically and ethnically diverse neuropsychologists in high-resource countries can provide education, training, and mentoring to colleagues from their country of origin to increase the availability of neuropsychological services around the world. Conversely, international colleagues can educate Western neuropsychologists on pertinent cultural factors for understanding and performing assessments with ethnic minorities. These collaborations can also facilitate the development of translated and normed Western tests, as well as indigenous tests.

Summary

There is an increased need for developing competence in cultural neuropsychology on both global and national levels. Many objectives need to be accomplished to meet needs, including increasing the numbers of ethnic minority providers to service ethnically and linguistically diverse minorities, developing better education and training models, increasing accessibility of education and training, increasing the number and availability of translated tests and norms, and increasing cultural neuropsychology research. Although there have been advancements in each of these areas, there is still much to accomplish to address healthcare disparities in neuropsychology for ethnic minorities. The year 2020 has been pivotal for cultural neuropsychology due to the technologies developed to provide services during the COVID-19 pandemic, increased awareness of institutional racism from the BLMM, and growing diversity in leadership. This has energized efforts for increasing the availability of competent neuropsychological services for ethnic minority patients.

This book contributes to the advancement of culturally competent neuropsychological services by providing pertinent cultural information for understanding patients from different ethnic groups as well as identifying testing resources. This information will be useful for developing a culturally informed conceptualization and context for collecting accurate data, interpreting data, and making useful recommendations. This resource can be used in both education and training, as well as guiding clinical practice.

References

1. World Health Organization. World health statistics 2019: monitoring health for the SDGs [Internet]. Geneva: World Health Organization; 2019 [cited 2020 Aug 22]. Available from: https://www.who.int/gho/publications/world_health_statistics/2019/en/
2. World Health Organization. Towards a dementia plan: a WHO guide [Internet]. France: World Health Organization; 2018 [cited 2020 Aug 22]. Available from: https://apps.who.int/iris/bitstream/handle/10665/272642/9789241514132-eng.pdf?ua=1

3. United Nations. The number of international migrants reaches 272 million, continuing an upward trend in all world regions, says UN [Internet]. New York (NY): United Nations; 2019 Sep 17 [cited 2020 Mar 6]. Available from: https://www.un.org/development/desa/en/news/population/international-migrant-stock-2019.html

4. Satinsky E, Fuhr DC, Woodward A, Sondorp E, Roberts B. Mental health care utilisation and access among refugees and asylum seekers in Europe: a systematic review. Health Pol. 2019 Sep;123(9):851–63.

5. U.S. Census Bureau. Quick Facts [Internet]. [place unknown]: United States Census Bureau; 2019 [cited 2020 Aug 29]. Available from: https://www.census.gov/quickfacts/fact/table/US/PST045219

6. U.S. Census Bureau. New Census Bureau Report Analyzes U.S. Population Projections [Internet]. [place unknown]: United States Census Bureau; 2015 Mar 3 [cited 2020 Aug 29]. Available from: https://www.census.gov/newsroom/press-releases/2015/cb15-tps16.html

7. COVID-19 Coronavirus Pandemic. [Internet]. 2021. Worldometer [cited 2021 Jan 29]. Available from: https://www.worldometers.info/coronavirus/

8. Wilson B, Betteridge S, Fish J. Neuropsychological consequences of Covid-19. Neuropsych Rehab. 2020 Sep 1;30(9):1625–8.

9. Troyer EA, Kohn JN, Hong S. Are we facing a crashing wave of neuropsychiatric sequelae of COVID-19? Neuropsychiatric symptoms and potential immunologic mechanisms. Brain Behav Imm. 2020 Apr 13;87:34–9.

10. Ponsford J. International growth of neuropsychology. Neuropsychology. 2017 Nov;31(8):921–33.

11. Sakamoto M. Neuropsychology in Japan: history, current challenges, and future prospects. Clin Neuropsychol. 2016 Nov;30(8):1278–95.

12. Boivin MJ, Giordani B. Neuropsychology of children in Africa: perspectives on risk and resilience. New York (NY): Springer; 2013.

13. Grote CL, Novitski JI. International perspectives on education, training, and practice in clinical neuropsychology: comparison across 14 countries around the world. Clin Neuropsychol. 2016;30(8):1380–88.

14. Ledoux C, Pilot E, Diaz E, Krafft T. Migrants' access to healthcare services within the European Union: a content analysis of policy documents in Ireland, Portugal and Spain. Glob Health. 2018 Jun 15;14(1):57.

15. Rivera-Mindt M, Byrd D, Saez P, Manly J. Increasing culturally competent neuropsychological services for ethnic minority populations: a call to action. Clin Neuropsychol. 2010 Apr;24(3):429–53.

16. APA Directory. Demographic Characteristics of Division 40 Members by Membership Status [Internet]. Washington (DC): American Psychological Association, Center for Workforce Studies. 2017. Available from: https://www.apa.org/about/division/officers/services/div-40-2017.pdf

17. Cole S, Barber E. The problem. In: Cole S, Barber E, editors. Increasing faculty diversity: the occupational choices of high achieving minority students. Cambridge (MA): Harvard University Press; 2003a. p. 1–38.

18. Cole S, Barber E. Role models, interaction with faculty, and career aspirations In: Cole S, Barber E, editors. Increasing faculty diversity: the occupational choices of high achieving minority students. Cambridge (MA): Harvard University Press; 2003b. p. 163–86.

19. Bieliauskas. The Houston conference on specialty education and training in clinical neuropsychology. Arch Clin Neuropsychol [Internet]. 1998 March 1 [cited 2020 Aug 29];13(2):160–6. Available from: https://academic.oup.com/acn/article/13/2/160/1745

20. American Academy of Clinical Neuropsychology, Board of Directors. American Academy of Clinical Neuropsychology (AACN) practice guidelines for neuropsychological assessment and consultation. Clin Neuropsychol. 2007 Mar 28;21:209–31.

21. American Psychological Association. Guidelines on multicultural education, training, research, practice, and organizational change for psychologists. Amer Psych. 2003;58:377–402.

22. Elbulok-Charcape MM, Rabin LA, Spadaccini AT, Barr WB. Trends in the neuropsychological assessment of ethnic/racial minorities: a survey of clinical neuropsychologists in the United States and Canada. Cult Divers Ethn Min Psych. 2014 Jul;20(3):353–61.

23. Lin, L, Stamm, K, Christidis, P. Demographics of the US psychology workforce. Washington (DC): American Psychological Association; 2018.

24. Guidotti-Breting LM, Towns SJ, Butts AM, Brett BL, Leaffer EB, Whiteside DM. 2020 COVID-19 American Academy of Clinical Neuropsychology (AACN) student affairs committee survey of neuropsychology trainees. Clin Neuropsychol. 2020 Aug 8;34(7–8):1284–313.

25. Domen, CH, Collins RL, Davis JJ. The APPCN multisite didactic initiative: development, benefits, and challenges. Clin Neuropsychol. 2021 Jul 2;35(1):115–32.

26. Michalski, DS, Cope, C, Fowler, GA. Graduate study in psychology summary report: admissions, applications, and acceptances. Washington (DC): American Psychological Association; 2019.

27. American Education Research Association; American Psychological Association; National Council on Measurement in Education (US). Standards for educational and psychological testing. 2nd ed. Washington (DC): American Education Research Association; 2014.

28. Greenfield PM. You can't take it with you: why ability assessments don't cross cultures. Am Psych. 1997;52(10):1115–24.

29. Fujii D. Conducting a culturally informed neuropsychological evaluation. Washington (DC): American Psychological Association; 2016. p. 281.

30. Fujii D. Developing a cultural context for conducting a neuropsychological evaluation with culturally diverse client: the ECLECTIC framework. Clin. Neuropsychol. 2018;32(8):1356–92.

31. Fujii D, editor. The neuropsychology of Asian Americans. New York (NY): Psychology Press; 2011 Jan 11. p. 324.

32. Davis JM, D'Amato RC, editors. Neuropsychology of Asians and Asian Americans: practical and theoretical considerations. New York (NY): Springer Science and Business Media; 2014. p. 325.

33. Uzzell BP, Ponton M, Ardila A, editors. International handbook of cross-cultural neuropsychology. Mahwah (NJ): Psychology Press; 2013. p. 408.

34. Ferraro FR, editor. Minority and cross-cultural aspects of neuropsychological assessment: enduring and emerging trends. 2nd ed. New York (NY): Psychology Press; 2016. p. 538.

35. Nicoladis E, Montanari S, editors. Bilingualism across the lifespan: factors moderating language proficiency. Washington (DC): American Psychology Association; 2016. p. 361.

36. Uomoto JM, editor. Multicultural neurorehabilitation: clinical principals for rehabilitation professionals. New York (NY): Springer Publishing Company; 2016. p. 336.

37. Pedraza O, editor. Clinical cultural neuroscience: an integrative approach to cross-cultural neuropsychology. New York (NY): Oxford University Press; 2019. p. 312.

38. Fujii D, Judd T, Morere D, Byrd D. Cultural and disability issues in neuropsychological assessment. In: Stucky K, Kirkwood M, Donders J, editors. Neuropsych Study Guide and Board Review. 2nd ed. New York (NY): Oxford University Press; 2020. p. 194.

39. Nelson AP, Roper BL, Slomine BS, Morrison C, Greher MR, Janusz J et al. Official position of the American Academy of Clinical Neuropsychology (AACN): guidelines for practicum training in clinical neuropsychology. Clin Neuropsychol. 2015 Oct 3;29(7):879–904.

40. Smith G, CNS. Education and training in clinical neuropsychology: recent developments and documents from the clinical neuropsychology synarchy. Arch Clin Neuropsychol. 2018 May 1;34(3):418–31.

41. Salinas, C, AACN R2050 Peer Consultation Network Project (2018). Cultural Neuropsychology Postdoctoral Training: Preliminary Results on Competency and Practice from APPCN Training Directors.

42. National Council on Interpreting in Health Care. National Certification for Healthcare Interpreters [Internet]. Washington (DC): National Council on Interpreting in Health Care; [cited 2020 Aug 30]. Available from: https://www.ncihc.org/certification

43. U.S. Bureau of Labor Statistics. Top 30 Fastest-Growing Jobs by 2020 [Internet]. [place unknown: publisher unknown]; 2020 [cited 2020 Sep 21]. Available from: https://www.bumc.bu.edu/gms/files/2012/02/Top-30-fastest.pdf

44. British Psychological Society. Working with Interpreters: Guidelines for Psychologists [Internet]. Leicester: British Psychology Society; 2017 Nov 20 [cited 2020 Mar 30]. Available from: https://www.bps.org.uk/news-and-policy/working-interpreters-guidelines-psychologists

45. Canadian Psychological Association. Canadian Code of Ethics for Psychologists, 4th ed. [Internet]. Ottawa (ON): Canadian Psychological Association; 2017 Jan [cited 2020 Mar 30]. Available from: https://cpa.ca/docs/File/Ethics/CPA_Code_2017_4thEd.pdf

46. Fujii D, Santos O, Malva LD. Interpreter-assisted neuropsychological assessment: clinical considerations. In: Evans J, Fernandez A, editors. Understanding cross-cultural neuropsychology: science, testing and challenges. New York (NY): Taylor and Francis (in press; Routledge).

47. International Test Commission (ITC). ITC Guidelines for Translating and Adapting Tests [Internet]. Lincoln (NE): International Test Commission; 2017 [cited 2020 Mar 22]. Available from: https://www.intestcom.org/page/16

48. Nasreddine ZS, Phillips NA, Bédirian V, Charbonneau S, Whitehead V, Collin I et al. The Montreal Cognitive Assessment, MoCA: a brief screening tool for mild cognitive impairment. J Am Ger Soc. 2005 Apr;53(4):695–9.

49. Paradis M. Bilingual aphasia test. Hillsdale (NJ): Lawrence Erlbaum Associates; 1987.

50. Franzen S, Papma JM, van den Berg E, Nielsen TR. Cross-cultural neuropsychological assessment in the European Union: a Delphi expert study. Arch Clin Neuropsychol. 2020 Oct 12; 36(5): 815–30.

51. Nielsen TR, Segers K, Vanderaspoilden V, Bekkhus-Wetterberg P, Minthon L, Pissiota A et al. Performance of middle-aged and elderly European minority and majority populations on a Cross-Cultural Neuropsychological Test Battery (CNTB). Clin Neuropsychol. 2018 Nov;32(8):1411–30.

52. Rivera-Mindt M, Marquine MJ, Aghvinian M, Paredes AM, Kamalyan L, Suárez P et al. The Neuropsychological Norms for the US-Mexico Border Region in Spanish (NP-NUMBRS) project: overview and considerations for life span research and evidence-based practice. Clin Neuropsychol. 2021 Jul 29;35(2):466–80.

53. Rivera D, Arango-Lasprilla JC. Methodology for the development of normative data for Spanish-speaking pediatric populations. NeuroRehabilitation. 2017;41(3):581–92.

54. Shuttleworth-Edwards AB, Van der Merwe AS. WAIS-III and WISC-IV South African cross-cultural normative data stratified for quality of education. In: Ferraro RF, editor. Minority and cross-cultural aspects of neuropsychological assessment: enduring and emerging trends. 2nd ed. New York (NY): Psychology Press; 2015. p. 72.

55. Gasquoine PG. Race-norming of neuropsychological tests. Neuropsych Rev. 2009 Jun 1;19(2):250.

56. Lynn R, Meisenberg G. National IQs calculated and validated for 108 nations. Intelligence. 2010 Jul–Aug;38(4): 353–60.

57. Lynn R, Vanhanen T. IQ and global inequality. Augusta (GA): Washington Summit Publishers; 2006. p. 442.

58. Guilmette TJ, Sweet JJ, Hebben N, Koltai D, Mahone EM, Spiegler BJ et al. American Academy of Clinical Neuropsychology consensus conference statement on uniform labeling of performance test scores. Clin Neuropsychol. 2020 Jan 10;34(3):437–53.

59. Bialystok E, Luk G, Peets KF, Yang S. Receptive vocabulary differences in monolingual and bilingual children. Bilingualism. 2010 Oct;13(4):525–31.

60. Multilingual People [Internet]. place unknown: ilanguages.org; [cited 2020 Sep 27]. Available from: http://www.ilanguages.org/bilingual.php#:~:text=Bilingual%3A%20A%20person%20using%20or%20able%20to%20use,of%20world%20population%20speak%20more%20than%204%20languages%29

61. Chiao JY. Cultural neuroscience: visualizing culture-gene influences on brain function. In: Decety J, Cacioppo J, editors. Oxford handbook of social neuroscience. New York (NY): Oxford University Press; 2011. p. 742–61.

62. Hedden T, Ketay S, Aron A, Markus HR, Gabrieli JD. Cultural influences on neural substrates of attentional control. Psychol Sci. 2008 Jan;19(1):12–7.

63. Nisbett RE, Masuda T. Culture and point of view. Proc Nat Acad of Sci. 2003 Sep;100(19):11163–70.

64. Cherner M, Marquine MJ, Umlauf A, Paredes AM, Rivera-Mindt M, Suárez P et al. Neuropsychological Norms for the US-Mexico Border Region in Spanish (NP-NUMBRS) project: methodology and sample characteristics. Clin Neuropsychol. 2021 Apr 22;35(2):253–68.

65. Guàrdia-Olmos J, Peró-Cebollero M, Rivera D, Arango-Lasprilla JC. Methodology for the development of normative data for ten Spanish-language neuropsychological tests in eleven Latin American countries. NeuroRehabilitation. 2015 Jan 1;37(4):493–9.

66. Cullum, CM, Hynan LS, Grosch M, Parikh M, Weiner MF. Teleneuropsychology: evidence for video teleconference-based neuropsychological assessment. JINS [Internet]. 2014 Oct 24 [cited 2020 Aug 29];20(10):1028–33. Available from: https://www.ncbi.nlm.nih.gov/pmc/articles/PMC4410096/ doi:10.1017/S1355617714000873.

B. Skills and Training

2 Multicultural Education and Training in Neuropsychology
Let's Talk About *Skill* Acquisition!

Orlando Sánchez and Tedd Judd

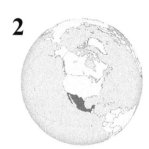
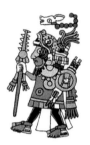

Taka ma ñayi nguiakoi ñayivi ñatu na ja'a tnu'u ja kusa'a ndeva'ña-i, su'uva kajito va'aña-i, yuka ku ja jiniñu'u ja kukototna-i. – *Ñuu Savi* (Mixteco) language

All human beings are born free and equal in dignity and rights. They are endowed with reason and conscience and should act towards one another in a spirit of [community].

(Universal Declaration of Human Rights, Article 1)

Section I: About This Chapter

This chapter is intended for neuropsychologists and neuropsychology trainees interested in the practical clinical application of Western neuropsychology to non-Western contexts. While we certainly do not presume to have all the answers to this complex dilemma, we offer at least a preliminary solution; a conceptual, clinical framework grounded in more than four decades of research relevant to multicultural education. In addition, the framework draws from the first author's insights as an indigenous *Ñuu Savi (Mixteco)* immigrant neuropsychologist, as well as the second author's expertise with more than 40 years of cross-cultural clinical neuropsychology experience working with underserved populations from around the world.

Context: Why Do I Lack the Skills to Work with Diverse Populations?

In the 21st century, the notion of delivering high-quality "culturally competent" care to humanity is a universally espoused value within healthcare professions, including psychology. Yet, bringing "culturally competent" care to fruition on a wide scale remains a daunting challenge. While it would seem that the independent and scientific discipline of psychology is well-positioned to meet the needs of diverse communities, in fact, most minority groups continue to be underserved and psychology continues to struggle to recruit, train, and place sufficient practitioners in these communities. Why? We propose that our education and training are among the primary barriers preventing us from meeting this challenge head-on. Specifically, these barriers include:

1 **Literature relevant to multicultural education is hidden, overlooked, partially acknowledged, and/or not easily accessible.** Basic empirical science relevant to multicultural education and training is scattered and broad. The literature on cultural competency is overwhelmingly vast within the United States alone and even more formidable in a global context of multicultural psychology, cultural psychology, international or global psychology, cross-cultural psychology, and transnational psychology. Though the literature base is enormous (and growing), it

DOI: 10.4324/9781003051862-4

lacks depth (e.g., consensus on constructs and theory development[1]). Overall, the literature on multicultural education requires periodic synthesis to facilitate access and effectively inform training and clinical practice in psychology.[1,2]

2 **Multicultural education and training remain an incoherent, "hodgepodge" of strategies with minimal focus on skill acquisition.** Education and training in general psychology, at least in the United States, are the foundations of clinical neuropsychology—the latter competencies building upon the former. While both general and subspecialty acknowledge *"Individual and cultural diversity"* as a core competency,[3–9] efforts are largely disconnected and the same appears true in other parts of the world.[10] Though some details concerning cross-cultural conceptual and practical elements have recently emerged in neuropsychology,[7,11] systematic skill training has yet to be described. We argue that, like other core elements in psychology, multicultural education requires an organized, developmental approach (i.e., graded complexity from graduate school to postgraduate training and beyond) ultimately designed to foster skills required for clinical assessment and intervention. We know of no such approach in psychology anywhere in the world. Currently, there is wide variability among graduate and postgraduate programs in the United States, and similar variability in other parts of the world.[12] Overall, multicultural education and training remains an incoherent, "hodgepodge" of strategies with minimal focus on skill acquisition. Available evidence suggests that programs almost exclusively focus on content-based knowledge (e.g., teaching broad facts about heterogenous racial/ethnic groups) and "awareness" (e.g., racism/discrimination, biases), but with minimal attention to education or training targeting specific, practical clinical skills that are desperately needed to address existing health disparities.[13–18]

3 **The concern with the politics of identity.** There is growing criticism within the United States that social science research is yielding constructs with inherent sociopolitical ideological biases.[19] Given the universal influence of Western psychology, this has implications for the field in other parts of the world. The concern and criticism are not only towards ideological bias in research but that this is negatively influencing multicultural education/training with the risk of it being viewed as another biased structure promoting a left-leaning political-ideological agenda under the guise of training.[19–21]

Overall, considering the aforementioned, it is no wonder that the majority of us lack the skills to effectively work with individuals who are markedly different than ourselves. While the issue is complex, one thing is certain, disparities in access to psychological and neuropsychological services will persist as long as the issue of training clinical multicultural *skills* remains unaddressed.

The Story behind the S-JMVAM

Before jumping into the empirical foundations of the Sánchez-Judd Minneapolis VA Model (S-JMVAM), allow us to share how this model emerged. Since the multicultural movement surged in the 1980s, Tedd Judd has been addressing healthcare disparities in a direct and practical manner. During that time, he has evaluated clients from approximately 90 countries with a special interest in the most marginalized populations including Amerindians (e.g., Makah, Lummi, Zapoteco, Maya, etc.) and refugees (e.g., Somali, Iraqi, Meskhetian Turk, Nepali-Bhutanese, etc.). In addition, Tedd has taught neuropsychology in 25 countries observing the varied cultures-of-neuropsychology, including their adaptations and applications in different cultural and language contexts. This experience produced many insights about Western psychology in non-Western contexts, which he subsequently began to share with others in our field, including trainees. Tedd's trainees have included immigrants and speakers of 17 different languages. Orlando Sánchez was one of these trainees and has been collaborating with Tedd for over ten years.

Orlando Sánchez was born in a small, impoverished indigenous (Mixteco) village in southern Mexico. In pursuit of the coveted "American dream," he and his family immigrated to the United States in the early 90s. While completing a basic formal education in the United States, Orlando simultaneously was immersed in his indigenous culture (e.g., learning indigenous philosophy and the art of living with wisdom in service of the community, living according to indigenous values/ principles, honoring indigenous traditions). Given his commitment to indigenous philosophy, as Orlando contemplated higher education, a career in psychology appeared an obvious fit. The ambition and desire were to learn from Western science and technology and use this knowledge to serve his community. Unfortunately, Orlando grew increasingly discouraged and disappointed in Western psychology and contemplated abandoning this endeavor. Fortunately, Orlando met Tedd in his second year of graduate school before officially withdrawing from his program and the rest is history.

In 2016, Orlando took the teachings from Tedd and, in partnership with the Minneapolis VA, piloted this model within their psychology training program. This subsequently informed and produced a more refined training curriculum with emphasis on skill acquisition.[22] Thus, in the absence of multicultural education and training in psychology specifically aimed at developing and promoting culturally informed clinical *skills*, the formal S-JMVAM was born.

The S-JMVAM

Sue and colleague's tripartite model (*Awareness, Knowledge,* and *Skill*)[23] has enjoyed widespread development in psychology and related disciplines, it has broadly informed multicultural education, and it has offered a useful foundation for multicultural neuropsychology. However, as previously stated, the general training currently offered (i.e., "hodgepodge" of strategies) is highly inadequate for the specific skills needed for competent multicultural neuropsychology. In response, we offer a conceptual, clinical framework (S-JMVAM) as a possible solution.

The S-JMVAM is a developmental, interdisciplinary model rooted in the pioneering works of Sue and colleagues. Briefly, in our model, we retain Sue's original categories (*Awareness, Knowledge,* and *Skill*) but redefine these with an eye towards more precise skill development. It is our belief that all three of these domains develop continuously throughout the professional lifespan. The *Awareness* component is thoroughly reviewed and discussed elsewhere in this book (see chapter by Dr. Swanda on using reflective self-awareness); consequently, this will not be reiterated here. Instead, we will focus on those components of *Knowledge* and *Skill* that are more specific to neuropsychology.

Foundational Knowledge Base

Ideally, trainees should develop a firm multicultural knowledge base before engaging in clinical practice. This knowledge base would enhance critical thinking, reasoning, problem-solving, and judgment with respect to cross-cultural work. In our model, this *Foundational Knowledge* is defined as encompassing three components:

1   **Science and history.** Trainees should be familiar with the history of cross-cultural psychology (late 1960s) and multiculturalism (1980s), relevant theories and constructs (e.g., acculturation), seminal works (e.g., Sue's Tripartite Model[23]), the science of multicultural education and training in psychology,[1] and the strengths/limitations of this broad body of

literature (see Table 2.1 for sample reading recommendations). As is true in every discipline and area of study, history and foundational scientific knowledge are the bedrock of "cultural competency."

Table 2.1 Sample of history and foundational scientific knowledge

Foundational knowledge
Benuto, L., Casas, J., & O' Donohue, W. (2018). Training culturally competent psychologists: A systematic review of the training outcome literature. *Training and Education in Professional Psychology 12*(3), 125–134. https://doi.org/10.1037/tep0000190
Shiraev, E. & Levy, D. A. (2021). *Cross-cultural psychology critical thinking and contemporary applications.* New York, NY & London: Routledge.
Smith, T. B. & Trimble, J. E. (2016). *Multicultural education/training and experience: A meta-analysis of surveys and outcome studies.* In T.B. Smith & J.E. Trimble: Foundations of multicultural psychology: Research to inform effective practice (pp. 21–47). Washington, DC: American Psychological Association, viii, p.308.
Sue, D. W., Bernier, J. B., Durran, M., Feinberg, L., Pedersen, P., Smith, E., & Vasquez-Nuttall, E. (1982). Position paper: Cross-cultural counseling competencies. *The Counseling Psychologist, 10*(2), 45–52.

2 **Recognizing ourselves as cultural beings.** This is the knowledge that serves to inform the *Awareness* component of cultural competency. Within neuropsychology, some of the most important components of this awareness relate to our interpersonal, family, and social values; perspectives on health, illness, and healing; patterns of communication, language, and literacy; and experiences of education, cognitive skills, and testing. By recognizing ourselves and others as cultural beings, we can enter the other's worldview and use our clinical expertise in a socially responsible manner to facilitate optimal evaluation and treatment in a collaborative manner (see Table 2.2 for sample reading recommendations and sample exercises).

3 **Clinical practice knowledge.** This includes, for example, the importance of researching a client's background, how to facilitate an effective clinical relationship, how to conduct a culturally competent clinical interview, how to use the DSM-5 cultural formulation, how to work effectively with interpreters, how to access and use cultural consultation, and how to use measures and norms with cultural competence.

We believe that this knowledge should be introduced early in the training sequence. We would never expect someone to be a competent psychologist/neuropsychologist after a couple of classes, seminars, workshops, and/or years of jumbled up, incoherent training, particularly training that is dissociated from *skill* development. The same is true for multicultural education; in the United States, a firm foundation in graduate school is key to developing clinical skills during practicum, internship, and beyond. Consequently, we strongly urge the field to adopt a systematic, coherent, focused, developmental approach to multicultural education and training. The S-JMVAM is an attempt at such approach and is very much in line with the movement towards competency-based education, training, and credentialing in psychology and neuropsychology.[3–9]

Clinical Practice (Skill Development)

Appropriate skillsets for multicultural neuropsychology training need to be worked out by our profession at large and will vary with the setting. We offer here a rough draft of 13 foundational skills domains. While each of these can be seen as skills that are important in all of clinical

Table 2.2 Sample identity development models and cultural awareness & sensitivity exercises

---

Recognizing ourselves as "cultural beings": Awareness & sensitivity exercises

---

Identity development models

- Hoffman, J. L., & Hoffman, J. L. S. (2006). Sculpting race: An innovative approach to teaching racial identity development. Presentation at the Western Regional Careers in Student Affairs Day, California State University, Fullerton. https://meh.religioused.org/RacialIdentityDevelopment.pdf
- Atkinson, D. R., Morten, G., & Sue, D. W. (1979). *A minority identity development model.* In: D. R. Atkinson, G. Morten, & D. W. Sue (Eds.), Counseling American minorities: A cross-cultural perspective. Dubuque, IA: William C. Brown.
- Cross, W. E. & Fhagen-Smith, P. (2001). In: C. L. Wijeyesinghe, B. W. Jackson III. (Eds.), New Perspectives on racial identity development (1st ed.; pp. 243–268). New York, NY: New York University Press.
- Helms, J. E. 1995. *An update of Helms's White and people of color racial identity models.* In: J. G. Ponterotto, J. M. Casas, L. A. Suzuki, & C. M. Alexander (Eds.), Handbook of multicultural counseling. Thousand Oaks, CA: Sage.
- Rowe, W., Bennett, S. K., & Atkinson, D. R. (1994). White racial identity models: A critique and alternative proposal. *The Counseling Psychologist, 22,*129–146.
- Ferdman, B. M. & Gallegos, P. I. (2001). *Racial identity development and Latinos in the United States.* In: C. L. Wijeyesinghe & B. W. Jackson, III (Eds.), New perspectives on racial identity development: A theoretical and practical anthology (pp. 32–66). New York, NY: New York University Press.
- Nadal, K. (2004). Filipino American identity development model. *Journal of Multicultural Counseling and Development, 32,* 45–62.
- Kim, J. (2001). *Asian American racial identity theory.* In: C. L. Wijeyesinghe & B. W. Jackson, III (Eds.), New perspectives on racial identity development: A theoretical and practical anthology (pp. 138–161). New York, NY: New York University Press.
- Horse, P. G. (2005). *Native American identity.* In: S. R. Jones & S. K Watt (Eds.), New directions for student services (pp. 61–68). Wiley Periodicals, Inc. https://doi.org/10.1002/ss.154
- Poston, W. S. C. (1990). The biracial identity development model: A needed addition. *Journal of Counseling and Development, 69,* 152–155.
- Rockquemore, K. & Laszloffy, T. A. (2005). Moving beyond tragedy: A multidimensional model of mixed-race identity, raising biracial children (1st ed.; pp. 1–17). Lanham, MD: AltaMira Press.
- Gibson, J. (2006). Disability and clinical competency: An introduction. *The California Psychologist, 39,* 6–10.
- Forber-Pratt, A. J., Merrin, G. J., Mueller, C. O., Price, L. R., & Kettrey, H. H. (in press). Initial factor exploration of disability identity. *Rehabilitation Psychology.* Advance online publication. https://www.ncbi.nlm.nih.gov/pubmed/31944783
- Lev, A. I. (2004) Transgender emergence: Therapeutic guidelines for working with gender-variant people and their families (1st ed.; p. 235). LCSW, CASAC. New York, NY: Haworth Clinical Practice Press.
- McNeill, B. W. (2001). An exercise in ethnic identity awareness. *Journal of Multicultural Counseling and Development, 29*(4), 274–279. https://doi.org/10.1002/j.2161-1912.2001.tb00470.x
- Pedersen, P. (2004). 110 experiences for multicultural learning. Washington, DC: American Psychological Association.
- Sandeen, E., Moore, K. M., & Swanda, R. M. (2018). Reflective local practice: A pragmatic framework for improving culturally competent practice in psychology. *Professional Psychology: Research and Practice, 49*(2), 142–150. https://doi.org/10.1037/pro0000183

---

psychology, each skill also has important and distinctive neuropsychological features (for a review of advanced skills, please refer to Fujii, 2016):

1 Researching a client's culture, language, and background, especially with respect to neuropsychological dimensions.
2 Working with an interpreter.
3 Establishing rapport across cultures.

4 Taking a cultural, language, education, migration, and acculturation history.
5 Taking a diagnostic history with few or no pertinent medical records available and from eval-uees and their family members with limited or no education and/or knowledge of medicine, including lack of familiarity with and/or distrust in the mainstream healthcare system.
6 Understanding and taking into account influences from language, culture, and education in testing, including test and norm selection and how to test individuals who are test-naive.
7 Understanding and taking into account cultural considerations in neurological health, mental health, symptoms, perceptions, and presentation, including culturally distinct mental health disorders, idioms of distress, and cultural limitations of the DSM-5.
8 Interpreting and integrating the findings resulting from culturally sensitive interviewing, test-ing, behavioral observations, and other sources of cultural and clinical information.
9 Taking culture into account in planning interventions.
10 Communicating findings and recommendations to diverse clients/families.
11 Communicating cultural considerations to other professionals in written and oral formats and through modeling of behavior.
12 Seeking and/or offering cultural consultation.
13 Advocating for the client and family (when needed).

Additionally, students or clinicians who intend to offer services in a language or languages other than the language of training may pursue some or all of the following:

1 Clinical competence in the target language.
2 Interpreter/translator skills.
3 Academic proficiency in the target language.
4 Accessing target language professional literature.

Each of these can be further specified into individual subskills that can be refined and mastered via education and training. Many of these skills can be taught initially through didactics and con-sultations with interpreters and cultural experts from various disciplines. Skill practice can then be trained through clinical exercises and role plays prior to deploying these skills with clients. All of these skills can also be readily targeted in clinical training by providing appropriate clinical experiences with culturally competent supervision, ongoing academic study, and clinical cultural consultation. As a profession in science and practice, neuropsychology has done little to develop preclinical exercises in multicultural neuropsychology; to define, describe, and train culturally competent supervision; and to develop models, networks, habits, and payment systems for multi-disciplinary cultural consultation.

Section II: Case Study

The following is an amalgam of case experiences derived from over 15 years of practicum training in cross-cultural psychology at refugee service centers. These experiences are described in narra-tive form to illustrate some clinical ways of training each of the skills listed above. While not all of the details below were present in a single case, all of them have occurred in this teaching with Somali clients, most of them multiple times. This presents a snapshot of teaching at the clinical training stage. These students had already received clinical psychology preclinical teaching in *Awareness and Knowledge*, as described above. They had preclinical training in all of the *Skills* listed above (these are the learning objectives of our cross-cultural psychology practicum). They had observed several evaluations and then gradually began participating in the evaluations to the level represented here. They have each also developed interpreter skills and a specialty in working in their own first languages with people of multiple ethnicities. Through learning with continual feedback, as described below, they later progressed from this level to independent practice to teaching other practicum students.

A Brief Cultural Background Review (Prior to the Clinical Encounter)

Background research is fundamental in preparing to see a client from an unfamiliar country, language, or culture. Neuropsychologically pertinent information includes[24]:

- Languages and language features (e.g., writing system)
- Neuroepidemiology
- Educational system
- Health care system (when pertinent)
- Recent history
- Social and family structures and roles
- Attitudes and beliefs regarding health, illness (causation and relief of disease), healing (traditional, religious, and Western), mental health, disability, idioms of distress
- Communication and interpersonal style
- Legal system (when pertinent)

Thanks to the digital revolution, we can now readily and rapidly access useful information about most people's cultural background, sometimes down to the specific village (for example, the first author once did a review of his village and was surprised to find a picture of his aunt's adobe house on a website showcasing the diversity of indigenous villages in Oaxaca, Mexico).

This initial review offers us a broad view of a client's cultural background and supplies hypotheses about their perspectives and experiences (See the Somalia chapter in the book for further country background for this case and details of care of Somalis. The present case presentation is focused on the teaching process rather than clinical specifics of Somalis). However, individual language use, education, migration, acculturation, employment, beliefs, and values must be explored thoroughly and directly with each client. Often subsequent cultural details that are revealed during the evaluation need to be further researched.

Case Referral

Kahlid is an approximately 35-year-old Somali refugee, married female homemaker with no formal secular education who was referred by her primary care provider for an assessment concerning her failure to learn English.

Students

Olga, originally from Belarus, is a 29-year-old trilingual (English/Belarusian/Russian) female in her 3rd year of doctoral training in clinical psychology. Mohamed, a professor from Saudi Arabia, is a 32-year-old bilingual (English/Arabic) male also in his 3rd year of doctoral training in clinical psychology (both are students in our cross-cultural psychology practicum). In addition, informally, both have had to function as interpreters for their respective families. Currently, both have studied interpreter ethics and professional standards with goals of becoming certified interpreters (e.g., their training has included watching online videos concerning interpreter use and practicing interpreter use skills with peers). Each student made distinctive contributions to the evaluation.

Preparation and Planning

Kahlid's medical records concerned obstetrics but were otherwise unremarkable. Both students learned about Somali refugees from several sources including:

- The Somali medical profile in ethnomed.org
- Somali language in omniglot.com
- About Somalia from reliable Internet searches

The appointment was at the refugee service center where Kahlid's family had received settlement services. We met with the interpreter, Rahmed, who was also a mental health therapist in the community mental health center portion of the refugee services. We reinforced our previous agreement with Rahmed—i.e., that her role as counselor would be separate and distinct from her role as interpreter within our evaluation process.[25] Given that Rahmed was a refugee herself, we had also previously discussed potential secondary traumatization in hearing refugee trauma stories. Rahmed briefed us about what little she knew about this family, including that Kahlid's husband, Omar, spoke functional English and was very protective of her. Consequently, we planned on giving extra attention to winning his trust. Our tentative plan was that:

- Initially, we would all talk together until sufficient rapport was established.
- We would then initiate logistics (i.e., confidentiality, etc.)
- We would then proceed with the interview (Joint Interview 1 and 2 below)
- We would then separate for confidential perspectives, to triangulate independent perspectives, and for testing Khalid:

  - Olga, with Rahmed as the interpreter, would interview and test Kahlid since Omar would likely be more agreeable to this (i.e., congruent with cultural customs, two women rather than men talking with his wife without his presence). Mohamed and Dr. Judd would interview Omar.

In addition, we decided that the students would use their first names with the family for warmth and interpersonal connection, while Dr. Judd would use the formal "Dr. Judd" to reinforce professional authority.

Rapport

Kahlid arrived with Omar and their youngest 1-year-old child (their other children were in school). As we settled into the room, Olga offered them tea while Dr. Judd played peek-a-boo with the child (Mohamed offered the child an age-appropriate toy). Since it was a snowy day, Mohamed initiated a conversation about how difficult it was for them to learn to deal with snow, a conversation that Rahmed, Omar, and, eventually, Kahlid joined in on. The conversation then progressed to a discussion about American cultural peculiarities, such as trying to make sense of Halloween and Thanksgiving. Olga then spoke a bit about her own toddler and the conversation turned to a discussion about babies. All of these topics generated laughter and a sense of connection, to the degree that we felt we had established sufficient rapport, so we proceeded to the evaluation logistics.

Mohamed explained the evaluation process, including that we would talk both together and separately. In addition, Mohamed apologized, on behalf of the team, for our not speaking Somali and asked their patience while doing our best to understand their experiences. Mohamed explained that we would do an exam with Kahlid to understand the health of her brain. He explained this as being somewhat like a doctor's exam and somewhat like the things she did in English class. Finally, Mohamed explained the standard disclosure elements including confidentiality and the roles of the individuals present (interpreter, students, and primary/supervising clinician).

Dr. Judd elaborated on what Mohamed explained as needed, partly to clarify and repeat and partly to accentuate his authority in the process. After everything was explained, Mohamed offered the disclosure forms—first to Omar, as a sign of respect in this male-dominant culture where there is an expectation that husbands will control or oversee their wives' interactions, and then to Kahlid so that she could mark her Xs, since she is illiterate, on the signature lines. With logistics completed, we proceeded to the clinical interviews.

Joint Interview 1

Olga began the interview by taking a cultural, language, and immigration history. She directed her questions to Kahlid, but Omar often answered and Kahlid deferred to him. Olga tolerated this for a while, but eventually, she said, "For this next question I would like to know what Kahlid knows about this." We learned that Kahlid did not know her own age and that her paperwork contained a birthdate (the conventional January 1) assigned by refugee personnel. She primarily spoke Somali with some MaiMai (which she learned as a child) and some Swahili (which she learned while living at the refugee camp). With respect to her immigration history, Kahlid and her sister (her primary caretaker) fled the war in Somalia on foot when Kahlid was approximately five years old (Kahlid became tearful as Omar shared this history). Consequently, Kahlid grew up in the Dadaab Refugee Camp in Kenya. While she did not attend "government school," she did attend Quranic school where she worked and attended part-time, from ages 5 through 8. Her work history included selling water for ablutions, basket and mat weaving, housekeeping, and childcare. During her time in Quranic school, it took her approximately three years to recite the first book, which is as far as she got (this was the extent of her education and she never learned to read). Kahlid had an arranged marriage at approximately age 13 and had her first of 6 children at age 14. Kahlid, Omar, and their children came to the United States as refugees five years prior to this interview. During her time in the United States, she mostly stayed home except for when attending English classes with Omar. While Omar benefited from English classes, she never made it past Level 1 over the course of three years.

Consolidation 1

Following the first portion of the interview (above), we took a break. During this time, the students researched the Dadaab refugee camp (e.g., https://www.unhcr.org/ke/dadaab-refugee-complex). They learned:

- That it is one of the largest refugee camps in the world with refugees predominantly from Somalia.
- That refugees in Dadaab learn Swahili as this is the uniting language across many tribal languages.
- That there are medical services but limited schooling, employment opportunities, inadequate security from crime and ongoing ethnic feuds, and limited ability to leave the camp.

Rahmed, who also lived in Dadaab, shared her experience with the students. In addition, Olga and Mohamed researched the MaiMai people and learned about their language and role in Somali society. Mohamed explained to Olga that the Quranic school is religious instruction for a few hours a week, that students memorize the Quran in classic Arabic, that the first book is very short, and that taking three years to learn the first book is atypical.

Joint Interview 2

After the break, to reinforce rapport, Dr. Judd, knowing about the clinic's basket weaving group, shared with Kahlid and Omar photos of a basket weaving demonstration he had encountered as a tourist in the Bolivian Amazon. Kahlid was pleased with this and discussed Somali weaving techniques with Rahmed. The students showed photos of Dadaab and Omar, Kahlid, and Rahmed shared their experience living in this camp. Kahlid looked away from some of the photos. Following this, the interview continued.

Omar and Kahlid both reported that she had attended English class regularly, studied diligently, and developed friendships with a few Somali women who also attended classes. Nevertheless, Kahlid could not remember what she studied beyond a few social phrases, individual letters, and isolated simple words. On inquiry, they reported that she had memory difficulties for conversations and everyday family events. They indicated that she does not go out alone because she is afraid of getting lost. Omar and her older children manage the finances, shopping, appointments, and medications. Kahlid attends mosque and has a few Somali women friends in their apartment complex. She enjoys video calls to her sister in Dadaab and can use autodial; she can also access YouTube and Facebook by icons but has not been able to learn other smartphone functions. Omar indicated that the family made sure someone supervised when she cooked because she often forgot things on the stove. Dr. Judd asked Omar if she was a good cook and he said, "Yes, very good." Dr. Judd then asked, "When are you inviting us all over to dinner?" (everyone laughed). Omar said, well, you can come if you want. You would love to meet our children. We then asked permission to call their oldest son, age 21, to confirm the history and they both agreed.

When Olga reviewed Kahlid's medical history she reported that she had been told that she had been kicked in the head by a camel when she was a child, but she did not know anything else about this. She had not received medical attention. She said that she had a scar and dent and indicated the left side of her head. We asked permission of her and of Omar to examine it and they said that only Olga would be allowed to see her without her head scarf. Olga reported from this that there was a scar under her scalp and a palpable skull dent over the left temporal area. Olga asked if she had had any major illnesses and they said no. Olga asked if she had had malaria, and Omar said, "Well, everyone gets malaria."

Consolidation 2

At that point in the interview, in the interest of time, we suggested that we would talk separately. We took a short break, refreshed out coffee and tea, Kahlid did a diaper change, and Dr. Judd approved Olga's plan for a directed interview and testing. Dr. Judd reminded her of how to do a malaria interview. Dr. Judd, Mohamed, Omar, and the baby went to another room.

Collateral Interviews (Dr. Judd, Mohamed, and Omar with His Child)

Omar's English was adequate for an interview, which was conducted by Mohamed. Omar reported that Kahlid had never had a good memory and that she experienced severe malaria about a year before they left Kenya. He said she had been hospitalized for two weeks, was delirious for a week, and that the doctor thought she might die. Overall, she had a slow recovery and, afterwards, her memory worsened. On inquiry, he also reported that long before he knew her, he had heard that she had been attacked in the refugee camp. He said that she sometimes awakened at night screaming, that she did not like to watch the news from Kenya or Somalia that included violence, and that she was afraid to go outside. He was fairly content with her housekeeping and parenting but wished that she were more able to connect with the community. He also wished that she would someday be employed. Following the interview with Omar, Mohamed called their eldest son and confirmed this history to further triangulate and validate our data.

Client Interview 1 (Olga, Rahmed, and Kahlid)

During this interview, Kahlid said she had been sick not long before they came to the United States, but she did not remember much about it. She did not know what her illness was and did not recognize the word for malaria. On directed inquiry, she remembered having a high fever and chills a couple of different times. She also remembered taking a very bitter medicine. Olga screened for and ruled out domestic violence.

Testing 1

Olga administered the Fuld Object Memory Evaluation,[26] a test involving memory for ten common objects. This test is reliably understood across cultures and is not sensitive to language or level of education but is sensitive to age and to memory loss. Kahlid was able to name the objects readily but used the MaiMai name for two of them and the Swahili name for one of them. Her learning curve was moderately impaired, as was her delayed recall, which was out of proportion to her initial learning. Her responses to a two-alternative, forced-choice recognition memory task for the ten items were rapid and accurate, suggesting good test effort and valid results.

Client Interview 2

During this interview, the following exchange occurred:

OLGA: *"I noticed that you got tearful when Omar was talking about your leaving Somalia. I know that this can be a difficult thing to talk about and I am sorry to ask you about such a difficult thing, but I really would like to understand what has happened to you so that we can help you to adjust to life in America."*

Tearfully, Kahlid shared that the Somali army invaded her village and killed her parents in front of her, but she was saved by her sister. She shared fragmentary, frightening memories of their long, dangerous walk to Kenya. Olga, using the "some people" construction she had been taught, said: *"Some people who have such experiences still carry it heavily in their hearts. Is that true for you?"* Similarly, she asked about dreams, flashbacks, avoidances, and the photos of Dadaab that she had turned away from earlier. Olga learned that Kahlid had been attacked in Dadaab at about age 11. She confirmed nightmares, flashbacks, and avoidances. Once these were confirmed, Olga judged that she had enough information for our purposes; she thanked Kahlid for her trust, changed the subject to children, and eventually called for a break.

Testing 2

We took a break and consolidated our findings, including checking on clinic resources with Rahmed. We all came together again and Dr. Judd improvised informal testing with Kahlid. She was able to read the letters of the English alphabet reliably, and these include all of the letters of the Somali alphabet. She was able to sound out short words in English. She was then presented with writing in Somali, which she had never attempted. To her delight, she was able to slowly sound out and understand short words in Somali.

Feedback

Dr. Judd introduced the feedback in order to give it the weight of his authority, but the students explained the results. Mohamed explained that Kahlid's slow learning was likely due to being kicked in the head by the camel and also because of the illness she had while in Dadaab (i.e., malaria that infected her brain). Mohamed explained that we would complete the immigration form to give her a medical exemption from learning English and United States history and civics for the US citizenship exam. Olga thanked Kahlid for her trust and explained that she carried a heavy burden on her heart from the war and her attack while living in Dadaab. Olga carefully explained that those experiences still cause pain and are keeping her from being able to adjust to American life. She explained that there is help available to lift that burden and suggested that Kahlid see Rahmed for psychotherapy. Mohamed repeated this offer, framing it in an Islamic worldview, which both Kahlid and Omar appreciated. Omar and Kahlid agreed that Kahlid would see Rahmed for psychotherapy. At Dr. Judd's invitation, Rahmed switched roles from interpreter to therapist and briefly explained what treatment would entail. In addition, Rahmed offered Kahlid the opportunity to join the clinic's Somali women's basket weaving and support group, which delighted Kahlid.

Dr. Judd then suggested that Kahlid had the potential to learn literacy in Somali and that this might be more realistic than learning English. He suggested that her older children might also eventually be able to teach her more Internet access using Somali, including the use of a translation application. Rahmed volunteered to include this in her treatment plan. The feedback was repetitive on all of these points, with questions answered. We thanked them for their trust and honesty and for the joy of bringing their baby along. Gratefully, Kahlid offered to take the teacups back to the kitchen and wash them for us; we thanked her but declined her kind offer.

Debriefing

At our debriefing, immediately following this 2½ hour appointment, Rahmed explained that Kahlid's Somali had a MaiMai accent with some MaiMai words mixed in. She had the Bantu appearance of her MaiMai heritage. These things could subject her to some discrimination in parts of the Somali community. We fine-tuned Olga and Mohamed's interpreter-use skills as well as our rapport- and trust-building strategies. Mohamed and Rahmed discussed some of the dynamics of arranged marriages and of Islamic worldviews, including how that would figure into Rahmed's therapy with Kahlid. She explained how she would use prayer and family involvement to work on anxiety and phobia desensitization; she assured us that she was experienced in pacing her therapy and that she would unpack Kahlid's war traumas and the trauma of the attack in Dadaab with a pacing that Kahlid could handle. We discussed possible diagnoses of PTSD and depression and the cultural limitations of DSM-5. We recommended that Rahmed record summaries of their session recommendations on Kahlid's cell phone and collaborate with her family in training her in accessing them to accommodate for Kahlid's memory impairment. Rahmed informed us that there is no Somali word for depression and little in the way of a cultural concept of depression.

We reviewed the cyclical fever and chills of malaria, the bitter taste of the treatment of quinine, and the impact of cerebral malaria falciparum. Mohamed, who is interested in neuropsychology, decided to read about it further. Dr. Judd explained how the transparent orthography of Somali contrasted with the opaque orthography of English and how that manifested in the informal reading testing we did. This also factored in our recommendation that Kahlid learn to read Somali.

We acknowledged that, when we were discussing children during rapport building, Olga had referred to her own wife as her husband. We also acknowledged that this suppression of her own identity was an appropriate and valid professional ethics decision made in the interests of building rapport and trust with the clients. We then acknowledged how we all had to suppress our feminist urges in order meet this couple where they were and serve them appropriately. In context, we reviewed the timing of when Olga asked Omar to allow Khalid to speak for herself, how and when to request to speak to their eldest son, how to ask and when to proceed to separate interviews, and the choice of having just Olga examine Kahlid's scar. Rahmed affirmed that our behavior and decision-making had been culturally sensitive and appropriate.

We discussed the secondary gain of citizenship and the potential for dishonesty. We reviewed our indicators of validity—independent confirmation of her history including failure to learn English with three years of good effort, the dent in her skull congruent with her history of childhood head injury, her plausible history of cerebral malaria, and her plausible test performance including on an informal performance validity measure.

We reviewed our process in our incidental discovery of her emotional trauma symptoms and our process of referral for treatment. We reviewed precautions in clearly identifying Rahmed's dual role as interpreter and therapist and when she was switching, the necessity of such roles in small language communities, and the advantage in this context that this couple had the opportunity to get to know her before making a decision, making therapy seem more familiar. We reviewed Olga's decisions about how far to go in eliciting Kahlid's memories of her emotional traumas so as to get necessary information while minimizing retraumatizing.

Report

In our report to her primary care provider, we recommended precautions regarding the choice of Somali interpreters to avoid possible discrimination against her as a MaiMai. We included recommendations concerning family involvement in her care because of her memory impairment. We recommended that Kahlid might be a candidate for medications such as prazosin, a beta blocker, and/or a selective serotonin reuptake inhibitor for trauma symptoms, but we suggested that medication might best be managed by the refugee clinic's psychiatric prescriber.

Follow-Up

On our next clinic visit, we enjoyed the Somali dessert that Khalid sent to us via Rahmed. In addition, we ran into her at the clinic six months later and she proudly displayed her citizenship certificate. She said via Rahmed, *"Now I can talk with Rahmed about what happened, because now I know they can't send me back."*

Section III: Lessons Learned

Although this amalgam case is relatively extreme with respect to the client's cultural distance from mainstream white US culture, it is nevertheless fairly typical of the Somali refugee population and has many features similar to many other refugee populations. This case description touches on the training of all 13 of the multicultural neuropsychology skills listed above. In our practicum, not every case touches on all 13 skills, but most cases touch on most of them, and the above description is reasonably typical of such case training experiences.

   Clinical training in neuropsychology often begins with the more extreme cases—severe traumatic brain injuries, severe strokes, more advanced dementias or severe developmental disorders. This allows the trainee to see neuropsychological phenomena when they are obvious—severe amnesia, aphasia, left neglect, disinhibition—so that they are better able to recognize these phenomena when they are less obvious—mild memory impairment or word-finding difficulties or mild distractibility. Similarly, training with clients who are culturally quite distant from the trainee such as non-English-speaking adult immigrants, allows for the recognition of, and sensitization to, cultural differences when they are more obvious. This facilitates recognizing them when they are more subtle, such as with English-speaking second or third-generation immigrants.

Takeaway Points

1 Neuropsychological cultural competencies include, but go well beyond, the cultural competencies of clinical psychology.
2 Prior knowledge and research about a language and culture are helpful for generating hypotheses and for preparing for modes of communication and rapport. Nevertheless, additional knowledge is typically needed and may be gained from the client, family, other informants, cultural experts, and further research. In the case reviewed here, additional knowledge included information about the MaiMai, Dadaab, Quranic school, arranged marriages, cerebral malaria falciparum, and basket weaving, which was acquired from Kahlid, Omar, Rahmed, Mohamed, and the Internet.
3 Neuropsychological assessment can involve educating and acculturating clients about things that may be culturally unfamiliar like confidentiality, testing, snow, Halloween, and psychotherapy. This process can contribute to trust and rapport.
4 Training for cultural competence is challenging, but it is also quite possible. It often requires departing from our usual clinical habits and reaching out to diverse patient and professional populations geographically, linguistically, and culturally.
5 There are multiple routes to the elusive cross-cultural rapport—respect, common ground, empathetic communication, spontaneity, flexibility, research, pacing and humor. Rapport is a factor in every contact and communication throughout the clinical encounter and beyond. Cultural humility is an important aspect, as well, and may need to be stated (e.g., one way is to apologize for not speaking their language or for bringing up sensitive topics).
6 Training cultural competence is facilitated by going to where the clients are: refugee and immigrant service centers, legal services, community clinics, community centers, and similar institutions, and even into homes, either directly or via teleneuropsychology.
7 Training cultural competence may involve reaching out to interpreters, cultural consultants, allied professionals, and culturally competent supervisors. These approaches can allow for more precise linguistic and cultural services.
8 Diverse trainees also require training in cultural neuropsychological competence, including regarding their own languages and cultures. Those who have learned their own language and culture as small children may not be aware of how these have formed their own belief systems.
9 Diverse trainees can contribute their own knowledge and skills with language and culture in the context of a learning community but should **not** be used as primary instructors of these skills unless they have been specifically trained to do so.
10 Exercising neuropsychological cultural competencies not only serve our legal and ethical obligations but also serve social justice. And finally, they are tremendously rewarding both personally and professionally.

References

1. Smith TB, Trimble JE. Multicultural education/training and experience: a meta-analysis of surveys and outcome studies. In: Smith TB, Trimble JE, editors. Foundations of multicultural psychology: research to inform effective practice. Washington (DC): American Psychological Association; 2016. p. viii, 21–47, 308.
2. Smith TB, Constantine MG, Dunn TW, Dinehart JM, Montoya JA. Multicultural education in the mental health professions: a meta-analytic review. J Couns Psychol [Internet]. 2006;53:132–45. Available from: http://dx.doi.org/10.1037/0022-0167.53.1.132
3. Fouad NA, Grus CL, Hatcher RL, Kaslow NJ, Hutchings PS, Madson, MB, et al. Competency benchmarks: a model for understanding and measuring competence in professional psychology across training levels. Train Edu Prof Psychol [Internet]. 2009;3(4, Suppl). Available from: https://doi.org/10.1037/a0015832
4. Hatcher RL, Fouad NA, Grus CL, Campbell LF, McCutcheon SR, Leahy KL. Competency benchmarks: practical steps toward a culture of competence. Train Edu Prof Psychol [Internet]. 2013;7(2):84–91. Available from: https://doi.org/10.1037/a0029401
5. Kaslow NJ. Competencies in professional psychology. Am Psychol [Internet]. 2004;59(8):774–81. Available from: https://doi.org/10.1037/0003-066x.59.8.774
6. Rubin NJ, Bebeau M, Leigh IW, Lichtenberg JW, Nelson PD, Portnoy S, et al. The competency movement within psychology: an historical perspective. Prof Psychol: Res Pract [Internet]. 2007;38(5):452–62. Available from: https://doi.org/10.1037/0735-7028.38.5.452
7. Heffelfinger AK, Janecek JK, Johnson J, Miller LE, Nelson A, Pulsipher DT. Competency-based assessment in clinical neuropsychology at the post-doctoral level: stages, milestones, and benchmarks as proposed by an APPCN work group, Clin Neuropsychol [Internet]. 2020. Available from: https://doi.org/10.1080/13854046.2020.1829070
8. Hessen E, Hokkanen L, Ponsford J, van Zandvoort M, Watts A, Evans J, et al. Core competencies in clinical neuropsychology training across the world. Clin Neuropsychol [Internet]. 2018;32(4):642–56. Available from: https://doi.org/10.1080/13854046.2017.1413210
9. Smith G. Education and training in clinical neuropsychology: recent developments and documents from the clinical neuropsychology synarchy. Arch Clin Neuropsychol [Internet]. 2018;34(3):418–31. Available from: https://doi.org/10.1093/arclin/acy075
10. Grote CL. Prologue to special issue of "International Perspectives on Education, Training and Practice in Clinical Neuropsychology." Clin Neuropsychol [Internet]. 2016;30(8):1151–3. Available from: https://doi.org/10.1080/13854046.2016.1218549
11. Fujii D. Conducting a culturally informed neuropsychological evaluation. Washington (DC): American Psychological Association; 2016.
12. Lee A, Khawaja N. Multicultural training experiences as predictors of psychology students' cultural competence. Aust Psychol [Internet]. 2012;48(3):209–16. Available from: https://doi.org/10.1111/j.1742-9544.2011.00063.x
13. Benuto L, Casas J, O'Donohue W. Training culturally competent psychologists: a systematic review of the training outcome literature. Train Edu Prof Psychol [Internet]. 2018;12(3):125–34. Available from: https://doi.org/10.1037/tep0000190
14. Carter RT. Back to the future in cultural competence training. Couns Psychol [Internet]. 2001;29:787–9. Available from: http://dx.doi.org/10.1177/0011000001296001
15. Reynolds AL. Using the multicultural change intervention matrix (MCIM) as a multicultural counseling training model. In: Pope-Davis DB, Coleman HLK, editors. Multicultural counseling competencies: assessment, education and training, and supervision [Internet]. Thousand Oaks (CA): Sage; 1997. p. 209–26. Available from: http://dx.doi.org/10.4135/9781452232072.n9
16. Reynolds AL. Understanding the perceptions and experiences of faculty who teach multicultural counseling courses: an exploratory study. Train Edu Prof Psychol [Internet]. 2011;5:167–74. Available from: http://dx.doi.org/10.1037/a0024613

17. Pieterse AL. Teaching antiracism in counselor training: reflections on a course. J Multicult Couns Dev [Internet]. 2009;37(3):141–52. Available from: https://doi.org/10.1002/j.2161-1912.2009.tb00098.x

18. Priester PE, Jones JE, Jackson-Bailey CM, Jana-Masri A, Jordan EX, Metz AJ. An analysis of content and instructional strategies in multicultural counseling courses. J Multicult Couns Dev. 2008;36:29–39.

19. Silander NC, Geczy B, Marks O, Mather RD. Implications of ideological bias in social psychology on clinical practice. Clin Psychol: Sci Pract [Internet]. 2020;27(2). Available from: https://doi.org/10.1111/cpsp.12312

20. Gallegos JS, Tindall C, Gallegos SA. The need for advancement in the conceptualization of cultural competence. Adv Soc Work [Internet]. 2018;9(1):51–62. Available from: https://doi.org/10.18060/214

21. Shepherd SM. Cultural awareness workshops: limitations and practical consequences. BMC Medical Educ [Internet]. 2019;19:14. Available from: https://doi.org/10.1186/s12909-018-1450-5

22. Minneapolis VA Health Care System. VA.gov: Veterans Affairs [Internet]. 2019 May 21. Available from: https://www.minneapolis.va.gov/education/psychology/internship/pre_div.asp

23. Sue DW, Bernier JB, Durran M, Feinberg L, Pedersen P, Smith E, et al. Position paper: cross-cultural counseling competencies. Couns Psychol. 1982;10(2):45–52.

24. Judd T, Beggs B. Cross-cultural forensic neuropsychological assessment. In: Barrett K, George WH, editors. Race, culture, psychology and law. Thousand Oaks, CA: Sage Press; 2005. p. 141–62.

25. Diamond LC, Moreno MR, Soto C, Otero-Sabogal R. Bilingual dual-role staff interpreters in the health care setting: factors associated with passing a language competency test. Int J Interpreter Educ [Internet]. 2012;4(1). Available from: https://doi.org/10.1016/s0925-9635(12)00146-x

26. Fuld PA. Fuld object memory evaluation. Wood Dale (IL): Stoelting; 1982.

C. Awareness of Self

3 Using Reflective Self-Awareness to Enhance Cultural Competence between Neuropsychologist and Client

Rex M. Swanda

Introduction

The state of New Mexico is a richly diverse cultural environment within the United States, known for a large number of distinct Native American tribes and pueblos that have inhabited the region for centuries, as well as descendants of the colonial Spanish, who were the earliest European settlers in North America. This chapter began as an attempt to characterize the challenges of neuropsychology practice in this diverse cultural environment. However, it became apparent along the way that the diversity of New Mexico, far from exceptional, may actually be typical of the diversity that is present in most regions if one is prepared to see it.

The most obvious goal of this chapter is to share a model of cultural competence training, based on Reflective Self-Awareness, that is intended to help a culturally informed neuropsychologist find the rich cultural diversity that I believe is present in every region of practice. By actively looking for that diversity and examining culturally based assumptions that can influence attitudes, emotions and behavior, the neuropsychologist is more likely to appreciate the diversity that surrounds us and less likely to commit unintended **cultural errors**.

My cultural path in neuropsychology was marked by my first job coordinating neuropsychological services at Bellevue Hospital in New York. This was a setting that served large numbers of immigrants from all around the world, so many of the referred patients spoke native languages other than English. It became clear almost immediately that no single neuropsychologist could possibly possess meaningful cultural information about all of the patients we were expected to serve. And even with a "language bank" of nearly 2,000 volunteers, we could not necessarily even communicate effectively with some patients.

Some of the most valuable lessons I learned through that experience had to do with the considerations that had to be faced when working with persons whose language and culture I did not know. I learned that it was important (i) to refine the referral question and clarify realistic expectations for the goals of the evaluation, (ii) to identify cultural and linguistic limitations in the assessment approach and materials that were available, (iii) to gather as much objectively documented history and medical information as possible, and (iv) to be as aware as possible of my own underlying cultural assumptions, knowing that those assumptions would potentially influence any clinical interactions and interpretation of the testing performance.

"Universal Precautions" and Reflective Self-Awareness

The years I worked in New York (1985 to 1991) were a critical time in the AIDS pandemic. The causal virus, HIV, had not yet been identified, and effective treatments were still on the horizon. Fear of contagion was creeping throughout the city, and increasing discrimination was being

DOI: 10.4324/9781003051862-6

leveled against already-marginalized groups that were sometimes labeled the "Four H's" (hemophiliacs, heroin addicts, homosexuals, and Haitians), all of whom were perceived to be agents of infection.[1] However, in 1985, the Centers for Disease Control (CDC) issued a set of public health guidelines called "Universal Precautions."[2] This new policy called for health care workers to treat all bodily fluids as potentially infectious. By following such policies, some of the discriminatory practices toward targeted groups gradually subsided since the public was taught to treat every patient the same, without knowing anything about their health status.

By the time I moved to New Mexico in 1991, I recognized that, even with the challenge of getting to know the major cultural communities in the state, I was never going to learn all I would want to know about the various sub-groups of Native American and Hispanic communities. By that point, however, I also realized that, even if I had knowledge of "typical" characteristics of persons from a specific cultural community, I would still have to learn from each specific client in what ways they were or were not typical of that culture. This point was driven home for me when I once asked a Navajo woman, in my most culturally sensitive manner, whether she thought traditional Navajo ways of healing would be helpful for addressing her issues. She replied, "No. My family is Baptist." In my mind, this cultural blunder will always represent a classic example of an unnecessary cultural error, which resulted from my own unexamined cultural assumption that all Navajo people would value traditional ways of healing. The assumption was based on a stereotype, of course. But the error drove home the importance of assuming that every interaction has potential cultural significance.

The cultural approach of "Universal Precautions" that I try to apply to the work of neuropsychology is to assume that every interaction has potential cultural significance. From a cultural perspective, then, I treat all patients the same, assuming that every patient has a rich and unique cultural identity that I cannot know unless they let me know. Whether the client is Hispanic, Native American, Anglo, Asian American, African American or any other ethnicity, the lesson I have learned in New Mexico is that, when I assume that all of my clients have interesting and unique cultural backgrounds, they are able to teach me about their interesting and unique cultural backgrounds.

Culturally Competent Practice in Neuropsychology

Neuropsychology still has a long road ahead to meet the challenge of fully integrating cultural competence into the routine practice of neuropsychology. However, the road to that destination is illuminated by increasing visibility of cultural diversity issues in educational forums and journals, as well as policy and advocacy work in the large professional organizations that represent neuropsychology. For example, the American Academy of Clinical Neuropsychology (AACN)[5] published Practice Guidelines for Neuropsychological Assessment and Consultation that specifically called attention to practice guidelines for addressing cultural and language issues in underserved and diverse populations. Those guidelines generally focused on the importance of taking unique cultural, language, and ability information into account and called attention to the risks associated with the administration and interpretation of tests with individuals for whom insufficient test adaptations, normative data, or validity studies exist. The same practice guidelines emphasize that neuropsychologists who agree to evaluate members of diverse populations should have experience in administering and interpreting procedures that are relevant for the patient in question, and they should take care to report on the methods and effectiveness of their efforts to communicate with the examinee. Interpreter-mediated communication should include culturally mediated meanings, affective tone, and nonverbal "body language" in addition to literal content.[5] Practical elements in the guidelines remind us that culturally competent neuropsychologists avoid using family members, friends, or other untrained individuals as interpreters and emphasize the importance of considering threats to validity that can be introduced by cultural bias in both translated and adapted instruments. Neuropsychologists are also reminded, when working with populations for whom tests have not been standardized and normed, to make use of direct observation, with particular consideration of adaptive functioning within the "real-world" community of the examinee.

Rivera-Mindt, Byrd, Saez and Manly[6] summarized a proposal for increasing culturally competent neuropsychological services for ethnic minority populations. This was based in part on Sue's[3] conceptualization of cultural competence that emphasizes (i) self-awareness of one's own assumptions, values, biases, and stereotypes about ethnic minorities and how such beliefs and attitudes could negatively impact the provision of neuropsychological services; (ii) knowledge and understanding of one's own worldview and that of the perspective and culture of one's clients; (iii) acquisition of specific and culturally appropriate skills for assessment, intervention and communication to effectively work with ethnic minority groups, and (iv) development of core cultural competencies at the organizational level, based on theories, practices, policies, and organizational structures that are responsive to all groups. Rivera-Mindt et al.[6] reviewed historical foundations and applicable ethical guidelines that are addressed in ethical standards having to do with boundaries of competence. Practical limitations were identified, having to do with the relatively small number of neuropsychologists who self-identify as culturally competent as well as other health disparities for ethnically diverse people. Recommendations were offered to remedy the "broken pipeline" of neuropsychologically trained professionals from ethnically diverse groups by expanding training opportunities at the early stages of professional development for neuropsychologists from diverse backgrounds. Four goals were identified including increasing multicultural awareness and knowledge within neuropsychology, increasing multicultural education and training, increasing multicultural neuropsychological research, and increasing provision of culturally competent neuropsychological services for ethnically diverse people.

More recently, Fujii[4] has introduced the ECLECTIC framework for conceptualizing different facets of culture that are pertinent for understanding a culturally diverse client and how these facets can impact performance on a neuropsychological evaluation. The components of the framework include E: Education and literacy; C: Culture and acculturation; L: Language; E: Economics; C: Communication; T: Testing situation: Comfort and motivation; I: Intelligence conceptualization; and C: Context of immigration.[4]

Increasing Self-Awareness of Cultural Assumptions

Sue's[3] multidimensional model of cultural competence reminds us that, as human beings, the attitudes, beliefs, biases, stereotypes and prejudices we hold are based on a foundation of underlying assumptions about the world. These assumptions reflect a worldview and perspective that is nurtured and grows out of the unique cultural matrix in which each individual develops and lives. This is the same cultural matrix through which information, attitudes and beliefs are filtered, consciously or not, with the potential to influence each individual's behavior, emotions and interactions with others in the environment of the real world.

These underlying assumptions about the world and about the people with whom we interact may be implicit or explicit, conscious or unconscious. They may be questioned or unquestioned, denied or embraced. But they are nonetheless ever-present, persistently influencing behavior and interactions, whether or not the individual is aware of their existence. It follows that the more we can be aware of our own underlying cultural assumptions, the better we might be able to manage our behavioral and emotional responses. If we can recognize culturally sensitive issues when they arise, we have a better chance of responding in a deliberate and intentional way that can lower the risk of unintended cultural errors.

Responsibility for Management of Cultural Factors within the Professional Relationship Rests with the Neuropsychologist

Responsibility for managing cultural factors in a professional relationship rests squarely in the hands of the neuropsychologist, who generally holds greater power in the relationship and has both a professional and ethical responsibility for integrating cultural competence into their practice.[4] Whether or not the neuropsychologist explicitly recognizes and is aware of any critical cultural assumptions that might influence their professional interactions, the neuropsychologist must still take responsibility for any *cultural errors* that develop by having failed to identify and clarify the unexamined assumptions. A culturally competent neuropsychologist, then, must bear responsibility for actively examining and identifying to the greatest extent possible any underlying cultural assumptions that might be relevant to an effective outcome in a professional interaction.

Reflective Local Practice

A specific training model is presented below, as well as some tools that are intended to add to the effort to increase multicultural awareness and knowledge as well as multicultural education and training in neuropsychology. This model is particularly focused on the expectation that a culturally competent neuropsychologist should be able to identify and be aware of underlying cultural assumptions that are likely to influence their professional interactions.

The name, Reflective Local Practice,[7] is a mnemonic for elements of a model that emphasizes awareness of underlying assumptions, attitudes and bias through reflective introspection. Knowledge of the local culture, traditions, and language of the region is encouraged, as well as the development of professional skills and communication that are needed for the culturally competent practice of neuropsychology.

Development of a Cultural Diversity Training Model

This model grew out of a cultural diversity training seminar for psychology interns and postdoctoral residents that was developed at the Albuquerque VA Medical Center over 20 years ago. The consortium-based psychology internship training program was accredited in 1993, in partnership with the local offices of Indian Health Service (IHS) and the University of New Mexico Medical Center. Working in collaboration with my colleague, Evelyn Sandeen, we initially designed a program of cultural diversity seminars that included a series of speakers who represented various ethnic and sociocultural groups from the local area. The series was well-received and helped trainees adjust successfully to rotations in the VA, University Hospital, and IHS settings that served the 1,000-year-old pueblo village of Acoma (Sky City), about 50 miles west of Albuquerque. However, after a few years, we felt our program was falling short of our goal for trainees to acquire a broader degree of cultural competence that would prepare them for culturally competent practice in any region of the country or world. We knew that many of our trainees would eventually move on to work in other regions, and we wanted to offer cultural diversity training that would help trainees hit the ground running, and find their cultural bearings, wherever they might land.

A review of our program helped us realize that our training model had primarily emphasized the *knowledge* and *skills* components of Sue's[3] multidimensional model of cultural competence, but frankly, we had neglected the important component of *self-awareness*. The seminar schedule had been filled with monthly presentations of *knowledge* and information by cultural "experts" who represented various cultural groups in the region. The training and supervision we had provided were designed to develop professional *skills* in interview, communication and interventions. But we did not have a systematic approach to emphasize *self-awareness* of culturally based assumptions. Our review concluded that the cultural diversity training we had provided up to that point had lacked any systematic or coherent approach for helping trainees explore and identify their internal sources of bias, prejudice and unexamined assumptions that might seep into the interactions of a professional relationship. We also identified the need to develop more effective tools for discussing difficult issues.

Goals for a Cultural Diversity Training Model

Based on our program review, we resolved to design a training model that would (i) be *relevant and adaptable* to serve any cultural group in any geographic region; (ii) *provide tools* that would help training participants improve culturally based communication and minimize unintended cultural errors; and (iii) help psychologists understand their *professional responsibility* for identifying and managing cultural factors in any professional interaction.

Six Assumptions of Reflective Local Practice

In addition to the goals set forth above, the Reflective Local Practice model is based on a set of six assumptions, all of which are discussed in Sandeen, Moore and Swanda.[7] These six assumptions are summarized here, with specific application to the practice of neuropsychology:

1   **Everyone has a culture.** Although it seems unnecessary to state that "Everyone has a culture," it is not unusual to realize in the course of the discussion that some training participants hold a very narrow sense of "culture," as if culture refers only to "others" who are different from themselves. Some training participants have wistfully expressed regret that they did not grow up within a rich and diverse culture. In my experience, the failure to appreciate the universality of culture is not usually a consciously formed belief but an unquestioned cultural assumption that comes from a place of naivete.

In New Mexico, discussion of cultural identity offers an opportunity to discuss the diverse and complex cultural identities that are represented in this state. If a neuropsychologist in this region wants to understand the cultural heritage of a client, they would be well-advised to listen carefully and ask delicately, not knowing what underlying emotions might be associated with the topic. For example, "Native Americans" in this state are represented by at least 23 sovereign tribes, including Navajo, Apache, and 19 distinct Pueblo tribes, who may or may not share significant cultural traditions or language. Among Spanish-speaking New Mexicans, those who identify as "Hispanic" commonly regard themselves as direct descendants of the Spanish **conquistadores**, many of whom proudly trace their family lineage many generations back to the earliest European settlers in North America. Mexican Americans usually identify with Mexican roots, even though their families might have lived several generations in the region. The terms "Latino" or "Chicano," when used in New Mexico, usually encompass geographically broader Spanish-speaking populations and are often used with connotations of political activism. Many New Mexicans also identify with mixed heritage, in combination with Pueblo, Navajo or other Native American tribes, although even within the same family, some members might embrace mixed heritage while others strongly identify with only one side of their culture. Some Hispanic New Mexicans have embraced the cultural identity of "hidden Jews" or "crypto-Jews," after learning that their ancestors had been persons of the Jewish faith who had fled Spain in the aftermath of the Spanish Inquisition.

2 **Individuals exist within a matrix of intersecting cultural identities.** This model emphasizes that cultural identity is based not only on racial and ethnic identity but also encompasses a complex matrix of intersecting biologically and socially defined roles, relationships, and affiliations. The term intersectionality was originally used in 1989 by Kimberle Crenshaw[8] to call attention to multiple overlapping, or intersecting, social identities that are associated with discrimination and oppression, especially among women of color. The concept of intersectionality has since been applied more broadly by others, including Cole,[9] who has discussed the concept in the context of research in psychology. In this Reflective Local Practice model of training, participants are asked to consider their own cultural identity in light of intersecting socio-economic factors, education, employment, religious affiliation, sexual and gender identity, as well as family roles (parent, child, sibling). We ask them to explore their own cultural identity through the lens of "family culture," such as mealtime traditions (who ate together, was there any discussion, and if so, what topics were acceptable or unacceptable for discussion), household rules, and family secrets. We also prompt participants to consider cultural characteristics that might have been instilled through developmental experience with any community and social groups with which they were affiliated.

The diversity of cultural identities in New Mexico also consists of a complex network of intersecting cultural identities. The description of Native American and Hispanic New Mexico above fails to acknowledge the many other ethnic groups that make up the rich diversity of this state, including the Anglo and African American communities, Asian Americans, and other Latin American cultural communities that may not fit neatly into any of those groups. Other distinct cultural communities in New Mexico include the LGBTQ+ community, as well as many veterans and active military service women and men, for whom military and veteran culture is their primary cultural identity. Communities of differently abled persons include, but are not limited to, persons with hearing impairment, as well as persons who live and work with spinal cord injuries. Most spiritual and religious identities are represented in the state, including Latter-Day Saints, many versions of Christianity, Judaism, Islam, and others. Harder to classify, but no less valid as a cultural identity include increasing numbers of people who might identify politically and culturally as liberal or progressive and show up for a Black Lives Matter protest, or those who identify with conservative, white supremacist or the gun culture of nationalist militia groups.

In our training, information about the diverse culture of New Mexico is presented by representatives of many of these cultural communities. We encourage trainees to get out into the community to learn about local culture through restaurants, festivals, music, Pueblo feast days and local museums. However, we also emphasize that the example of their approach to cultural exploration in New Mexico is intended to serve as a template that can enhance their appreciation for future cultural experiences in any other setting.

3 **Culture is ever-changing.** Social and political changes are ongoing in local communities, the nation and around the world, most of which impact the cultural identities of individuals in some way. Changes in an individual's underlying attitudes and beliefs can be related to age and changing economic status of an individual, while national or world events, such as the current world-wide pandemic, might result in significant shifts in cultural attitudes and beliefs among many individuals or across entire cultural groups.

4 **Bias is universal.** A fundamental part of this cultural diversity training model encourages training participants to accept that bias, stereotyping, and formation of prejudicial attitudes are normal outcomes of the human struggle to develop schemas and make sense of the world. These normal, implicit processes of grouping and categorizing begin in our earliest

development and continue throughout our lives. However, the insidious aspect of bias, prejudice, cultural blindness and other cultural assumptions is that they are woven so tightly into the fabric of our cultural selves that we often cannot even be aware of their existence, much less their origins, unless we consciously turn our attention to look for what is there. Consequently, this training model recommends that neuropsychologists who are committed to cultural competence should use some of the tools that are described below to develop professional habits that can help them consciously explore underlying attitudes and assumptions in order to more explicitly take potential sources of bias and prejudice into account.

5 **An understanding of group power structures and history is a crucial foundation for cultural competence.** Although there is a tendency to view bias, prejudice, and discrimination through the lens of race and ethnicity, we encourage training participants to consider the effects of power and powerlessness as the foundational basis for **white privilege**, bias and discrimination. In the state of New Mexico, for example, discrimination and prejudice can be found among cultural groups with superficially related ethnic identities. A person from a generations-old Hispanic family might express prejudice against first-generation "Mexican-Americans," with the same complaints (e.g., "They will take our jobs") that are often leveled against immigrants in many other societies, regardless of race or ethnicity. Many examples can be found around the world, in which persons from related ethnic communities display prejudice or discriminate against persons of different religious or political beliefs, usually in association with the relative power of the oppressor in relation to the powerlessness of the oppressed. *Colorism* is not uncommon, in which persons with relatively darker skin tone experience prejudice or discrimination from others within the same ethnic community. Persons who identify as LGBTQ+ around the world have certainly experienced the effects of prejudice and discrimination at the hands of persons who otherwise share significant cultural identities of race and ethnicity.

6 **Cultural competence is a foundational aspect for the ethical practice of neuropsychology.** Basic ethical principles of beneficence and nonmaleficence call for neuropsychologists to do no harm, and a general goal of cultural competence in this Reflective Local Practice model is to avoid cultural errors that might inadvertently bring harm to a professional relationship. Integration of cultural competence into neuropsychology practice should be considered a core standard of practice, especially in light of AACN's 2007 publication of practice guidelines that specifically addressed underserved and diverse populations.[5] Those guidelines have put the field of neuropsychology on notice that there is an ethical obligation to practice in a culturally competent manner.

Hot Spots, Blind Spots, and Soft Spots

Identifying Barriers and Resistance to Necessary But Difficult Cultural Discussions

In order to help training participants take responsibility for identifying and managing cultural factors in their professional interactions, we knew it would be important to identify barriers and resistance that would be likely to arise in the discussion of difficult issues. Silence or reluctance to engage is a common barrier to the productivity of difficult but necessary cultural discussions. Whether the reluctance to engage is driven by fear (e.g., fear of sounding foolish or expressing inappropriate or socially undesirable statements) or lack of effective communication skills, an important goal of this Reflective Local Practice training model has been to provide some tools to facilitate communication in discussions of challenging cultural issues.

Tools for Facilitating Difficult But Necessary Discussions

In order to lessen the impact of defensive, shy, or fear-based reactions to discussions in cultural diversity training, we wanted to come up with a more neutral vocabulary that participants could use to talk about strong emotional responses that often emerge as a natural part of any cultural discussion.

We laid the groundwork for introspection and self-disclosure in our discussions by emphasizing in our six assumptions that *bias is universal.* As human beings, we reflect the product of our cultural influences, which include bias, prejudice and stereotypes, all of which are human cognitive tools that are used to categorize and bring order and perspective to the chaotic world into which we are born.

With a nod to the power of language, we also reasoned that if we could find a less emotionally evocative language with which to communicate about strong emotions, we might be able to help training participants engage more effectively in these "difficult but necessary" cultural conversations. With this goal in mind, we adopted the terms *hot spots, blind spots,* and *soft spots* to help training participants be more aware of culturally based assumptions that have the potential to influence their behavior, emotions and interpersonal interactions and to facilitate the expression of those culturally related concerns in group discussion.

Hot Spots are areas of strong emotional sensitivity, often borne out of trauma or developmental experiences, which have the potential to evoke strong emotional responses. In Sandeen, Moore, and Swanda,[7] we write that "Hot spots may arise when persons who have experienced powerlessness in certain areas of their lives have understandably strong emotion associated with that dimension." We also note that "Strong emotion is a normal reaction to having been powerless, oppressed, or harmed." Some common examples of hot spots include:

- A person of color avoids reacting to perceived slights and microaggressions while having a drink at a bar but simmers internally, with racing thoughts and fears that any overt response might result in a bad outcome. The hot spot involves feelings of powerlessness and oppression that are related to their perspective of historic bias and discrimination toward the ethnically diverse aspect of his or her cultural identity.
- A gay professional is momentarily distracted, wondering what his client thinks about him after she describes her new hair stylist with the comment, "He's so flamboyant – you know, 'that way!'" The hot spot, in this case, involves instinctive fear of being discovered and feelings of powerlessness associated with the sexual orientation aspect of his cultural identity.
- A woman considers whether she should speak to Human Resources after her supervisor comments that he really likes it when she dresses this way. She is torn between her interest in putting a stop to personal comments and fear that it would hurt her chances for a desired change in her work assignment. The hot spot here involves feelings of pent-up anger, resentment and powerlessness associated with her supervisor's condescending attitude and objectification of the female aspect of her cultural identity.

By normalizing and humanizing the experience of strong emotions, training participants seem much more receptive to the idea of introspectively examining their inner emotional self in order to identify their own "hot spots." In the context of cultural diversity training, the goal is not to embark on a therapeutic experience but to encourage participants to engage in the reflective experience of scanning their inner emotional self for "hot spots," which they are not necessarily expected to share with the group. Participants typically respond quickly and intuitively to the term, and in later discussion, it has not been unusual for a training participant to share that a discussion comment had tapped into a "hot spot." The term normalizes the presence of strong emotional triggers and offers a rational way to refer to or think about the trauma associated with those triggers.

Blind Spots are found in those aspects of life that are taken for granted by an individual or a class of people that have never had to confront a challenge or a barrier in that area, usually due to higher levels of privilege, power or authority in an environment of unequal power. In Sandeen, Moore and Swanda,[7] we wrote that "Blind spots refer to those situations in which a psychologist is unaware of relevant cultural information regarding the client because of unexamined assumptions related to the psychologist's own background." We added that "Blind spots tend to occur in dimensions of experience in which the person has held relative power."

- Many of our training participants, who were raised with an expectation for achieving a college education, have been able to acknowledge their own blind spots having to do with education, in failing to appreciate the struggle that many of their clients face to finish high school, let alone go on to college, especially in an era of skyrocketing student debt.
- One of our trainees once shared the shame they felt upon discovering how "blind" they had been to the challenges faced by a client who had incurred a third "no show" appointment. After entering a termination of treatment note, due to the "no shows," the intern revealed that they had "assumed" and taken for granted that the client had convenient transportation when, in fact, the client had to arrange for someone else to look after a relative with dementia and a pre-school child, while allowing about an hour and a half each way to negotiate a series of bus lines. In this case, a culturally competent approach might have avoided the blind spot of assuming that our clients have the financial means and support to arrange for easy transportation with coverage for family care needs.

Soft Spots refer to those instances when unexamined assumptions lead to deviations from usual practice, usually having to do with lowered expectations or overidentification with a client. Soft spots often reflect a perceived power differential in either direction. A person who is perceived as holding more power might feel sympathy for a less powerful person or might make special accommodations for a person who is perceived to be more powerful. Soft spots can be subtle and difficult to identify but may be present when a professional is considering altering their usual practice in a way that might violate professional boundaries or pose ethical risks. The following examples involve scenarios in which cultural factors may or may not be obvious central issues but illustrate the role that differential power relationships can play in professional decision-making.

- A neuropsychologist, who ordinarily sees clients only in the office, would be advised to introspectively check for "soft spots" in their underlying attitudes, beliefs and assumptions if they agreed to make an exception and instead meet at a coffee shop for an initial "interview" with a client who was perceived to be wealthy and powerful.
- A prescribing provider should consider whether any unexplored "soft spots" might contribute to their decision to "make an exception" to continue a prescription for Valium for a patient who reminds her of a beloved aunt who had suffered from a "nervous disorder."
- A psychology instructor realizes that he is inclined to find a way to justify a passing grade for a very engaging young Hispanic man, who is the first person in his family to finish high school and attend college, even though he has performed below objective standards for passing. The instructor wisely takes a step back to consider whether his own internal biases and sympathies (soft spots) might be contributing to his decision-making process.

Applying Reflective Self-Awareness to Your Professional Practice

Like most of our development throughout training and professional practice, the process of incorporating new ideas and skills usually begins by consciously and explicitly considering and evaluating those new ideas. If the idea of reflective self-awareness is intriguing enough to explore further, then the next step would be to find ways to incorporate those ideas and skills and apply them as a routine part of your practice. We all have our own unique styles of learning and growing professionally. But, if you think that "reflective self-awareness" might have value for improving cultural competence in your practice of neuropsychology, please consider the following three suggestions for incorporating reflective self-awareness into your practice routine.

Perform a Cultural Self-Assessment

A matrix of cultural influences is presented in Table 3.1 to help identify some of the multiple, overlapping aspects of our own cultural identities as neuropsychologists. As an exercise in cultural self-assessment, examine the cells of the matrix in Table 3.1 and identify the various dimensions that you would consider to be important aspects of your own cultural identity. Some people might identify one or two dimensions that strongly contribute to their cultural identity, while other persons might select 6 or 7 dimensions as important aspects of their cultural identity.

As discussed earlier in this chapter, "power" and "powerlessness" are thought in this model to be critical modifiers of the various dimensions of cultural identity.[7] To better understand the way that power modifies the cultural experience that is associated with each of these dimensions, rate each of the dimensions you selected according to the degree of power that you would associate with that aspect of your cultural identity. Keep in mind that "power" in this exercise refers to the degree to which a person has felt more or less powerful in each of the dimensions.

Table 3.1 Intersectional matrix: Dimensions of cultural identity

Social class	*Sexual orientation*	*Gender identity*	*Education level*
Family role	Looks/body type	Geographic origin	Veteran status
Profession/work/retirement	Political affiliation	Religion/spirituality	Health/disability
Survivor status	Race	Ethnicity	Age

Source: Adapted from Sandeen, Moore, and Swanda.[7]

Assign ratings of power to each of the dimensions that contribute to your cultural identity:

- (+) powerful = your experiences in this dimension have given you power and privilege over others; this may predispose you to a BLIND SPOT or, under certain circumstances, a SOFT SPOT
- (0) neutral = your experiences in this dimension have been neutral regarding power over others (are you sure?)
- (−/+) mixed = your experiences in this dimension have both given you power over others and others have had power over you; this may lead you to inconsistent reactions
- (−) powerless = your experiences in this dimension have put you in a one-down position relative to others; this may predispose you to a HOT SPOT or if shared with your client, a SOFT SPOT

We have assigned self-ratings of power that range from "Powerful" (+), "Neutral" (0), "Mixed" (+/−), and "Powerless" (−). Each of these ratings of power, especially on the extreme ends of "powerful" and "powerless," are likely to be associated with the various "spots" that have been discussed above. Persons who have experienced less power in some dimensions of cultural identity would be more likely to identify "hot spots" within those dimensions.

Consider an example of a "hot spot," which tends to be associated with feelings of powerlessness, helplessness or trauma in certain dimensions:

Board certified neuropsychologist Gloria Martinez was elated when the department chair called her in to tell her that she had been selected to take on the leadership role for a challenging clinical service, with a significant increase in pay and benefits. She had worked for such a long time to reach this goal, and this was one of her best days in a long time, being congratulated by so many colleagues. As she came down a hallway, however, she heard an unseen but familiar voice from around a corner comment that, "It must sure be nice to benefit from affirmative action." Dr. Martinez immediately felt crushed and deflated and decided to skip meeting her colleagues for a celebratory Happy Hour, because she thought none of them would understand. A few weeks later, she found herself in a cultural diversity training, reflecting on a matrix of aspects of cultural identity. She had rated several cultural dimensions as "Powerful," including dimensions of Education, Profession, Spirituality and her Family Roles as a responsible daughter, a strong mother, and a loving wife. She had identified another aspect of her cultural identity as "Hispanic" and wanted to mark Powerful, when she thought of the pride she felt for her traditional culture. But when she thought about the broader socio-economic structure of the country, and her personal experiences as an occasional target of racial discrimination, bias, and microaggressions, she had to admit to herself that she would rate any race or ethnicity besides white as "less powerful." She suddenly recalled the recent incident of micro-aggression, when the words of one person had had the effect of dampening her joy on what should have been one of the best days of her life. In that moment, she understood how the feelings of powerlessness she had felt as a target of discrimination and bias over the years had come to represent a "hot spot" within the matrix of her cultural identity. She resolved to use her increased self-awareness of that "hot spot" to anticipate and better manage situations that might arise in the future. She considered alternative responses, such as confronting a "micro-aggressor," moving ahead with positive plans, and seeking support, and she began to feel as if she could reclaim her sense of self-esteem. She resolved to continue to find ways to take care of herself in the future.

Persons who rate themselves as more powerful in certain dimensions may be predisposed to experience "blind spots" in those areas:

Neuropsychologist Ted Smith rated dimensions of "Education level" and "Profession/Work" as "Powerful" aspects of his cultural identity, because he is proud that he has met his goals for an advanced degree and he is aware that he has attained higher levels of education than most of the people he knows. He also feels fortunate to work in a profession he loves. After performing this Cultural Self-Assessment exercise, however, he began to think about a client who had reported that she had recently completed an Associate's degree. He realized with chagrin that he had followed up in the interview by asking whether she had any plans to "finish" her schooling with a Bachelor's degree. He worried that this question might have conveyed an attitude of discounting her achievement, as if her Associates degree was not "good enough." Upon reflection, he realized that his response probably did represent a "blind spot" in his assumptions, and an attitude of bias. He was able to acknowledge that the phrasing in his question reflected unexplored cultural assumptions that 1) of course, anyone would naturally have a goal of completing as much education as possible, and 2) anyone (in his worldview, at least) would be capable of meeting the significant financial and time demands that additional education might require. He resolved to take steps in the future to avoid repeating this potential "cultural error" by revising his interview template to include more culturally-sensitive questions. Instead of asking how many years of education they had completed, he would ask clients to describe their goals in education or work and how far they had progressed toward meeting those goas. Rather than making unwarranted assumptions about their goals, he thought he could follow up by asking clients if they face or anticipate any barriers that would get in the way of meeting their goals.

Another scenario provides examples of hot spots, blind spots, and soft spots that are associated with different dimensions for the same individual:

Frank Thomas left school in 11th grade, and went on to build a successful business with 50 employees. In a cultural diversity training exercise, he completed a matrix of cultural identity, indicating that he felt less powerful on the dimension of education. In fact, he was aware that he would usually shrink away from discussions having to do with past school experiences. However, as a leader in the business community, he assigned a very powerful rating on the dimension of Profession/Work. During discussion, he thought that he might identify the dimension of education in his own cultural identity as a "hot spot," in which he feels less powerful compared to most of his associates. He also recalled a couple of times in the past when he had angrily reacted to someone "with a fancy degree." When he considered the dimension of work/profession, however, he realized that he had exhibited a "blind spot" toward others in the past who were struggling to find work in times of economic distress. Without previously realizing where his attitude was coming from, he could see how unsympathetic he must have sounded, by making comments that he expects people to "make it on their own," and "pull themselves up by the bootstraps," just like he had to do. However, he thought that he had acted in a sympathetic way that might have represented a "soft spot" by passing over a highly educated job applicant and instead, "giving a break" to a person who, like himself, had struggled through school. He didn't know whether that had been the right thing to do, because his usual hiring policy was to take education into consideration, but he had to admit that this person had impressed him because he reminded him of himself.

Provocative Questions

Another way to explore various dimensions of cultural identity is to consider questions about culturally based values and assumptions that were probably formed and reinforced through early experiences within the family and cultural community in which a person was raised. The article by Sandeen, Moore and Swanda[7] provides a link to supplemental training materials that include a long list of "Provocative Questions" that have been used for discussion in cultural diversity training. Some examples of those questions include:

- What was the attitude toward education in your family?
- Describe an experience when you became acutely aware of cultural differences between yourself and those around you.
- Describe an experience when you became aware of cultural differences between how you were raised and how you had developed as an adult.
- Describe a professional experience in which you made a "cultural error."

- Describe a prejudice or bias that you acquired in childhood.
- Describe a time when you felt shame about some aspect of your family of origin.
- Describe a time when you felt hurt or damaged by cultural blindness on someone else's part.
- Did your parent enjoy his/her work?
- What were your parents frightened of? How did you know this?
- How was emotion handled in your family? Which emotions were "allowed" and which were not?
- What was your family's attitude toward the armed services? Were there veterans in your family?
- What group did your parents talk bad about behind closed doors? What was the "cover" or "core" issue they did not like about this group?
- Are there rituals or customs that you had as a child that you miss today? Any rituals or customs that you are glad to have shed?
- What was dinnertime like in your family? Who cooked, if anyone? Were you all together? Were there discussions or arguments or mostly silence?

These questions are designed to evoke reminders of past experiences that a neuropsychologist might not typically think about in the realm of "culture." But where else would our values, prejudices, biases and other attitudes come from? And the very reason these questions are posed is to provoke consideration of unexplored cultural assumptions, to identify those assumptions, to better understand what the assumptions represent, and to explicitly decide how to express the assumptions. This is the main goal of reflective self-awareness, to make implicit assumptions explicit and to explore previously unexamined assumptions.

Establish a Habit

For those neuropsychologists who are interested in developing a more culturally competent professional practice, I recommend starting with one small behavioral change that will establish a new habit. For example, neuropsychologists frequently deal with templates and forms for data collection, summarizing results and reporting conclusions. I suggest that the route to increased self-awareness can be as simple as making a few strategic changes to templates that are routinely used in professional practice. For example, in a previous scenario dealing with "hot spots" about a person's education, it was suggested that questions about education and occupation could be altered to emphasize a client's goals and barriers to those goals. This kind of a small but intentional change to a form might serve as a sufficient reminder that would reverberate throughout the rest of a clinical interview. One intentional change to an interview question might serve as a starting point to remind the neuropsychologist to think a little more explicitly about the cultural assumptions that underlie other questions. This change can have the effect of helping the neuropsychologist to be more sensitive to "blind spots" or to watch for culturally significant comments and questions that might otherwise have the potential for offending or discounting.

Summary

As a concluding reminder, this model of cultural competence suggests that increased self-awareness through reflection on unexplored cultural assumptions can improve a neuropsychologist's cultural competence and enhance cultural understanding between the neuropsychologist and client. Although it will always be an advantage to gather as much information as possible about the cultural traditions and practices of our clients, the neuropsychologist's level of cultural competence can also benefit from any opportunity to engage in reflective self-awareness. The more self-aware we can be of our own cultural identity and cultural assumptions, the more sensitive we can be toward others. By observing these cultural "Universal Precautions" and routinely examining the assumptions we bring to interactions with every client, the more successful we will be in engaging with all clients in culturally competent practice.

Glossary

Conquistadores.   Literally, "conquerors" refers to explorers and soldiers of the Spanish and Portuguese empires who brought colonialism to many parts of the world, especially including present-day Spanish and Portuguese-speaking areas of North America, South America, and the Philippines.

Cultural error.   Similar to microaggressions, cultural errors involve indirect or unintentionally offensive behaviors or remarks made toward persons of a different culture. Cultural errors typically reflect lack of cultural awareness and result when unquestioned cultural assumptions are acted upon.

White privilege.   Advantages in social and economic power that are automatically conferred on white persons that are not shared by persons of color in an inequitable social structure.

References

1. Gallo RC. A reflection on HIV/AIDS research after 25 years. Retrovirology. 2006 Oct 20;3(72):1–7.
2. Centers for Disease Control. (1985). Recommendations for preventing transmission of infection with human T-lymphotropic virus type III/lymphadenopathy-associated virus in the workplace [Internet]. [Place unknown]: Morbidity and Mortality Weekly Report; 1985 Nov 15 [cited 2021 Mar 23]. Available from: https://www.cdc.gov/mmwr/preview/mmwrhtml/00033093.htm
3. Sue DW. Multidimensional facets of cultural competence. Couns Psych. 2001;29:790–821.
4. Fujii D. Developing a cultural context for conducting a neuropsychological evaluation with a culturally diverse client: the ECLECTIC framework. Clin Neuropsych. 2018 Nov;32(8):1356–92.
5. Board of Directors. American Academy of Clinical Neuropsychology (AACN) practice guidelines for neuropsychological assessment and consultation. Clin Neuropsych. 2007 Mar 28; 21(2):209–31.
6. Rivera-Mindt M, Byrd D, Saez P, Manly J. Increasing culturally competent neuropsychological services for ethnic minority populations: a call to action. Clin Neuropsych. 2010 Apr;24(3):429–53.
7. Sandeen E, Moore KM, Swanda RM. Reflective local practice: a pragmatic framework for improving culturally competent practice in psychology. Prof Psych: Res and Prac. 2018 Apr;49:142–50.
8. Adewunmi B. Kimberlé Crenshaw on intersectionality: "I wanted to come up with an everyday metaphor that anyone could use" [Internet]. [Place unknown]: New Statesman; 2014 Apr 2 [cited 2021 Mar 23]. Available from: https://www.newstatesman.com/lifestyle/2014/04/kimberl-crenshaw-intersectionality-i-wanted-come-everyday-metaphor-anyone-could
9. Cole ER. Intersectionality and research in psychology. Am Psych. 2009 Apr;64(3):170–80.

D. Awareness of Others

4 Liberating the Narratives of BIPOC Neuropsychologists

Unpacking Microaggressions through Lived Experiences

Anita Herrera Hamilton, Shaquanna Brown,
Velissa Johnson, and Sagar Lad

> I remember, as a child, before we would go into a store, my mother would say, "Don't get in here and embarrass me in front of these White people." That has been ingrained in me and I bring that into the room with me in these predominantly White spaces.
>
> (Neuropsychology postdoctoral fellow)

> I started cleaning houses on Saturday mornings when I was twelve and remember how people looked at me … through me. And now I have a Ph.D., and I'm board certified. But there are times when I feel like I am right back to cleaning houses … allowed to work hard but required to stay quiet and compliant. All that education and yet to some colleagues, patients and administrators I'm a "domestic" … an academic domestic.
>
> (Neuropsychologist)

As neuropsychologists, we are unified by our passion for brain-behavior relationships, service of clinical populations, and dedication to scholarship. Embedded in our collective mission are assumptions of academic integrity, enlightenment, and **equity**. Yet, many Black, Indigenous, and People of Color (BIPOC) neuropsychologists encounter professional experiences incongruent with the equitable values and honorable missions of our field and institutions. The convergence of **colorblind** attitudes, neoliberal values, and assumptions of ahistorical scientific neutrality has significantly impacted academic, institutional, programmatic, and administrative aspects of medicine and healthcare.[1,2] Similar inequities are likely experienced by BIPOC neuropsychologists,[1,3,4] although the frequency, scale, and impact are relatively unexamined and remain unclear.

Systemic and institutional inequities, frequently obvious to BIPOC neuropsychologists, are often mystifying to their dominant culture colleagues. These discrepant perspectives may be due, in part, to the decline of blatant acts of workplace discrimination. Although racism persists, blatant **discriminatory** acts have been replaced by more covert and ambiguous manifestations of discrimination, such as **microaggressions**,[1,5,6] which are more reflective of the fluid and evolving consciousness of society. This is perhaps more evident in sophisticated social contexts, such as academia.

Although studies are emerging regarding BIPOC discrimination and outcomes related to academics, there is increasing literature indicating that **systemic racism** significantly contributes to occupational health disparities.[4] According to Okechukuwu,[4] workplace injustices have been associated with three outcomes including psychological (e.g., anxiety and depression) and physical health (e.g., increased blood pressure, headaches and sleep disturbance), health behavior (increased alcohol intake and smoking) and job outcomes (e.g., increased absence from work and restriction of information or services related to advancement). Workplace bullying and sexual harassment were associated with posttraumatic stress disorder (PTSD[4]). While these studies

DOI: 10.4324/9781003051862-8

reveal broad workplace injustices and health disparities, studies targeting various levels of education and expertise within specific careers are needed.

Despite increasing recognition of **structural racism** in psychology, academia and academic medicine,[2,7,8] there has been a lack of scientific inquiry into the experience of systemic racism and **inequity** within the field of neuropsychology. This chapter aims to amplify the voices of BIPOC neuropsychologists and neuropsychology trainees, illuminating the **inequitable, oppressive, intolerant**, discriminatory, and often systemic practices that maintain power and privilege imbalances.

We used semi-structured interviews to collect data regarding personal experiences of identity-based discrimination and systemic racism. We hope that this chapter will inspire meaningful conversations that advance the implementation of policies that specifically address the gendered and racialized experiences of BIPOC in our field.

History and Terminology

"I can't breathe." "Say her name." These collective mantras forged from the murders of George Floyd and Breonna Taylor reflect a 21st-century racism, long-integrated (and thriving) within public systems created and funded for community welfare in the United States. Marches, rallies, social media, live news feeds, smartphone video and body cam footage jolted us individually and collectively into a deeper awareness of systemic racism woven into 21st-century American government, law enforcement, healthcare, and academia, including medicine and neuropsychology. Scientific methods and classifications not only reflected racist views but were used by dominant culture scientists, some of whom directly influenced the field of neuropsychology.[9]

As national shock turns to reflection, individual (e.g., "What is my role?") and collective (e.g., "What can we do?") questions have emerged. For the neuropsychological community, as academicians, diagnosticians, and custodians of mental health, we recognize that effective intervention within our spheres of institutional and clinical influence first requires an appreciation for the etiology of systemic and **institutional racism** infiltrating our field.

While addressing race and race-related disparities are more "en vogue," within the context of psychological scientific inquiry, the denial of disparities and inequities within academic and healthcare institutions persists.[1,5,6] To rise among the ranks of dominant culture academia, BIPOC professionals must often **assimilate**, simultaneously minimizing or denying the occurrence and impact of identity-based discrimination. Within this context, the academic success of BIPOC professionals engenders an adaptive dissociation of experience or individual epistemology of unknowing.[2] Relevant to this point is the substantial body of research implicating dissociation as a long-term consequence of traumatic stress and an important factor in the development of trauma-related disorders.[1,2]

Microaggressions

Lukianoff[10] characterized microaggressions as the catastrophization of being offended, implying that BIPOC is somehow responsible for the acts of racism they experience or are characterologically flawed (e.g., overly sensitive) if they are offended by the act. Other scholars have questioned the conceptual clarity of microaggressions and argued that research on the topic is not yet mature enough to draw conclusions.[11]

However, we take Sue's view[3] that microaggressions are: (a) constant and continual in the lives of BIPOC, (b) cumulative, representing a lifelong burden of stress, (c) continuous reminders of second-class status in society, and (d) symbolic of systemic injustices at the bedrock of dominant culture values (e.g., freedom) and institutions (e.g., government and education) (p. 130). As such, "micro" acts of discrimination are often experienced as "macro" acts of discrimination impacting career trajectory, professionalism, productivity, personal and professional development, physical and mental health, identity and well-being. As a result, the use of the term "micro" is meant to refer to "everyday or frequent" acts of discrimination rather than implying that these behaviors are insignificant or minor.

Racial microaggressions are defined as brief and commonplace daily verbal, behavioral, or environmental indignities, whether intentional or unintentional, that communicate hostile derogatory or negative racial slights and insults toward people of color.[12] Microaggressions include **microinvalidations** (e.g., forms of discrimination perceived by the dominant culture as subtle but effectively continue the subjugation of BIPOC individuals), **microinsults** (e.g., ambiguous insults), and **microassaults** (e.g., personal attacks that fit with conceptualizations of traditional racism).[1]

In short, microaggressions are not isolated negative events or hardships, but each microaggression adds to a lifelong pattern of marginalized or denied personal agency.[3] The target is under constant demands to assert mental toughness and to re-assert and re-claim personal dignity. For many, the threat is unpredictable and can be experienced within any context, including professional and personal relationships previously experienced as equitable, further adding to the stress, psychological exhaustion and placing BIPOC professionals' health at risk.

Borrowing from Liberation Psychology, which seeks to obtain and disseminate the narratives of oppressed and marginalized communities,[2] the aim of this chapter is to use the personal narratives of BIPOC neuropsychologists and neuropsychology trainees to begin to "unrepress" the silenced voices of academic neuropsychology through a tone of inquiry. By normalizing diverse narratives, the goal is to forge alternative perspectives of scholarship, professionalism, practice and achievement, which informs future policy, healthcare, and power allocation.

Lived Experiences of BIPOC

We recruited neuropsychologists and neuropsychology trainees (i.e., graduate students, predoctoral interns, and postdoctoral fellows) from Listservs for professional organizations (e.g., American Academy of Clinical Neuropsychology (AACN-List), American Board of Clinical Neuropsychology (ABCN), Asian American Psychological Association (AAPA), Asian Neuropsychological Association (ANA), Hispanic Neuropsychological Society (HNS), International Mail List for Pediatrics Neuropsychology (PEDS-NPSY), Massachusetts Neuropsychological Society (MNS), National Academy of Neuropsychology (NAN), Society for Black Neuropsychology (SBN), and Society for Clinical Neuropsychology (ANST). Eligibility included age 18 and older and English speaking. Respondents provided verbal consent to participate in an interview.

Semi-structured qualitative interviews were conducted via virtual face-to-face technologies (e.g., Zoom) and phone calls. The growing body of research on microaggressions, racism, color blindness, discrimination in the workforce, and disparities in academic medicine provided a lens through which the interview was developed.[1,3,4,8,13–21] More specifically, the interview included questions from the Racism and Life Experiences Scale-Brief (RALES-B),[22] the Racial and Ethnic Microaggression Scale (REMS),[17] the Assessment of Racial Microaggressions in Academic Settings Scale (ARMAS), and the work of Sue and colleagues.[23] Interviews took approximately 60 to 120 minutes to complete. Respondents were instructed to indicate the number of times that a microaggression occurred throughout their career as a neuropsychologist or neuropsychological trainee. Questions were shaped by respondents' responses, such that respondents reporting microaggressions were asked to provide additional detail about their experiences in order to gain insight on how they experienced acts of discrimination, racism, and microaggressions throughout their training and career.

Of respondents (n = 12), the majority self-identified as female (n = 11, 91.6%), with ages ranging from 26 to 46 years (M = 36.78, SD = 6.01). The sample was ethnically/racially diverse, with 44.4% Black or African American, 33.3% Asian, 11.1% Hispanic or Latino, and 11.1% Biracial. The sample was also diverse with regard to career stages, with 66.7% early-career, 11.1% mid-career, 11.1% predoctoral student, and 11.1% postdoctoral fellow or resident. With respect to work settings, 77.8% of the respondents reported working in an academic/university hospital, 11.1% in a VA or government facility, 22.2% in private practice, and 11.1% in a corporate setting. There was the option to select as many settings as applicable. A large proportion (77.8%) reported that their institution consisted of 2–5 neuropsychologists and 22.2% reported working with 10+ neuropsychologists at their institution.

Forms of Microaggression

Respondents were interviewed regarding types of microaggressions experienced in the workplace, including microassaults, microinsults, and microinvalidations.

To date, our interviews have yielded rich quantitative and qualitative data. Most respondents reported experiencing microaggressions (78%), with microinsults and microinvalidations reported more frequently (67% and 89%, respectively) than microassaults (33.3%). Qualitatively, the career stage emerged as a prominent factor with respect to microassaults only, such that respondents reported being the target of microassaults from academicians most often during their training, whereas microassaults experienced in subsequent career stages most often occurred during patient interactions. Nevertheless, in both cases, respondents reported feeling powerless in holding the offender responsible for their actions.

The following includes verbatim excerpts from interviews.

Microassaults are blatant statements or actions with clear intent.[23]

> I remember having an A+ on a report and when the professor ... called out my name and I went to grab the report, he said, "Oh! You're not X." I said yes and he said, "Oh, I didn't know you were Black." On the second instance, I remember getting a C ... I went back to the same professor and asked about some clarification ... he told me, "I can't have a Black person having the highest grades in my class."

Themes and subthemes	Interview quotes related to microassaults
Race-based assumptions	
Attack on intellect	• I was graded lower when the professor knew that I was Black, and the only reason I can say that with confidence is that they actually verbalized that to me. So, ... I tried to make sure that the professors never saw me if that was possible.
Assumptions of inferior status	• When I was actually supervising a fellow .... she was racist, to put it lightly ... she was constantly questioning my credentials ... questioning my authority. Some concrete examples would be not showing up on time for our meetings when she would show up on time for meetings with my other colleagues, not coming in prepared .... resistant to feedback, [and] questioning and comparing my recommendations to that of my fellow colleagues. Actually, being called a "monster" to my face.
Assumptions about family structure	• I actually had someone say, "You mentioned your father, do you know him?" They assume that because I am Black, I come from a single-parent matriarchal home. My parents have been married for 40 years. I know my White colleagues do not get asked if they know their fathers, and there isn't this shock when they talk about their fathers.

Assumptions about citizenship status	• It feels like I'm an outsider and I don't belong … more subtle events, like people asking me and no one else about citizenship status. Without knowing if I'm a permanent citizen or permanent resident or not … people will bring this up, like, … to do a postdoc, you need to, like, apply for a green card … and start to explain this line of information to me, which is not something I asked.

Microinsults are actions that convey insensitivity or rudeness or directly demean a person's racioethnic heritage, such as mistaking a person of color for a service worker.[23] Though regarded as a "subtle" form of discrimination, microinsults are also potentially damaging to the target, posing a threat to mental well-being.[1,24]

> One of the biggest things I have had to face is this assumption that I don't deserve to be where I am. There are comments about affirmative action or how things are more lenient. This has actually been the main driving force for pursuing board certification … board certification was the one thing people can't take away from me. There is no quota. The standards are the same for everyone. There are objective guidelines … I needed to get boarded for myself. I needed to know that I belong and I wasn't just handed my position or degree.

Themes and subthemes	*Interview quotes related to microinsults*
Denounced, devalued, and insulted	
Disparaging remarks	• One Saturday, my White supervisor told me and another practicum student, also a Black woman, that we should have stopped at our bachelor's degrees because we were "not going to get very far." It felt very intentional. Ironically enough, his daughter was also in our PsyD program – earning her second doctorate. When we brought that up, he was like, "She'll be fine." My body knew it was racially charged, but my mind was still trying to make sense of it.
Backhanded "compliments"	• I recently started directing a neuropsych program in a new hospital division, and one of the lead nurses came up to me in the clinic to tell me that the Chief really liked me and how surprised he was that I was so smart. Her wide smile told me that I was supposed to take this as a compliment.
Accusations of unprofessional behavior	• I was working as a psychometrist at a private practice … the patient, a White woman, arrived and she walked in the room and said I smelled like weed. [She] said to me, "this country is the way it is because of people like you." [She] told me that she didn't want to move forward with the testing … [My supervisor] told me, "We really need to get this testing done. What I would like for you to do is just apologize to her- just say you apologize to her for anything you could have possibly done to offend her." Even during testing, the patient threw papers at me and made other comments and it felt horrible. I cried the entire way home.

Microinvalidations include behaviors that minimize or marginalize the competence of BIPOC professionals while often denying the importance of race and of personal racism (e.g., the myth of societal **meritocracy**).[1] Of note, our findings suggest that BIPOC neuropsychologists are more likely to experience microinvalidations compared to microinsults in the workplace.

> When sharing my personal racism experience in the field with a colleague, there was minimalization of my experiences – it can't just be your name why clients aren't calling you from the list – they probably lived closer. Or you look young that's why they give your trainees more eye contact than you – don't worry about this little stuff too much.

Themes and subthemes	Interview quotes related to microinvalidations
Professional development and perceived competence	
Inadequate mentorship •	I always felt like I had to fight for what I had. I had to really make an effort to network. I made contacts on my own and was not given contacts, yet I noticed that some of my White colleagues were. I was fortunate to secure great training, but I felt like it was from my own doing.
Credentials disregarded •	I once had parents in inpatient refuse to call me Doctor. One of the Caucasian psychologists went into the patient's room right before me and was called doctor without issue. When I came in, I was asked if I had an MD. I was then told that I shouldn't be allowed to call myself doctor, even though the psychologist who went in before me also had a PhD. After I did the feedback, the father finally called me "doctor." Almost emphasizing it. It was like I had to prove my expertise. Once he saw that I actually knew what I was talking about, he was willing to call me doctor.

Overtly disturbing and cruel, the racist undertones of microassaults are obvious to the target.[1] In contrast, microinsults and invalidations are ambiguous, socially subtle forms of microaggressions. As Offerman et al.[1] point out, in some ways, microinsults and microinvalidations are more severe in that they: (a) often go unaddressed, despite often causing the target emotional/physiological distress; (b) are minimized/normalized given that they are more likely to be viewed as a misunderstanding or personal matter; (c) occur more frequently than microassaults; (d) are experienced by the target as racism, yet the lack of recognition and support by dominant culture observers triggers self-doubt and self-criticism within the target. Cumulatively or in isolation, each of these factors undermines or erodes professional performance, well-being, and morale, as well as personal identity and self-competence.

Microalienations. Interestingly, a new theme emerged from the interview data, which we have tentatively termed as **microalienation**. Unlike the existing microaggression subtypes, microalienations are acts of omission (e.g., failing to provide trainees of color with opportunities for research engagement) that are seemingly more difficult to quantify, but by respondents' reports, no less frequent, relevant or harmful to BIPOC neuropsychologists and neuropsychology trainees. Indeed, respondents reported that microalienations impacted their professional and personal development and well-being.

Themes and subthemes	Interview quotes related to microalienations
Thwarted belongingness and employment	
Underrepresentation and isolation	• Yes, feels like I'm an outsider and I don't belong. Never included.
Inequity in opportunities	• I always felt like I had to fight for what I had. I had to really make an effort to network. I made contacts on my own and was not given contacts, yet I noticed that some of my White colleagues were.
	• I was initially denied a position but was subsequently hired after one of the neurologists fought to open up the position for me. He questioned why a different neuropsychologist was selected over me when that person had less experience with neurological syndromes. I think the prevailing response in those situations was that selection is based on "fit," but what does that mean exactly?

Sexism, Racism, and Intersectionality

Intersectionality acknowledges how unique aspects of gender, race, class, and even physical appearance create different modes of discrimination and privilege. In reference to intersectionality,

Kimberlé Crenshaw states, "All inequality is not created equal."[25] This statement highlights that overlapping identities can compound experiences of discrimination. For example, poor mental health and work outcomes among female employees are associated with combined experiences of sexist and racist discrimination, including harassment and microaggressions.[1,18,26] As such, it is important to recognize concurrent forms of oppression to understand the depth of inequities and associated contexts.

Themes and subthemes	Interview quotes
Sexual harassment, unsupportive work environments, and power imbalances	
Stalking and sexual misconduct	• As a trainee, I was being sexually harassed ... I was a practicum student, and he was an intern. And when I reported it to my supervisor at the program, they told me that I should consult with other women in the field because they would know how to deal with it. And then when I told the director of the program at the practicum site ... the woman literally told me to come in and shut the door and told me to keep my mouth shut, and I would need to learn how to live with this to get by. I documented everything, and I even had text messages that he had sent to me. I had multiple witnesses who observed it. He was coming up and trying to rub my back. A lot of vulgar comments ... even my grad program, when I reported it, was very dismissive until I actually had to threaten legal action and all they did was move me to a different site. But they allowed him to finish and become a psychologist.
Intersectionality of identities	
Intersection of race and gender	• A supervisor once said, "You look great in that skirt, do you run a lot?" I just froze. He got embarrassed and rarely talked to me again socially, and became really critical of my work. Looking back ... I realized that this dynamic was different for me as a woman of color. My White female colleagues were allowed to ignore or reject a proposition from a White male supervisor without consequences. When I did, I was treated with passive aggression, and in two cases, transferred. Of course, I would never get a letter of recommendation. I figured out by the end of my doctoral program that ... it was easier to be the unattractive, nerdy Latinx trainee and get by than risk insulting them and jeopardizing my career.
Intersection of race, sex, and ability	• I was diagnosed with a chronic illness three months after starting postdoc. The faculty informed me that my contract would not be renewed for a second year because the intersection between my medical treatment and COVID-19 made the task of training me "insurmountable." My treating physician wrote a letter, which I provided to the faculty. The letter noted that even in the context of COVID-19, my medical treatment did not preclude me from performing the essential functions of my job. Only then did the faculty offer me a second-year contract. It taught me that being a female ethnic minority with a disability is three strikes. I left the contract and my dreams of becoming a neuropsychologist behind.

Personal Impact and Coping

Gaining insight into how respondents were affected by or coped with microaggressions was a particularly relevant area of interest given the profession of our sample. Our preliminary results revealed that microaggressions have a negative impact on health, with respondents reporting elevated mental health difficulties (50%), disruption to well-being (67%), adverse impact on personal relationships (78%), and negative work outcomes (33%) as consequences of microaggressions. Additionally, respondents expressed feelings of exhaustion as the respondent below:

> They've made me exhausted honestly. I just feel tired. Sometimes I feel like I can't keep fighting this fight, but I also don't see any way out of it because the fight isn't over. I do feel a responsibility, particularly to women of color coming up behind me, to keep making the argument, to keep showing up, to keep pointing out instances of systemic racism, both obvious and subtle. But I do feel very tired.

Most respondents reported that they sought treatment (67%), such as psychotherapy, psychiatry, or chaplaincy, because of their microaggression experiences. Additionally, several participants reported efforts to overcompensate by working longer hours and taking on additional responsibilities. Respondents often noted that this attempt to fend off stereotypes through workaholism further compounded the negative impact on their professional and personal lives (e.g., lack of sleep, burnout, and poorer relationship quality with partners and children). Respondents' reported patterns of coping varied in both strategy (e.g., problem-focused and avoidance-oriented coping strategies) and formality (e.g., seeking support from friends and/or relatives to psychopharmacology and psychotherapy). Of note, supportive dominant culture allies and minority-based institutional resources were noted to serve as important resources for managing microaggression-related distress and concerns.

> Currently, I am involved in a mentorship program that my hospital has for Black doctors. I'm so fortunate to have this outlet. It gives me a space to discuss my feelings, barriers, and develop strategies with a senior physician. She doesn't understand the field of neuropsychology, but she gets the impact of prejudice/discrimination. It also helps to talk to family and friends about what I am going through.

In some cases, participants reported that discussing and reliving their experiences of microaggressions during the semi-structured interview unearthed specific internalized feelings that have gone unaddressed and untreated.

Protective Factors

Of the few protective factors identified by respondents, the only male participant emphasized the impact of sex.

> Being a male gave me privilege...especially on units where they know me, (and) gave me advantage which a female would not be able to enjoy.

This same respondent and others noted the importance of dominant culture allies and supervisors, particularly males, as well as affiliations with well-renowned clinicians, researchers, or institutions in mediating experiences of microaggressions. While powerful, dominant culture allies are uniquely positioned to provide support to BIPOC colleagues, this dynamic also illustrates the power of *implicit systemic bias* in which the BIPOC professional is somewhat dependent on dominant culture colleagues for career credibility. As such, the power differential between BIPOC neuropsychologists and neuropsychological trainees can be further intensified. Additionally, pressure to assimilate and accommodate (e.g., not challenge, or speak up about microaggressions) to the needs of a dominant culture or more senior colleague is likely greater as well. The implication is that while affiliations with dominant culture allies may be a protective factor, within some contexts, the professional development and career trajectory of BIPOC neuropsychologists and neuropsychology trainees may also be dependent on the power of an alliance with a dominant culture colleague, rather than experience and/or expertise.

Given the vulnerability of BIPOC neuropsychologists and neuropsychological trainees, the role of the dominant culture colleague as a protective factor is two-fold. First, it is important for dominant culture colleagues to validate (e.g., provide **microaffirmations**) the BIPOC professional's experiences of microaggression. To do so, dominant culture colleagues may have to pursue more psychoeducation and be willing to expand their points of view, perhaps even their worldview.

Within the professional community and institution, dominant culture colleagues, particularly males, are uniquely and strategically positioned to advocate for BIPOC colleagues, ensuring that appropriate experience and expertise are attributed to their BIPOC colleagues. The latter will be particularly challenging, particularly if, by doing so, the dominant culture colleague may have to resign an aspect of professional power.

Several respondents cited institutional protective factors, including having a group of colleagues (e.g., mentorship programs and diversity-related committees or organizations) that validate their experiences of discrimination. Respondents reported that receiving validation from their colleagues positively influenced their mood and sense of belonging. In addition, to support within professional settings, several respondents cited the support of their relatives and friends was as a protective factor.

While the need for **microinterventions**[3] was reported by nearly all respondents, the importance of context in the development of microintervention frameworks is paramount in determining effectiveness and outcomes. In short, *how* microinterventions are implemented is likely as important, if not more important, than *what* type of microinterventions is used. To make the invisible visible, microinterventions will need to be context-driven, fluid, adaptive, and administered by individuals and institutions that value emotional intelligence, reward collaboration over hierarchy, and appreciate the intersectional complexity of microaggressions to enhance institutional equity.

Conclusions and Future Directions

Our preliminary findings, which are consistent with previous research examining microaggressions among medical professionals, provide compelling evidence that microaggressions pervade the workplace of BIPOC neuropsychologists and neuropsychology trainees, placing these individuals at risk for adverse health, work, and relationship outcomes.

Results revealed that microaggressions are commonly experienced by neuropsychologists and neuropsychology trainees and that microinvalidations and microinsults are more frequent than microassaults. The prevalence of vague and subtle microaggressions highlights Sue et al., views that the strategic goal of the microintervention is to make the "invisible visible"[3] (p. 134). While many of our respondents reported enduring microinsults and microinvalidations in isolation and often without any recognition of offense, microintervention frameworks[3] emphasize the need for acknowledging and disarming the microaggression in "real time" (e.g., validation, microaffirmations) and educating the offender. Individual microinterventions will need to be supported by institutional leadership and policies to ensure BIPOC career development and advancement. While frameworks for addressing microaggressions have been proposed,[3] as the literature and our findings attest, more work is needed in this area.

Regardless of microintervention, an understanding of context is critical to outcomes. Factors that need to be considered are the following: How is the offender addressed (e.g., publicly or privately)?[1] Is this an isolated event, a pattern of behavior, or part of systemic institution culture? and[4] Can the target's professional relationship with the offender place them at risk for negative outcomes?

Unfortunately, there is always the potential risk that microinterventions can be met with negative consequences or passive retaliation (immediately or in the future) that can jeopardize career development, opportunities, health and welfare. Notably, microaggression intervention strategies should give serious consideration to the effects of interlocking identities and the physical and mental health impact on BIPOC in processing their experiences, coping, and seeking out support.

Additionally, our findings suggest that intersectionality is an important lens through which BIPOC neuropsychologists and neuropsychology trainees attempt to understand and make meaning of microaggressions. This aspirational level of active coping might be one of the driving forces behind treatment seeking, as most respondents reported that they sought treatment to address their microaggression-related distress and concerns. Taken together, these findings beg the question of whether and how intersectionality is addressed within the therapeutic context. Researchers have emphasized the therapeutic utility of discussing therapist/client intersectionality in the context of treatment, noting that intersectionality may have a significant impact on the therapeutic alliance depending on the way in which it is addressed or avoided.[27] Discussions about intersectionality might be particularly salient for clients presenting with discrimination-related distress or concerns. We refer interested readers to the corresponding reference for more in-depth information, including recommendations on how to structure conversations about intersectionality with clients.[27]

A limitation of this study is selection bias, as individuals who had more significant or frequent experiences microaggressions may have been more likely to self-select to participate. Of note, however, our female to male ratio (11 females; 1 male) is consistent with previous findings suggesting that female-identifying individuals are more vulnerable to the impact of institutional racism and intersectional inequities.[4,28] Generalizability is also a limitation of the current study. Although inequity is experienced globally, our respondents are highly educated professionals residing in North America. As such, their inequitable experiences reflect a narrow institutional context and may not generalize to other countries or careers. Recruitment and analysis of interview data is ongoing. Although our investigation is centered on collecting the narratives of BIPOC neuropsychologists and neuropsychology trainees at risk of repression, our goal is to expand our sample to include dominant culture neuropsychologists and neuropsychology trainees to investigate how they identify with and respond to witnessed microaggressions and the impact such experiences might have on their personal and professional development.

We hope this undertaking will steer us toward a comprehensive understanding of the impact discrimination has on our field, aiding in the development of micro- and macrointerventions that aim to reduce interpersonal and institutional discrimination. These efforts potentially help to safeguard and ensure the professional development of BIPOC neuropsychologists as we move the discipline toward a more equitable future. Success will be measured not only as BIPOC neuropsychologists become leaders among their BIPOC peers but leaders in the field of neuropsychology at large. This will provide a more representative reflection of the populations we serve as well as the underrepresented populations in need of our services.

Glossary

This section will define terms used in throughout the chapter. For more detailed information, readers are referred to the cited literature.

Assimilate. To make similar; to give up one's native ethnic beliefs and adopt those of the host culture.

Colorblind. An ideal in which skin color is considered insignificant.

Discriminatory. Showing an unfair or prejudicial distinction, especially when bias is related to age, color, national origin, religion, sex, etc.

Equity.   The quality of being fair and impartial.

Inequity/inequitable.   Lack of fairness; injustice.

Intersectionality.   Acknowledges how unique aspects of gender, race, class, and physical appearance create different modes of discrimination and privilege, with compounded experiences of discrimination.[25]

Intolerant.   Unable or unwilling to endure others' views, beliefs, or behaviors.

Meritocracy.   Social system in which success and status in life depend primarily on an individual's talents, abilities, and effort.

Microaffirmations.   Small acts or tiny acts of opening doors that can be public or private, often unconscious but effective in offering gestures of inclusion, success, or care.

Microaggressions.   Everyday verbal, nonverbal, and environmental slights or insults, whether intentional or unintentional, which communicate hostile, derogatory, or negative messages to a target person(s) based solely upon their marginalized group membership.[3,12,23]

Microalienation.   Form of discrimination by the dominant culture that actively, overtly and/or subtly excludes, omits, or isolates an individual.

Microassaults.   Acts of discrimination that are overtly disturbing and cruel to the recipient.[1,12]

Microinsults.   Actions that convey insensitivity or rudeness or directly demean a person's racioethnic heritage.[1,24]

Microinterventions.   Everyday words or deeds, whether intentional or unintentional, that communicates to targets of microaggression messages of validation, value, affirmation, support, encouragement, and reassurance.[3]

Microinvalidations.   Subtle form of discrimination that excludes, negates, or nullifies the experiential reality of a person from a marginalization group.[1]

Oppressive.   Unjust or cruel exercise of authority or power.

Racial microaggression.   Brief and commonplace daily verbal, behavioral, or environmental indignities, whether intentional or unintentional that communicate hostile derogatory or negative racial slights and insults toward people of color.[12]

Structural racism.   Macro-level conditions, such as residential segregation and institutional policies, that limit opportunities, resources, power, and well-being of individuals and populations based on race/ethnicity and other statuses, included but not limited to gender, sexual orientation, gender identity, ability status, religion, physical characteristics, health conditions, or English proficiency.[7,8]

Systemic racism (also known as institutional racism).   Form of racism that is embedded as normal practice, such as rules, practices, and customs that are rooted in laws, society, or an organization.

References

1. Offermann LR, Basford TE, Graebner R, Jaffer S, De Graaf SB, Kaminsky SE. See no evil: color blindness and perceptions of subtle racial discrimination in the workplace. Cultur Divers Ethnic Minor Psychol. 2014;20(4):499–507.
2. Adams G, Dobles I, Gómez LH, Kurtiş T, Molina LE. Decolonizing psychological science: introduction to the special thematic section. J Soc Polit Psychol. 2015 Aug 21;3(1):213–38.
3. Sue DW, Alsaidi S, Awad MN, Glaeser E, Calle CZ, Mendez N. Disarming racial microaggressions: microintervention strategies for targets, White allies, and bystanders. Am Psychol. 2019 Jan;74(1):128–42.
4. Okechukwu CA, Souza K, Davis KD, de Castro AB. Discrimination, harassment, abuse, and bullying in the workplace: contribution of workplace injustice to occupational health disparities. Am J Ind Med. 2014 May;57(5):573–86.
5. Dipboye R, Collela A. Discrimination at work: the psychological and organizational bases. 2005.

6. Dovidio JF, Gaertner SL. Aversive racism and selection decisions: 1989 and 1999. Psychol Sci. 2000 Jul 1;11(4):315–9.

7. Serafini K, Coyer C, Brown Speights J, Donovan D, Guh J, Washington J, et al. Racism as experienced by physicians of color in the health care setting. Fam Med. 2020 Apr 3;52(4):282–7.

8. Torres MB, Salles A, Cochran A. Recognizing and reacting to microaggressions in medicine and surgery. JAMA Surg. 2019 Sep 1;154(9):868.

9. Broca P, Blake CC, Carter C. On the phenomena of hybridity in the genus Homo [Internet]. London: Longman, Green, Longman, & Roberts; 1864. Available from: https://www.biodiversitylibrary.org/item/68441

10. Lukianoff G, Haidt J. The coddling of the American mind. The Atlantic. 2015;316(2):42–52.

11. Lilienfeld SO. Microaggressions: strong claims, inadequate evidence. Perspect Psychol Sci. 2017 Jan 1;12(1):138–69.

12. Sue DW. The challenges of becoming a white ally. Couns Psychol. 2017 Jul 1;45(5):706–16.

13. Bailey ZD, Krieger N, Agénor M, Graves J, Linos N, Bassett MT. Structural racism and health inequities in the USA: evidence and interventions. The Lancet. 2017 Apr;389(10077):1453–63.

14. Halley MC, Rustagi AS, Torres JS, Linos E, Plaut V, Mangurian C, et al. Physician mothers' experience of workplace discrimination: a qualitative analysis. BMJ. 2018 Dec 12;363:k4926.

15. Harrison C, Tanner KD. Language matters: considering microaggressions in science. CBE—Life Sci Educ. 2018 Mar;17(1):fe4.

16. Kuroki M. Perceived racial discrimination in the workplace and body weight among the unemployed. Biodemography Soc Biol. 2017 Oct 2;63(4):324–31.

17. Nadal KL. The racial and ethnic microaggressions scale (REMS): construction, reliability, and validity. J Couns Psychol. 2011;58(4):470–80.

18. Velez BL, Cox R, Polihronakis CJ, Moradi B. Discrimination, work outcomes, and mental health among women of color: the protective role of womanist attitudes. J Couns Psychol. 2018 Mar;65(2):178–93.

19. Williams DR. Stress and the mental health of populations of color: advancing our understanding of race-related stressors. J Health Soc Behav. 2018 Dec;59(4):466–85.

20. Williams MT. Psychology cannot afford to ignore the many harms caused by microaggressions. Perspect Psychol Sci. 2020 Jan;15(1):38–43.

21. Rodríguez JE, Campbell KM, Pololi LH. Addressing disparities in academic medicine: what of the minority tax? BMC Med Educ. 2015 Dec;15(1):6.

22. Utsey SO. Assessing the stressful effects of racism: a review of instrumentation. J Black Psychol. 1998 Aug;24(3):269–88.

23. Sue DW, Capodilupo CM, Torino GC, Bucceri JM, Holder AMB, Nadal KL, et al. Racial microaggressions in everyday life: implications for clinical practice. Am Psychol [Internet]. 2007 May–Jun;62(4):271–86. Available from: https://doi.org/10.1037/0003-066X.62.4.271

24. Noh S, Kaspar V, Wickrama KAS. Overt and subtle racial discrimination and mental health: preliminary findings for Korean immigrants. Am J Public Health. 2007 Jul;97(7):1269–74.

25. Crenshaw KW. On intersectionality: essential writings. NY: The New Press; 2017.

26. Sojo VE, Wood RE, Genat AE. Harmful workplace experiences and women's occupational well-being: a meta-analysis. Psychol Women Q. 2015 Aug 27;40(1):10–40.

27. Pettyjohn ME, Tseng C, Blow, AJ. Therapeutic utility of discussing therapist/client intersectionality in treatment: when and how? Fam Process. 2020;59:313–27.

28. Kelly EL. Discrimination against caregivers? Gendered family responsibilities, employer practices, and work rewards. In: Handbook of employment discrimination research. New York (NY): Springer; 2005. p. 353–74.

E. Action

5 Stepping into Action

The Role of Neuropsychologists in Social Justice Advocacy

Mirella Díaz-Santos, Kendra Anderson, Michelle Miranda, Christina Wong, Janet J. Yañez, and Farzin Irani

Psychologists take reasonable steps to avoid harming their clients/patients, students, supervisees, research participants, organizational clients, and others with whom they work, and to minimize harm where it is foreseeable and unavoidable.

(APA, 2017)

Neuropsychology is political.

(Suarez, 2021)

Introduction

In the United States, the murders of George Floyd, Breonna Taylor, Rayshard Brooks, and so many others by police officers and civilians, as well as the synergistic double pandemic of COVID-19 and racial inequities,[1] have propelled issues of justice, equity, diversity, and inclusion to the forefront of national and organizational initiatives and dialogues. Regional, national, and international neuropsychology conferences and publications are increasingly including didactics, discussion spaces, and papers on these topics. Even so, how many of us (neuropsychologists) still struggle with unsettled feelings about injustice? Is raising awareness of these topics enough? Is passive learning without any action acceptable? Could our silence continue to maintain injustice? How many of us even really understand what advocacy is and what it could look like in neuropsychology? And perhaps most importantly, how many of us wonder whether our field should play a more active role in social justice advocacy?

This chapter is a call for neuropsychologists to step into action as social change agents. We focus on US-based race-relations due to our awareness of the historical context and systemic structures in the United States. We simultaneously invite our international neuropsychology colleagues to also consider their respective roles in social justice advocacy. We review advocacy-related historical and ethical considerations in neuropsychology in North America and highlight some reasons *why* neuropsychologists generally avoid engaging in advocacy and *what* the realities are that deter neuropsychologists from social justice advocacy in particular. We then provide specific ways on *how* neuropsychologists can transition from advocacy awareness to action. We propose a shift in frame of reference toward a *transformational learning* approach that emphasizes how we know. We use an *ecological systems* framework toward advocacy to suggest opportunities for neuropsychologists to dismantle inequities across microsystems, mesosystems, exosystems, and macrosystems. Concrete suggestions and examples of how neuropsychologists can engage in bite-sized, larger scaled, and transformative advocacy efforts are included. Lastly, we point to *where* equity and advocacy can lead neuropsychology, i.e., toward transformational justice and social responsibility in neuropsychology (SRN).

DOI: 10.4324/9781003051862-10

Advocacy Is Clearly Mandated in Competency and Ethical Guidelines

APA's 2011 competency benchmarks for professional practice include measures of advocacy involving empowerment and systems change at the practicum, internship, and postdoctoral levels. This advocacy benchmark is defined as taking "actions targeting the impact of social, political, economic or cultural factors to promote change at the individual (client), institutional, and/or systems level."[2]

In the field of neuropsychology, advocacy is also a relevant functional competency area in clinical neuropsychology training models across the world.[3] Some neuropsychologists have tried to encourage advocacy related to forensic neuropsychology practice,[4] public sector changes in the veteran's administration,[5] influence policies impacting reimbursements and favorable practice climates for neuropsychologists[6,7] and to increase awareness about other aspects of neuropsychological practice (see 2010 Special Issue on advocacy in The Clinical Neuropsychologist). Yet, neuropsychology and psychology have been slow to create actionable change related to promoting human rights for all. Analysis of the history of the American Psychological Association (APA) reveals that social justice advocacy has been neglected, despite the illusion of the field being built on universal human rights principles.[8]

One barrier for neuropsychologists to step into becoming active social change advocates in collaboration with marginalized and minoritized communities[9] could be the misperception that there is no explicit ethical mandate for psychologists to engage in social justice advocacy. Yet, the APA ethics code[10] Human Relations standard ensures that we avoid unfair discrimination (3.01) and harm to the public (3.04). Aspirational principles also ask us to "recognize that fairness and justice entitle all persons access to and benefit from the contributions of psychology and to equal quality in the processes, procedures, and services being conducted by psychologists" (Principle D: Justice). We additionally have an obligation to safeguard the welfare and rights of those we serve (Principle A: Beneficence and Nonmaleficence) and to be aware of our professional and scientific responsibilities to the specific communities in which we work (Principle B: Fidelity and Responsibility). This calls on us to recognize the socio-economic hardships, health care disparities, and systemic racism faced by the communities we serve; examine and change our own personal racial biases; and remove institutional and social barriers that impede neuropsychologists' academic, career, or personal-social development.[11] Yet, neuropsychologists avoid engaging in social justice advocacy despite a clear mandate to do so from our own ethical code and competency guidelines.

Why Do Neuropsychologists Generally Avoid Engaging in Advocacy?

Historically, there has been hesitancy from psychologists to engage in advocacy efforts broadly, which could be related to a lack of awareness about public policy issues and perceived lack of knowledge to discuss these issues competently.[12] Additional rationalizations for neuropsychologists to avoid engaging in advocacy may involve excuses such as "it's not in my backyard," "nothing is wrong, so we do not need to act," "others are taking care of it," "I can't make a difference," "I don't have time," "I don't know how to get involved," and "advocacy is uncomfortable because it is emotional, not scientific."[6] There may also be a lack of understanding of a clear pathway for advocacy or "advocagnosia."[13]

Practice guidelines already exist to enable neuropsychologists to advocate effectively. Many scholars who work with culturally diverse populations have made tangible recommendations about the provision of neuropsychological evaluations to more diverse cultural communities[14,15] (2010 Special Issue on advocacy in The Clinical Neuropsychologist). Yet, such recommendations have yet to be widely adopted as a gold standard or mainstream "best practice."

Buttressing individual providers' unawareness and discomfort, there is a systemic or cultural avoidance of social justice advocacy within the field. Neuropsychology as a specialty has taken on the values of the larger system it is embedded in (i.e., healthcare, science, academia). The culture of neuropsychology remains political, patriarchal, individualistic, largely made up of members who are not from underrepresented groups, and uses Western values as the gold standard.[16–19] As a result, the field is inadvertently perpetuating and maintaining the same systems of oppression that underscore health disparities (e.g., diagnostic, treatment) in marginalized and minoritized communities.

What Are the Realities Deterring Neuropsychologists from Engaging in Social Justice Advocacy?

Bias

Racism and cultural incompetence threaten the health of patients and providers. The United States Centers for Disease Control in April 2021 finally named racism as a public health threat.[20,21] However, as a predominantly white, gendered-binary, Catholic, middle-high class, monolingual, highly educated, and able-centered discipline,[17,18] neuropsychology continues to rely on largely monolingual, mono-cultural neuropsychological assessment strategies and providers, which is likely to make it irrelevant in the healthcare marketplace by the year 2050 (e.g., Relevance 2050 Initiative of the American Academy of Clinical Neuropsychology[22]).

Being satisfied with the status quo, or with halfway measures toward culturally competent practices, exemplifies racial bias. It is important to recognize that the pervasive inequality mindset and practices may be masked by a façade of equal rights and access that continues to perpetuate known health disparities. Many still state that a minimal acknowledgment of cultural competencies without consistent, meaningful change is "the best they can do," and when pressed may follow with, "Well, this is better than nothing." Words like these have a history rooted in longstanding racial and cultural inequality of wealth and power. "Something is better than nothing" or the British version, "for better is half a loaf than no bread," dates back to the book, "The Proverbs of John Heywood: Being the 'Proverbs' of that Author Printed 1546." John Heywood, a Roman Catholic in England, fled to Belgium when Elizabeth I (a Protestant) took the crown in 1564. A similar proverb made it in the United States when Madison and Jefferson were discussing the Constitution between 1788 and 1789: "If we cannot secure all our rights, let us secure what we can." This was approximately 168 years after the inception of chattel slavery in Virginia by a Dutch ship to the nascent British colonies when slavery was legal. We, as neuropsychologists, must acknowledge the roots of our own narratives when justifying our inactions toward equity and social justice.

Tax and Trauma

The same inequities that are present in the broader US society are also present in the disproportionate burden carried among our marginalized and minoritized colleagues. These inequities have been described as "the minority tax," which is the tax of extra responsibilities placed on minoritized faculty in the name of efforts to achieve diversity.[23] This is when neuropsychologists from underrepresented and marginalized groups end up spending more time working on efforts related to equity, diversity, and inclusion because they feel obligated (or targeted by their own institutional leaders) to address disparities in the communities they represent or value serving these communities.[23] However, this work may not always be valued by their institutions or considered as promotion-earning work.[23] This leaves these providers and researchers overburdened as they may still need to meet demands of their institutions while trying to serve underserved communities. This tax is not only unfair, but the burden itself is a form of racism that exacerbates disparities in the field.

In addition, colleagues who experience daily micro/macroaggressions, oppression, and the constant barrage of current events where people from our communities are losing their lives through hate crimes, police brutality, and gun violence are at increased risk for experiencing psychological harm or *ethno-racial trauma*.[24] Chavez-Duenas, Adames, Perez-Chavez, and Salas[24] define ethno-racial trauma as "the individual and/or collective psychological distress and fear of danger that results from experiencing or witnessing discrimination, threats of harm, violence, and intimidation directed at ethno-racial minority groups. This form of trauma stems from a legacy of oppressive laws, policies, and practices" (p. 49). Increasing awareness of the extra burden and trauma being inflicted on neuropsychologists from underrepresented groups and equitable allocation of financial resources (including base salary and startup packages) are the first steps that can lead the field toward taking action for creating equity.

Differing Perspectives

In the past year, many in our field have made a pledge toward equity and social justice (see 2021 Special Issue on White Privilege in The Clinical Neuropsychologist). Others in health care have continued to struggle with acknowledging, naming, and accepting the structural racism that has given some the privilege of even denying its very existence. A recent example is the Journal of the American Medical Association's 2021 Podcast on "Structural Racism for Doctors – What Is It?" where two white men physicians debated the existence of structural racism under the claim that no physician is racist. The podcast has since been withdrawn after a massive backlash from the medical community (https://jamanetwork.com/journals/jama/pages/audio-18587774).

Within the context of these arguments, there appears to be one common thread: The concept of equity is constantly contested and susceptible to different interpretations. Equity is used synonymously to refer to "fair," "just," and "impartial." Some define it as "fair and respectful treatment of all people." Based on these interpretations, it will seem that many of us are engaging in equitable practices while pledging to raise our awareness of our own prejudices, implicit bias, and covert-overt micro and macro-aggressions/transgressions, and individual racism. Yet, these interpretations of "equity" are lacking since equity is supposed to target actions toward structures that disproportionately allocate wealth and power to privileged groups.[25]

Unfortunately, these differing perspectives in conversations often become polarized and dissolve quickly into conflicts between those with opposing views, which escalate toward "cancel culture" (that is, the tendency to avoid engagement altogether and stop listening to alternative perspectives). Unsurprisingly, we as a field have rarely transited to a reciprocal "reflective discourse/dialogue" perhaps based on our own fears of being labeled incompetent and/or racist.[26,27]

Many have raised discomfort and expressed disapproval of neuropsychology becoming "political" and, consequently, voluntarily removing themselves from the critical dialogues. Silence, withdrawal, and inaction are actions that sustain systems of oppression, giving some the privilege to deny that oppression even exists. To make progress, honest dialogues need to occur. We need to avoid tendencies to disengage from difficult dialogues and silence important reflective conversations about equity, diversity, and inclusion. Valuable social justice-related conversations are often directed "back-channel" or toward "cultural neuropsychology" forums alone. This could be viewed as modern iterations of historical "cultural erasure and cultural genocide" when dominant cultures of oppressors and colonizers insidiously attempt to negate, suppress, remove, and ultimately erase the voices and lived experiences of "subordinate" cultures/groups from history.[28] By systematically isolating the voices of those from underrepresented communities, the social control of wealth and power gets maintained by a small elite group, and "cultural neuropsychology" remains siloed. At a systems level, those in power can benefit from continuing to create policies that defend their own interests, thus maintaining and furthering access to power without consideration of all voices and perspectives.[29] This does not serve all neuropsychologists and the communities we serve. Instead, we need to create and embrace safe spaces to reckon with our collective discontent (e.g., shame, guilt, and fear in response to internal biases) as such reckoning is imperative to our collective liberation from the toxicities of racism, as well as to the relevance of our field.[22]

How Can Neuropsychologists Step into Action?

We questioned *why* the field of neuropsychology has been slow to meaningfully integrate advocacy and social justice practices despite calls to action[19] and awareness of methods to increase advocacy in neuropsychological practice.[6] Now we turn to *how* do we transition from knowledge acquisition and awareness to intentional action by leaders and majority of neuropsychologists instead of just a few. How do we transition from being diagnosticians to becoming agents of social change?

Transformational Learning

One pathway lies in reflecting upon how we teach advocacy and equity, diversity, and inclusion practices in neuropsychology. While commitments of the current political and field-specific movements toward equity, diversity, and inclusion are encouraging, our collective approach toward social justice and advocacy remains *transmissional* with an emphasis on improving *what* we know through webinars, trainings, and superficial conversations.[30,31] A "transmissional" approach is one that conveys information but doesn't give neuropsychologists a framework for processing or understanding what they are learning or applying it to their own preconceptions or to their everyday practice.

Yet, sustainable integration of social justice advocacy is most effective when learning is *transformational*, with an emphasis on changing *how* we know.[32,31] The transition from advocacy awareness to action will require a fundamental shift in our "frame of reference," in which we critically analyze the concepts, values, and associations that define the worldview of our field through transformative learning.[31] For example, the deleterious impact of socio-economic and health inequities on cognition has been well-documented.[33,34] Yet, little practical guidance exists on *how* neuropsychologists can incorporate this information into their day-to-day practice, such as how to align their clinical interview questions, test selection, and report recommendations with principles of equity and social justice.

Our existing *frames of reference* are "structures of assumptions through which we understand our experiences,"[35] (p. 5) and serve as the catalyst to our actions. To date, the frame of reference for neuropsychology has largely been oriented toward dominant culture, which has manifested as a lack of inclusivity and diversity in our clinical and research practices, normative data, and training curricula. Thus, considering the theory of transformative learning may offer insight regarding how to move neuropsychology toward intentional, transformative change in equity, inclusion, and social justice advocacy.

Mezirow[30] asserts that the process of transforming frames of reference begins with "disorienting dilemma(s) that challenges an individual's current worldview, followed by self-examination and critical assessment of previously held assumptions and values" (p. 22). Individuals then engage in "reflective discourse" by sharing their discontent (e.g., shame, guilt, and fear in response to internal biases) and evolving perspective with others for reciprocal validation.[30,32] That is, *transformational learning is relational and collectivist by nature and cannot be accomplished through individual, one-off efforts.*[32] Next, learners explore new ways of being (roles) and relationships that are better aligned with their new perspective and develop a plan to garner the requisite competence and skills to test these new roles. Finally, individuals build self-confidence in their new frame of reference by integrating it with their lived experience. *Action is the ultimate reflection of true transformation* (see Mezirow[30] and Kitchenham[36] for a comprehensive review).

The parallels of Mezirow's work to the current status of advocacy in the field of neuropsychology are uncanny. We have witnessed this very process through our collective experience of the double pandemic of COVID-19 and racial inequity (disorienting dilemmas) that challenged American ideologies of meritocracy and universalism. These events served as a catalyst for neuropsychologists to examine their contributions to maintaining the status quo (self-examination). Now, more than ever, trainees, researchers, and providers have been engaging in dialogue (reflective discourse) about next steps to take to adopt antiracist policies and dismantle structural racism in the field. Action-oriented courses on allyship and bystander training have proliferated. We have reached a critical decision crossroad, though. Where are we going from here? The next step to enact transformational change is to integrate our new frame of reference with lived experiences. Now, it is imperative that we "walk the talk." Transformational learning, collectivism, and social action are inextricably linked. Indeed, "education without social action is a one-sided value because it has no true power potential. Social action without education is a weak expression of pure energy. Deeds uninformed by educated thought can take false directions"[37] (p. 164).

Social justice advocacy is a collective responsibility to which we must all contribute; otherwise it will not fully manifest into meaningful change. It is time for neuropsychologists to fully step into our "true power potential" by actively engaging in social justice activism in solidarity or risk leading our field in the direction of irrelevance.[22] To this end, the following section outlines tangible strategies to get involved in social justice advocacy. We utilize Bronfenbrenner's[38] ecological systems framework (microsystem, mesosystem, exosystem, and macrosystem levels) to provide a graded, developmental approach for transitioning to a social change agent.

A Systems Approach to Advocacy

How an individual relates to and is influenced by their immediate environment and greater social contexts can be examined at the microsystem, mesosystem, exosystem, and macrosystem levels.[38] Factors at each of these levels influence each other and contribute to inequalities in healthcare services and outcomes.[39]

The *microsystem* level advocacy focuses on knowledge of the relationship between individual patients and their immediate environment, including their family, friends, colleagues, place of work, and religious institutions.[40] *Mesosystem* advocacy involves addressing inherent, reciprocal connections among an individual's microsystems. For example, a patient may no longer be able to work due to a neurological condition, which might increase financial stressors and conflict within the family microsystem. *Exosystem* advocacy is oriented toward enacting change in large-scale systems that may indirectly affect the patient, such as at the organizational, state, regional, and federal levels. Finally, *macrosystem* advocacy targets addressing the overarching societal and cultural ideologies, such as the predominance of individualism within US culture, that perpetuate bias and disparities.

Opportunities for neuropsychologists to engage in the process of dismantling inequities across variables such as race, ethnicity, gender, religion, sexuality, disability status at each of these levels are described below (see Figure 5.1).

Bite-Sized Advocacy: Advocating at the Micro- and Mesosystem Levels

For those who may feel overwhelmed by the process of engaging in social justice advocacy, a sustainable approach may be to start with "bite-sized" advocacy by incorporating advocacy into everyday actions in your clinical and research practices. Goodman et al.[41] proposed six key elements in social justice advocacy: (i) ongoing self-examination, (ii) sharing power, (iii) giving voice, (iv) facilitating conscious raising, (v) building strengths with patients, and (vi) equipping patients

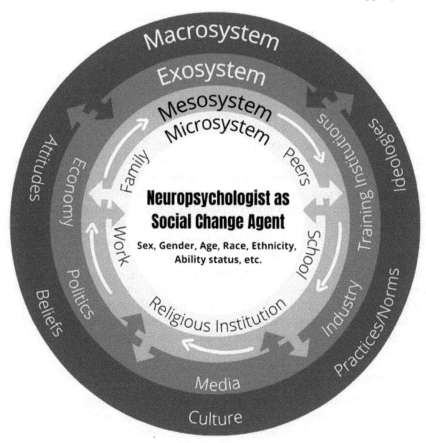

Figure 5.1 System approach to advocacy in neuropsychology

Source: Adapted from Bronfenbrenner's (1979) ecological systems theory

with tools that promote social change. Examples of how to implement this model to incorporate social justice advocacy in clinical service and research are included below.

Self-Examination

Neuropsychologists are encouraged to engage in ongoing self-examination and cultivate self-awareness, as these practices are often cited as the first steps to making meaningful progress toward becoming a social change agent.[6] It is important to identify our own privileges within intersectional identities, reflect on what we have been taught to believe about ourselves and our worlds, and learn how inequities are formed and maintained.[42] For instance, prior to meeting with a patient, some self-reflective questions to consider may include: (i) What assumptions might I have about the patient? (ii) Do I have the appropriate knowledge base to effectively serve this patient (e.g., knowledgeable about appropriate norms or linguistic expertise)? (iii) Would the patient be best served by consulting with a colleague or referring to another provider? Regarding self-examination of broader advocacy efforts, Ratts and Ford[43] developed the Advocacy Competencies Self-Assessment Survey© (ACSA) for assessing one's advocacy competency across domains of patient empowerment, patient advocacy, community collaboration, system advocacy, public information, and social/political advocacy. Assessing strengths and areas of growth is critical, as this knowledge informs where to "anchor" your efforts in advocacy for maximum impact.

Sharing Power

It is important to develop a critical consciousness about power differentials that exist between patients and providers, supervisors and trainees, managers and staff, investigators, and research participants. Tyler et al.[44] suggest that neuropsychologists be equipped to identify the impact of social determinants of health (SDoH: https://www.cdc.gov/socialdeterminants/index.htm) in patients' healthcare. Neuropsychologists may be the first to identify unmet needs, witness the effects of inequities, unjust policies, and barriers to access adequate health care. When possible, neuropsychologists can then use their power to identify disparities and obtain resources for their patients. One such example is illustrated by the Spanish TeleNP Assessment and Research (STAR) Consortium,[45] which rapidly formed to guide and support neuropsychologists serving Hispanic/LatinX populations during the COVID-19 pandemic. Specific barriers to telehealth identified in these communities included not having required equipment (e.g., computer, internet access) or a quiet space to have a private discussion or complete testing, and lack of technical knowledge.[46] Highlighting these needs has promoted advocacy within healthcare and research institutions to address these barriers by providing technology and patient education/support, effectively increasing access to teleneuropsychology services by underserved communities.

Consciousness Raising and Giving Voice

Consciousness raising involves raising awareness of the role of racism, sexism, discrimination, socio-economic, and other cultural factors that impact well-being, while *giving voice* entails providing a safe and nonjudgmental platform for patients to share narratives about their lives, questions, and goals.[41] For example, within the assessment process, neuropsychologists might facilitate discussion during the clinical interview about societal factors impacting patients' well-being and functioning and include these factors in the social history of the report. Cultural differences including linguistic barriers may prevent patients from accessing care or receiving equitable care. Subsequently, giving voice would involve amplifying the patient's narrative to improve accessibility of healthcare services to diverse communities. This may include advocating for materials to be provided in multiple languages and providing interpretive services at no cost to the patient. Similarly, in the context of research, consent forms and research measures should be offered in commonly spoken languages within the recruitment area. Hiring outreach and research coordinators and having principal investigators who are familiar with diverse groups and understand different cultural views about participating in research can help improve the experience for the participant and increase the diversity of research cohorts. Further, empowering communities to take the lead in shaping research design and participant recruitment within their community is another way to give voice and agency.

Building Strengths and Equipping Patients with Tools

Focusing on the strengths of patients is critical in social justice advocacy at the level of direct patient care. In the context of the neuropsychological evaluation, neuropsychologists could elicit patients' and their family's strengths by asking about cultural protective factors during the clinical interview, giving self-report measures that specifically query about positive aspects of their support systems (e.g., Positive Aspects of Caregiving Questionnaire[47]), and directly discussing patient's strengths evidenced on testing during the feedback session. During the course of an evaluation, sharing power may manifest as a neuropsychologist providing a patient with educational resources and directly assisting her/him/them in navigating the social safety net in the healthcare system and community. Taking care to build connections with non-profit organizations and state agencies is another way to alleviate burdens through partnerships, with the ultimate intention of empowering patients and their families to become advocates in their healthcare.

Large Scale Advocacy: Advocating at the Exosystem Level

Neuropsychologists and our professional organizations are involved in exosystem level advocacy via promoting legislation and policies that improve access to healthcare services and address needs of underserved communities. This work may involve practice organizations advocating for neuropsychological and psychological services to be included in healthcare coverage plans. Given the complexity of navigating local, regional, and national policies, the benefits of *coordinated advocacy* are demonstrated by the Inter-Organizational Practice Committee (IOPC), which was formed in 2012 and consists of practice chairs of several national neuropsychology organizations.[8] The IOPC published a model of 360 Degree Advocacy that includes the IOPC, national neuropsychology organizations, state, provincial, or territorial associations (SPTAs), regional neuropsychology organizations, and the American Psychological Association Practice Organization (APAPO).

At the federal level, the APAPO has highly impacted the Current Procedural Terminology (CPT) coding system and facilitated neuropsychologists' involvement in the CPT Editorial Panel (i.e., Drs. Antonio E. Puente and Neil Pliskin). Advocacy for healthcare coverage of neuropsychological testing and other services still has a long way to go. From a social justice perspective, the lack of reimbursement for the additional time and effort required for culturally informed neuropsychological evaluations may contribute to providers not engaging in this type of work. Rather than accepting the constraints of the current healthcare system, we need to bring these issues to the forefront of advocacy agendas and push for changing the larger systems in which we function in order to provide equitable care to our patients. One option may be to advocate for billing systems to include additional add-on codes for reimbursement of cultural complexity reimbursements. Another incentive could be licensing boards providing continuing education credits for literature reviews required for culturally responsive evaluations.

Neuropsychologists can also impact federal-level policies related to access to care by responding to calls for action. For example, APA organized a call to action of members to amplify the message to support permanent Medicare coverage of audio-only tele-behavioral health services and to co-sponsor the Tele-Mental Health Improvement Act (S. 660[48]) in the Senate. For these types of requests, templated responses (with the option to add in personal examples) and information about contacting one's representatives make contributing to advocacy efforts easier for members. High response rates demonstrate that our field will not tolerate policies that limit access to care for many ethnic/racial minoritized communities. Neuropsychologists are encouraged to take the initiative to write, call, or make contact with their representatives and, as a constituent, voice support for measures that have the potential to improve the lives of underserved or oppressed individuals. We have a duty to contribute to our collective voice at the federal level and can no longer ignore these requests. Becoming an active member, joining legislative and advocacy committees, and running for leadership positions in state-level psychology organizations are identified as some of the most effective ways to create meaningful change to benefit neuropsychology practice and our patients. Most professional organizations in neuropsychology have ethnic minority and/or advocacy committees with core missions to improve access to quality neuropsychological services for underserved individuals (see Table 5.1).

Table 5.1 Professional organizations and committees addressing inequality in neuropsychology

American Psychological Association (APA)	Society of Clinical Neuropsychology—APA Division 40 (SCN)	SCN Division 40 Ethnic & Minority Affairs Subcommittee	National Academy of Neuropsychology (NAN)—Culture and Diversity Committee
International Neuropsychological Society (INS)—Culture Special Interest Group	American Academy of Clinical Neuropsychology (AACN)—Relevance 2050 Initiative	Society for Black Neuropsychology (SBN)	Hispanic Neuropsychological Society (HNS)— Social Justice and Advocacy Committee
Asian Neuropsychological Association (ANA)— Advocacy Committee	Cultural Neuropsychology Council (CNC)	Queer Neuropsychological Society (QNS)	

In addition to advocacy for access to healthcare and favorable practice climates, neuropsychologists can and should play a role in addressing larger issues of social justice. For example, culturally united sister organizations that have emerged recently include the Asian Neuropsychological Association (ANA), Society for Black Neuropsychology (SBN), and Hispanic Neuropsychological Society (HNS). These groups have joined together on several initiatives to address systemic racism and social justice issues within neuropsychology and beyond. In response to the tragic deaths of George Floyd, Breonna Taylor, and many others, these organizations made official statements to be resolute in efforts to fight against systemic racism and racial health inequities. Other actionable steps have included encouraging members to support the Justice in Policing Act (H.R. 1720[49]) and resist Immigration and Customs Enforcement policies that affect the international community within the United States. SBN, HNS, and ANA also collaborated on providing powerful culturally relevant webinars (e.g., cultural humility, addressing microaggressions, advocacy in neuropsychology). Spurred by SBN leadership, these three sister organizations along with the National Academy of Neuropsychology (NAN), submitted statements calling upon State and Federal legislative bodies to ban the death penalty for offenses committed prior to age 21. As neuropsychologists, we were uniquely positioned to comment on this issue based on our expertise in brain development research. Other examples of neuropsychological organizations joining larger advocacy efforts include the ANA Advocacy Committee working with Stop AAPI Hate, an advocacy group for Asian Americans and Pacific Islanders, to provide resources for addressing racism, bullying, harassment, and trauma of youth and adults, which escalated during the COVID-19 pandemic. The Queer Neuropsychological Society is the newest collaborative partner for cultural identity based groups in the field.

Transformative Advocacy: Advocating at the Macrosystem Level

If the specialty of clinical neuropsychology would like to affect real, impactful, and lasting change, it will need to consider the culture of its own field. As discussed earlier, neuropsychology has taken on the mainstream culture of the academic system in which it is embedded. If we take a look at the history of academia, we will see that the culture of universities was inherited from European universities and was based on hierarchies, elitism, and exclusion.[50] The United States, like other countries such as New Zealand, then superimposed their own pioneering culture onto this inherited culture and added individualism, toughness, and physical prowess.[50] These are characteristics of a patriarchal society, where senior-level males have dominion over junior-level males and are allied by the descent in the male line.[51] This culture and system maintains racism, sexism, prejudice, and oppression, which is harming our colleagues, students, and patients/clients. One alternative structure for the field would be to transition to a matriarchal culture that is founded on an egalitarian system, as opposed to a hierarchy, where cooperation, collaboration, community, collectivism, and nurturing are paramount values.[52]

The main statement is that there is a desperate need to create change. It may take a long time to get to this level of change in our field; however, this type of real change is imperative in order to not only retain our colleagues from underrepresented groups and encourage/attract students from underrepresented groups to be a part of this field, but also to provide the type of services our diverse patients and clients deserve. In order to initiate this kind of change, the leadership in our field and each individual will need to do their part.

Tangible steps that can be taken include:

- Individuals in leadership roles who model behaviors that are in line with matriarchal values such as inclusive decision-making, transparency, and consistency.
- Creating a vision that includes social justice and advocacy at all levels in the field, from graduate programs, to training sites, to professional spaces.
- Improving the culture of institutions for diverse faculty and trainees by diversifying the workforce to decrease isolation experienced by many individuals from underrepresented groups.
- Changing current promotion systems in academic institutions that emphasize and reward research productivity above all other activities, while advocacy work often goes unrecognized, and remains constantly devalued in promotion

Table 5.2 summarizes the steps involved in advocacy at each level.

Where Can Equity and Advocacy Lead Neuropsychology?

We have honestly discussed *what, why, and how* neuropsychology can integrate advocacy and social justice practices. We turn now toward answering the question, *where* can equity and advocacy lead neuropsychology? The answer is toward transformational justice and greater social responsibility.

Transformational Justice

A framework is urgently needed for our collective shift in frame of reference. Transformational justice is a well-known framework in the field of criminology designed to create change in social systems. Specifically, transformative justice "is defined as transformative change that emphasizes local agency and resources, the prioritization of process rather than preconceived outcomes and the challenging of unequal and intersection power relationships and structures of exclusion at both the local and the global level"[53] (p. 340). It shifts the focus from reducing health disparities (i.e., restorative justice) to transforming the roots of the harm (i.e., structural "isms"). One example in neuropsychology is the treatment recommendations for a patient diagnosed with diabetes from a low-income, underserved, marginalized, and minoritized community. A typical recommendation is to modify the diet to be more aligned with the Mediterranean diet. Although an evidence-informed treatment recommendation, it inadvertently obscures the structures (racial segregation, red-lining, increase prevalence of fast-food chains, and liquor stores) sustaining this medical condition. Partnering with community organizations to advocate for increased numbers of affordable grocery stores and parks is instead a transformative action toward equity and social justice for the patient and their community. Other examples include the intention of ending conditions such as poverty, trauma, isolation, heterosexism, cis-sexism, xenophobia, white supremacy, misogyny, ableism, mass incarceration, forced displacement, residential segregation (including gentrification) and slavery.

The slow movement toward equity and social justice within psychology is also likely driven in part by the unchanged composition of our structural leadership. Historically, many fields, including neuropsychology, have engaged in *restorative justice*,[54,55] where the onus is on the individual,

Table 5.2 Steps to advocacy in neuropsychology at each level

Micro- and mesosystems level	
Self-examination and self-awareness	• Complete the Advocacy Competencies Self-Assessment Survey©
	• Understand your own identity development and intersectionality of identity
	• Identify your own privileges (e.g., educational, gender, race, etc.)
	• Reflect on your beliefs, values, assumptions, and worldview
	• Learn how inequities are formed and maintained
	• Consider power differentials between patients, providers, and institutions
Education and training	• Students: Request instruction and guidance on incorporating advocacy into your training and professional development
	• Faculty: Create a curriculum that includes principles of social justice and involvement in advocacy work
	• Attend presentations and seek continuing education on advocacy and socially responsive neuropsychology
Patient care	• Identify unmet needs, unjust policies, and barriers to adequate care for your patients
	• Develop understanding of your patients' social, cultural, community environment
	• For assessments, seek options for testing in preferred language, use appropriate norms, and include strengths/protective factors
	• During feedback, provide patients with resources in their community and education to navigate the health system
Access to services	• Provide informational materials and interpretive services in different languages
	• Educate treatment providers on the importance of using interpretive services and avoid using family members to replace interpreters
	• Offer options for low-cost healthcare for those in financial need
	• Provide transportation, lodging, community resources, respite, and childcare if needed
	• Offer telehealth options and address technology barriers
Community involvement	• Provide outreach and community education to increased patient awareness of neuropsychology and how to gain access to services
	• Build relationships and trust with community-based organizations
Exosystem level	
Professional organizations	• Become an active member in national, state, and/or regional organizations in psychology and neuropsychology
	• Join a cultural neuropsychology organization and/or advocacy and social justice committee
	• Serve as a mentor and/or sponsor students from under-represented groups to attend conferences
Training guidelines and accreditation	• Urge APA to include social justice and advocacy competencies for program and training site accreditation
Healthcare coverage	• Advocate for add on codes for cultural complexity reimbursements to improve access to services
Policy and legislation	• Respond to calls for action to contact representatives to support healthcare access and social justice policies
	• Build relationships with representatives in your district and keep them informed of relevant issues
	• Provide expert opinion to policy makers to improve access for patients and address disparities
Macrosystem level	
Culture of the field	• Model behaviors consistent with matriarchal values (e.g., collaboration, community, collectivism, and nurturing)
	• Make efforts to diversify workforce and support recruitment and retention of diverse trainees
	• Reward advocacy work through promotions, bonuses/raises, and time release from other responsibilities
	• Provide support (e.g., self-care opportunities) to trainees and colleagues who are actively engaging in advocacy

and the primary focus is on human violations and the need for healing and restoration of individuals and relationships. The transformative justice movement ignited by Ruth Morris in the late 1990s challenged such restorative justice approaches because it did not address issues of oppression, injustices, social inequities, and the sociopolitical and economic context driving the conflicts.[56]

The movement of advocacy in neuropsychology more recently reflects the transition from restorative justice to transformative justice. This has been depicted in our colleagues from underrepresented communities creating support spaces and trying to reclaim power. Unity among new cultural neuropsychology groups such as SBN, ANA, HNS, and QNS promotes systemic change by elevating voices and lived experiences of marginalized and minoritized communities. Through this approach, transformative justice resists the "one-size justice" fits all justice across space and time. It embraces the process and its continual iterations as more individuals join the movement. If the world is to be transformed, we need everyone to transform and everyone to be voluntarily involved in critical dialogue together. We understand that not everyone wants to engage in transformative justice. We also understand that their engagement means social status and financial loss. However, we also understand that not engaging in this transformative justice movement will increase irrelevance of the field.

Social Responsibility in Neuropsychology

Relatedly, the field can earnestly implement an ethical framework of SRN that suggests that "each person, organization, and institution have an inherent responsibility to act in a manner that promotes the positive growth of, and protects the rights of every individual"[57] (p. 17). When the field can move toward a more equitable and collectivistic culture and share the responsibility of diversity, social justice, and advocacy work, we can reduce harm, support the success of all members, and provide the quality of care that our patients/clients, trainees and research participants deserve.

Conclusion

Neuropsychology has the opportunity to learn from other fields (i.e., community psychology, counseling psychology, nursing, public health, sociology, anthropology) and to blaze a new trail that can effectively protect, include, and nurture all of its constituents equitably rather than equally. This chapter integrated transformative learning and transformative justice frameworks to anchor equity and social responsibility in neuropsychology while highlighting step-by-step suggestions for neuropsychologists on how to engage in advocacy work on a consistent, daily basis. We intentionally seek to raise critical consciousness, or conscientization, in which we as individuals become aware of, acknowledge, and reckon with the pervasive history of structures predetermining the lived experiences and conditions of both the oppressor and the oppressed.[58-60] Only then can we engage in an interactive process in which true reflection leads to transformative action,[54] specifically directed at transforming structures of oppression. The time has come for neuropsychologists to step into our roles as social change agents alongside underserved and historically marginalized communities.

Lilla Watson, an Aboriginal elder, activist, and educator from Queensland, Australia, used these words to capture the "why and how": *"If you have come to help me, you are wasting your time. If you have come because your liberation is bound up with mine, then let us work together."* Our role as social agents is not to save people and show them the way to salvation. Our role is to save ourselves from the perceptions and attitudes perpetuating colonial and capitalistic mentalities that are corroding our teachings, science, and practice. The time is now to be awakened and take action. Our own humanity depends on it.

References

1. Addo IY. Double pandemic: racial discrimination amid coronavirus disease 2019. Soc Sci Humanit Open. 2020;2(1):100074. doi: 10.1016/j.ssaho.2020.100074
2. American Psychological Association (APA). Revised competency benchmarks for professional psychology. Washington (DC): American Psychological Association; 2011 [cited 2021 Apr 25]. Available from: http://www.apa.org/ed/graduate/competency.aspx
3. Hessen E, Hokkanen L, Ponsford J, Zandvoort M, Watts A, Evans J et al. Core competencies in clinical neuropsychology training across the world. Clin Neuropsychol. 2018 May [cited 2021 Apr 25];32(4):642–56. Available from: https://pubmed.ncbi.nlm.nih.gov/29214891/
4. Ruffalo CA. Advocacy in the forensic practice of neuropsychology. In: Franklin RD, editor. Prediction in forensic and neuropsychology: sound statistical practice. 1st ed. New York (NY): Psychology Press; 2003. p. 5–27.
5. Goldstein G. Advocacy for neuropsychology in the public sector: the VA experience. Clin Neuropsychol. 2010 Apr 6 [cited 2021 Apr 25];24(3):401–16. Available from: https://www.tandfonline.com/doi/abs/10.1080/13854040903313597
6. Howe L, Sweet J, Bauer R. Advocacy 101: a step beyond complaining. How the individual practitioner can become involved and make a difference. Clin Neuropsychol. 2010 Apr [cited 2021 Apr 25];24(3):373–90. Available from: https://pubmed.ncbi.nlm.nih.gov/19859856/https://pubmed.ncbi.nlm.nih.gov/19859856/
7. Postal K, Wynkoop T, Caillouet B, Most R, Roebuck-Spencer T, Westerveld M et al. 360 degree advocacy: a model for high impact advocacy in a rapidly changing healthcare marketplace. Clin Neuropsychol. 2014 Feb 17 [cited 2021 Apr 25];28(2):167–80. Available from: https://www.tandfonline.com/doi/full/10.1080/13854046.2014.885087
8. Leong F, Pickren W, Vasquez M. APA efforts in promoting human rights and social justice. Am Psych. 2017 Nov [cited 2021 Apr 25];72(8):788–90. Available from: https://pubmed.ncbi.nlm.nih.gov/29172580/
9. Harper SR. Am I my brother's teacher? Black under-graduates, racial socialization, and peer pedagogies in predominantly White postsecondary contexts. Rev Res Educ. 2013;37:183–211. doi:10.3102/0091732X12471300
10. American Psychological Association (APA). Ethical principles of psychologists and code of conduct. Washington (DC): American Psychological Association; 2017 [cited 2021 Apr 25]. Available from: http://www.apa.org/ethics/code/
11. Lee C. Counselors as agents for social change. In: Lee CC, Walz GR, editors. Social action: a mandate for counselors. 1st ed. Alexandria (VA): American Counseling Association; 1988. p. 3–16.
12. Heinowitz AE, Brown KR, Langsam LC, Arcidiacono SJ, Baker PL, Badaan NH et al. Identifying perceived personal barriers to public policy advocacy within psychology. Prof Psych Res Pract. 2012 Jul 2 [cited 2021 Apr 25];43(4):372–78. Available from: https://studydaddy.com/attachment/113872/document%28154%29.pdf
13. Bauer R. President's message. Newsletter 40. 2006;24(1):26.
14. Ferraro FR, editor. Minority and cross-cultural aspects of neuropsychological assessment: enduring and emerging trends. 2nd ed. New York (NY): Psychology Press; 2016. p. 538.
15. Fujii D. Conducting a culturally informed neuropsychological evaluation. Washington (DC): American Psychological Association; 2016. p. 281.
16. Diaz-Santos M. *Decolonizing neuropsychology research with (alongside) the underserved* [Powerpoint slides]. International Neuropsychological Society Conference. 2021.
17. Manly, J. Centering social justice and public health in neuropsychology. International Neuropsychological Society Conference. 2021 Feb.
18. Suarez, P. Decolonizing neuropsychology [PowerPoint slides]. International Neuropsychological Society Conference. 2021 Feb.
19. Rivera-Mindt M, Byrd D, Saez P, Manly J. Increasing culturally competent neuropsychological services for ethnic minority populations: a call to action. Clin Neuropsychol. 2010 Apr [cited 2021 Apr 25];24(3):429–53. Available from: https://pubmed.ncbi.nlm.nih.gov/20373222/

20. Ford CL, Griffth DM, Bruce MA, Gilbert KL. Racism: science & tools for the public health professional. 1st ed. American Public Health Association Press; 2019. p. 616. https://doi.org/10.2105/9780875533049

21. Jones CP. Toward the science and practice of anti-racism: launching a national campaign against racism. Ethn Dis. 2018 Aug 9 [cited 2021 Apr 25];28(suppl 1):231–4. Available from: https://www.ncbi.nlm.nih.gov/pmc/articles/PMC6092166/

22. Postal K. President's annual state of the academy report. Clin Neuropsychol. 2018 Jan [cited 2021 Apr 25];32(1):1–9. Available from: https://doi.org/10.13854046.2017.1406993

23. Rodriguez JE, Campbell KM, Pololi LH. Addressing disparities in academic medicine: what of the minority tax? BMC Med Ed. 2015 Feb 1 [cited 2021 Apr 25];15(6):1–5. Available from: https://doi.org/10.1186/s12909-015-0290-9

24. Chavez-Dueñas NY, Adames HY, Perez-Chavez JG, Salas SP. Healing ethno-racial trauma in Latinx immigrant communities: cultivating hope, resistance, and action. Am Psych. 2019 Jan [cited 2021 Apr 25];74(1):49–62. Available from: https://psycnet.apa.org/fulltext/2019-01033-005.pdf

25. Wilkerson, I. Caste: the origins of our discontents. New York (NY): Random House; 2020. ISBN 978-0-593-23025-1

26. DiAngelo R. White fragility: why it's so hard for White people to talk about racism. 1st ed. Boston (MA): Beacon Press; 2018. p. 192.

27. Kendi IX. How to be an antiracist. 1st ed. New York (NY): One World; 2019. p. 320.

28. Zinn H. A people's history of the United States: 1492–present. Harper Perennial Modern Classics; 2005. ISBN 0-06-083865-5.

29. Bernard TJ, Snipes JB, Gerould AL. Vold's theoretical criminology. 6th ed. New York (NY): Oxford University Press; 2009. p. 384.

30. Mezirow J. Learning to think like an adult: core concepts of transformation theory. In: Merzirow J, editor. Learning as transformation: critical perspectives on a theory in progress. 1st ed. San Francisco (CA): Jossey-Bass; 2000. p. 3–33.

31. Goodman LA, Liang B, Helms JE, Latta RE, Sparks E, Weintraub SR. Training counseling psychologists as social justice agents: feminist and multicultural principles in action. Couns Psych. 2004 Nov 1 [cited 2021 Apr 25];32(6):793–836. https://doi.org/10.1177/0011000004268802

32. Baumgarter L. An update on transformational learning. New Dir Adult Cont Educ. 2002 Feb 26 [cited 2021 Apr 25];89:15–25. Available from: https://onlinelibrary.wiley.com/doi/abs/10.1002/ace.4

33. Zahodne LB, Manly JJ, Smith J, Seeman T, Lachman ME. Socioeconomic, health, and psychosocial mediators of racial disparities in cognition in early, middle, and late adulthood. Psychol Aging. 2017 Mar;32(2):118–30. doi:10.1037/pag0000154, PMID: 28287782; PMCID: PMC5369602.

34. National Academies of Sciences, Engineering, and Medicine; Health and Medicine Division; Board on Population Health and Public Health Practice; Nicholson A, editors. Brain health across the life span: proceedings of a workshop. Washington (DC): National Academies Press (US); 2020 Mar 31.

35. Mezirow, J. Transformative learning: theory to practice. In: Cranton P, editor. Transformative learning in action: insights from practice — new directions for adult and continuing education. 1st ed. Hoboken (NJ): Jossey-Bass; 1997. p. 5–12. Available from: https://www.ecolas.eu/eng/wp-content/uploads/2015/10/Mezirow-Transformative-Learning.pdf

36. Kitchenham A. The evolution of John Mezirow's transformative learning theory. J Transform Ed. 2008 Apr 1 [cited 2021 Apr 25];6(2):104–23. Available from: https://journals.sagepub.com/doi/abs/10.1177/1541344608322678

37. King ML. Where are we going? In: King ML, editor. Where do we go from here? Chaos or community. 1st ed. Boston (MA): Beacon Press; 1968. p. 143–75.

38. Bronfenbrenner U. The ecology of human development: experiments by nature and design. 1st ed. Cambridge (MA): Harvard University Press; 1979. p. 352.

39. Richter M, Dragano N. Micro, macro, but what about meso? The institutional context of health inequalities. Int J Public Health. 2018 Mar [cited 2021 Apr 25];63(2):163–4. Available from: https://pubmed.ncbi.nlm.nih.gov/29250722/

40. Marshall-Lee ED, Hinger C, Popovic R, Miller Roberts TC, Prempeh L. Social justice advocacy in mental health services: consumer, community, training, and policy perspectives. Psych Serv. 2019 Apr 18 [cited 2021 Apr 25];17(S1):12–21. Available from: https://psycnet.apa.org/record/2019-20177-001

41. Goodman LA, Liang B, Helms JE, Latta RE, Sparks E, Weintraub SR. Training counseling psychologists as social justice agents: feminist and multicultural principles in action. Couns Psych. 2004 Nov 1 [cited 2021 Apr 25];32(6):793–836. Available from: https://journals.sagepub.com/doi/10.1177/0011000004268802

42. Singh S. I am who I need to be: reflections on parental identity development from a father of a child with disabilities. Dis Soc. 2019 Mar 25 [cited 2021 Apr 25];34(5):837–41. Available from: https://www.tandfonline.com/doi/full/10.1080/09687599.2019.1589754

43. Ratts MJ, Ford A. Advocacy Competencies Self-Assessment (ACSA) Survey: a tool for measuring advocacy competence. In: Ratts MJ, Toporek RL, Lewis JA, editors. ACA advocacy competencies: a social justice framework for counselors. 1st ed. Alexandria (VA): American Counseling Association; 2010. p. 21–6.

44. Tyler ET. Aligning public health, health care, law and policy: medical-legal partnership as a multilevel response to the social determinants of health. J Health Biomedical L. 2012 Jun 5;8:211. Available from: http://docs.rwu.edu/law_feinstein_sp/2

45. Spanish TeleNP Assessment & Research Consortium. TeleNP for Spanish speakers in the time of COVID-19: benefits, challenges, and practical considerations. Webinar session presented at: Taquitos de Sesos Webinar; 2020 Apr 27; Zoom.

46. Arias F, Safi DE, Miranda M, Carrión CI, Diaz Santos AL, Armendariz V et al. Teleneuropsychology for monolingual and bilingual Spanish-speaking adults in the time of COVID-19: rationale, professional considerations, and resources. Arch Clin Neuropsychol. 2020 Nov 19 [cited 2021 Apr 25];35(8):1249–65. doi:10.1093/arclin/acaa100

47. Tarlow BJ, Wisniewski SR, Belle SH, Rubert M, Ory MG, Gallagher-Thompson D. Positive aspects of caregiving: contributions of the REACH project to the development of new measures for Alzheimer's caregiving. Res Aging. 2004 Jul [cited 2021 Apr 25];26(4):429–53.

48. Tele-Mental Health Improvement Act, S. 660, 117th Cong. 2021.

49. George Floyd Justice in Policing Act of 2020, H.R. 7120, 116th Cong. 2020.

50. Munford R, Rumball S. Women in university power structures. In: Kearney ML, editor. Women, power, and the academy: from rhetoric to reality. New York (NY): UNESCO; 2000. p. 91–9.

51. Uberoi P. Problems with patriarchy: conceptual issues in anthropology and feminism. Soc Bul. 1995 Sep 1 [cited 2021 Apr 25];44(2):195–221. Available from: https://journals.sagepub.com/doi/10.1177/0038022919950204

52. Taylor FL. *Decolonizing academia* [PowerPoint slides]. University of Utah Diversity, Equity, and Inclusion series. 2021.

53. Gready P, Robins S. From transitional to transformative justice: a new agenda for practice. Int J Trans Jus. 2014 Nov;8(3):339–61. Available from: https://academic.oup.com/ijtj/article-abstract/8/3/339/2912084

54. Claassen R. Restorative justice principles and evaluation continuums. Paper presented at National Center for Peacemaking and Conflict Resolution; 1995 May; Fresno Pacific College. 6p. Available from: http://restorativejustice.org/rj-library/restorative-justice-principles-and-evaluation-continuums/1084/#sthash.ggljPTzc.dpbs

55. Zehr H. Justice paradigm shift? Values and visions in the reform process. Med Quart. 1995 [cited 2021 Apr 25];12(3):207–16. Available from: https://onlinelibrary.wiley.com/doi/abs/10.1002/crq.3900120303

56. Morris, R. (2000). Stories of transformative justice. Toronto (CA): Canadian Scholar's Press.

57. Suarez P, Casas R, Lechuga D, Cagigas X. Socially responsible neuropsychology in action: another opportunity for California to lead the way. The Calif Psychol (Fall Ed.). 2016;49(4):16–8.

58. Freire P, Ramos MB. Pedagogy of the oppressed. 1st ed. New York (NY): Herder and Herder; 1970. p. 186.

59. Watts RJ, Williams NC, Jagers RJ. Sociopolitical development. Am J Comm Psych. 2003 Mar;31:185–94. Available from: https://link.springer.com/article/10.1023/A:1023091024140

60. Mosley DV, Hargons CN, Meiller C, Angyal B, Wheeler P, Davis C et al. Critical consciousness of anti-black racism: a practical model to prevent and resist racial trauma. J Couns Psych. 2021 Jan [cited 2021 Apr 25];68(1):1–16. Available from: https://pubmed.ncbi.nlm.nih.gov/32212758/

Part II

Case Studies

A. North: America (Canada and United States)

Black American

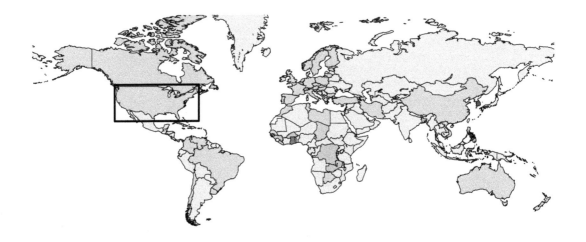

6 Culturally Sensitive Neuropsychological Assessment in Black Americans

Vonetta M. Dotson and Anthony Y. Stringer

Section I: Background Information

Terminology and Perspective

A variety of terms have been used to describe Americans of African descent throughout history, including Negro, Afro American, Black, and African American. Currently, Black and African American are the most commonly used terms, with individual differences in the preferred term. In this chapter, we will use the term Black American to broadly refer to persons of African ancestry living in the United States. This includes both Hispanic and non-Hispanic Black individuals and encompasses immigrants who have not only come from Africa but also from other regions including the Caribbean, Central America, and Europe.

Our perspective is that of African American neuropsychologists working as scientist-practitioners in academic settings in the southeast United States (Atlanta, Georgia).

People

The Black population of the United States is diverse and includes descendants of enslaved people, descendants of immigrants, and recently arrived immigrants. Black Americans make up approximately 14% of the national population, according to 2019 estimates.[1] Of the 46.8 million people in the United States who identified as Black in 2019, 87% identified as solely non-Hispanic Black, 8% as non-Hispanic Black and another race, and 5% as Hispanic Black. Immigrants make up approximately 10% of the Black population in the United States, most of whom are from African or Caribbean countries. Black Americans tend to live in the south, with 56% of the Black population living in the south in 2019.

History of Inequality and Racism

The Black American experience has been shaped by historical and current racism and discrimination. Most Black Americans can trace their lineage to Africans who were kidnapped in their native lands and sent to the Americas through the transatlantic slave trade from the sixteenth to the nineteenth century. After emancipation, black codes and Jim Crow laws continued to limit the freedom of Black Americans by hindering occupational opportunities, housing, education, voting rights, and healthcare.[2] The Civil Rights Act of 1964 ended legalized segregation and prohibited discrimination based on race, color, religion, sex, and national origin but did not eliminate the many laws and policies built into fundamental structures of our society (e.g., redlining, backed by the Federal Housing Administration, that prohibited Black Americans from buying

DOI: 10.4324/9781003051862-13

homes in suburbs and building equity). Longstanding racial disparities in the criminal justice system, ranging from policing and pretrial detention to sentencing and parole outcomes, have widespread impacts on Black American life at the individual and community level.[3,4] By depleting resources and social capital, biases in the criminal justice system affect emotional and physical health, family structure, employability, and housing.[5] These deeply entrenched laws and policies persist and perpetuate economic, educational, and health disparities, including neuropsychological outcomes, in the Black community.

In addition to these direct effects of racism and discrimination, vicarious threat and trauma experienced by Black Americans have been shown to impact physical and mental health.[6] Studies also show experiences of everyday discrimination, including microaggressions, are associated with negative physical and emotional consequences for Black Americans.[7,8]

Education

Educational opportunities for Black Americans have increased over time, but disparities still exist. The percentage of Black adults with at least a college degree rose from 15% in 2000 to 23% in 2019,[1] paralleling the 9-point increase from 24% to 33% in the entire US population in the same time period. The numbers are higher in Black immigrants (28%), and Black immigrants from Africa are actually more likely than the general US population to have a college degree or higher.[9] However, Black Americans remain underrepresented in elite universities, such as Harvard and Brown. At all levels, educational attainment is lower in the Black community compared to the non-Hispanic white population.[10] For example, 87.2% of Blacks compared to 93.3% of non-Hispanic whites had at least a high school diploma in 2019.

The quality of education is a particularly important issue when it comes to neuropsychological assessment. In the United States, learning opportunities vary dramatically depending on social status. Unequal access to key educational resources, including funding, skilled teachers, quality curriculum, and optimal class size, contribute to race differences in educational outcomes.[11] Biased treatment by teachers also contributes to disparities. For example, Black students receive more disciplinary actions such as being suspended or expelled and are less likely to be recommended for gifted-education programs, even after adjusting for relevant factors such as standardized test scores.[12] Research has consistently shown that quality of education, often measured by single-word reading ability, impacts cognitive performance across the lifespan and explains much of the race-related differences in cognitive function.[12–14]

Socio-Economic Status

Socio-economic status (SES) is an important consideration in the assessment of Black Americans. Across indicators of SES, such as education, household income, wealth, and home-ownership, Blacks are disadvantaged. For example, according to 2019 estimates from the US Census Bureau,[15] the median income for non-Hispanic Black households was $43,771, compared to $71,664 for non-Hispanic white households. Compared to non-Hispanic whites, Black Americans are more than twice as likely to live in poverty (21.2% vs. 9%) and to be unemployed (7.7% vs. 3.7% in 2019)—disparities that have been compounded in the time of the COVID-19 pandemic. An important factor in these economic disparities is the consistent devaluation of assets in Black neighborhoods, which hinders the accumulation of wealth for Black homeowners. For example, according to the Brookings Institution, homes of similar quality are valued on average $48,000 lower in majority-Black compared to majority-white neighborhoods.[16] Another factor is race differences in single-parent households. About 30% of Black households are headed by a woman with no partner present, over three times what we see in white households (9%).[17] SES is an important mediator of racial disparities in physical and mental health[18,19] and has been linked to various markers of brain health.[20]

Role of Religion

The church has historically played a significant role in the Black American community.[21,22] Black Americans are more likely than any[22] other racial or ethnic group in the United States to engage in religious activities, such as attending church services.[23] Approximately three-fourths of Black Americans consider religion to be very important in their lives, and half report attending church services at least once a week. However, there are generational differences. Only 28% of younger Blacks report attending church at least weekly.[24] Black older adults are more likely than their younger counterparts to participate in religious activities outside of church services and to attend Black congregations.[24]

The church has been an important agent of change and resilience in the Black community, often serving as a primary, and even sole, source of safety, education, and support. As such, it is not surprising that research shows many Black Americans turn to ministers for mental health concerns more often than mental health professionals or physicians.[25,26] Studies have shown that church attendance and social support from church networks can be a protective factor against depressive and anxiety symptoms, substance use disorders, suicide, and overall psychological distress.[27–30]

Health Status

Heart disease, cancer, and stroke are the leading causes of death in the Black American community. While the prevalence of these conditions has decreased over the last two decades,[31] rates are still high and racial disparities remain. Approximately 44% of Black men and 48% of Black women have some form of cardiovascular disease.[32] Compared to whites, Black Americans are more likely to die from a variety of medical conditions, including stroke, cardiovascular disease, diabetes, cancer, HIV/AIDS, and pneumonia.[31] Racial disparities are also prominent during the COVID-19 pandemic, as Black Americans are more likely to suffer severe illness and COVID-related death compared to whites,[33] in part due to the higher prevalence of preexisting conditions that complicate the course of the disease. Similar to disparities in other health outcomes, these differences have been attributed to social determinants, such as inequalities in health care access, unemployment, and poverty.[34]

Mental Health Views

Black Americans carry a greater burden of psychological symptoms compared to the general population.[35] Despite a lower prevalence of psychological disorders in many studies, the severity, chronicity, and negative sequelae of psychological conditions are higher in Black Americans.[36–38] Of note, subthreshold symptoms, such as feelings of sadness and hopelessness, have been shown to be more prevalent in Blacks.[32] In addition, there are age differences, such as a higher prevalence of depression in Black older adults compared to non-Hispanic white older adults. Moreover, reports[39] of rising rates in the Black community of serious mental illness and suicidal ideation, plans, and attempts over recent years highlight the importance of screening for psychological symptoms in the neuropsychological assessment of Black Americans.

Rates of mental health services use in the Black community is less than half the rate in whites, with an estimated one-third of Black Americans with a diagnosed psychological disorder receiving professional treatment.[40] This under-treatment can be attributed to a number of factors, including discrimination and bias in the healthcare system and cultural views of mental health.[41,42] Stigma of mental illness can deter Black Americans from seeking help due to concerns their family and friends will see them as "crazy."[43] Other factors contributing to low mental health service use include lack of insurance or under-insurance, lack of mental health literacy, cultural mistrust of medical and mental health professionals, and discrimination.[44,45]

Neuropsychological Approach

Normative differences in neuropsychological test performance in Black and white samples are known to occur in the absence of neurological disease,[14] leading some neuropsychologists to advocate the use of race-based norms to avoid false-positive bias in test diagnostic interpretation.[46] The most common race-based normative systems for use in the United States are the Revised Comprehensive Norms for an Expanded Halstead-Reitan Battery: Demographically Adjusted Neuropsychological Norms for African American and Caucasian Adults,[47] which cover the adult age span, and the Mayo Clinic norms for Black older adults.[48] An alternative approach utilizes multiple regression techniques that combine race and other factors with a known correlation with test performance to derive an expected test score that can be compared to the score obtained on the test. Discrepancies between predicted and obtained scores theoretically should reflect factors outside of race and other variables in the prediction equation. This approach has been utilized to predict intelligence test scores[49] and has potential for adoption for predicting other areas of cognitive functioning.

These approaches are race-inclusive and should not be considered "race-neutral" as they share unintended and potentially harmful consequences in the way they handle race as a factor in clinical decision-making. While initially intended to decrease the likelihood of false-positive diagnostic error (e.g., misclassifying a Black patient as having dementia as a result of using Caucasian norms), both approaches create a higher hurdle for Black Americans to exceed, compared to whites, to qualify for compensation in forensic contexts.[50] Both approaches also risk further entrenching racist stereotypes about Blacks and other US minority populations. Race often becomes a proxy for numerous other harder to measure factors including prenatal care, nutritional status, educational quality, extracurricular opportunities, expectations that influence examinee performance, biases in examiner interpretation of performance, health status, access to and intensity of healthcare services, the impact of environmental stressors (including racism), socio-economic status, etc. Research suggests literacy and other factors readily account for differences between racial groups in neuropsychological performance.[51]

Unfortunately, the challenge of collecting data on the many variables that may account for racial differences in cognitive performance has led neuropsychologists to settle for the "convenience" of race as a proxy for the presumptive impact of socio-economic inequity. Consequently, a healthy Black American from an upper socio-economic class with an Ivy League education may be predicted to perform worse than a non-Hispanic White at the same or a more disadvantaged rung in society, an incongruous expectation arising regardless of whether race-based norms or race-inclusive multiple regression approaches are utilized.

Test norms are an important consideration, but a recent review article[52] calls to attention other racist practices in psychological assessment that affect the Black community and other minoritized groups, such as the use of racist stimuli in testing material. For example, the inclusion of the noose in the Boston Naming Test not only carries the potential for a negative psychological impact on Black examinees, but it can also negatively impact test performance due to stereotype threat, and it can contribute to mistrust in the healthcare system. Clearly, an important priority for the field of neuropsychology is to not only diversify the field to meet the needs of an increasingly diverse American society but also to directly address and end racist practices that have largely gone unquestioned in the field.

Section II: Case Study — "Seeing the Bigger Picture in Race, Resilience and Examiner Expectation"

The following case illustration will highlight some, though not all, of the issues introduced in Section I. Possible identifying information and several aspects of history and presentation have been changed to protect patient identity and privacy.

Presenting Concerns

Patient A.B. (not actual initials) was a 44-year-old, right-handed, Black male who was seen for neuropsychological examination because of progressively worsening memory problems. He came to medical attention approximately six months prior to the neuropsychological examination because of complaints of headaches, blurred vision, and memory difficulty. Magnetic resonance imaging (MRI) identified a pituitary adenoma, and A.B. subsequently underwent a trans-sphenoidal (i.e., through the nose, sphenoid bone, and sphenoidal cavity) resection, a common approach to treating pituitary tumors. Surgery resolved his blurred vision and decreased the frequency of his headaches but precipitated the onset of hypogonadism and worsened memory problems.

Language Proficiency, Educational, and Vocational History

A.B. was fluent in standard English and did not speak any other languages. A.B. completed high school with "C" average grades. He denied any history of grade failure, learning disability, attention deficit diagnosis, and school suspensions or expulsions. A.B. served in the US Army for 22 years, working in logistical operations. He served in active combat during Operations Desert Storm and Iraqi Freedom. In the years since his army discharge, A.B. worked in logistics and purchasing departments in the civilian aerospace and defense industry. He was on medical leave from his job at the time of his evaluation because of his worsening memory problems after surgery. Co-workers complained that he forgot work assignments. He began taking detailed notes to compensate for his memory failures but eventually had to stop work because of his poor performance. He remained hopeful of returning to work if his memory improved.

Psychological History

A.B.'s childhood was traumatic. At age 12, he witnessed his father kill his mother and then commit suicide. A.B. was currently married and lived with his wife of 13 years in a private residence. He had no children.

During combat deployment, he frequently witnessed violence and death, events that he continued to reexperience in nightmares and flashbacks. For example, after returning from his last deployment, there had been multiple incidents in which he believed he heard soldiers screaming. The last flashback was 2 to 3 months prior to his neuropsychological examination. After returning from combat, A.B. had a 21-day Veterans Administration psychiatric hospitalization for posttraumatic stress disorder (PTSD).

A.B. additionally acknowledged problems with anger management. In the two years prior to his neuropsychological examination, he had become physically violent twice, though neither incident resulted in injury to others or arrest. A.B. endorsed past suicidal ideation with a plan for ending his life when he first returned from Iraq. He also reported suicidal ideation after his tumor diagnosis but denied having any plan for acting on these thoughts. At the time of his examination, A.B. denied suicidal ideation, plan, or intent. He did report past episodes when he exhibited manic symptoms, including a decreased need for sleep, feelings of grandiosity, pressured speech, increased activity, irritability, and agitation. During these episodes, he averaged 4 to 5 hours of sleep a night with the use of a sleep aid but often went without sleep entirely.

Finally, A.B. acknowledged consuming 2–3 alcoholic beverages an average of 3–4 times weekly prior to his tumor surgery but reported no consumption in the past six months. He denied ever having problems at home, work, or in his community related to alcohol consumption and reported no other drug or tobacco use.

Additional Health History

A.B. suffered one diagnosed and a second suspected concussion during his military service. The first occurred 23 years prior to the examination during a parachute jump when he lost his balance when landing, fell and hit his head. He was unconscious for a few minutes and experienced a post-traumatic amnesia of approximately 10 minutes but no retrograde amnesia. He was diagnosed with a concussion and hospitalized overnight for observation. The second suspected concussion occurred three years prior to the neuropsychological examination when he hit his head on a wall following a blast detonation. He did not suffer a loss of consciousness but felt dazed for several minutes. He did not seek medical evaluation or treatment following this second incident. A.B. did not experience any residual cognitive problems following either incident.

At the time of his evaluation, A.B. additionally had hyperlipidemia and hypertension. A recent blood test detected elevations in the liver enzymes aspartate and alanine aminotransferase. His medications included over-the-counter pain relievers for his occasional headaches; prazosin for hypertension; simvastatin for hyperlipidemia, vardenafil for erectile dysfunction; testosterone hormone supplementation; and sertraline, quetiapine fumarate, lorazepam, and risperidone for mood and sleep regulation.

Daily Functioning

A.B. was independent in basic activities of daily living (ADLs) but had difficulty with more complex activities because of poor memory. He had trouble remembering routes, computer passwords, and prospective tasks such as appointments, errands, and bill payment due dates. His wife took over bill payments and provided reminders for appointments and to take medications.

Behavioral Observations

Rapport was easy to establish and maintain. A.B. was friendly and cooperative throughout the evaluation. He provided good eye contact but demonstrated an anxious affect. He appropriately engaged in and initiated casual conversation. He worked at an appropriate pace. While he was able to maintain his attention throughout testing, he had difficulty sitting still and frequently shook his legs and shifted in his seat. He was also mildly impulsive, sometimes starting tasks before instructions were completed. The Victoria Symptom Validity Test (VSVT[53]) was administered to more objectively gauge motivation and validity of testing. On the VSVT, A.B. scored within the valid range for items that appear "easy" (23 out of 24 correct) and on items that appear "difficult" (18 out of 24 correct). Thus, A.B. appeared to put forth adequate effort.

Test Results

Test Score Classification

Severity classifications vary across individual neuropsychologists. While the mild range of impairment is sometimes defined as beginning at 1.5 or even two standard deviations below average, if we require a further one standard deviation test score drop to change impairment classification, moderate range performance will fall three standard deviations below average (99.7th percentile) so that performance is worse than 99.7% of the normative group. Severe range performance will then be worse than 99.9% of the normative sample. In effect, the moderate and severe classifications become functionally meaningless. For this reason, in this chapter test scores that are one, two, and three standard deviations below average are respectively labeled mild, moderate, and severe impairment. As a result, the mild range of impairment corresponds to the 16th percentile, the moderate range to the 5th percentile, and the severe range to the 1st percentile, preserving a functionally useful and interpretable distinction between these impairment classifications.

Attention

A.B. was alert and interactive throughout the examination. He was able to sustain his attention over time and was not distracted by background noise. The span of verbal information that he could process was average, as was his ability to simultaneously listen to incoming information and mentally manipulate it so that he could report it in reverse sequence. Similarly, visual processing span was average, as was his ability to simultaneously pay attention to visual sequences and reverse their order. Overall, A.B. showed intact attention.

Perception

On visual field testing, A.B. was unable to perceive stimuli in the upper right quadrant of his left eye. Responses to unilateral and bilateral simultaneous stimulation in visual, auditory, and tactile modalities were within expected limits. Visual acuity was *20/20* OD and *20/25* OS without corrective lenses. Line bisection and color perception were intact. Basic visual form perception was assessed with the Object Decision Test,[54] which requires the patient to correctly choose which of four plausible appearing black silhouettes is a real object. Normed in Great Britain, the test refers to objects by names less familiar to people in the United States (e.g., "pram," "lorry"). The patient, however, does not have to identify objects by name. Nonetheless, the test includes some objects that could be insufficiently familiar to people in the United States to be identified by silhouette alone (e.g., oilcan, teapot). A.B.'s form perception fell in the mildly impaired range based on British norms. A.B.'s ability to match and discriminate complex visual stimuli on the Benton Facial Recognition Test,[55] which uses Caucasian faces exclusively, was mildly impaired.

In contrast, A.B. performed better on most spatial perception tests. He was fully intact in his stereoscopic depth perception, judgment of the orientation of lines in space, his ability to picture mentally how a complex stimulus would look after it was rotated in space, and his ability to determine the number of rectangular blocks needed to build various pictured three-dimensional geometric structures. The only spatial ability showing mild impairment was judgement of the relative positions of points in space, also assessed with a British normed test that is part of the same test battery as the Object Decision Test.[54]

Finally, recognition of presumed familiar stimuli was fully intact. Specifically, A.B. accurately identified the characteristic color of various objects named to him (e.g., that grass is green, charcoal is black). He also accurately identified stimuli shown to him including fingers (e.g., thumb, index finger), famous people (e.g., US presidents Barack Obama and Gerald Ford), and landmarks (e.g., the Washington Monument).

Psychomotion

A.B.'s resting gaze was central, he showed no impersistence in maintaining the fixation of his gaze in either lateral direction, and he was able to shift his gaze in all directions upon command. Grip strength was intact bilaterally. Speed of alternating hand movements (pronation and supination) was within expected limits bilaterally. Performance on a speeded manual finger-tapping task was within expected limits (based on age and sex) for his left hand but was in the mildly impaired range for his dominant right hand. Speed was intact with his left hand on a fine motor dexterity task where A.B. was asked to quickly place small pegs into differentially oriented holes, but speed on this task was mildly impaired with his right hand. He accurately performed a novel sequence of hand movements (i.e., repeatedly putting his hands in fist, edge-down, and palm-down positions) and tandem reciprocal movements (e.g., showing one finger when the examiner showed two, and vice versa).

There were no signs of perseveration in A.B.'s copies of triple loop figures. He accurately reached for targets with each hand. He readily pantomimed previously learned movements involving facial muscles (e.g., sniffing a flower), hands (e.g., turning a key in a lock), or use of hands to perform a habitually linked series of movement (e.g., sealing a letter in an envelope and placing a stamp in the correct location). A.B.'s drawings of simple geometric figures from a model, however, were mildly impaired with his right hand but intact with his left hand. His drawing of a more complex figure with the right hand, however, was within the average range for his age.

Language and Calculation

A.B.'s conversational speech was fluent, with normal articulation, prosody, grammar, and syntax. Confrontation naming utilizing low-frequency objects was intact. He had no difficulty with the mechanics of writing. He accurately read numbers and arithmetic signs and had no trouble performing basic mental addition, subtraction, multiplication, and division.

Learning and Memory

Visuospatial memory was assessed using the Tombaugh[56] administration of the Taylor Complex Figure. This test required A.B. to draw a complex figure from memory, with the expectation that he would recall an increasing number of details with each timed exposure to the figure over four learning trials. He performed in the mildly impaired range for immediate recall. He demonstrated variability across learning trials, and his performance was ultimately mildly impaired by the fourth learning trial. On all recall trials, A.B. maintained the overall gestalt of the complex figure, with his performance only lowered by the number of details that he included. After a 15-minute delay, he again performed in the mildly impaired range for recall of the figure, although he retained all the details that were recalled on the most recent learning trial.

Verbal memory was assessed with the California Verbal Learning Test,[57] which consists of five learning trials of a 16-word list, followed by short and long delay recall trials. Immediate recall was average, with six words recalled. A.B. recalled five words when an alternate list was presented, also in the average range. He recalled 12 of 16 words at the end of the fifth presentation (performance in the average range). After a short delay, A.B. recalled nine words, performance in the average range. After a 20-minute delay, he performed in the mildly impaired range, recalling 8 of 16 words. He did not seem to benefit from semantic cuing. A.B. avoided repeating words he had already recalled on a given trial, and he also did not intrude extraneous words that were not from the list presented to him. When asked only to recognize words from the list, distinguishing them from distractors, A.B. correctly identified only 11 of 16 words and made two false-positive errors. This put his recognition score in the severely impaired range; however, his recognition was still superior to his delayed recall. When asked to choose between a word from the target list and an obviously incorrect word, he did not make any errors, suggesting that he was not attempting to feign memory difficulties.

A.B.'s verbal memory abilities were also assessed using the Logical Memory subtest of the Wechsler Memory Scale—3rd Edition,[58] which consists of two short stories that are learned respectively over one or two trials and recalled after a 30-minute delay. His ability to acquire the details of the stories was high average, and his ability to remember the details of the stories after a delay was average.

Problem Solving and Reasoning

A.B. was fully oriented to person, place, time, and situation. He was administered a short form of the Wisconsin Card Sorting Test[59] to assess problem solving and the ability to maintain cognitive sets across changing stimulus conditions. The test included periodic verbal queries about possible sorting strategies, and A.B. identified all three alternate sorting strategies at the beginning, middle, and end of the test. He achieved six sorts of the cards, a performance in the average range. He avoided repetition and set loss errors. We next administered the Short Category Test.[60] This test is designed to assess complex concept formation and abstract categorizing. A.B. performed in the mildly impaired range on this test.

Intellectual Functioning and Academics

On the Wechsler Abbreviated Scale of Intelligence 2nd Edition (WASI[61]), A.B. obtained a Verbal IQ of 98 (45th percentile; average range), Performance IQ of 87 (19th percentile; low average range), and Full Scale IQ of 91. His Full Scale IQ placed him at the 27th percentile as compared to same-age peers. An estimate of A.B.'s likely premorbid intellectual functioning was calculated using demographic and educational background and oral reading performance on the Wechsler Test of Adult Reading (WTAR[62]). The WTAR yielded estimates of premorbid Verbal, Performance, and Full Scale IQ scores in the Low Average Range. A.B.'s currently measured intellectual test performance from the WASI was at or above these premorbid estimates.

Emotion and Behavior

A.B.'s affect was anxious. He reported problems with depression, PTSD, and anger management, as documented above. A.B. completed the Minnesota Multiphasic Personality Inventory-Restructured Format (MMPI[63]) to assess his current emotional functioning and personality characteristics. While his pattern of responses suggests that he approached the test in a consistent manner, his profile indicates that he likely over-reported and exaggerated psychopathology. Given this, his profile was invalid and considered an overestimate of current psychopathology. His response pattern is most likely a cry for help and an indication of significant emotional distress.

Diagnostic Impressions

Neuropsychological examination revealed intact attention. Basic visual perceptual testing revealed an upper right quadrant field cut confined to his left eye. A field cut in only one eye would have to result from a preoptic chiasm lesion. The proximity of the pituitary to the optic pathway makes it likely this was an unintended consequence of surgery. A.B.'s good visual acuity, even in the left eye (i.e., 20/25 without corrective lenses) and his intact performance on a range of perceptual measures with equally demanding visual requirements, suggests the mild impairment on the Object Decision[54] and Benton Facial Recognition[55] tests was not due to this minor visual field cut.

Cultural factors must be considered in interpreting these two visual perceptual tests. The Object Decision Test[54] uses British norms and includes stimuli that the patient may never (e.g., a yacht) or relatively rarely (e.g., an oilcan and teapot) have personally encountered. While potentially identifiable when shown in full detail, depiction in black silhouette shorn of all feature cues requires greater than casual familiarity with these objects, especially when needing to distinguish the objects from equally plausible appearing foils. Similarly, the use of Caucasian faces alone to judge perceptual ability on the Benton Facial Recognition Test may create a greater challenge for Black Americans.

A.B.'s intact performance on multiple spatial tests that do not use culture-specific stimuli adds to the suspicion that the above findings may reflect the impact of culture on test performance. Indeed, the only perceptual test not utilizing culture-specific stimuli, on which A.B. scored below the intact range, was a measure requiring judgment of position in visual space. While this test also uses British norms, it is not as clear why nation of origin would impact perception of spatial position. Given the potential remapping of visual coordinates in the cortex following onset of blindness in one eye quadrant, this finding may reflect a neuropsychological deficit rather than the confounding influences of culture and normative bias.

Black Americans born and reared in the United States are likely to be more acculturated to the traditionally dominant white subculture than a more recent US immigrant. A.B.'s 22 years in the military likely added to his acculturation given the emphasis on US patriotic symbols in the army. Hence, A.B. readily performed tests intended to detect agnosia using stimuli such as the faces of US presidents and pictures of US monuments. A.B. showed no evidence of agnosia to any category of stimuli. He showed intact strength, speed, and coordination in his left hand but had a mild decrease in fine motor speed in the right hand. He had a good ability to plan, sequence, and cognitively regulate movements. No difficulties with oral language or mental calculations were noted. A.B. had mild difficulty learning visuospatial information with repetition, but he retained what he learned over a 15-minute delay and primarily showed a limited acquisition of detail. Verbal learning was intact for both lists and meaningfully organized narratives, though he did show mild difficulty retaining list information. While A.B. recognized more list items than he could freely recall, normatively his recognition performance was in the severe range. The fact that verbal memory was better with narratives, than with lists, suggests he benefitted from having information semantically organized and meaningfully integrated.

Performance varied across measures of reasoning and problem solving. A.B. demonstrated a good ability to perceive alternative problem-solving strategies and was both flexible and systematic in applying those strategies. He had mild difficulty, however, with categorical reasoning such that he could not always identify the target principle for grouping stimuli. An estimate of premorbid functioning that included race and reading performance as predictors yielded intellectual scores that were either comparable to or lower than A.B.'s actual obtained IQ scores, illustrating the challenge of using such approaches with Black Americans. A successful military and civilian career working in logistics and purchasing, including time in the typically high-demand aerospace industry, requires at least average intellectual functioning, if not higher. A.B.'s Full Scale IQ is at the bottom of the Average Range and likely is lowered by his relatively poorer scoring on the perceptual and timed motor tests contributing to the Performance IQ. Hence, rather than concluding that IQ scores are better than expected based on the race-inclusive prediction, historical information suggests current functioning could be lowered.

A.B. experienced traumatic events during childhood and subsequently during his military service and appeared to meet criteria for PTSD. Additionally, he has had both manic and depressive episodes, consistent with Bipolar I Disorder. At the time of his examination, his psychological distress was so high that he invalidated his MMPI[63] through symptom over-endorsement, a response pattern interpreted as a cry for help. These psychiatric disorders, however, predate the onset of his acute cognitive impairment and do not provide a viable explanation for his neuropsychological profile.

The neuropsychological examination documented cognitive impairments that were concordant with the decrease in adaptive functioning at home, work, and in community settings, warranting a diagnosis of Major Neurocognitive Disorder. The most probable etiology is the one most proximate to the onset of his cognitive complaints, namely the pituitary adenoma and subsequent surgical resection. The visual field cut is most clearly related to this etiology; however, mild deficits in right-hand speed and categorical reasoning may further implicate trauma to superiorly adjacent frontal lobe regions. The dissociation between mildly lower memory for lists that require the patient to generate an organizational strategy and intact memory for already semantically organized information may also be explainable by left frontal lobe involvement. Poorer recall of detail than gestalt is more common with left hemisphere pathology and does not detract from this proposed functional localization. This parsimonious explanation notwithstanding, the impact of two mild concussive episodes, PTSD, bipolar disorder, and a history of psychological trauma beginning in childhood cannot be excluded as contributors to this patient's current presentation.

Feedback and Follow-Up

A.B. and his wife attended a feedback session with the examiner. The results of the examination were reviewed. They were encouraged that the cognitive impairments were overall mild and potentially addressable through a program of cognitive rehabilitation that focused on teaching practical, compensatory strategies for the effects of these impairments on everyday functioning. A.B. was also encouraged to utilize mental health services available through his local Veteran's Administration (VA) Medical Center, and with his permission, a written report was subsequently sent to his psychiatrist and psychologist.

Cognitive rehabilitation was instituted approximately one month following the examination, consisting of weekly, one-on-one sessions with a therapist. The primary focus was on training A.B. in memory compensation strategies that he could use at work. A.B. remained emotionally stable during this time and consistent in attending individual and group counseling sessions through the VA. A.B. was discharged from cognitive rehabilitation after approximately 12 weeks, and at that time was considering an attempt to return to work part-time on a trial basis.

Section III: Lessons Learned

Race-inclusive Normative Interpretation

Patient A.B. illustrates the challenge arising from race-inclusive predictions of premorbid function. A successful career in logistics in both the military and private industry is incongruous with the WTAR premorbid estimate of low average intellectual functioning. Despite A.B.'s history of multiple concussions, pituitary adenoma, PTSD, and bipolar disorder and his inability to perform his work up to the required minimum standard, comparison of current intellectual functioning with the premorbid estimate fails to detect any functional change. In this circumstance, a false negative outcome arguably is worse than a false-positive result. If we conclude there has been no meaningful functional decline, are disability benefits justified, and should we proceed with cognitive rehabilitation? While these decisions obviously do not hinge on a single result in a neuropsychological examination, intellectual test scores are sometimes used as an overall index of level of functioning and may set an expectation for how well a patient should perform in other cognitive domains that are correlated with intelligence, including memory and executive function. If we accept that A.B. has always been intellectually low average, do the mild memory deficits represent a decline or his baseline level of function? There is no universally applicable or infallible guideline when considering whether to use race-inclusive normative or predictive approaches with Black American patients, and clinicians are advised to proceed in full knowledge of the complex interpretative challenges involved.[64]

> Race-based norms and multiple regression approaches that include race as a prediction variable have the potential advantage of decreasing false-positive diagnostic errors. Neither are race-neutral in that they both lead to potentially deleterious consequences for Black Americans, including the possibility of a false negative conclusion, denial of benefits, and failure to treat. In recognition of the advantages and disadvantages of these approaches, we recommend comparing how interpretation of a Black American patient's test scores might change with and without the use of race-inclusive normative approaches, consideration of the potential harms that might result depending upon the choice to use or not to use race-inclusive approaches, and explicit discussion and justification of the clinician's decision in each instance.

Academic vs. Functional Achievement

Black Americans have lower academic achievement compared to white Americans regardless of whether this is measured in years of education and degrees obtained or school performance at a given level of education.[65] Consequently, use of academic achievement will lead to a lower expectation of performance for Black Americans, creating a similar problem to what has already been described for race-inclusive normative approaches. Use of academic achievement to estimate premorbid functioning ignores many racial inequities, including historical and ongoing differences across racial groups in academic advising, quality of education, and college preparation,[66] college and university admissions,[67] and the economic resources made available to pay for education.[68] As already noted, race becomes a convenient, though imprecise proxy for the effect of these many hard-to-measure variables and their impact on premorbid performance.

In developing a fuller picture of the premorbid status of Black patients, it is useful to consider functioning within other settings and institutions that allow patients more opportunity for self-efficacy and self-actualization. This may include vocational or occupational achievements, though Black Americans may face many of the same inequities here as in academic institutions. The patient's standing within the Black family as matriarch, patriarch, or reliable sibling; and accomplishments within church settings as choir singer, musician, lay preacher, deacon, pastoral care volunteer, etc., may all provide a more complete impression of a Black patient's premorbid functioning with less distortion from endemic racial biases and inequities. Even when church participation is limited, Black Americans may belong to fraternities, sororities, and a variety of social clubs and sports leagues that make available opportunities for personal achievement and provide the neuropsychologist with information on premorbid functioning supplemental to achievement in academic institutions.

With respect to A.B., though academic achievement was marginal and limited, his successful military and civilian careers provide a useful counterpoint to what might otherwise be low expectations for his neuropsychological performance.

> In evaluating the usefulness of education as a predictor of performance, neuropsychologists should consider factors that may differentially impact Black Americans' academic achievement. When potential biases and inequities may have affected academic achievement, neuropsychologists should seek additional sources of information on premorbid functioning, including occupational accomplishments, social standing in the Black family, and achievement in church and other community settings.

Functional Resilience and Prognosis

A similar point can be made with regards to setting expectations for improvement for Black patients. Contemporary life is generally regarded as stressful; however, bearing the brunt of institutional racism and racial microaggression adds an extra layer of tension and stress. Black Americans who not only survive but, in fact, manage to thrive under such conditions demonstrate a level of emotional strength and psychological resourcefulness that should not be ignored.

A.B. amply illustrates the importance of paying attention to the functional resilience of Black patients. He has a number of negative prognostic indicators, including early exposure to trauma, multiple concussions, and multiple psychiatric diagnoses. This has all certainly taken a toll, yet he had successful military and civilian careers, maintained a stable marriage, and never developed a postconcussive syndrome despite the potential secondary gain inherent in the awarding of service-connected disability benefits within the US VA system. Resilience in the face of so many challenges might justify greater optimism about prognosis in this case. Once diagnosed and in rehabilitation, A.B. did indeed progress to the point that a return to work became a realistic possibility. If we were to say that A.B. exceeded expectations in his eventual functional outcome we may be guilty of having set unrealistically low expectations, without duly considering all he has survived.

> Demonstrable functional resilience in the face of personal and societal challenges justifies an optimistic prognosis and supports the martialling of resources to treat Black patients even in the context of a complex clinical presentation.

Pathognomonic Performance

Not all neuropsychological tests yield a normally distributed distribution of scores. While intellectual functioning measures yield score distributions that are either normally distributed or are corrected to approximate a normal distribution, we do not expect a test of hemispatial neglect or aphasia, for example, to yield such a score distribution. Some neuropsychological tests are designed to detect the presence of performance that does not occur in healthy, nonneurological populations. We do not see marked directional biases in line bisection or a failure to follow one-step commands in healthy populations irrespective of their racial composition.

The importance of such pathognomonic signs is evident in A.B.'s neuropsychological profile. The right upper quadrant field cut in the left eye only is a clear sign of neurosurgical trauma that lends localizing confidence when considering the pattern of performance on other neuropsychological tests. Our ability to arrive at a parsimonious functional localization is greatly enhanced by this unambiguous clinical sign. While contemporary neuropsychologists may focus more on the sophisticated psychometric instrumentation that distinguishes our field from related medical disciplines, pathognomonic indicators are less likely to be influenced by cultural factors and can serve as important interpretive guides in assessing Black patients.

> Inclusion of tests that yield results that are pathognomonic of neuropsychological disorder is an advantage in assessing Black patients as such tests are less susceptible to the effect of the myriad variables subsumed under the proxy of race.

Cultural Influences on "Hold" and Pathognomonic Test Performance

In contrast to neuropsychological tests that detect pathognomonic patterns are so-called "hold" tests that are relatively resistant to the influence of neurological disease. Reading performance, for example, typically is spared when primary oral and written language areas in the dominant cerebral hemisphere are not damaged.* Reading tests therefore are often used as a means of estimating premorbid ability in areas with little apparent relationship to reading. For example, oral reading performance combined with demographic data is used to predict Performance IQ.[49] This is also not a "race-neutral" approach. To the extent that race is a proxy for culture, it is important to note that Black Americans may pronounce words differently than white Americans, reflecting unique familial and regional variability in word pronunciation. This is especially true when the reading tests include irregular words whose pronunciation cannot be derived from the rules of American English phonology and, hence, must be learned entirely through imitation of others or generalization from words possessing a similar orthography.

A related problem arises on pathognomonic tests. Agnosia, or the inability to recognize familiar stimuli, does not occur in nonneurological populations. Yet detecting agnosia requires stimuli to be familiar. This problem is sometimes overcome by using stimuli from the patient's life (e.g., pictures of close relatives to detect facial agnosia), yet this abandons standardization across individuals. The other option is to use stimuli presumed to be familiar to most people. Faces of recent presidents, for example, may be substituted for family members, or pictures of famous landmarks may replace pictures of locations within a patient's home to standardize detection of face or topographical agnosia. Black Americans may differ, however, from Caucasians in their familiarity with various stimuli. Often the perspective and experience of a white test developer or white patient is centered in the design of such tests.

While much of the white American population over a particular age may recognize Ronald Reagan, the Eiffel Tower, or the music of Neil Diamond, Black Americans of the same age may not, so that inclusion of these stimuli may confuse a lack of premorbid familiarity with a postmorbid agnosia. American society has a growing mixture of subcultures. Being born and reared in America does not guarantee equal assimilation into the white Anglo-Saxon Protestant subculture that has traditionally been considered dominant. Formal measures of acculturation with

---

*This is an oversimplification for purposes of discussion, as reading performance is susceptible to the influence of many nonlinguistic factors, including attention and sensory perception.

an established relationship to neuropsychological test performance are generally not available so that most examiners will be forced to rely on more informal methods of querying to determine premorbid familiarity with categories of test stimuli.

A.B. was intact in his performance across multiple tests of stimulus recognition. If, however, he had failed to recognize presidents or landmarks, it would have been essential to query his degree of prior exposure. The impact of cultural familiarity was most evident, however, in his perceptual test performance. There was a clear difference in his performance on perceptual tests that relied on culture-specific or race-specific stimuli compared to tests that used more abstract stimuli. In addition, we have already noted the low estimate of premorbid intellectual functioning on the WTAR, a test that entirely conflates standard English pronunciation with reading ability (i.e., one may read and correctly interpret a word even if it is not pronounced in standard English). The possibility that this low premorbid estimate arose in part due to nonstandard pronunciation during reading cannot be excluded.

Neuropsychologists must consider the Black patient's familiarity with "standard" English oral and written word pronunciation when attempting to use reading performance as a hold measure for estimating premorbid ability.

In addition, the degree of acculturation, whether measured formally or estimated informally, into the traditionally dominant white Anglo-Saxon Protestant subculture must be considered in the evaluation of Black Americans when neuropsychological tests include stimuli whose exposure may vary across racial or cultural groups. In the absence of formal, validated acculturation measures, testing of limits should include querying Black Americans regarding their familiarity with stimuli (or stimulus categories) included in tests.

The Need for an Expanded Toolkit

Finally, the question should be asked, why include tests with a potential cultural bias or inappropriate norms in the assessment of Black patients? The unfortunate answer is that relying entirely on tests demonstrably uninfluenced by culture or with normative databases that include a representative sample of Black Americans will limit the comprehensiveness of the assessment. It may be just as inequitable to not attempt a full and complete assessment of the Black patient as it is to incorporate problematic test instruments in the overall battery. This highlights the critical need for an expanded test toolkit. Given the growing cultural and ethnic diversity of the US population and the infrastructure available to each of the major US test development companies, the failure to expand our clinical toolkit over the next decade will be a telling indictment of neuropsychology as a clinical profession. Where we are as a diagnostic profession is neither where we should be, nor hopefully where we will be, in the coming years. Expanding out toolkit of culturally appropriate neuropsychological tests should be the top priority for the entire clinical profession.

References

1. Center PR. The growing diversity of Black America. 2021.
2. Progress CfA. Systematic inequality and economic opportunity. 2019.
3. Barnert ES, Perry R, Morris RE. Juvenile incarceration and health. Acad Pediatr. 2016;16(2):99–109.
4. Binswanger IA, Redmond N, Steiner JF, Hicks LS. Health disparities and the criminal justice system: an agenda for further research and action. J Urban Health. 2012;89(1):98–107.

5. Hinton E, Henderson L, Reed C. An unjust burden: The disparate treatment of Black Americans in the criminal justice system [Internet]. 2018. Available from: https://www.vera.org/publications/for-the-record-unjust-burden

6. Laurencin CT, Walker JM. Racial profiling is a public health and health disparities issue. J Racial Ethn Health Disparities. 2020;7(3):393–7.

7. Williams MT, Kanter JW, Ching THW. Anxiety, stress, and trauma symptoms in African Americans: negative affectivity does not explain the relationship between microaggressions and psychopathology. J Racial Ethn Health Disparities. 2018;5(5):919–27.

8. Zeiders KH, Landor AM, Flores M, Brown A. Microaggressions and diurnal cortisol: examining within-person associations among African-American and Latino young adults. J Adolesc Health. 2018;63(4):482–8.

9. Center PR. Key facts about black immigrants in the U.S. 2018.

10. States U, Services DoHaH. Profile: Black/African Americans. 2021.

11. Weir K. Inequality at school. Monit Psychol. 2016;47(10):42.

12. Nicholson-Crotty S, Grissom JA, Nicholson-Crotty J, Redding C. Disentangling the causal mechanisms of representative bureaucracy: evidence from assignment of students to gifted programs. J Public Adm Res Theory. 2016;26(4):745–57.

13. Manly JJ. Deconstructing race and ethnicity: implications for measurement of health outcomes. Med Care. 2006;44(11 Suppl 3):S10–6.

14. Sisco S, Gross AL, Shih RA, Sachs BC, Glymour MM, Bangen KJ, et al. The role of early-life educational quality and literacy in explaining racial disparities in cognition in late life. J Gerontol B Psychol Sci Soc Sci. 2015;70(4):557–67.

15. Semega J, Kollar, M., Shrider EA, Creamer JF. Income and poverty in the United States: 2019 (P60–270). U.S. Census Bureau, Current Population Reports. pp. P60–270.

16. Perry AM, Rothwell J, Harshbarger D. The devaluation of assets in Black neighborhoods: the case of residential property [Internet]. Brookings Institution; 2018. Available from: https://www.brookings.edu/research/devaluation-of-assets-in-black-neighborhoods/

17. Census US, Bureau. 2011–2015 ACS 5-year estimates. 2019.

18. Fiscella K, Williams DR. Health disparities based on socioeconomic inequities: implications for urban health care. Acad Med. 2004;79(12):1139–47.

19. Stormacq C, Van den Broucke S, Wosinski J. Does health literacy mediate the relationship between socioeconomic status and health disparities? Integrative review. Health Promot Int. 2019;34(5):e1–17.

20. Farah MJ. Socioeconomic status and the brain: prospects for neuroscience-informed policy. Nat Rev Neurosci. 2018;19(7):428–38.

21. Giger JN, Appel SJ, Davidhizar R, Davis C. Church and spirituality in the lives of the African American community. J Transcult Nurs. 2008;19(4):375–83.

22. Lincoln CE, Mamiya LH, editors. The religious dimension: toward a sociology of black churches. In: The Black Church in the African American experience [Internet]. New York (NY): Duke University Press; 1990. p. 1–19. Available from: https://doi.org/10.1515/9780822381648-003

23. Center PR. Black Americans are more likely than overall public to be Christian, Protestant. 2018.

24. Nguyen AW. Religion and mental health in racial and ethnic minority populations: a review of the literature. Innov Aging. 2020;4(5):igaa035.

25. Chatters LM, Taylor RJ, Lincoln KD, Schroepfer T. Patterns of informal support from family and church members among African Americans. J Black Stud. 2002;33(1):66–85.

26. Young JL, Griffith EE, Williams DR. The integral role of pastoral counseling by African-American clergy in community mental health. Psychiatr Serv. 2003;54(5):688–92.

27. Chatters LM, Nguyen AW, Taylor RJ, Hope MO. Church and family support networks and depressive symptoms among African Americans: findings from the National Survey of American Life. J Community Psychol. 2018;46(4):403–17.

28. Himle JA, Taylor RJ, Chatters LM. Religious involvement and obsessive compulsive disorder among African Americans and Black Caribbeans. J Anxiety Disord. 2012;26(4):502–10.

29. Taylor RJ, Chatters LM, Joe S. Religious involvement and suicidal behavior among African Americans and Black Caribbeans. J Nerv Ment Dis. 2011;199(7):478–86.
30. Robinson JA, Bolton JM, Rasic D, Sareen J. Exploring the relationship between religious service attendance, mental disorders, and suicidality among different ethnic groups: results from a nationally representative survey. Depress Anxiety. 2012;29(11):983–90.
31. Cunningham TJ, Croft JB, Liu Y, Lu H, Eke PI, Giles WH. Vital signs: racial disparities in age-specific mortality among Blacks or African Americans—United States, 1999–2015. MMWR Morb Mortal Wkly Rep. 2017;66(17):444–56.
32. Disease Cf, Prevention Ca. Summary health statistics: National Health Interview Survey: 2017. 2019.
33. Zelner J, Trangucci R, Naraharisetti R, Cao A, Malosh R, Broen K, et al. Racial disparities in coronavirus disease 2019 (COVID-19) mortality are driven by unequal infection risks. Clin Infect Dis. 2021;72(5):e88–95.
34. Aleligne YK, Appiah D, Ebong IA. Racial disparities in coronavirus disease 2019 (COVID-19) outcomes. Curr Opin Cardiol. 2021;36(3):360–6.
35. Brody DJ, Pratt LA, Hughes JP. Prevalence of depression among adults aged 20 and over: United States, 2013–2016. NCHS Data Brief. 2018;303:1–8.
36. Bailey RK, Blackmon HL, Stevens FL. Major depressive disorder in the African American population: meeting the challenges of stigma, misdiagnosis, and treatment disparities. J Natl Med Assoc. 2009;101(11):1084–9.
37. Bailey RK, Patel M, Barker NC, Ali S, Jabeen S. Major depressive disorder in the African American population. J Natl Med Assoc. 2011;103(7):548–57.
38. Williams DR, González HM, Neighbors H, Nesse R, Abelson JM, Sweetman J, et al. Prevalence and distribution of major depressive disorder in African Americans, Caribbean blacks, and non-Hispanic whites: results from the National Survey of American Life. Arch Gen Psychiatry. 2007;64(3):305–15.
39. Services SAaMH, Administration. National survey on drug use and health (NSDUH): African Americans. 2018.
40. Services SAaMH, Administration. Racial/ethnic differences in mental health service use among adults. HHS Publication No. SMA-15-4906. S. A. M. H. S. A. 2015.
41. Psychiatric A, Association. Mental health disparities: African Americans. 2017.
42. Strakowski SM, Keck PE, Arnold LM, Collins J, Wilson RM, Fleck DE, et al. Ethnicity and diagnosis in patients with affective disorders. J Clin Psychiatry. 2003;64(7):747–54.
43. Ward EC, Wiltshire JC, Detry MA, Brown RL. African American men and women's attitude toward mental illness, perceptions of stigma, and preferred coping behaviors. Nurs Res. 2013;62(3):185–94.
44. Alang SM. Mental health care among blacks in America: confronting racism and constructing solutions. Health Serv Res. 2019;54(2):346–55.
45. Maura J, Weisman de Mamani A. Mental health disparities, treatment engagement, and attrition among racial/ethnic minorities with severe mental illness: a review. J Clin Psychol Med Settings. 2017;24(3–4):187–210.
46. Norman MA, Moore DJ, Taylor M, Franklin D, Cysique L, Ake C, et al. Demographically corrected norms for African Americans and Caucasians on the Hopkins Verbal Learning Test-Revised, Brief Visuospatial Memory Test-Revised, Stroop Color and Word Test, and Wisconsin Card Sorting Test 64-Card Version. J Clin Exp Neuropsychol. 2011;33(7):793–804.
47. Heaton RK, Miller SW, Taylor MJ, Grant I. Revised comprehensive norms for an expanded Halstead Reitan battery: demographically adjusted neuropsychological norms for African American and Caucasian adults. Lutz (FL): Psychological Assessment Resources; 2004.
48. Lucas JA, Ivnik RJ, Smith GE, Ferman TJ, Willis FB, Petersen RC, et al. Mayo's Older African Americans Normative Studies: norms for Boston Naming Test, Controlled Oral Word Association, Category Fluency, Animal Naming, Token Test, WRAT-3 Reading, Trail Making Test, Stroop Test, and Judgment of Line Orientation. Clin Neuropsychol. 2005;19(2):243–69.
49. Psychological T, Corporation. Test of premorbid functioning: advanced clinical solutions for use with the WAIS-IV and WMS-IV. San Antonio, Texas. 2009.

50. Possin KL, Tsoy E, Windon CC. Perils of race-based norms in cognitive testing: the case of former NFL players. JAMA Neurol. 2021;78(4):377–8.

51. Manly JJ, Jacobs DM, Touradji P, Small SA, Stern Y. Reading level attenuates differences in neuropsychological test performance between African American and White elders. J Int Neuropsychol Soc. 2002;8(3):341–8.

52. Byrd DA, Rivera Mindt MM, Clark US, Clarke Y, Thames AD, Gammada EZ, et al. Creating an anti-racist psychology by addressing professional complicity in psychological assessment. Psychol Assess. 2021;33(3):279–85.

53. Slick DJ, Hopp G, Strauss E, Thompson GB. Victoria Symptom Validity Test: Professional manual. Psychological Assessment Resources; 1997.

54. Warrington EK, James M. The visual object and space perception battery. Bury St. Edmunds: Thames Valley Test Company; 1991.

55. Benton AL, Sivan AB, deS. Hansher K, Varney NR, Spreen O. Contributions to neuropsychological assessment a clinical manual. 2nd ed. New York (NY): Oxford University Press; 1994.

56. Tombaugh TN, Faulkner P, Schmidt JP. A new procedure for administering the Taylor complex figure: normative data over a 60-year age span. Clin Neuropsychol. 1992;6(1):63–79.

57. Delis CD, Kramer JH, Kaplan E, Ober BA. California verbal learning test-third edition. San Antonio (TX): Pearson; 2017.

58. Wechsler D. The Wechsler memory scale-fourth edition (WMS-IV). San Antonio (TX): Pearson Assessments; 2009.

59. Stringer AY. A guide to adult neuropsychological diagnosis. Philadelphia (PA): F. A. Davis; 1996.

60. Wetzel L, Boll TJ. Manual for the short category test. Los Angeles (CA): Western Psychological Services; 1987.

61. Wechsler D. Wechsler abbreviated scale of intelligence (2nd Edition) (WASI-II). San Antonio (TX): NCS Pearson; 2011.

62. Wechsler D. Test of adult reading: WTAR. San Antonio (TX): Pearson; 2001.

63. Ben-Porath Y, Tellegen A. The Minnesota multiphasic personality inventory restructured format. San Antonio (TX): Pearson; 2008.

64. Manly JJ. Advantages and disadvantages of separate norms for African Americans. Clin Neuropsychol. 2005;19(2):270–5.

65. Aud S, Hussar W, Planty M, Snyder T, Bianco K, Fox M, et al. The Condition of Education 2010 (NCES 2010-028). Washington (DC): National Center for Education Statistics, Institute of Education Sciences; 2010.

66. States U, Department of Education OoCR. Civil rights data collection data snapshot: college and career readiness [Internet]. 2014. Available from: http://ocrdata.ed.gov/Downloads/CRDC-College-and-Career-Readiness-Snapshot.pdf

67. Musu-Gillette L, Robinson J, McFarland J, KewalRamani A, Zhang A, Wilkinson-Flicker S. Status and trends in the education of racial and ethnic groups 2016 (NCES 2016-007) [Internet]. Washington (DC): U.S. Department of Education, National Center for Education Statistics; 2016. Available from: http://nces.ed.gov/pubsearch

68. Libassi CJ. The neglected college race gap: racial disparities among college completers [Internet]. 2018. Available from: https://www.americanprogress.org/issues/education-postsecondary/reports/2018/05/23/451186.

Coast Salish Native American

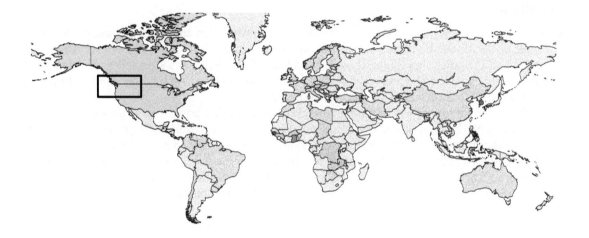

7 Neuropsychology in Coast Salish Native American Contexts

Tedd Judd and Eagle Bear

Introduction

JUDD: When I received the invitation from Dr. Irani to write this chapter I thought of the principle of "Nothing about me without me" and so I realized that I wanted a Native American coauthor. I recalled that Eagle Runs Around Bear (Eagle Bear)[1] is a storyteller who wants the story of his people to be preserved for his people and to be known by others and so I invited him to be my coauthor. Fortunately, he accepted.

Part of my biography is in the Guatemala chapter of this book. I have grown up with an interest in Native Americans, in a house with Navajo rugs, Kachina dolls, photographs, many books about Native Americans, and with summer family visits to reservations mostly in the US Southwest. The Pacific Northwest has been my home for the past 40 years, and I have gotten to know many of the local tribes through visits, powwows, festivals, music, friendships, and clinical work, including a contract with the clinic of the remote Makah Tribe, with biannual visits.

EAGLE BEAR: My great, great grandfather was the man you call Chief Seattle. He was Duwamish. I grew up Lummi, but my family was banished from the reservation because my mother struck and killed a child with her car on the reservation in 1945. I have land on the reservation but still we have to live in Marietta (a run-down village that often floods across the Nooksack River from the reservation). When I was a boy and bears still came to Portage Island (a wooded island that is part of the reservation and can be reached on foot at low tide) there was a bear and I ran all of the way around it, and so they gave me the name of Runs Around Bear. I spent a lot of my time from age 6 to 10 at my elders drumming, singing, dancing, listening, and remembering.

When I was growing up there was a lot of alcohol and not a lot of love. I suffered from that and couldn't understand it. My guiding spirit voice first came to me when I was 4 years old and has helped me through since that time. I had a vision. I flew to my parents and the door flew open and they were surprised and I told them I wanted them to stop drinking. When I first did my ceremony at age 20 I stayed awake for 3½ days. When I started to fall asleep I flew. I flew out of my body in my 4th month of ceremony and flew over Lummi. I have had visions forever.

Prelude: Eagle Bear: Oral Improvised Poem-Song

Just hoping the memory of our people when we are a family and community,
When we have love and understanding and how we hear and remember
With the Indian our grandmother moon
Reminds us it's good to stay in tune

DOI: 10.4324/9781003051862-15

With the Creator of all things and the message each creation brings.
With the Indian this is our way of life
And not just a tomahawk bow and knife
With training in everything we use
So we won't be careless and abuse
With the Indian this way of life became hard
Because by a new way we were scarred
With many left to wonder
Why such a good way went asunder
With the Indian we only have one choice
That is to continue listening to ancestor's voice
No matter how hopeless things be around us
Our Creator will always surround us
With the Indian we'll forever continue on
In the old ways that help keep us strong
For we have a spirit within our heart
That will help us to do our part
With the Indian we all must stand together
In the ways that help us remember
We are Mother Earth and we should always share in her birth
And her birth is to give us life
Give us some peace and calm and hope and faith
And some trust definitely some trust
Honesty truth respect and above all
To honor all those that have went before us
Honor who we are withing the eyes of Creation
The strong gotta be strong
Me, I'm out there every day that's what I was made for
To be part of that voice
So others can make a choice to rejoice.

Section I: Background Information

Terminology

The Indigenous peoples of North America are extremely diverse linguistically and culturally. Many of these Indigenous peoples identify primarily with their own group, tribe, language, or reservation more than with a common Indigenous identity. In formal settings, especially intertribal encounters, speakers usually introduce themselves with their tribes and clans and often with their lineage, sometimes going back several generations. When viewed collectively, Indigenous peoples are most commonly called Native Americans and Native Alaskans in the United States and First Nations in Canada. "Indian" is often used (sometimes NDN in social media) and occasionally objected to as pejorative. There are also many insulting and pejorative terms and images, some of which, at this writing, are still used as names of sports teams, in spite of vociferous objections by Native peoples.[2]

This chapter will focus on Native Americans in the United States, and particularly the Coast Salish people of the Pacific Northwest around the Salish Sea (Puget Sound, Straights of Georgia, Straights of San Juan de Fuca). And this will be especially the Lummi, Eagle Bear's people.

While Native Americans usually identify most strongly with their tribe, mixed heritage is common. For example, the Métis are a French-First Nations cultural group of about a half million people in central Canada and the northern United States who speak a French-Cree creole. Tribal mixtures are also common, and it is common to encounter someone who will say, "I'm X tribe," but later they may elaborate, "Actually, my mother is Y tribe" or "but I was raised or spent summers on the Z reservation."

It is usually best for clinicians to ask about heritage and identity, listen patiently and make note of such lineages, and feel honored when Native clients are willing to share their full identity.

Geography

European and other peoples in North America have displaced many Native American tribes from their accustomed territories, sometimes multiple times. They have typically been given reservations that are a small fraction of the size of their original territory and often far from their original territory. Clinicians are advised to learn the histories of the particular groups and tribes they work with. There is a Native American flavor of humor that can be gently teasing, yet pointed, and it is reflected in this chapter, including in the following: "They took away our land and gave us new land that they said we could have as long as the water flows and the grass grows. But they broke that promise and gave us new land that they said we could have as long as the water flows and the grass grows. But they broke that promise, too, and gave us land where no water flows and no grass grows."

> When an Indian laughs, it's because they are applying a fresh layer of medicine on an open wound.[3]

Most Coast Salish people have not been fully displaced but have been consolidated onto remnants of their original territories through mid-nineteenth-century treaties with the US government. Sometimes this means that tribes that were distinctive, perhaps hostile to one another, and may even have spoken different dialects or languages were placed together on the same reservation. Historically the Lummi territory spanned the US-Canada border. The Lummi reservation[4] is in the United States, but the tribe has special treaty rights with respect to border crossing. The reservation was illegally reduced in size several generations ago, but Lummi treaty fishing rights in those waters persisted, and those rights allowed the Lummi to block the construction of what was proposed to be the world's largest coal port for shipping Montana coal to Asia. Conflicts over fishing rights and other treaty rights have perpetuated tensions between Coast Salish people and others in the area, including some conflicts between tribes.

History

Most Native American tribes have oral histories that reach back from events that may correspond to written histories or anthropological records through to mythologies, as is the case for most societies (e.g., the Iliad, the Bhagavad Gita, the Holy Bible, the Popol Vuh). Some aspects of oral histories are public, and others may be more closely guarded and unknown to outsiders. For those who are strongly identified with their tribes, these oral histories may strongly shape their worldview and their engagement with others including outsiders, health care, and neuropsychologists (just as the texts cited above strongly shape their corresponding societies). Nontribal neuropsychologists need not—indeed, often cannot—know these histories intimately, but some familiarity with the oral history of the specific tribe is helpful for serving that tribe.

EAGLE BEAR: The written history is "his story," not our story.

The distinctive prehistories and written histories of the many tribes are beyond the scope of this chapter, but neuropsychologists serving a local reservation, tribe, or community are encouraged to study the history of that tribe. Most tribes were decimated by infectious epidemics and wars following the arrival of Europeans.[5] Tribes have typically had strong spiritual, cultural, and technological ties to their territories, and displacement was highly disruptive to that. Most US tribes have Reservations and First Nations in Canada have Reserves. Tribal treaties are formally just below the US Constitution in authority, but this typically has not been the case in practice. Gross treaty violations by the federal and local governments and nontribal populations have been experienced by almost every tribe. Most treaties grant land rights, often hunting and fishing rights, health care and education rights, and exemption from many state and local laws. Treaties often grant local governance for various legal functions, social services, etc., but tribal government structures are often outwardly imposed. The federal government at times used a "quantum blood" standard to determine who qualified as Native and as members of a specific tribe. Most tribes now determine their own membership. Approaches vary widely from tribe to tribe and are often contentious, especially regarding access to services and communal property. Neuropsychologists are encouraged to visit the websites of the local tribes they serve and to visit the reservations themselves, including the tribal governments, clinics, schools, social services, museums, casinos, and those cultural events that are open to the public in order to familiarize themselves with the tribe.

EAGLE BEAR: We don't just have teepees. [Coast Salish people did not traditionally use teepees at all.]
JUDD: On one such visit, my son and I were at the Lummi Stommish canoe races wearing distinctive red voter registration t-shirts. My son asked the powwow Master of Ceremonies to announce the voter registration. He obligingly announced, "If anyone isn't registered to vote, go see the white boy in the red t-shirt ... or was that the red boy in the white t-shirt?"

Some tribes do not have treaties or federal recognition. Some such groups persist in maintaining their identities and structures, and many have undergone decades-long onerous legal struggles to gain federal recognition.

EAGLE BEAR: Intermarriages kept the peace. My great, great grandfather was the man you call Chief Seattle. He was Duwamish. He gave your city its name. But my people on that side, the Duwamish people, don't have tribal recognition. You recognize us when you use our names and our land and city but you don't recognize that we are still here. We've all been denied the truth through religion, education, famine, war, greed, hate, drugs, and alcohol. Our history, our identity, our intimacy comes from being intimate with the creation. That means knowing when to berry pick, where to dig clams, where and when to fish, and so on. Peoples' character is expressed in their totems and what stories songs and medicine you have.

Men are born ignorant, not stupid. They are made stupid by education.

(Bertrand Russell)

During the 19th and much of the 20th century the governments of the United States and Canada maintained policies of cultural assimilation, often enforced through residential schools that were harshly punitive of native language use and cultural practices, quasi-military in structure, and often deadly.[6] Intergenerational residential school trauma is still a major theme of Native mental health.

EAGLE BEAR: I still cry over it; my heart is still broke over it. For me it's all children; all have been denied.

Coast Salish people lived mostly in villages by the sea and rivers for more than a millennium and were able to be partly sedentary hunter-gathers because of the richness of the region. They traditionally used canoes for fishing, sealing, and whaling and also hunted on land. Rich runs of salmon were a staple. Intertribal warfare was not unusual. White people and later others arrived throughout the 19th century, preceded by smallpox and other epidemics. There were skirmishes with the whites but no major wars. Most Coast Salish tribes now have reservations centered around their original villages. Old rivalries have been reduced but live on in tribal school sports leagues and occasional fishing rights lawsuits and struggles over tribal clinic resources and administration. Collaboration has evolved, however, through cultural revivals such as the powwow circuit, canoe races, and the annual canoe journey,[7] in which each summer each coastal tribe sends one or more canoe "families" as much as 400 miles on the open and inland sea to a single reservation that hosts the week-long gathering of over 100 canoes that may carry up to 20 paddlers.

Languages

There were hundreds of Native North American languages and dialects, with great linguistic diversity. A handful of languages are healthy and maintained, while many are extinct, at risk, or endangered.[8,9] Other than elderly Navajo (Diné), it is rare to find Native North Americans who are monolingual in their tribal language. There were about 14 Coast Salish languages, and most of these are now extremely endangered or extinct. There are attempts to maintain and revive them, as is also the case for many other Native languages. The Salish Sea area is one of the world's hotbeds of endangered languages.

JUDD: I had occasion to evaluate an elderly instructor in one of the local endangered languages after they had a mild stroke with mild aphasia. Needless to say, there were no standardized aphasia tests in that language available. Instead, the process involved aphasia evaluation in English and then informal evaluation assisted by the client's adult child (also an instructor) in the native language. Focus was on the instructional materials that they used in the preschool and the tribal college. We settled on a strategy of home rehabilitation through repeated story telling using the instructional materials. The child also worked to record and document further language knowledge. The intervention also involved negotiations with school administration to allow the instructor to resume teaching with a reduced load and accommodations, especially for energy budgeting. I felt a tremendous responsibility in trying to help preserve and recover not just a person's language, but a people's language.

Communication

I don't tell my shit to white people.

(Tessa's Dance)[10]

Communication styles may vary across tribes and depending upon acculturation. Many Native Americans are skilled at code switching from tribal to mainstream communication styles. Even where tribal languages are extinct, there are residual dialectical differences within English that reflect those languages and some dialectical differences that cross many tribes. Authors such as Louise Erdrich, Sherman Alexie, and the Missouri Cherokee descendant novelist, musician, and neuropsychologist, David Walker (http://www.davidedwardwalker.com/index.html), have captured much of these dialectical differences in their writing.

EAGLE BEAR: Show respect for elders by listening, hearing, and understanding what they said before answering. Consider deeply the things they have said.

Most pertinent to neuropsychology, Native Americans are often very comfortable with silence. They may have few words and may speak slowly until they are ready. They may have a circular and repetitive narrative style, often deepening the meaning and detail and disclosure with each repetition as trust is built and understanding is established. Elders are especially to be respected and not hurried. At least among the Coast Salish, they are invariably honored and given full respect, first in the processions, and the best seating at tribal events. This participation may prevail well into mid-stages of dementia, strokes, and similar disability.

JUDD: My wife (Roberta DeBoard, PhD) worked as a school psychologist at the Lummi Tribal School. The children were often boisterous, to say the least. But when an elder would come for a cultural lesson they all quieted down and were very attentive. Elders are regularly bused from the tribal assisted living/nursing home, Little Bear, to the place of honor in the front row of school assemblies.

JUDD: I attended the opening ceremony for an international UNESCO conference in Seattle. The organizer was officiously rushing around with a clipboard, trying to keep everything on schedule. The first speaker was a Coast Salish elder, scheduled for 5 minutes, to welcome the conference, recognizing that it was being held on historically native territory. She talked, and talked … and talked. She absolutely ignored all signals to cut it short and attempts to intervene until she was done with her say. And that was just the way it was going to be.

Education

Cultural education in many tribes such as the Lummi occurs primarily through extended families, especially through sharing and living together. Mother and daughter time together is very important to communicate and learn to work. Cultural education also occurs through other tribal organizations and institutions. Smokehouse is a secret society in many Coast Salish tribes that is heavily engaged with adolescent coming-of-age training, initiation, spirit quest, and community commitment. Tribal fishing industries and boats also build communities and culture. There are also organizations and cottage industries that maintain crafts, music, dance, costume, healing practices, ceremonies, and celebrations. There are also many Indian Shaker Churches on Coast Salish reservations, a blend of Salish, Catholic, and Protestant beliefs and practices that include healing ceremonies that may induce shaking (unrelated to the US East Coast Shaker churches).[11]

EAGLE BEAR: I spent a lot of my time from age 6 to 10 at my elders drumming, singing, dancing, listening, and remembering.

Tribes and reservations that are large enough may have their own schools, especially elementary schools, that may be under tribal or school district administration. There is typically a priority for having tribal staff, when possible. Curriculum often includes cultural materials and sometimes language. Tribal schools are often underfunded. Sports are often popular and an important focus. The Lummi high school has a dormitory for teens who want to finish high school but are having difficulties with their home life. It is not unusual for Native students to encounter discrimination, cultural incomprehension, and bullying in mainstream schools off the reservation.[12] A common pejorative that students use against Native children in the schools around the Lummi reservation is "dummy Lummi."

There are 37 tribal colleges and universities in the United States, serving 27,000 students from 250 tribal nations.[13] The Northwest Indian College (https://www.nwic.edu/) has its main campus on the Lummi Reservation, with six satellite campuses on Coast Salish and inland (Nez Perce) reservations. It offers Bachelors of Arts degrees in Native Studies Leadership, Tribal Governance and Business Management, Native Environmental Science, and Community Advocates and Responsive Education in Human Service.

Literacy

Literacy in tribal languages is generally low with the exception of a few of the larger tribes. Many languages have writing systems, many of them using variants of the Latin alphabet. There may be signage and limited literature, but tribal languages are more often practiced orally. As a population, Native Americans generally lag behind the general population in their level of English literacy skills.

Values and Customs

Values and customs vary widely by tribe. The Northwest Indian College provides a succinct statement of values common in the US Northwest tribes, presented in the Lummi language:

- *Səla-lexʷ:* Our strength comes from the old people. From them we receive our teachings and knowledge and the advice we need for our daily lives.
- *Schtəngəxʷən:* We are responsible to protect our territory. This means we take care of our land and water and everything that is on it and in it.
- *Xwləmi-chosən:* Our culture is our language. We should strengthen and maintain our language.
- *Leng-e-sot:* We take care of ourselves, watch out for ourselves and love and take care of one another.
- *Xaalh:* Life balance/sacred

Health

Although there is much variation in culture and experience, Native Americans currently share, for the most part, a number of cultural experiences and history due primarily to the impact of the colonization of the Americas by Europeans. Among characteristics that are most neuropsychologically relevant are[14]:

1 Poverty or, at least, lower income than the general population.
2 Distinctive, internationally recognized human rights as Indigenous peoples that are poorly enforced.[15]
3 Worse overall health than the general population and lower access and quality of health care services.[16]
4 Worse brain health than the general population.
5 Chronic turbulent relationships with centralized societal systems such as governmental health care, education, social welfare, and justice systems.

6 Distinctive views of disability, health, healing, and familial/social relationships; these affect how they are individually and collectively impacted by brain illnesses and disabilities as well as how they interface with professional neuropsychology in both clinical application and research. There has been very little neuropsychological research or understanding of this distinctiveness.

7 Relatively few neuropsychological services available and little professional knowledge of how to apply neuropsychology to these populations.[17]

8 Indigenous epidemiology that is often distinctive due to genetics, distinctive exposures to pathogens and toxins, diet, racism, etc.[18-21]

9 Distinctive pharmacogenetics.[22]

10 Culturally distinctive perception of and coping with neuropsychological disabilities.

11 Designated communal tribal lands and separate tribal government, legal systems and courts, health care systems, vocational rehabilitation, industries, and education systems.

In the United States, the Indian Health Service (IHS), usually a treaty right, has a mixed history in the appropriateness, cultural sensitivity, and acceptance of its services. Discrimination from health care services (IHS and others) is still a common and influential experience.[23]

Mental Health View

Most tribes readily acknowledge the public health data that indicates tragically high levels of depression, anxiety, PTSD, suicide, domestic violence, substance abuse, traumatic brain injury (TBI), cerebrovascular disease, learning disorders, and other conditions in most Native populations. At the same time, each of these conditions may be viewed differently from a Native worldview. In general, they are likely to be seen primarily in their social context and with multiple social causes, rather than from the individualistic, personal-failings perspective that is more prevalent in the general US population and in much of the framing of professional psychology. Local Native worldviews may even radically depart from outside conceptualizations. For example, some tribal members say that their tribes do not have any dementia. They acknowledge that elders may lose various skills and abilities, but they continue to be regarded as valued, honored, and integrated members of their communities rather than as marginalized people who are ill.

Assessment Needs

Administratively, Native American neuropsychology assessment needs are not much different from other US resident assessment needs in that they are interfacing with many of the same or similar institutions: Health care, education, injured workers, child welfare, criminal justice, civil proceedings, competencies, vocational rehabilitation, etc. However, many of these functions may be answering to tribal agencies that may have distinctive rules and ways of operating. Neuropsychologists would be well advised to determine if they will be answering to tribal agencies and to familiarize themselves with these institutions and their procedures before engaging in this work.

Neuropsychological research on Native Americans is sparse and not well-differentiated by tribe, region, or language.[17] Available research often calls into question the applicability of conventional English neuropsychological tests and norms to Native American populations, with Native Americans typically showing stronger performances on visual-perceptual tasks (sometimes stronger than white comparison groups) and weaker performances on English verbal tasks.[17]

Neuropsychology does not have a high profile in many Native American communities and institutions. Tribal institutions and individuals are quite accustomed to being misunderstood and mistreated in many ways by outsiders. While superficial friendliness and generosity toward outsiders are common and welcome attitudes, it takes time, patience, listening, goodwill, and sensitivity to build trusting and effective working relationships. A holistic, pragmatic, and culturally sensitive vision of what neuropsychology can offer will typically serve better than an individualistic, high-tech, cognitivist, universalist approach.

Migration

International migration is uncommon for Native Americans except for those tribes that have historically straddled the Canadian, Mexican, and Russian borders. Intertribal and inter-reservation travel and marriage is common, and it is common to live in the rural areas surrounding reservations. Urban migration is also common. It is common that urban migrants will retain ties to their tribe and reservation.

Acculturation

As noted above, Native Americans have a wide range of cultural identities. Since most are now native English speakers and often have access to mainstream institutions and education, many may be highly acculturated to mainstream culture. Many learn to "pass" and hide their indigenousness when convenient. Many will code switch from one identity to another. It is likely that such individuals will present themselves in their acculturated identity to the non-Native neuropsychologist, but this may not tell the whole story.

JUDD: I saw a Native couple for therapy for coping with the TBI of one partner. While they had both grown up on the reservation, they had received their education off of the rez, lived off rez for many years, and both had masters degrees and highly responsible non-tribal employment. I proceeded as if with a white couple, but soon came to realize that their expectations for their marital relationship and for their relationships with their extended family and tribe were profoundly Native. This also applied to their understanding of their own emotional needs and the intergenerational causes of those needs. I had to adjust my explanations and operate from a position of mutual problem solving rather than clinical authority.

Section II: Case Study — "Making it Through the Spiraling Fire Tunnel"

Identification and Referral

At the time of the evaluation in May 2000, Robert Lawrence was a 46-year-old, Lummi, single, 10th grade and GED-educated, unemployed, multiskilled laborer who was referred by his primary care provider of the Lummi Tribal Health Center for a neuropsychological assessment of a TBI with particular reference to eligibility for disability. No medical records were made available.

Interview

History of the Present Illness

Mr. Lawrence said that on January 24, 1979, he was assaulted by six guys with hammers and knives while in Walla Walla State Penitentiary. He described this as a manipulation by the prison administration, who turned some of the "lifers" into vigilantes. His spirit helper had told him three times not to go into lifer's park. It told him, "F*** those crazy people and f*** this place. Why don't you go in the hole and think about going home?" But he told the spirit he wasn't afraid of anything. The lifers attacked him and his spirit told him not to fight back. He got struck by a hammer in the right parietal area. He saw himself going through a spiraling fire tunnel. He kept asking his spirit how to reach their spirits. He was hit in the head with the claw part of the hammer and his hands were hit many times. "I stayed conscious and aware of me getting beat. When hit with the hammer it caved my head in. When this happened, my spirit was lifted into a giant fire that was moving like a tornado, but slower. I twirled around two times and came back to my body and I immediately began a prayer. I said, 'I'm praying to you, Great Spirit, please don't hurt me anymore.'" They thought he was dead and felt that he was not breathing and had no pulse, but he was still conscious and listening to them. He now sees this as having been dead and coming back. As they left he saw a white cloud leave with them. Then he felt Jesus' spirit come and heal him.

He was taken to the nearby hospital. He remembers seeing his parents praying for him in the Emergency Room. He saw energy waves from his gut going between him and his mother. He woke up from anesthesia before they operated to tell the doctor to save his hair. He had had a skull fracture in the right parietal area, and he had the skull fragments removed and the wound debrided. Later he had an acrylic plate placed. He also had surgery on his right hand.

Background

"God has been pretty gracious to me so that I have not had to suffer much, I've never had to ask for help. This was given to me in a vision in 1974. I was on a self-destruct suicide mission, feeling that I had been abused and my father never said he loved me. But in 1974 I started having visions and they came true within 2 days. I didn't understand the gifts we people had in dreams and visions to guide us. I was never taught how to love myself or to plan for my future. We got dehumanized by boarding schools to get civilized. These are the stories we hear about only in family circles growing up. My father beat me, the schoolteachers beat me when I was growing up. I couldn't tell my father. I ran away from home. I heard that the police were looking for me so I turned myself in, but they just took me back home. In prison nobody cared for me, either. I didn't get help. They didn't have child abuse programs then. The spirit people told me my heart was full of punctured holes but we're going to try to help you. From when I was little I remember being on the floor with the beer bottles all around. I remember feeling 'How come my parents aren't talking to me, just drinking?' They talk about not being able to pray in school, but why don't they teach them about self-talk and feelings and how to be a good parent? It's all in my autobiography, I'm writing a book. I get paid $300/hour to do lectures and workshops about these things. To me the most important things are the internal things."

Spontaneous Complaints

Mr. Lawrence reported that he had sharp, shock, stabbing, or throbbing pain in his head where the plate is or where the black spot is. Sometimes it was in the back of his head, his spine, or behind his eyes. Sometimes it also went to his ears, especially the right, and felt sensitive, or as if his glands were swollen. The pain was especially intense when he was emotional. He also felt that the left side of his body was tightening up.

His girlfriend said he had troubles at night sometimes with sharp movements and quivers. Sometimes she had to wake him because he was having spasms.

He said that his memory had gotten worse. If he did not write things down he would forget them. He was feeling more tired lately. He had had a job from time to time, but his prison record made it hard for him to get jobs.

He had to make an extra effort to remember that he had a left side and to use it. He felt that its coordination was not good. His girlfriend told him that she thought he needed a tranquilizer because of his expectations for other people. He felt that she didn't really understand him or care to, and so he was upset at that suggestion. He was on epilepsy pills after the injury, but he quit them because they were making him worse. He took them for a couple of months but got feelings of things shooting down his left side. When he quit them those feelings went away, but he still got them periodically.

Coping

When the pain got bad he would put his hand on his head to remind him of the spirit, and he would pray. He carried a notebook to help his memory.

Previous Medical History

Dislocation surgeries on each shoulder, 1970, 1971. Knife wound exploratory surgery in the stomach, 1973. Multiple TBIs from fights, the last in 1995.

History of Traumatic Experiences

Mr. Lawrence said that his father used to beat him up and abuse him mentally. He felt emotionally abused in school by teachers, especially with racism. He remembered being called a dumb Indian, and so on. He felt trapped in prison and had dreams that he was going to be assaulted again and dreams of being shot and feeling the bullet go into his brain and going back into the fire tunnel. The dreams had been less frequent since leaving prison. When he had those feelings along with pain he felt that he was close to having a heart attack again. He could feel anxious at that time and feel that he was slipping away, and he would say his prayers. He thought this would happen especially when he would get emotional. This could happen almost every day, or less frequently.

Alcohol and Drug Use

Mr. Lawrence reported that alcohol has been a problem all of his life. He was sober when he was in prison. He got back into it when he got out and used his relationship as an excuse to drink. He had alcohol treatment at Thunderbird House (Native American residential substance abuse treatment center) in Seattle, graduating 10 months prior to the evaluation with ongoing care at Lummi Care. He was particularly mindful that he should not drink because of his injury. He had used cannabis and a little bit of everything else. He felt that there was still something missing from treatment, or perhaps he should have stayed in Thunderbird House longer.

Psychosocial Situation

Mr. Lawrence lived with his mother and brother. He broke up with his girlfriend the previous month. He already sang a mourning song for that and so felt resolved about it. They had been together six years.

Family History

Mr. Lawrence's mother had 13 children altogether, and he was number 5. Five of those 13 died young.

Pertinent Results of Review of Neuropsychological Systems

Mr. Lawrence sometimes has difficulty staying focused. He had had difficulty getting going on a beading project recently. He felt that he is perhaps impulsive. He said he could plan well for writing and was learning more about planning for other things.

At age four at his uncle's funeral, he was impressed by the speakers and wanted to learn to speak publicly himself. He had hoped that his father would guide him in this but he did not. He learned to be a writer out of his desire to be a public speaker. In 1980, he had a vision of his grandmother guiding him toward expressing his experiences. A wind of spirits took her two days later. He used to type but can no longer do so with his left hand. He used to use a computer to write, but no longer had a computer. The teacher in prison would not work with him on computers.

He felt that his visual-spatial skills were OK. He showed a fancy beaded wristband he made which he designed without sketches with much symbolism in it.

He reported that he had to focus more on his balance. High places bothered him, mostly because of his left side getting tight. His left side was weaker, less coordinated, and not as sensitive, such as having something in his left hand and not realizing it. He was very sensitive to loud noise and startled easily. His left side would jump to noise, but not his right. His gait was uneven.

He tried to stay cheerful and to be a peacemaker but would get depressed at times. He was depressed about not being able to get a job and about his breakup with his girlfriend. He drank in the past in part because he was depressed. He had had suicidal thoughts. He thought of drinking as a suicidal, self-destructive act. He had difficulty falling asleep. He had a hard time eating commodity foods (surplus foods supplied by the federal government) and felt malnourished but had an appetite for a balanced diet. He was often bothered by intense anxiety, often associated with pain. He acknowledged an anger problem, including physical fights, especially in prison.

He often had visions or heard voices, but he was clear in his description that these were spiritual experiences distinct from the reality shared with others and not full-blown hallucinations. These experiences are certainly within the norm for his culture and not suggestive of a psychotic process.

Review of Functions

He finished the 10th grade, then got his GED at Community College in 1971. He has studied on his own and studied a few quarters at Northwest Indian College. He had done furniture factory work, custodian, cook, janitorial, construction, fishing, and assembly line. His longest job had been 3–4 months. He was in prison for 22 years for armed robbery and related charges and was then pardoned because of having been convicted on false testimony. He had a poetry and photography book in preparation.

He knew how to drive but lost his license for a DUI in 1997.

He believed in the "Chief of Many Names," whom he saw as Native spirits but also as Jesus. He had a religious experience at age four, which the elders told him was the tree spirits. He grew up in the Catholic Church, as well. The spirit of Jesus first spoke to him in 1980.

Informant's Perspective

His mother reported that she was quite concerned about him because of his headaches. She reported that his left hand got shaky sometimes. She saw him as being depressed once in a while. She noted seeing him holding back the desire to cry. She reported that he made friends easily and got along well in the community. She felt that he had difficulty with anger in the past, such as punching holes in the wall.

Behavioral Observations

Attitude

Mr. Lawrence was attentive, cooperative, and quite open and talkative. He had an attitude of looking for help. He was wearing casual clothing, including a cedar visor and leather cell phone pouch that he made, and carrying a native drum.

Speech, Language

His speech was normal in articulation, tone, rate, word-finding, and coherence. He has a finely developed sense of narrative and drama, like a good storyteller. He also makes good eye contact, sometimes piercing. When speaking about spiritual matters he switched into an oratory style. His comprehension of test instructions was normal. His handwriting was legible, coherent, and organized on the page, and correct in spelling, grammar, and punctuation above the level expected for his education.

Self-Awareness

Mr. Lawrence was aware of the quality of his test performance.

Effort, Validity

Mr. Lawrence gave a good effort on the tests and tolerated frustration well. This was a valid testing.

EAGLE BEAR: After being dehumanized to become civilized by lies and denied my human rights to become a human being my life has been one of heartache and pain. And this is why I am so thankful for Tedd Judd. In the beginning I was uncertain about what kind of person he might be and whether he would believe me when I talked to him about this voice I heard since I was four years of age. This voice stayed with me until now and helped guide me many times.

JUDD: When I first met Eagle Bear I expected that he would be reluctant to trust and to tell me his story and I was prepared to be patient. I expected that he would speak slowly and would not be very specific or expressive. I was wrong ... mostly. He was highly articulate and expressive, spoke fast, and was eager to tell most of his story and to trust me with it. But there were parts that were still difficult, that could not be shared, and things he could not trust me with. Some of these came out later in therapy.

When I heard his life story and his education and employment I expected that on testing he would perform in the low normal range on our tests, but with visual-spatial impairments from his right parietal injury. I was wrong.

When I checked his birthdate I noticed that he and I were born within a few months of each other. I could not help but feel how different our life paths had been through the accident of the circumstances of our births. And I also felt a generational affinity of our birth cohort, growing up through some of the same national and world events shaping our development.

The stated purpose of the evaluation concerned eligibility for disability (State and SSI). But I came to realize that Robert was searching for understanding and meaning regarding his brain injury and help with coping with it and that his physician and other care providers were also looking for direction as to how to best serve him. So I chose screening testing that could look for both strengths and weaknesses and that would also focus on areas of particular concern. I chose Wechsler subtests, Rey Figure, verbal fluency, and sensory and motor screening.

Results

Mr. Lawrence performed in the superior range on speed of information processing and working memory. His Block Design score was in the low normal range, lower than is to be expected for someone of his background. His approach involved difficulties with his perception of the designs, as expected with a right parietal lesion, but very good and systematic problem-solving strategies for overcoming these difficulties. As a consequence, he gained only one bonus point for speed and got two designs correct after the time limit. His Similarities score was average, consistent with his education. His memory performances were above average, with particularly strong memory for faces. There was slight "confabulation" on his story memory, suggesting that he tends to interpret and process deeply when recalling narrative. His word list memory was precise and in the superior range. His copy of the Rey figure was ultimately well organized, but he arrived at it through a piecemeal strategy and corrections. His recalls were better organized through a more global strategy and were within the normal range. He named 27 animals in one minute, with very strong verbal fluency. His specific responses reflected his cultural perspective: Eagle, falcon, raven, crow, hawk, pelican, brant goose, mallard, pintail duck, black duck, sea otter, coyote, deer, elk, cougar, bear, skunk, opossum, porcupine, grouse, pheasant, seagull, whale, mountain goat, parrot, snake, salmon. (parrot is the only one that is not from his regional environment).

He was mildly impaired in left-hand tactile perception. Right-hand coin rotation was fast normal, but it took him 47 seconds to perform 10 rotations with his left hand, which included 5 drops of the coin, at which point the test was discontinued due to frustration.

Conclusions

Mr. Lawrence had a traumatic brain injury due to an assault in 1979 that resulted in a skull fracture over the right parietal area. He has had multiple other closed traumatic head injuries. As a consequence, he had a left hemiparesis and a subtle left hemisensory deficit, with mild left neglect. In spite of this severe injury, however, he showed high normal to superior intellectual functioning. He was particularly gifted in verbal expression. The only cognitive difficulty evident from this screening evaluation was a weakness in visual-spatial perception. He had compensated well for this weakness with good problem-solving skills so that he was able to design complex beadwork without sketches, for example.

Mr. Lawrence was physically and emotionally abused as a child. He had had many traumatic experiences, including numerous assaults as an adult. He had spent 22 years in prison, convicted on false testimony. He had been alcoholic, depressed, and suicidal. He had had difficulties with anger. Counterbalancing this extreme traumatization, he had a strong spiritual grounding, several channels of artistic expression, tenacious motivation, and a somewhat tenuous but committed sobriety. He showed extraordinary resilience in now wanting to tell his story through writing, speaking, and song, with a message of forgiveness, peacemaking, cultural preservation, and respect for elders, children, and the environment.

For administrative purposes, I gave him these Western diagnoses: posttraumatic stress disorder, major depressive disorder, moderate, recurrent, alcohol abuse, in remission.

Recommendations

I recommended psychotherapy through the Lummi Tribal Health Center so as to be culturally appropriate or through mentoring with a tribal elder. I recommended client-centered, minimally directive therapy, especially at the outset, staying within his spiritual framework, avoiding psychobabble, attention to long-term issues and trauma, and reinforcing sobriety and healthy relationships. I offered to consult with his therapist/mentor or to be his therapist if the referral didn't work out. I recommended consideration of a selective serotonin reuptake inhibitor targeting depression and anxiety.

1 I recommended physical therapy to maintain the flexibility of his left side.
2 I noted that he did not have cognitive impairments that would be likely to qualify for disability on that basis alone but recommended that his hemiplegia, PTSD, depression, and anxiety be considered.
3 I recommended the Northwest Indian Vocational Rehabilitation Program to explore his potential as a writer, teacher, and related activities as a cultural resource or youth counselor or coach at the Lummi Tribal School.

Feedback

I reviewed these findings and recommendations with Mr. Lawrence, and he was appreciative. I gave him some direction for dealing with TBI impulsive anger.

Follow-Up

JUDD: Two years after the evaluation he called me and wanted to see me for therapy. He was in therapy at the tribal clinic and after discussion we agreed that it would be sufficient for him to continue with that established relationship.

Two years after that my wife and I encountered him in his craft booth at Stommish, the annual sea canoe races and powwow on the reservation. We bought a pair of cedar bark earrings he had made. A few months later he called me and asked to see me for therapy. There were some things he wanted to talk about that he felt that he could not talk about in the tribal clinic. I contacted his therapist who agreed to this. He began seeing me to deal with issues with family and tribal government. My file logs 28 psychotherapy sessions over 4 years, the last one being 12 years ago. But the file also logs about three times that number of contacts. He did not drive at that time and public transportation from the rez into town was so infrequent that it wound up being an all-day affair. There were a lot of rescheduled appointments and phone appointments. I was in touch with his prescriber about medications, his girlfriend as collateral to his treatment, social workers about disability, and vocational rehabilitation counselors. His girlfriend was white, although quite acculturated to Coast Salish ways. Nevertheless, their cultural differences in expectations for relationships were substantial and a focus of therapy. And I continue to run into him in the community at festivals and civil rights demonstrations.

Through all of this I paid close attention to balance the professional ethic of maintaining professionally traditional boundaries of the therapeutic relationship with more relaxed, culturally-sensitive Native expectations of the therapeutic relationship. There are advantages to each. For example, in my consultations to another tribe that is distant and isolated I have encountered many clients who would prefer to drive 90 minutes each way for their psychotherapy rather than be seen going to the tribal clinic. And there have been issues of cognitive disability and professional competence of tribal employees where they welcomed my outside evaluation because I was not allied with either side in the tribal politics surrounding the decision. So the outsider is sometimes a role of benefit. On the other hand, people from the tribe almost always understand the context and relationships and appropriateness of behavior and dangers and resources much better than I do. And the tribe is often a much better source of authority.

One of the most challenging aspects of the therapeutic relationship for me was to gain enough trust that he would feel that I could hear out his anger and would validate it, yet still be able to confront and challenge him to find productive and not destructive ways to act on that anger through his art, teaching, and storytelling. This involved our mutual dissection of his feelings and actions to determine what was justified and what not, and what was reflective of impulsive anger resulting from his TBI. At one discouraged moment he said that nothing could be done about the dehumanization and destruction of their culture that has come with "civilization." I reframed this into the ways he can try to choose what aspects of the new culture to accept, and he accepted the reframing.

We made use of his spiritual practices such as his power song to help him with his emotional control. The Coast Salish have many metamorphosis myths that are acted out in dances using transformation masks, in which one animal spirit mask opens up to reveal another animal spirit within. We used this imagery to help him to transform from his angry self to a loving, happy self. He struggled with his pain from his injuries, with the temptation to self-medicate, and with the humiliation of not being believed by clinic doctors, which he experienced as racism and discrimination because of his incarceration history. For pain management he decided to call on his eagle spirit to be very observant of pain and to ask himself if there is anything it was trying to tell him about what he needed to do to keep it from getting worse. He could then use his warrior spirit to ignore the pain and move above it.

He told me his names: Eagle Runs Around Bear. Eagle Bear. Two Fires. Comes with the Wind.

I gave careful consideration to the ethics of asking Eagle Bear to participate in this writing. It had been 8 years since we had had any official professional connection and 12 years since our last therapy session. After ethics consultation I decided that asking him was congruent with what I knew of his life goals. I assured him that his participation was entirely voluntary and that he would have full control over what portions of his story he chose to reveal. I decided to pay him for his contribution so as not to exploit his knowledge and skill, but to tell him of this only after undertaking the agreement so as not to leave him feeling that he was under the obligation of employment. Because of COVID-19 we had to work outdoors, so we met to work in the parking lot of a retail store where he busks with his drum. He has a smart phone but not a computer, so he wrote longhand and I scanned and transcribed his writing or took down his words.

Section III: Lessons Learned

- Background cultural knowledge is very helpful in working with Native Americans. While there are many commonalities among tribes and much intertribal interaction, the differences between tribes are equally important. It is very important for clinicians to get to know the local tribes that they will serve. This is best done through a mix of academic learning and direct experience. Since most tribes are strongly identified with their locations, it is particularly important to visit.
- Background knowledge is important, but individuals are individuals, and it is important to take time to understand their ancestry, acculturation, identities, social connections, and connections to tribes and tribal organizations and groups. Such information may emerge only slowly as trust is built.
- Many Native Americans, especially those with ties to their reservations, have strong, extended, and persisting connections with extended family and with tribal, cultural, spiritual, and governmental communities and institutions. These connections have positive and negative aspects and are critical to take into account when considering how brain disabilities may be manifested, understood, and dealt with.
- Many people who identify as or can be identified as Native American have pervasive and persisting experiences of racism that are traumatic and multigenerational. Relationships may be problematic and at least initially nontrusting with nontribal organizations and services, including health care, education, courts, child and elder welfare, vocational services, and neuropsychology.

- Many Native Americans have strong spiritual belief systems that are often syncretic, incorporating elements of local tribal spiritual beliefs and practices along with outside influences. These may or may not relate to identifiable spiritual communities and organizations. They often weigh heavily in their understanding of medical and mental problems, solutions, and treatments.
- Native Americans may have visions, hear voices, or have tremblings that are sought-after spiritual experiences, culturally congruent, positive, and not due to psychosis or somatization disorders.
- Native narrative and dialogue styles are variable and distinctive from mainstream medical and mental health styles.
- Native formal educational experiences and experiences of testing are wide-ranging and variable. Conventional US English tests and norms cannot be applied with full confidence.

COVID-19 Addendum

The COVID-19 pandemic has been devastating to Indigenous populations in the United States and around the world, often hitting them much harder than neighboring populations. The reasons for this particular health disparity are many, some of them noted above. They are being studied and better information will be available by the time this chapter is published. But the cultural toll has been even more disparate, with many of the elder repositories of culture, history, language, wisdom, and guidance being forever taken from us. It is likely that a handful of the world's 7,000+ languages have gone extinct due to this pandemic.

There is a bright spot in this. Many US tribes have been leaders in the vaccination program and have successfully vaccinated most of their members ahead of much of the rest of the United States. Given the history of epidemics on this continent, there is reason for reflection that yesterday, as I write this (February 28, 2021) the Lummi Tribe held a vaccination clinic in their casino for the teachers and staff of the neighboring Ferndale School District. Chairman Lawrence Solomon said, "Since time immemorial, our past and current leaders always think about the future of our people. We continue that responsibility today by giving our children everything they need to live a healthy life. Which means we must act as good neighbors, work together with our surrounding governments, to take care of our children, and to take care of each other.… In 1855, our ancestors signed the Point Elliot Treaty with the United States government, which states that our people will receive healthcare, including vaccinations. Therefore today, as a sovereign nation, we have the unique ability as a government to establish our own policies and prioritization of the vaccines we receive from the Indian Health Service."[24]

References

1. Eagle Bear. 2019. Available from: https://www.facebook.com/profile.php?id=100031495866693. https://www.facebook.com/100031495866693/videos/284685929257934/ https://www.facebook.com/100031495866693/videos/pcb.283509652708895/283508866042307/
2. Davis-Delano LR, Gone JP, Fryberg SA. The psychosocial effects of Native American mascots: a comprehensive review of empirical research findings. Race Ethn Educ [Internet]. 2020;23:613–633. Available from: https://doi.org/10.1080/13613324.2020.1772221
3. Whitehead J. Jonny Appleseed. Vancouver, Canada: Arsenal Pulp Press; 2018.
4. Lummi Nation [Internet]. 2020. Available from: https://www.lummi-nsn.gov/Website.php?PageID=388, downloaded 12/12/20.
5. Koch A, Brierley C, Maslin MM, Lewis SL. Earth system impacts of the European arrival and Great Dying in the Americas after 1492. Quat Sci Rev [Internet]. 2019;207:13–36. Available from: https://doi.org/10.1016/j.quascirev.2018.12.004

6. Churchill W. Kill the Indian, save the man: the genocidal impact of American Indian residential schools. San Francisco (CA): City Lights Publishers; 2004.

7. Tla'amin Nation. 2021. Available from: https://www.tlaaminnation.com/tribal-journeys-2021/, downloaded 2/28/21.

8. *Endangered Languages Project*. n.d. Retrieved 2020 June 24. Available from: http://www.endangered-languages.com/

9. Native American Language Net. Preserving and promoting Indigenous American Indian languages. n.d. Retrieved 2020 June 24. Available from: http://www.native-languages.org/

10. Walker D. Tessa's Dance [Internet]. Seattle (WA): Thoughtful Publishing; 2012. Available from: http://www.davidedwardwalker.com/index.html

11. Wright E. Indian Shaker Church [Internet]. 2016. Available from: https://www.thecanadianencyclopedia.ca/en/article/shaker-religion, downloaded 4/24/21.

12. Johnston-Goodstar K, Roholt RV. "Our kids aren't dropping out; they're being pushed out": Native American students and racial microaggressions in schools. J Ethn Cult Divers Soc Work [Internet]. 2017;26(1–2), 30–47. Available from: https://doi.org/10.1080/15313204.2016.1263818

13. American Indian Higher Education Consortium [Internet]. Available from: http://www.aihec.org/, downloaded 12/30/20.

14. Ardila A, Judd T, Sanchez O, Verney S. Submitted, 2021. Neuropsychology of the Indigenous Peoples of the Americas.

15. United Nations. United Nations Declaration on the Rights of Indigenous Peoples [Internet]. 2007. Available from: https://www.un.org/development/desa/indigenouspeoples/wp-content/uploads/sites/19/2018/11/UNDRIP_E_web.pdf

16. United Nations. State of the World's Indigenous Peoples: Indigenous Peoples' Access to Health Services [Internet]. UN; 2016. Available from: https://www.un-ilibrary.org/public-health/state-of-the-world-s-Indigenous-peoples_7914b045-en

17. Verney SP, Bennett J, Hamilton JM. Cultural considerations in the neuropsychological assessment of American Indians/Alaska natives. In: Ferraro FR, editor. Minority and cross-cultural aspects of neuropsychological assessment: enduring and emerging trends. 2nd ed. New York (NY) and London: Psychology Press; 2015.

18. Gordon PH, Mehal JM, Holman RC, Rowland AS, Cheek JE. Parkinson's disease among American Indians and Alaska natives: a nationwide prevalence study. Mov Disord. 2012;27(11):1456–9.

19. Gracey M, King M. Indigenous health part 1: determinants and disease patterns. Lancet [Internet]. 2009;374(9683):65–75. Available from: https://doi.org/10.1016/S0140-6736(09)60914-4

20. Lakhani A, Townsend C, Bishara J. Traumatic brain injury amongst Indigenous people: a systematic review. Brain Inj [Internet]. 2017;31(13–14), 1718–30. Available from: https://doi.org/10.1080/02699052.2017.1374468

21. Suchy-Dicey A, Shibata D, Cholerton B, Nelson L, Calhoun D, Ali T, et al. Cognitive correlates of MRI-defined cerebral vascular injury and atrophy in elderly American Indians: the strong heart study. J Int Neuropsychol Soc [Internet]. 2020;26(3):263–75. Available from: https://doi.org/10.1017/S1355617719001073

22. Henderson LM, Claw KG, Woodahl EL, Robinson RF, Boyer BB, Burke W, et al. P450 pharmacogenetics in Indigenous North American populations. J Pers Med. 2018;8(1):9.

23. Findling MG, Casey LS, Fryberg SA, Hafner S, Blendon RJ, Benson JM, et al. Discrimination in the United States: experiences of Native Americans. Health Serv Res [Internet]. 2019;54(S2):1431–41. Available from: https://doi.org/10.1111/1475-6773.13224

24. Lummi Nation. Lummi Nation Announces COVID-19 Mass Vaccination Event Saturday, February 27, 2021 [Internet]. 2021. Available from: https://campussuite-storage.s3.amazonaws.com/prod/1530651/06c11be8-7bab-11e7-bf32-124f7febbf4a/2232684/eba32a3c-7868-11eb-8f1b-0a9002c40a47/file/COVID-19%20vaccine%20distribution.pdf, downloaded 2/28/21.

Indigenous Canadian

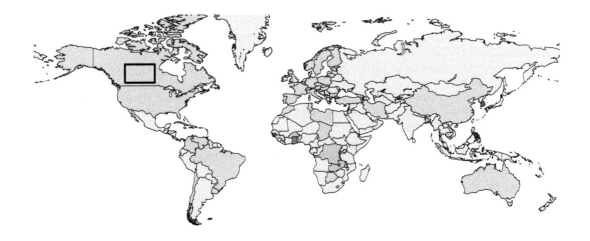

8 Neuropsychological Assessment with Indigenous Peoples in Saskatchewan

Megan E. O'Connell, Ivan Panyavin, Lisa Bourke-Bearskin, Jennifer Walker, and Carrie Bourassa

Section I: Background Information

Sociocultural Context and Perspective

The lead author and clinician practicing in the area of clinical neuropsychology (MEO) is a first-generation White settler on her father's side and second-generation settler on her mother's side. Despite working with humility to learn to be an Indigenous ally in Treaty 6 Territory and the Homeland of the Métis, as a clinician, MEO must be aware that she comes from a position of power and privilege and is, therefore, more at risk of perpetuating colonial practices. This introduction is an example of reflection and positioning of oneself,[1] which begins the process of self-awareness and is one of the core steps involved in providing culturally safe clinical care.[2] Cultural safety is a process, beginning with self-awareness, then involves seeking cultural sensitivity and cultural competency, and culminates in an environment of culturally safe clinical care.[3] In this definition, cultural safety for Indigenous Peoples goes beyond cultural competency[4] to being culturally secure and trauma informed regarding the continued violence and harm burdened by Indigenous Peoples. Clinical psychologists and clinical neuropsychologists are trained to constantly engage in reflective practices, but they might be more likely to focus this reflection on personal biases or countertransference reactions.

Colonial Context for Indigenous Peoples

When working with Indigenous Peoples, it is important to understand the history of colonialism and this history's past, present, and future impacts on Indigenous Peoples.[1,5,6] For those who are unaware, Canada, as an independent nation and as a dominion of Britain, has engaged in longstanding policies and practices to disenfranchise the independence, land ownership, and self-determination of the First Nations, Inuit, and Métis Peoples who have been inhabiting the geographic areas of North America for tens of thousands of years, which has implications for the health of Indigenous Peoples.[5,7] In Canada, a concerted government effort in forced assimilation and cultural genocide included forced relocation onto reserve lands and forced attendance at residential schools, settings where abuses of children, including those involving interpersonal violence, were common.[5,8] The country is attempting to heal by following the recommendations of the Truth and Reconciliation Commission[9] and its limitations,[10] but the impacts of intergenerational trauma, past and present racism persist.[11–14] The perspectives of Indigenous Peoples for psychological health must be understood from this holistic perspective—the current client conceptualization in the context of the past, the present, and the colonial context.[15] Understanding this history will foster awareness of the power of language, terminology, and Rights. As a clinical

DOI: 10.4324/9781003051862-17

neuropsychologist, you cannot determine if you provided culturally safe care; only your clients can determine this.[16] Knowing this requires humility, an open mind, and willingness to elicit feedback. Stated another way, the power for determining culturally safe care does not lie with the clinical neuropsychologist; rather the clinical neuropsychologist must strive to provide an environment that fosters cultural safety in clinical practice.

Geography and People

The province of Saskatchewan (one of ten provinces and three territories that make up the North American country of Canada) is home to 1,178,681 individuals.[17] Saskatchewan is a geographically vast area, occupying 651,900 km² (251,700 mi²). Consequently, nearly 60% of the population resides in small to medium population centers and rural municipalities.[18] Historically, individuals residing outside the major population centers have experienced a lack of access to specialist medical care.[19] Of the population of Saskatchewan, 13.5% self-identify as Indigenous,[20] which includes First Nations, Métis, and Inuit Peoples, with each comprising much variability in culture and language. For example, there are 74 First Nations in Saskatchewan: 10 Salteaux Nations, 7 Dene Nations, 8 Nakota/Lakota/Dakota Sioux Nations, and 49 Cree Nations.[20] Each First Nation has its own governance structures, and the First Nations governance structures interact with the provincial and federal colonial government systems. Préfontaine[21] described the origins of the word Métis as "mixed," Métis Peoples are a unique cultural and linguistic group whose ancestry includes members from various First Nations (commonly thought of as Cree or Salteaux but includes many Nations) and European settlers (from countries in Western Europe, notably France and Scotland, but also some from Eastern European regions).

Language

All Indigenous languages in Canada are at risk of extinction yet are considered to be protective factors for health.[22] There are over 60 Indigenous languages spoken in Canada.[23] For example, the Cree, who are the most widespread of Canada's First Nations Peoples, speak five main dialects of the Cree language.[24] The Saskatchewan Indigenous Cultural Centre[25] supports language projects in Plains Cree, Woodland Cree, Swampy Cree, Nakota, Dakota, Dene, Lakota, and Saulteaux.[26] Michif, which is the traditional language of the Métis, is also spoken in Saskatchewan.[23] The threat of language loss is a growing concern, given the historical context of residential schooling and consequent lack of exposure of children to their ancestral language. However, community efforts to revive Indigenous languages are underway, with the establishment of immersion programs for students across the province and the growing demand for language education at times outpacing available teacher supply.[27] The local health region has Cree interpreters available, but this is only one of the many languages spoken, and the clinic setting MEO and IP work within is not within the health region and so does not have access to these resources. The revitalization of the Language Act Bill C-91 reaffirms Indigenous rights as a fundamental issue that will help to ensure the survival of traditional knowledge systems, including language,[28] and hopefully interpretation services will be more accessible in the future.

Culture

The cultural, spiritual, and educational backgrounds of the Indigenous Peoples of Saskatchewan are as diverse as the languages spoken. Culture is a lived experience; the way people communicate and interact with one another and builds on the premise that culture is shared norms, values, and customs that influence the way health and wellness is established.[5] Each First Nation has its own identity and community-based history of interaction with settler populations.[29] According to Stonechild[29] some commonalities in traditional views include a belief that humans are one part of the interdependent circle of life, which also includes plant, animal, and (seemingly) inanimate features of nature. Each part of this circle of life includes a spiritual dimension, and wellbeing is achieved by relating to all facets of the circle of life; the aim of some ceremonies is to gain a better relationship with the spiritual dimension. Colonization has led to some integration of Indigenous spiritual beliefs with Christian beliefs. For example, Métis Peoples are varied in their religious and spiritual views, and some practice a mix of Christian and Indigenous spiritualism, others are Roman Catholic, and others practice various denominations of Protestantism.[30]

Education

Indigenous Peoples of Saskatchewan have either directly experienced or have experiences via intergenerational transmission of the traumas experienced from the attempted cultural genocide with residential schools.[29] The last residential school closed in 1996 in Saskatchewan. Educational policies ranged from isolation and assimilation in the residential school system to the present day which has more partnership-based approaches with First Nations, Métis, and government bodies.[31] Due to the trauma associated with residential schools, asking about educational attainment, a common question for intake interviews in neuropsychology, can be a challenging area to discuss. Data are available from Statistics Canada detailing that over half of Indigenous Peoples have post-secondary qualifications, with higher levels of education for younger than for older cohorts.[32] Nevertheless, the Indigenous Peoples of Saskatchewan experience an education gap relative to non-Indigenous Saskatchewanians, which has implications for workforce participation and lifetime earnings.[33] The education gap is higher for Indigenous Peoples residing in rural settings than for those residing in urban settings.[34] The education gap is being addressed with numerous Indigenous-specific educational programs. For example, the University of Saskatchewan has numerous initiatives to attract and retain Indigenous students, including small classes for Indigenous students with instructors who are culturally safe and engagement in cultural practices. Although as a group most Indigenous Peoples in Canada have achieved a high school diploma, estimates from 2016 were that 52% of Inuit Peoples, 32% of First Nations Peoples living off reserves, and 25% of Métis Peoples had less than a high school diploma.[34]

Communication

Our practice is informed by the research findings and personal experience and advice/suggestions of colleagues, patients, and family members from Indigenous backgrounds. Recommendations frequently found in the literature highlight the importance of establishing initial rapport—starting with personal introductions, which are suggested to be less formal—and interpersonal comfort in the context of clinical setting, which ought to reduce possible discomfort and mistrust.[35,36] First-hand experience of working with individuals from the Indigenous communities—particularly from those who are also involved in health care provision (e.g., nurses, medical doctors, social workers, etc.) —has provided the following tips for communication to establish a better therapeutic alliance and facilitate relational practice. Initial contact should be focused on establishing trust between the clinician and the patient. Relational practice involves genuineness and open communication. Our informal interview with an Indigenous caregiver who is also a healthcare provider suggested that male clinicians are advised to consider removing their necktie, rolling up the shirt sleeves in order to appear less "clinical" and "buttoned-up" and more open and receptive.

Nonverbal communication and body language are similarly important, with a consequent suggestion of being on a client's level—"sit and listen"—potentially foregoing scribbling and note-taking in order to focus on rapport-building and being present in the moment. An important insight regarding verbal communication was provided by an Indigenous nurse from an Indigenous Northern community: "if they agree to everything you say and ask by saying yeah, aha, yep–they are probably not really listening to you." The clinician should be cautious not to interpret the lack of direct eye contact as a sign of avoidance or disrespect; in fact, gaze avoidance is likely an indication of the opposite. An offer of "tea and snack" (a cup of tea, crackers, a slice of toast) to the patient and their family is a warm gesture that may serve as a solid first step in establishing a good working relationship. If the patient or their family, as a sign of respect or appreciation, offer a gift, the clinician is advised to accept it, as doing otherwise can be considered an insult. Health care practitioners oftentimes inform the family that they may not personally keep the gift (such as a beaver pelt)—instead asking the family's permission to display their token of appreciation in the common area of the Health Clinic for everyone to enjoy.

Disparities in Health Conditions

The arrival of colonial settlers and the displacement of Indigenous Peoples from their traditional ancestral bases has resulted in ongoing cultural, spiritual, emotional, and physical violence, with consequent negative health outcomes, disparities, and inequities.[5,37] These are evident across a number of metrics of particular relevance for neuropsychologists. Indigenous Peoples have higher rates of health problems than settler populations. These include, but are not limited to, infectious disease burdens, diabetes, hypertension, cardiovascular, and chronic renal disease, as well as diseases caused by environmental contamination, cigarette smoking, and substance use.[38] Few data exist related to Saskatchewan, but fewer First Nations Peoples have a primary healthcare provider than for settler populations in Saskatchewan.[39] First Nations in-patients tended to be younger than settler in-patients in Saskatchewan.[39]

Dementia in Indigenous Peoples

Partially due to health disparities the rates of dementia are higher, and in recent years have increased at a faster rate among Indigenous Peoples in Alberta, Canada.[40] Moreover, dementia tended to be diagnosed at a younger age in Indigenous Peoples, and the most common etiology was vascular, and males were more likely to have dementia, which is in contrast to the etiology and sex and gender profile of dementia in settler populations.[40] Not only does the epidemiological profile of dementia look different in Indigenous Peoples relative to settler populations, but Indigenous Peoples also have different views of dementia than those from the dominant culture. A 2020 review of the research on Indigenous Peoples and dementia[41] found that dementia was more often seen as a part of life versus as a biomedical disease, which appears to reflect a lack of stigma about dementia. This view is also reflected in views of some symptoms in a positive way (e.g., hallucinations could be viewed as demonstrating a strong connection with the spiritual dimension) and views of dementia as a disease that is Western.[41]

Neuropsychological Approach

Standardized testing, such as is the cornerstone of clinical neuropsychological practice, can work against providing culturally safe practices and perpetuate colonialism for the following three reasons: (1) the role of tester and testee perpetuates colonialist power dynamics and can be contrary to relational practices, (2) use of standardized testing that is not appropriate, either in the normative comparison standards or has not been explored for measurement invariance can lead to misidentification of cognitive status, and (3) use of standardized tests that are not culturally appropriate can lead to inadequate engagement with the testing process and underestimate cognitive ability. Development of culturally appropriate assessment procedures is a long and involved process for collaborative design and establishing evidence for psychometric properties, a process that has not been completed for many neuropsychological tests across cultures and has not been completed for Indigenous Peoples. There have, however, been gains made in the development of cognitive screening tools for Indigenous Peoples.

Due to lack of evidence for validity of cognitive screening tests when used with different cultural groups,[42] a team of researchers, community partners, expert language speakers, Elders, and clinicians collaborated[43] to develop the Canadian Indigenous Cognitive Assessment[43] tool. The CICA was adapted from the Kimberley Indigenous Cognitive Assessment, a culturally grounded cognitive assessment tool developed with Aboriginal communities in Northern Australia.[44] The adaptation process involved not only language translation and language interpretation but also cultural translation, with an iterative process of feedback about how the adaptation for language or cultural reasons could impact how cognition was measured. Evidence for validity of the CICA is in the process of being published but has been presented at an international conference.[45,46]

The clinical setting MEO and IP tend to work within is an interprofessional memory clinic. The one-stop diagnostic Rural and Remote Memory Clinic (RRMC) model was devised to reduce travel burden for rural and remote residents of the province[47]; consequently, the model includes a single full-day assessment with diagnosis provided by the end of day, and the authors MEO and IP practice clinically in this setting. The RRMC is an interprofessional clinic with a neuropsychology team, a neurologist, a nurse, a physical therapist, and a registered dietitian when available. To achieve the aim of providing a diagnosis to families by the end of the day, numerous changes were required to the typical practices of these health care professionals. Foremost, the clinic nurse sends each family requisitions for blood work to rule out potential medical causes of the cognitive impairment and an electrocardiogram to assess for potential contraindications for anticholinesterase medications. Families complete consent procedures, a medical history, and medication review with the clinic nurse. This information is provided to the interprofessional team, who subsequently joins the family for a joint interview (neurology, neuropsychology, and physical therapy). The interprofessional joint interview has the advantage of being time efficient but also allows families to share their stories only once and allows all team members to hear the clinical history.

After the joint interview, the patient completes a neurological exam while the family stays with the rest of the team. A typically presenting patient to the clinic attends a neuropsychological assessment, which is a brief battery of approximately two hours that assesses the domains of premorbid cognitive status (Advanced Clinical Systems (ACS) word reading),[48] suboptimal effort (for those under age 65 ACS Word Choice[48]; for all California Verbal Learning Test-II (CVLT-II) forced choice[49]; ACS/Weschler Adult Intelligence Scale-IV (WAIS-IV) Reliable Digit Span[48]; ACS/Weschler Memory Scale-IV (WMS-IV) Logical Memory Recognition),[48] language (Short Form Boston Naming Test (BNT[50]); Token Test,[51] visuospatial processing (WMS-IV Block Design[48]); Brief Visuospatial Memory Test-Revised (BVMT-R[52]) if needed Repeatable Battery of Neuropsychological Status Line Orientation,[53] attention/speed of mental processing (WAIS-IV Digit Span and Coding[48]); Delis Kaplan Executive Function System (DKEFS[54]); Trails Visual Scanning, Letter & Number Sequencing, Motor Sequencing; DKEFS Interference Colour & Word Naming),[54] semantic memory (Short Form BNT; CVLT-II Semantic Clustering; and if needed Point & Repeat test[55]); DKEFS Category Fluency), episodic memory (BVMT-R; CVLT-II short form; WMS-IV Logical Memory), executive function (DKEFS Letter Fluency, Category Fluency,

Switching; DKEFS Interference Inhibition & Inhibition/Switching; DKEFS Trails Number/ Letter Switching), and social cognition (Social Norms Questionnaire[56]). There are no normative data for Indigenous Peoples for the tests in this battery, and no data on measurement equivalence for these tests when given to Indigenous Peoples. The CICA is included in the RRMC battery, but due to its preliminary evidence for validity (at the time of this chapter writing, evidence for validity has not been published), it is included as an optional research task and is not used clinically. In the *Clinical Engagement with Indigenous Clients* section of the chapter, we discuss how or if we use the above-mentioned tests with Indigenous peoples presenting to the memory clinic.

Further assessment in the clinic includes interview with the family while the client is performing the neuropsychological battery and administration of standardized scales of function, behavior, and mood. Finally, the RRMC team meets and discusses the profession-specific findings (the neurologist interprets the medical workup), and the neurologist and neuropsychologist come to a consensus diagnosis. The team contributes to an interprofessional letter with recommendations. The neurologist and neuropsychologist meet with the family and communicate the diagnosis, recommendations, and plan for management and follow-up. This process occurs for two families on clinic day: The intake and feedback interviews are staggered, and while one family is performing the neuropsychology assessment the other family is receiving the physical therapy assessment. Follow-up occurs as needed and is provided by the neurologist using Telehealth. One year post initial assessment all families return to the RRMC for a half-day assessment by neuropsychology and physical therapy; further assessment and feedback of the in-person assessments is provided by Telehealth with the neurologist. Subsequent in-person assessments are provided only for a sub-set of patients: (1) whose diagnosis remains ambiguous, (2) patients who are diagnosed with mild cognitive impairment, (3) patients for whom their presentation of dementia is atypical.

Clinical Engagement with Indigenous Clients

Working with Indigenous Peoples as patients in the RRMC requires careful consideration because the structures and procedures of the RRMC are not, in themselves, culturally safe. Foremost, the RRMC model uses standardized scales that could be culturally and psychometrically inappropriate. Neuropsychological tests are compared with published comparison standards that are age and sex stratified, and for some tests also stratified by education. No known neuropsychological normative comparison standards exist for the Indigenous Peoples of Canada, and no known evidence on measurement invariance of neuropsychological tests for Indigenous Peoples has been reported, and data on differential item functioning or measurement invariance is needed for clinical use.[57,58] It is a clinical decision that takes great care—should we administer standardized tests at all? Villarreal[59] described the tensions between culturally appropriate assessment with Indigenous Peoples and need for standardization—and we described many of the practices involved in standardized assessment, particularly neuropsychological assessment as colonizing practices. Cultural appropriateness is one factor, but we also see people with few years of education, which can result in underestimates of neuropsychological test performance.[60] Would administration do more harm than good? If an Indigenous Person with zero years of formal education performs poorly, can we trust that poor performance on this standardized test to reflect cognitive functioning, at least to some degree? If unsure, it is best to choose not to administer such tests and use interview data predominantly. Alternatively, assessment procedures are administered but interpreted qualitatively.[61] Westerman and Wettinger[62] describe issues to consider when determining if psychological assessment with Indigenous Peoples is valid, including not only the content of what is assessed but also the methods used to assess. If test procedures are modified, it threatens the validity of the neuropsychological tests. An additional consideration is lack of appropriate normative comparison standards: Even if assessment processes are consistent with standardized procedures, interpretation of tests is nonstandardized due to inappropriate normative comparison standards. Postal and colleagues[63] created a framework used for deciding when deviation from standardized administration of neuropsychological tests is warranted based on a consideration of numerous factors, including incremental validity for the pandemic, which we have adapted for consideration of appropriate neuropsychological assessment with Indigenous older adults. If test administration is nonstandardized (either by virtue of administration procedures or normative comparisons) we consider whether the testing would add incremental validity, and if not, we choose to weigh our diagnostic process on the clinical history from interview with patient and collateral informants. This clinical decision is based on an understanding of the colonial nature of standardized assessment and the importance of increasing cultural safety in the context of diagnostic assessments when working with Indigenous Peoples.

Relational practices to help facilitate the process of a culturally safe clinical assessment involve an open discussion with the person who is participating in the assessment and with the family. The RRMC is set up to mimic a home-like environment. Each family gets a private room with some amenities for the day. The couches are commonly used for naps, they have a locking cupboard to keep possessions, and a computer and internet access are provided. Families are provided coffee or tea and shown the kitchenette where they can help themselves to additional drinks and asked to "make themselves at home." Although we do this for all families, MEO makes an attempt to personally offer coffee or tea with Indigenous families, even if the clinic nurse has already provided the first cup.

As clinicians, MEO and IP make few assumptions and check in with the family and, if appropriate, the person being assessed for dementia. Although MEO might make decisions that the neuropsychological tests might be inappropriate, she checks her decisions with the families, and there are numerous other standardized scales we administer for mood, behavior, and function at the RRMC. Indigenous Peoples vary widely in formal education, occupational attainment, and immersion/exposure to the dominant culture in Canada. Sometimes it is appropriate to administer these standardized tests and use the existing normative comparison standards and provide caveats for the interpretation of such tests in the written report and triangulate neuropsychological testing data with interview data and other standardized scales measuring function. Sometimes we administer the aforementioned neuropsychological battery, and sometimes we administer none of the standardized tests. MEO asks herself—can she trust that a very low score would reflect impairment, or would she wonder if it was due to lack of cultural appropriateness of the tests or lack of exposure to formal education, or both—if she is not sure, she chooses NOT to administer the typical battery of tests and uses interview data predominantly. MEO believes if you cannot be relatively confident in what the test performance means, it is more ethical to avoid administration of this neuropsychological test. Participating in a neuropsychological assessment is rarely enjoyable, and if the resulting test scores are highly suspect, this process does not adequality honor your patients' time and effort. This is a decision made on a case-by-case basis and whenever possible in consultation with the family.

Section II: Case Study — "A Lesson in Cultural Humility"

As an illustrative case, the following clinical assessment is provided, but this is a generated composite of presentations across patients. Henry Stony (not an RRMC patient's name) is an 80-year-old man who has lived in Île-à-la-Crosse for his entire life. Île-à-la-Crosse is a 5-hour drive north of the clinic in Saskatoon one-way, and Henry arrived by medical taxi at the RRMC. He speaks

Cree at home, and the variant of Cree he speaks is a mix of Plains Cree (spoken in the south) and Michif (a mix of French and Cree), which is common to several northern SK communities. He understands aural English and speaks some, but does not read or write, with a report of no years of formal education. He reported that his parents hid him from the government agents who tried to take him away from his home and his community for forced attendance at residential schools. He worked for most of his life as a trapper and guide and only recently gave up guiding the summer before the current appointment. Henry never married and currently lives alone. Henry is physically healthy (past medical and mental health history is negative for any diseases/disorders), takes no Western medications, and drinks medicinal teas to help with his sleep. He reports no current sleep disturbance, and his only problems remain in the domain of memory—forgetting names of people he knows but recognizing their faces. Henry has no surviving siblings, and he attended the appointment with his 19-year-old nephew, John. John is not genetically related to Henry, nor is he a longstanding member of the Île-à-la-Crosse community. He grew up in Saskatoon and was transplanted to Île-à-la-Crosse as a teenager. He was a neighbor of Henry's in Île-à-la-Crosse, and they adopted each other. Although John currently lives in Saskatoon to attend University, he keeps in touch with Henry remotely and feels he can act as a collateral informant. John's first language is English, but he is fluent in Plains Cree, and not Michif.

During interview Henry presents with moderate to severe hearing loss, but it is challenging to figure out if impaired comprehension is due to hearing acuity or the fact that he speaks in Cree most often, and the interview is conducted in English. We discuss with the family whether we should try working through any language barrier together. The lack of formal interpretation services is a limitation of our clinic setting and the one-day assessment model. Our interviews are family interviews so the ethical pitfalls of using family for interviews is somewhat lessened by the group nature of this method of interviewing. If, however, we have to perform some testing through translation we engage in a lengthy discussion about the pitfalls of this approach. The ethical quandary of not providing services versus the ethical issues of using a family member must be considered. The clinic setting does not have access to a translation service, and the logistics of incorporating a translation service for a one-day clinic model where we would not know a translator might be helpful until after we have started the assessment is another consideration. In Henry's case, asking him to travel the 5 hours back home only to travel back to the clinic at a time when a professional interpreter was available would not be an ethical choice. After discussing the pitfalls of using John for interpretation when needed, we decide to proceed.

John spontaneously begins to repeat what we ask Henry and then translate into Cree, and Henry appears animated and can answer questions in English with a low volume and Cree accent, but he elaborates very little. Henry displays more generative output in English when describing where he grew up and how he worked on the land. He denied any known developmental delays, and John reveals that Henry worked as a well-known and respected guide in the North. We ask Henry if he thinks he can do a physical exam with the doctor in English or would he prefer to have John come translate, and he jokes that he can as long as he won't get poked. While Henry and the neurologist are working together, the neuropsychology team speaks alone with John, who reveals that members of the community have expressed worries about Henry because they have noticed he has a hard time remembering people, and he keeps joking about how they've changed, and that is why he can't remember them. John recently discovered that Henry has been forgetting to pay bills, and he worked to set up automatic payments for Henry. Finally, John described a recent episode where Henry appeared to get lost in the bush. Although Henry denies he was lost and laughs off the incident, apparently the community was mobilized to search for him due to the minus 40-degree Celsius temperatures. This episode was a huge shock for the community given the large extent of Henry's longstanding trapline, his leadership in guiding, and his well-respected general knowledge of the land. John is concerned for his uncle's welfare since he is unsure about what is going on. John is in touch with his mother who is Henry's neighbor, and she helps John keep tabs on Henry during the 4 months of the school term when John is unable to see Henry. They feel Henry's problems go well beyond his marked hearing loss.

Our premorbid estimate of Henry is restricted to his developmental and occupational history, given the lack of formal education and inappropriateness of the word reading test in this context. We estimated Henry's premorbid ability was in the average range. We also decide that we would ask him questions about his mood rather than try to give him our standardized scale that requires a high level of reading fluency. We decide that most, if not all, of the standardized scales would likely be inappropriate for Henry, but in order to provide medications under the government formulary we need scores for a commonly used cognitive screening test. We decide to work with Henry on this screening test and subsequently make decisions about the rest of the assessment. We discuss with Henry and John the problems with the tests we give—they are culture bound and make assumptions about things taught in school. We discuss how these tests do not ask about his areas of extensive knowledge and ask things that might seem silly to him or not seem relevant to him or his life. We state that there is one test that the neurologist might need and we could give it a try together and see how it goes. We ask Henry if he thinks we should try it alone or should we try it in Cree and have John help with translation. Henry and John think it is a good idea to do this together and we can start in English and try in Cree as well. We begin the test in English. Henry does not answer the first question, and we decide to try this in Cree. Henry agrees, stating that he can hear Cree better—we joke that maybe he can hear John's deep voice better than the high voice of MEO. The three of us discuss the challenges with having John do the translation, and we discuss the lack of formal translation services available to us. They both agree we can give this a try.

MEO discusses with John how hard it will be to not elaborate on a question or an answer, and the purpose of these questions is to see how Henry can do on his own. We discuss how this process can feel odd because MEO will be making eye contact with Henry, but John will be speaking. MEO asks questions and John translates the question, Henry answers, and John translates. This occurs for much of the cognitive screening test, but on occasion Henry answers a question in English before John can translate. Once, John and Henry spoke back and forth in Cree, but the question was brief and the anticipated answer was also brief. I asked what was happening, noting the length of their discussion for such a brief question (recalling that it can be hard for family not to explain a question or elaborate on this). It turns out Henry responded with a word John was unfamiliar with due to difference in dialect and he was clarifying. We finish the cognitive screening task and discuss what Henry thought of it; he said it was ok but was a bit silly.

Henry had marked difficulty with this screening task, and given the collateral reports of decline in daily function we decide that further testing was not needed from a diagnostic viewpoint. That is, the incremental validity that could be provided by additional standardized testing was determined to be low, so we decided to limit our standardized testing with Henry to maximize the cultural safety of the clinical assessment. While Henry performs the physical therapy assessment, after a collaborative discussion about the appropriateness, John fills out some standardized scales about Henry's functioning, and we get permission to speak with John's mother over the phone given that she has been acting as more of the primary care provider now that John has moved to Saskatoon. She reports she is now providing Henry with meals because he was not cooking and had moldy food in the fridge, and she is needing to prompt him to bathe. She is scared that he will get lost again and not be able to find his way back home.

After Henry participates in a neuroimaging exam, the team meets to discuss the results from the comprehensive blood panel (requisition mailed before clinic day), the neuroimaging, the neurology exam, and the neuropsychology assessment. The physical exam procedures are all within normal limits. Much of the diagnostic process is based on clinical interviews and collateral interviews, which is not ideal. Nevertheless, the team understands that standardized assessments under inappropriate conditions make it impossible to tell if poor performance is due to the inappropriate assessment procedures, the lack of standardization due to translation, or reflect poor cognitive performance. The neurologist and neuropsychologist decide there is enough information to suggest a clinical diagnosis of dementia. We speak with Henry and John to discuss this diagnosis and its implications and discuss how we will be communicating a management plan with Henry's primary care provider. After the neurologist leaves, the neuropsychology team spends time debriefing with Henry and John about the diagnosis and the assessment process. Recommendations are provided for Henry, John, and Henry's primary care provider, which includes linkages with local homecare resources. Our clinic is 5 hours away and must rely on the local resources for postdiagnostic care.

We find it common to see patients presenting with overt cognitive impairments who could have been diagnosed in primary care. Ideally, we design a remote clinic where we can support the diagnostic procedures for primary care providers, saving the interprofessional assessment procedures of the RRMC for the most difficult to diagnose. The lack of neuroimaging facilities in the North makes a plan for a fully remote memory clinic challenging, and we continue with our current model because the assessment is completed in one day, which reduces travel time. We use relational practices and focus on interpersonal connection in an attempt to counter the highly medicalized nature of the RRMC, which could be seen as a setting that perpetuates colonial practices. Finally, we are aware of the limited contribution that standardized neuropsychological testing can have for people like Henry. The development of the CICA[44] is one way to help primary care providers obtain information on cognition for Indigenous Peoples, but this is only a screening test. It is, however, a model for how to develop a culturally appropriate cognitive assessment tool that could be used for neuropsychological tests in the future (see https://www.i-caare.ca/cica-tool). Foremost, tests need to be co-designed rather than led by non-Indigenous clinicians. Tests need to be iteratively trialed with cultural and language experts. Finally, exploring evidence for the psychometric properties of these newly developed tests needs to be established.

Section III: Lessons Learned

- The historical context of colonialism and residential schools, as well as cultural and linguistic differences, necessitate the need for more competent cultural clinical practice, which can lead to culturally safe care for Indigenous Peoples.
- Neuropsychology clinicians from Indigenous backgrounds are needed.
- Clinicians from non-Indigenous backgrounds are urged to make every attempt to conceptualize their clients' physical and psychological health needs from a holistic perspective, that is, in the context of the past, the present, as well as the colonial contexts.
- Culturally safe clinical assessment approaches can be developed by working with Indigenous Peoples such as been done with the CICA. While possible to do with neuropsychological tests, it is important that development of these tests prioritize co-design with the community rather than design led by non-Indigenous clinicians. Additional research on the psychometric properties would subsequently be needed before clinical use.
- Traditional neuropsychological assessment involves a balance between validity of test interpretation (either due to nonstandardized administration or nonstandardized application of normative comparison standards) with cultural safety. On a client-by-client basis, one needs to consider context (cultural context, language, education, colonial practices of the region

and its history, and the colonial experiences by your client) that could impact cultural safety. Although likely true for all cultural and linguistic groups, this clinical decision to maximize cultural safety is critical when working with Indigenous Peoples in Saskatchewan, given their intergenerational experiences, personal history, present, and future experiences with colonizing practices. As the client context increases in its distance from the dominant settler culture, the need for modifications to create a culturally safe assessment increase. These modifications decrease the validity of the test data (see Figure 8.1). We argue when balancing between validity and cultural safety clinicians should consider the incremental validity of the neuropsychological testing, that is, how critical is the testing information to the aim of the assessment. Can the aims of the assessment be achieved without them? Are deviations from standardization so large as to threaten all validity underlying test interpretation? If the answer to either of these

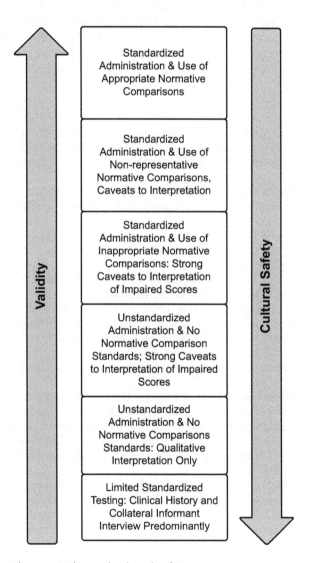

Figure 8.1 Validity of test interpretation and cultural safety

questions is yes, consider avoiding perpetuating a colonizing practice. In conclusion, we suggest standardized assessments are not necessarily culturally safe for some clients and should be used only when the incremental validity is high.

Maps (public domain): https://ian.macky.net/pat/map/ca/sk/sk_blu.gif
(https://ian.macky.net/pat/map/ca/sk/sk.html)[64]
(https://commons.wikimedia.org/wiki/File:Saskatchewan,_Canada.svg)[65]
(http://www.yellowmaps.com/map/saskatchewan-outline-map-589.htm)[66]

Acknowledgments

The writing of this chapter was supported and partially funded by funding from Team 15 on Rural Dementia Care (MEO & IP) in the Canadian Consortium on Neurodegeneration in Aging (CCNA) and Team 18 on Indigenous Dementia Care (MEO, JW, & LBB). CCNA is supported by a grant from the Canadian Institutes of Health Research (CIHR) with funding from several partners including CIHR Institute of Indigenous Peoples' Health, the Saskatchewan Health Research Foundation, the Centre for Aging and Brain Health, and the Alzheimer Society of Canada.

References

1. Brascoupé S, Waters, C. Cultural safety: exploring the application of the concept of cultural safety to Aboriginal health and community wellness. Int J Indig Health. 2009;5(2):6–41.
2. Papps E, Ramsden I. Cultural safety in nursing: the New Zealand experience. Int J Qual Health Care. 1996;8(5):491–7.
3. Health NCCfA. Towards Cultural Safety for Métis: an Introduction for Heath Care Providers [Internet]. 2013. Available from: https://www.ccnsa-nccah.ca/docs/emerging/FS-CulturalSafetyMetis-MetisCentre-EN.pdf
4. Curtis E, Jones R, Tipene-Leach D, Walker C, Loring B, Paine S, et al. Why cultural safety rather than cultural competency is required to achieve health equity: a literature review and recommended definition. Int J Equity Health. 2019;18(1):1–17.
5. Kirmayer LJ, Brass GM, Tait CL. The mental health of Aboriginal peoples: transformations of identity and community. Can J Psychiatry. 2000;45(7):607–16.
6. Kirmayer L, Simpson C, Cargo M. Healing traditions: culture, community and mental health promotion with Canadian Aboriginal peoples. Australas Psychiatry. 2003;11(supl):S15–23.
7. Greenwood M, de Leeuw S, Lindsay N. Challenges in health equity for Indigenous peoples in Canada. Lancet. 2018;319(10131):1645–8.
8. Sinclair R. Identity lost and found: lessons from the sixties scoop. First Peoples Child Fam Rev. 2007;3(1):65–82.
9. Truth and Reconciliation Commission of Canada. Honouring the truth, reconciling for the future: Summary of the final report of the Truth and Reconciliation Commission of Canada. 2015; iv, p. 382.
10. Niezen R. Truth and indignation Canada's Truth and Reconciliation Commission on Indian residential schools [Internet]. North York (NY), Ontario: University of Toronto Press; 2017. Available from: http://myaccess.library.utoronto.ca/login?url=http://books.scholarsportal.info/uri/ebooks/ebooks3/utpress/2018-03-27/1/9781487594404.
11. Bourassa C, McKay-McNabb K, Hampton M. Racism, sexism, and colonialism: the impact on the health of Aboriginal women in Canada. Can Woman Stud. 2004;24(1):23–9.
12. Evans M, Hole R, Berg LD, Hutchinson P, Sookraj D. Common insights, differing methodologies: toward a fusion of Indigenous methodologies, participatory action research, and white studies in an urban Aboriginal research agenda. Qual Inq. 2009;15(5):893–910.

13. Jacklin K, Pace JE, Warry W. Informal dementia caregiving among Indigenous communities in Ontario, Canada. Care Manag J. 2015;16(2):106–20.

14. Rice ES, Haynes E, Royce P, Thompson S. Social media and digital technology use among Indigenous young people in Australia: a literature review. Int J Equity Health. 2016;15:81–91.

15. Gould B, MacQuarrie C, O'Connell ME, Bourassa C. Mental wellness needs of two Indigenous communities: bases for culturally competent clinical services. Canadian Psychology/Psychologie Canadienne. 2020.

16. DeAngelis T. What should you do if a case is outside your skill set? Monit Psychol. 2018;49(05):30.

17. Saskatchewan Quarterly Population Report: Second Quarter 2020. Saskatchewan Bureau of Statistics; 2020.

18. Duffin E. Population distribution of Saskatchewan, Canada, in 2016, by rural/urban type [Internet]. 2019. Available from: https://www.statista.com/statistics/608710/population-distribution-of-saskatchewan-by-rural-urban-type/

19. Karunanayake CP, Rennie DC, Hagel L, Lawson J, Janzen B, Pickett W, et al. Access to specialist care in rural Saskatchewan: the Saskatchewan Rural Health Study. Healthcare. 2015;3(1):84–99.

20. Anderson A. Indigenous Population Trends [Internet]. n.d. Available from: https://teaching.usask.ca/indigenoussk/import/indigenous_population_trends.php

21. Préfontaine DR. Métis Communities. Indigenous Saskatchewan Encyclopedia. Regina (CA): University of Regina Press; n.d.

22. McIvor O, Napoleon A, Dickie KM. Language and culture as protective factors for at-risk communities. Int J Indig Health. 2013;5(1):6–25.

23. Aboriginal languages in Canada [Internet]. 2018. Available from: https://www12.statcan.gc.ca/census-recensement/2011/as-sa/98-314-x/98-314-x2011003_3-eng.cfm

24. Ratt S. Mâci-nêhiyawêwin: Beginning Cree. Regina (CA): University of Regina Press; 2018.

25. Guarnieri B, Adorni F, Musicco M, Appollonio I, Bonanni E, Caffarra P, et al. Prevalence of sleep disturbances in mild cognitive impairment and dementing disorders: a multicenter Italian clinical cross-sectional study on 431 patients. Dement Geriatr Cogn Disord. 2012;33(1):50–8.

26. Saskatchewan Indigenous Cultural Centre. n.d. Available from: https://sicc.sk.ca

27. Vescera Z. Demand for Cree-language education outpaces teacher supply. Saskatoon StarPhoenix. 2019. https://thestarphoenix.com/news/local-news/demand-for-cree-language-education-outpaces-teacher-supply

28. Assembly of First Nations. A Guide to: An Act respecting Indigenous languages: A Tool for First Nations Language Revitalization. 2019.

29. Stonechild B. Indigenous peoples of Saskatchewan. Indigenous Saskatchewan Encyclopedia. Regina (CA): University of Regina Press; 2005.

30. Préfontaine DR, Paquin T, Young P. Métis Spiritualism [Internet]. 2003. Available from: http://www.metismuseum.ca/media/db/00727

31. Bellegarde S, LaFontaine T. Indigenous Education Policy. Indigenous Saskatchewan encyclopedia. Regina (CA): University of Regina Press; 2005.

32. Statistics Canada. The educational attainment of Aboriginal peoples in Canada 2011 July 25, 2018 [Internet]. 2021. Available from: https://www12.statcan.gc.ca/nhs-enm/2011/as-sa/99-012-x/99-012-x2011003_3-eng.cfm

33. Howe E. Bridging the Aboriginal Education Gap in Saskatchewan. Gabriel Dumont Institute; 2011.

34. OECD. Chapter 2. Profile of indigenous Canada [Internet]. In: Reviews ORP, editor. Linking indigenous communities with regional development in Canada. Paris: OECD Publishing; 2020 Jan 21 [cited 3 Mar 2021]. p. 67–134. doi:10.1787/fa0f60c6-en

35. King J, Fletcher-Janzen E. Neuropsychological assessment and intervention with Native Americans. In: Fletcher-Janzen E, Strickland TL, Reynolds CR, editors. Handbook of cross-cultural neuropsychology. New York (NY): Springer; 2000. p. 105–22.

36. Verney SP, Bennett J, Hamilton JM, Ferraro F. Cultural considerations in the neuropsychological assessment of American Indians/Alaska Natives. Minority and Cross-Cultural Aspects of Neuropsychological Assessment: enduring and emerging trends. 2015;2:115–58.

37. Miller JR. Lethal legacy: current native controversies in Canada. Toronto (CA): McClelland & Stewart Ltd.; 2004.

38. Canada IaNA. A demographic and socio-economic portrait of Aboriginal populations in Canada. Ottawa (CA): Indian and Northern Affairs; 2009.

39. Lafond G, Haver CRA, McLeod V, Clarke S, Horsburgh B, McLeod KM. Characteristics and residence of First Nations patients and their use of health care services in Saskatchewan, Canada: informing First Nations and Métis Health Services. J Eval Clin Pract. 2017;23(2):294–300.

40. Jacklin KM, Walker JD, Shawande M. The emergence of dementia as a health concern among First Nations populations in Alberta, Canada. Can J Public Health. 2013;104(1):e39–44.

41. Jacklin K, Walker J. Cultural understandings of dementia in Indigenous Peoples: a qualitative evidence synthesis. Can J Aging. 2020;39(2):220–34.

42. O'Driscoll C, Shaikh, M. Cross-cultural applicability of the Montreal Cognitive Assessment (MoCA): a systematic review. J Alzheimer's Dis. 2017;58(3):789–801.

43. Bogdanov S, Naismith S, Lah S. Sleep outcomes following sleep-hygiene-related interventions for individuals with traumatic brain injury: a systematic review. Brain Injury. 2017;31(4):422–33.

44. Jacklin K, Pitawanakwat K, Blind M, O'Connell ME, Walker J, Lemieux AM, et al. Developing the Canadian Indigenous Cognitive Assessment for use with Indigenous older Anishinaabe adults in Ontario, Canada. Innov Aging. 2020;4(4):igaa038.

45. Walker J, O'Connell, ME, Crowshoe L, Jacklin K, Boeheme G, Hogan D, et al. Adaptation of the Canadian Indigenous Cognitive Assessment in three provinces and evidence for validity. AAIC 2020 Conference Featured Research; 2020.

46. O'Connell ME, Walker J, Jacklin K, Bourassa C, Kirk A, Hogan DB, et al. Classification accuracy of the English version of the Canadian Indigenous Cognitive Assessment (CICA) in a majority culture memory clinic sample. AAIC 2020 Conference; 2020.

47. Morgan D, Crossley M, Kirk A, D'Arcy C, Stewart N, Biem J, et al. Improving access to dementia care: development and evaluation of a rural and remote memory clinic. Aging Ment Health. 2009;13(1):17–30.

48. Wechsler D. Advanced Clinical Solutions for WAIS®-IV and WMS®-IV: Clinical and Interpretive Manual. Pearson; 2009.

49. Delis DC, Kramer JH, Kaplan E, Ober BA. The California Verbal Learning Test. 2nd ed. Psychological Corporation; 2000.

50. Mack WJ, Freed DM, Williams BW, Henderson VW. Boston Naming Test: shortened versions for use in Alzheimer's disease. J Gerontol. 1992;47(3):154–8.

51. Benton AL, Hamsher KD, Sivan AB. Manual for the Multilingual Aphasia Examination. AJA Associates; 1994.

52. Benedict RHB. Brief Visuospatial Memory Test—Revised: Professional Manual. Psychological Assessment Resources, Inc.; 1997.

53. Randolph C. RBANS: Repeatable Battery for the Assessment of Neuropsychological Status. Psychological Corporation; 1998.

54. Delis DC, Kaplan E, Kramer JH. Delis-Kaplan Executive Function System® (D-KEFS®): Examiner's Manual: flexibility of thinking, concept formation, problem solving, planning, creativity, impulse control, inhibition. Pearson; 2001.

55. Hodges JR, Martinos M, Woollams AM, Patterson K, Adlam ALR. Repeat and point: differentiating semantic dementia from progressive non-fluent aphasia. Cortex. 2008;44(9):1265–70.

56. Panchal H, Paholpak P, Lee G, Carr A, Barsuglia JP, Mather M, et al. Neuropsychological and neuroanatomical correlates of the social norms questionnaire in frontotemporal dementia versus Alzheimer's disease. Am J Alzheimer's Dis Other Dement. 2016;31(4):326–32.

57. Pedraza O, Mungas D. Measurement in cross-cultural neuropsychology. Neuropsychol Rev. 2008; 18(3):184–93.

58. Avila JF, Rentería MA, Witkiewitz K, Verney SP, Vonk JMJ, Manly JJ. Measurement invariance of neuropsychological measures of cognitive aging across race/ethnicity by sex/gender groups. Neuropsychology. 2020;34(1):3–14.

59. Villarreal ET. Evaluation of the learning of Indigenous students in Latin America. Challenges of measurement and interpretation in contexts of cultural diversity and social inequality. Revista mexicana de investigación educativa. 2006;11(28):225–68.

60. Franzen S, van den Berg E, Goudsmit M, Jurgens CK, Van De Wiel L, Kalkisim Y, et al. A systematic review of neuropsychological tests for the assessment of dementia in non-Western, low-educated or illiterate populations. J Int Neuropsychol Soc. 2020;26:331–51.

61. Thompson JC, Stopford CL, Snowden JS, Neary D. Qualitative neuropsychological performance characteristics in frontotemporal dementia and Alzheimer's disease. J Neurol Neurosurg Psychiatry. 2005;76(7):920–7.

62. Westerman T, & Wettinger M. Psychological Assessment and Intervention [Internet]. Psychologically Speaking. 1997. Available from: https://indigenouspsychservices.com.au/wp-content/uploads/2018/10/Psychological-Assessment-of-Aboriginal-People-Assessment.pdf

63. Postal KS, Bilder RM, Lanca M, Aase DM, Barisa M, Holland AA, et al. Inter organizational practice committee guidance/recommendation for models of care during the novel coronavirus pandemic. Arch Clin Neuropsychol. 2021;36(1):17–28.

64. Public Domain Maps of Saskatchewan; n.d.

65. File:Saskatchewan, Canada.svg; 2008.

66. Outline Government Map of Saskatchewan; n.d.

B. Arab World

Overview

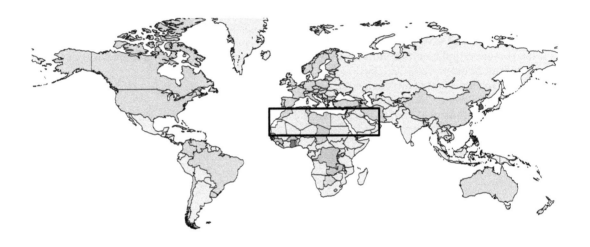

9   Cultural Considerations in Neuropsychological Assessment of Arab Populations

Ahmed F. Fasfous and Julia C. Daugherty

Context for the Arab World

Terminology and Perspective

In this chapter, we refer to people of the *Arab world*. Due to the fact that this term is highly simplified, lacking a true reflection of the vast diversity encompassed by Arab countries, we will attempt to illuminate the richness and heterogeneity of its people and cultures through brief descriptions of socio-economic discrepancies, language/dialects, culture, and geography. These descriptions are not meant to be exhaustive. Instead, they serve as an abbreviated introduction to the many cultures that make up this region to help practitioners and researchers identify specific cultural considerations when working with this population in the context of neuropsychological evaluation and care.

As such, we will focus on the clinical implications of cultural variables on neuropsychological assessment. From a clinical perspective, we will speak to certain differences between sub-cultural groups in the Arab world and how they should be considered in neuropsychological procedures.

Geography

The Arab world is made up of 22 countries, and of these, 12 are in Asia (Saudi Arabia, Bahrain, United Arab Emirates, Iraq, Jordan, Kuwait, Lebanon, Oman, Palestine, Qatar, Syria, Yemen), and 10 of which are found in Africa (Algeria, Comoros, Egypt, Djibouti, Libya, Mauritania, Morocco, Sudan, Somalia, and Tunisia). The Arab world is divided into four main geopolitical areas[1]: the Fertile Crescent (Iraq, Jordan, Lebanon, Syria, and Palestine), the Nile Valley (Egypt and Sudan), the Gulf states (Bahrain, Kuwait, Oman, Qatar, Saudi Arabia, and the United Arab Emirates), and the Maghreb (Algeria, Libya, Morocco, Mauritania, and Tunisia). There are four additional countries in the Arab world that have not been included in these four geopolitical areas. These countries geographically pertain to the Gulf of Aden (Djibouti, Somalia, and Yemen) and the Indian Ocean (Comoros Islands). Despite the geographical proximity between these countries in each geographical region, customs and traditions may differ from one country to another.

People

The term Arab is related to a specific region of the world. Most people in the region extending from the coast of Northern Africa to the Arabian Gulf refer to themselves as Arabs.[2,3] The Arab population is made up of over 400 million people,[4] representing around 5% of the global population. While Arab populations in the modern world are, generally speaking, considered to share

DOI: 10.4324/9781003051862-19

similar linguistic, historical, cultural background and genetic roots,[1,2] Arab ethnic identity is considered one of the most difficult to define. There are a variety of minority groups that have different ethnicities (such as the Kurds in Iraq or the Berbers in Morocco), and there may be social and familial mixing with other groups.[2] With regard to other population demographics, there are many discrepancies in terms of population density and age stratification. For example, in Egypt there are more than 100 million inhabitants, while in Qatar there are less than a million.[4] In terms of age characteristics, the majority of the population are either young adults or children.[5]

Immigration and Relocation

Over the history of the Arab world, there have been numerous emigration and relocation patterns marked by strife over land and resources. In more recent years, most of these relocations involved Syrians and Palestinians[6] who fled their countries in search of refuge. In fact, there are over two million people living in refugee camps in Palestine, over 700,000 Syrians and two million Palestinian refugees living in Jordan (nearly 40% of the total population), and one million Syrians and 470,000 Palestinian refugees living in Lebanon (close to 25% of the total population).[6] Of special relevance to those of us who work in neuropsychological outreach, these paramount shifts have placed many people at a greater risk of suffering mental health problems,[7,8] including neuropsychological difficulties.[9,10]

There have also been other important international immigration patterns, such as the migration of Arabs to North America. In the United States, it is estimated that there are around 3.7 million Arab Americans.[11] Despite the significance of this growth, many practitioners face difficulties in understanding how the culture of this population may influence health-related behaviors and consequently affect treatment.[2] In fact, some suggest that there is a prevailing idea that Arab patients should assimilate and adjust to the Western perspective of health care and disease,[2] which may exacerbate the disconnect between patients and practitioners. In this respect, more research and cross-culturally sensitive tools may help to ease this important gap.

Language and Communication

Throughout the 22 countries making up the Arab world, people typically read and write in Classic Arabic and its colloquial form, Modern Standard Arabic (MSA). Due to the fact that these forms of Arabic are often used for Arabic books, newspapers and major television shows, they are considered to be more neutral and are less geographically specific.[12] Nonetheless, each country has its own dialect(s), which in large part can be considered an informal variation of the classical Arabic language. These dialects, while stemming from the same root, are so diverse that they may even be incomprehensible for people speaking different dialects. In fact, the vernacular of each country, or even of each region within countries, differs so greatly from Classical Arabic that learning one could resemble learning a new language.[13] For example, the historical influence of different empires and civilizations has made an everlasting impression on the different variations of Arabic, as is the case in the Egyptian dialect, which has been influenced by the Coptic.[14]

Multilingualism is an additional factor that is also fundamental to language and communication in the Arab world. As a historical consequence of Western colonization and occupation (e.g., Morocco, Algeria), there is a high percentage of bilingual or multilingual individuals.[15,16] Many patois have adapted to these external influences, such as the French influence in Levant spoken in Lebanon and Morocco. Further, many schools and universities instruct in multiple languages, including English and French.

Socio-Economic Status, Education, and Literacy

Beyond linguistic differences, there are also many discrepancies between nations and regions in economic status as well as educational systems. These factors are all inextricably connected, as those who complete their high school degree tend to have more advanced Arabic comprehension and speaking skills than those with fewer years of education or less formal training.[17,18] Due to the fact that each educational system varies greatly by country in terms of quality, content, and teaching strategies, when conducting neuropsychological assessment it is essential to consider more than just the number of years studied when assessing level of education.[19] For example, in some countries it is not obligatory to attend preschool, and as such many children do not begin schooling until age 6. There may also be differences across countries and regions in terms of literacy rates. According to the World Bank,[20,21] 85% of men and 80% of women between 15 and 24 years of age are literate in the Arab world. Quality of education may largely be influenced by the socio-economic status (SES) of the region, as this can determine the caliber of training for professors, the infrastructure of school facilities, and the number of students per classroom. SES varies greatly from country to country, ranging from areas of high income due to natural resources (Gulf States) to more impoverished areas such as Sudan. Due to these differences, some have recommended factoring in both the quality of education as well as the level[22,23] and SES factors.

Religion

In the Arab world, a variety of religions are practiced. Islam, however, is the most practiced religion in the Arab world and the second most practiced religion in the world.[24] Followers of Islam, known as Muslims, believe that there is only one God and that Muhammad is the messenger of God's word, as is taught through the Quran. Often times the terms *Muslim world* and *Arabic world* are used interchangeably. It is important to make a distinction, however, as there are Muslim nations that do not pertain to the Arab world, such as Turkey, Afghanistan, and Pakistan.

Mental Health Views

The field of mental health in the Arab world faces significant barriers due to the stigma surrounding mental health disorders.[25] In our experience, people tend to seek services in severe cases and prefer receiving medicine over psychotherapy. Further, people living in the Arab world are more likely to report psychosomatic symptoms, such as headaches and stomach ailments.[26] The conversation surrounding the topic of mental health is also taboo and sensitive. Anecdotally, we once had the family of a patient ask that we not reveal our professional background to the patient so as not to alarm him.

Current State of Neuropsychology in the Arab World

Neuropsychology as a Science and Discipline in the Arab World

There is a clear bias in the amount of globally representative psychological research,[27,28] with the vast majority of research representing only 5% of the world population.[29] One way to avoid this bias and to improve our knowledge about the impact of cultural variables on neuropsychological performance is to study new cultures. Although clinical neuropsychology is not well developed in the Arab world, the number of neuropsychological studies has recently been increasing.

A systematic review conducted by Fasfous and colleagues[30] about the status of Neuropsychology in the Arab world revealed three major challenges: the scarcity of neuropsychological studies in the Arab world, the limited number of neuropsychological tests available for Arab populations, and the misuse of neuropsychological tests in research and practices. More recently, in a review of methodological practices for psychological testing in the Arab world, authors highlight that the majority (89%) of available tests have been translated or adapted from English using methods that are incompatible with the latest guidelines and standards.[31]

Neuropsychological Test Development and Validation in the Arab World

Despite the fact that the number of Arabic people in the world is far greater than the number of inhabitants in the United States, the majority of neuropsychological research and tests have been developed and validated in the United States. Further, many of those that have been normed and produced within the Arab world have not followed standard procedures for test translation and adaptation, making the true number of available tests much smaller.[30,31] In fact, of the 117 neuropsychological measures identified in the Arab world, only 57 provided normative scores. Of these 57 tests, 53 followed at least 3 of the principal criteria for test adaptation and validation, constituting only 55% of published neuropsychological measures.[30] It appears as though certain regions are following standard protocol for test adaptation more than others, as cognitive tests used in Jordanian publications represented 63% of those identified, followed by Lebanon (53%) and Libya (50%).

The amount of research in the Arab world has followed a similar pattern.[30] During the past years, there has been only an approximate rate of 7.7 publications per year of studies using cognitive measures with Arabic speakers, many of which were conducted in Egypt and nearly half a century ago. Fortunately, it seems that the number of publications is on the rise, beginning with 22 publications between 1961 and 1989 and later 204 from 2011 to 2015. Nonetheless, these studies are not all representative of the Arab context. The majority of these studies have been and continue to be conducted in Egypt, which took the lead with 45% of the studies included in the systematic review. Following Egypt, other countries such as Saudi Arabia and Tunisia have contributed a significant proportion as well (8.9% and 7.8%, respectively). Cross-country differences found in publication rates and test adaptation protocol may be related to the number of universities and the level of medical training offered at these institutions. These findings reflect the great need for the adaptation and validation of tests for new cultures[32,33] and a need for transparency regarding which tests are available for clinicians and researchers working with Arab individuals.

As previously detailed, there are a plethora of cultural biases on these tests that may impede an accurate diagnosis when used with the Arab population. The lack of tests not only hinders the development of Neuropsychology as a scientific discipline but also has a detrimental impact on patients with brain damage, both those living in their country of origin as well as those who have emigrated from the Arab world. In a review of the literature on available cognitive tests for Arab individuals, we found that there was a large variation in the quality of test adaptation. On the one hand, the adaptation of the MMSE in Tunisia[34] and Lebanon[35,36] met many of the criteria outlined by van de Vijver and Hambleton[37] as well as the standards for test development and adaptation.[38,39] These authors included back translations and piloting and even assessed the cultural adaption of both verbal and non-verbal measures.

On the contrary, other authors conducted a direct translation of some measures, which resulted in meaningless sentences in Arabic and a loss of construct validity. There is a general consensus that direct translations are not sufficient for the adaptation of psychological and neuropsychological tests which have been developed in and for another cultural context.[23,32] As such, the linguistic and cultural adaptations are fundamental to verifying the validity and reliability of the new version.[32] Many of the tests (e.g., Cambridge Cognitive Examination (CAMCOG), German Test

Battery of Attentional Performance for Children (KITAP), Arabic version of the Stroop Test, Motor-Free Visual Perception Test-Revised (MVPT-R)) have undergone a simple translation to Arabic without adapting the measures and validating the test for the Arabic population. Only seven of the identified 19 Arabic tests have been adequately adapted, including psychometric properties of validity, reliability and normative scores. For additional information about psychometric properties, cultural adaptation, and adequately adapted neuropsychological tests that could be properly used with Arabs, readers can refer to supplementary material published in Fasfous et al.[30] and Zeinoun et al.[31]

With these examples in mind, we believe that test validity and reliability are not sufficient, and tests must be carefully adapted for cultural differences in addition to following specific protocol for test translation. Critically, we have found that people of different cultures use different cognitive abilities to carry out the same task,[40] suggesting that there may be underlying cultural differences in the way we process information. With this in mind, we cannot assume that a test designed for a specific cognitive task is measuring the same skill-set in another population, even if the outcome in performance is similar. Construct validity may be useful when comparing the relevance of a task to measuring specific abilities.

Culturally Sensitive Training for Professionals in Neuropsychology

In addition to developing and validating culturally informed instruments for cognitive evaluation, it is imperative to bolster specialized training in the field of cross-cultural neuropsychology. This work is necessary both for professionals living in the Arab world, as well as neuropsychologists outside of the Arab world who may test patients of Arab origin. For the latter, it would be helpful for practicing professionals to have easy access to cultural information relevant to neuropsychological performance in Arabic individuals.

Most graduate programs in the Arab world do not include a specialization in neuropsychology, and those who wish to gain specific training must study outside the Arab world. As a consequence, the evaluation of neuropsychological impairment caused by brain injury or dementia is principally managed by neurologists and psychiatrists. Nonetheless, as time has gone on, there has been a significant growth in post-graduate psychologists who are specialized in evaluations. As a result, there has been an appropriate shift in who administers cognitive tests, and trained psychologists have begun to acquire more and more responsibility in this sector.

As new programs in graduate-level psychology continue to emerge in the Arab world, efforts should be made to emphasize the importance of valid cognitive testing in their training. These programs may consider developing a board of accreditation, similar to that of the American Board of Professional Psychology/American Board of Clinical Neuropsychology, to ensure a minimum standardization in the level of training for professionals. This would ideally be organized in unison with all Arab countries, so that each region would be able to contribute to determining standard protocol for teaching, practicing, and adhering to standard international guidelines for neuropsychological assessments, such as those by the American Educational Research Association[38,41] and the International Test Commission.[32] Establishing a board may also give way to organizing seminars and conferences in Arab countries so that professionals and academics may exchange information and further promote a cross-culturally sensitive protocol. Promoting international exchange could also potentially lead to the creation of professional groups for neuropsychological testing, leading to improved cross-cultural test adaptation, development and validation. Through these collaborations, Arabic speaking neuropsychologists may also be able to connect with linguists to create Arabic word-databases in order to develop language-based cognitive measures, such as vocabulary or wordlist memory tasks. Offering a platform to Arabic speaking neuropsychologists would allow professionals to share their experience about every-day practice and the different strategies they use for local populations. This could potentially lead to an open-access depository of translated tests and localized normative scores.

While development of accreditation boards and exchanges requires much coordination and time, there have been some notable efforts in this direction. One such example is the "Neurodevelopmental Care for Refugees (NeuCare)" which was launched in 2020 in order to design and implement a higher diploma program about neurodevelopment focused on refugee children for professionals involved in their care. The course, which is currently being developed at universities in Palestine (Bethlehem University and Hebron University) and Jordan (the University of Petra and Al-Yarmouk University) includes modules about brain and neuropsychological development, detection of neuropsychological problems, and cross-culturally sensitive instruments for detection. Further, it includes a teaching module to guarantee the sustainability of the project by means of qualifying students as trainers for new course editions. Due to a dearth of professionals trained in psychology, students will also be recruited from the departments of Social Work and Education to be trained in the latest advances on neurodevelopment applied to refugee children. In order to avoid competence conflicts with national professional regulations, qualifications based on competences will be adopted and modules will have different profiles for psychologists, social workers and teachers. The NeuCare project is thus a pioneering push in the way of universalizing a cross-culturally sensitive and standardized protocol of neuropsychological care in the public sphere of the Arab world.

Considerations for Neuropsychological Assessment in Arab Populations

While research dedicated to the specific cultural biases of neuropsychological tests for Arabic individuals is still nascent, findings in the existing literature may help to guide researchers and practitioners in detecting some of the central concerns. Below we will highlight some of the cultural uniquities found in cognitive test performance with Arabic individuals pulling from both empirical and anecdotal evidence.

Construct Relevance

After a plethora of studies demonstrating differences in neuropsychological testing between individuals of diverse cultures, the question arises as to whether we are measuring what we are claiming to measure. In other words, does the executive functioning task that was created in North America also measure executive functioning in Jordanians, even after it has been translated to Arabic? In one of our studies, we found that a Spanish and a Moroccan sample used different neuropsychological processes to achieve the same task on a test for non-verbal intelligence. If we apply these results to the field of Cross-Cultural Neuropsychology, perhaps we should begin with determining the concept of cognitive functions (for example, What is intelligence according to the members of this culture?), and only after should we develop the tools necessary to measure these constructs.

These questions resurface some of the oldest and central dilemmas of neuropsychological testing, which is critical to ensuring "fairness," as termed by the Standards for Educational and Psychological Tests.[41] In the absence of a sufficient number of cognitive tests that can ensure construct relevance to the Arab world, it is essential that researchers and practitioners inform themselves about these specific differences so that they may take extra precautions during testing. In practice, whenever possible, practitioners should select and use tests that have adequate construct validity to avoid this problem (for more information about available tests with adequate construct validity for Arab populations, see Zeinoun et al.[31] Further, neuropsychologists should follow APA recommendations when providing psychological services for individuals from different cultural backgrounds. Along these lines, there are different alternatives for standardized neuropsychological testing which could offer a more holistic view on cognitive performance in Arab populations. For example, Naturalistic testing (i.e., assessing behavior in a natural setting) could serve as an alternative method of measuring psychological variables.[42] Multiple and collateral interviews (such as parents, friends, teachers) may also offer pertinent qualitative information to understand the patient's status in their historical context. Ideally, the practitioner will be able to apply a mixed-methods approach, in which both qualitative and quantitative variables are interpreted. Mixed-method strategies may help clarify the construct being assessed and offer salient information relative to the patient's behavior and performance in his/her cultural context. Moreover, applying and comparing more than one neuropsychological test to measure the same function could help practitioners in validating their results.

Test Familiarity

As is widely noted in the literature, test comfort and familiarity are important predictors of neuropsychological performance.[23,43] Familiarity with standardized testing is especially relevant in the Arab world, considering the general population is not as accustomed to taking timed and standardized tests as compared to people in other countries, such as the United States. We will highlight some of the main concerns of test familiarity and why they are relevant to testing with Arab individuals.

In one of our studies, 80% of the Moroccan and 20% of the Spanish participants reported having never taken a psychological test.[41] In this same study, we found differences between the two groups on cognitive measures, and we hypothesized that the difference in familiarity may have impacted in the group performance.[44] One possible explanation is that Moroccans relied more on complex executive functioning skills as compared to Spaniards when performing a non-verbal intelligence task due to the fact that they are not familiar with this type of test. This coincides with previous studies, which have demonstrated that processing novel stimuli is related to increased cognitive control and activation of the prefrontal cortex.[45-7]. In other words, the Moroccan sample may have coped with the unfamiliar task by recruiting complex neuropsychological processes. This example highlights the impact of test familiarity on test performance.

Considering these findings, it may be useful for practitioners to ensure that patients clearly understand the test instructions and spend ample time in the sample trials prior to beginning the evaluation. Practitioners could also inquire about the patient's subjective experience with standardized timed testing to gauge how this may influence their performance.

Patient History

Since the number and quality of neuropsychological tests available for Arab populations are limited, all evaluations should include an extensive qualitative analysis about the individual's history and background. Considering the strong social ties between friends and family in the Arab world, it may be helpful to gather information from those who are involved in the patient's day to day care. On the other hand, it is important to note that many children in the Arab world have been exposed to distinct environmental insults that can affect their neurodevelopment. Among these factors is the exposure to war violence (e.g., Palestine and Iraq) or poverty and malnutrition, (e.g., Mauritania and Somalia). These factors have been related to neurodevelopmental problems.[48,49] This may develop during childhood and adolescence and later have influence throughout life, including impact on academic performance, professional status and mental health during adulthood.[50] As such, inquiring about these relevant details may be important when determining the possible causal mechanisms for alterations among patients.

Language Considerations

There are various factors to examine when considering the potential effect of language on cognitive performance in Arabic individuals. Beyond the aforementioned characteristics involving multilingualism and "code-switching," the Arabic script poses important differences from English and many Western languages in which most cognitive tests have been originally developed. One of these variables is the direction of the script, as Arabic is written and read from right to left. Some studies have shown that the direction of attentional biases can develop differently depending on these two ways of writing.[51] Further, another study has shown that the perception of time, including in which direction the past and the future move, is related to the direction in which one writes.[52] This reveals another subtle yet potentially decisive factor in neuropsychological performance of Arabic individuals, as multiple cognitive domains may be influenced by this directionality. As such, it is important for practitioners to consider the direction of the stimulus being presented when assessing Arab populations. For example, in tests measuring attention (such as the "cancelation task"), speed of processing, and reaction time, stimuli are often presented from left to right. Wherever possible, it is preferable for practitioners to apply tests that have adapted the direction to read from right to left, or to present stimuli on the right side, in an effort to reduce directional biases.

In addition to direction, the length of the words may also influence scores. Arabic dialects are often shorter than the Classic form of Arabic, and it is possible that individuals are able to name fewer words if they must do so in Classic Arabic because it takes them longer to pronounce all of them. Along these lines, other research comparing children from Lebanon and Holland found that differences in a digit task disappeared when controlling for the pronunciation speed. In light of these differences, practitioners should give precedence to assessing the patient in his or her native dialect when applying verbal tests such as verbal memory and fluency.

In addition, careful consideration must be taken with *how* neuropsychological tests are translated. As previously mentioned, there are many different dialects in the Arab world, some of which are incomprehensible to others. Further, some individuals may speak an Arabic dialect, but may not fully understand the formal Classic Arabic. As such, we recommend that when validating or adapting a new test, researchers and practitioners strictly follow the International Test Commission guidelines for test translation and adaptation. When carrying out these procedures, we also advise including an expert panel of individuals from different countries who are also experienced in psychological testing. A diverse representation of experts in cognitive assessment will help ensure that construct validity is being maintained and that the translated version is as culturally sensitive as possible. An example of an adequate adaptation and translation is the English verbal fluency test, FAS. Instead of using the same three letters to assess verbal fluency as are used in the English version (FAS), the Arabic version has included three letters (WRG) for which there is a comparable level of frequency in the verbal and written Arabic language.[53] It may be helpful for practitioners to pay special attention to how adaptations were made before applying them to ensure they have followed a similar protocol.

Bilingualism

There is extensive evidence that bilingualism can affect neuropsychological functioning and performance.[54,55] Due to a long history of colonization and Western occupation in the Arab world, there is a high percentage of bilingual or multilingual individuals (e.g., Morocco, Tunisia, Lebanon). As a consequence, individuals living in largely multilingual areas often resort to 'code-switching' (i.e., alternating between different languages within the same phrase or conversation). These authentic modes of communication surface the novel need for multilingual assessments, especially considering the scientific evidence that bilingualism is relevant to test and norm selection.[55,56] As anecdotal evidence of this phenomenon, we are facing particular difficulty in adapting certain neuropsychological measures for the Moroccan population. In addition to differences in preferred language by region, within regions individuals often mix multiple languages into their speech and have even integrated numbers into their script to accommodate vowel sounds that are not easily pronounced or reflected in the traditional Arabic language.

As we mentioned before, another important factor is the Arabic dialect, which in many cases could be considered as a second language. Instructions, performance, and norms could vary between classic Arabic and dialect. In fact, we have found in our clinical experience that children and adults perform better on fluency tests when using the dialect language. The literature has also reflected performance differences rooted in language. In a cross-cultural study conducted by Shebani et al.[57] to compare memory performance between Dutch and Arab children from Libya, they found that Dutch children outscored Arab children. However, when word length and pronunciation speed were controlled, the difference disappeared.

Considering the implications that bilingual- or multilingualism can have on neuropsychological performance, there are several approaches practitioners may take in order to reduce linguistic biases based. First, it is preferable for multilingual neuropsychologists to assess multilingual clients, as they are better equipped to resolve doubts about testing protocol and material. Further, it may be helpful for practitioners to assess language proficiency or to ask the participant in which language he or she feels most comfortable. This information can inform test selection, where practitioners may give precedence to tests available in the preferred language. On the other hand, practitioners may also consider applying multiple tests in different languages to evaluate the same function, especially when they face challenges in finding tests that are adequately validated and culturally adapted.

Timed Tests

In line with the importance of test familiarity, there are also cultural differences in terms of having to complete a certain task within a given amount of time. In some Arabic cultures, such as in Morocco, teachers often organize the school day according to how well children have grasped the subject and will not move on to the next topic until it has been fully comprehended by all. Further, students are usually given as much time as they need to complete exams. As such, when presented with timed testing demands, these individuals may not feel the same urgency, may experience more pressure or stress, or may not be able to organize their time in a fashion that would allow them to complete the task successfully. In line with these, we have found cultural differences between Moroccans and other cultural groups on timed tests that were once deemed to be "culture-free." In the case of the CCTT, Moroccan children took significantly longer than average North American children to complete the tasks.[58] The difference was so great that if we were to apply the North American normative scores to our sample, they would have appeared to be in the clinically impaired range (even after controlling for age, education level, and gender). Cross-cultural differences in timed testing have also been found in other cultures that do not share the same perception of time.[59] Due to these apparent discrepancies on the basis of time constraints, we urge practitioners to keep this in mind when interpreting the results of neuropsychological testing. It may not be that the patient is not able to correctly complete the task, but rather his/her past experience has taught her to complete it differently (i.e., giving precedence to variables other than speed).

Considering the cultural differences in time perception, practitioners may consider selecting both timed and non-timed tests to evaluate the same domains. Further, they may even measure the patient's subjective experience of time in order to understand how it may influence their test performance. To the best of our knowledge, there is only one measure (COTI-33) to assess this variable.[60] While this measure is currently not available in Arabic, is it currently being translated and cross-cultural adapted for Arabic populations. Finally, as previously mentioned, it is important for practitioners to ensure that patients comprehend test instructions. Spending extra time on sample trials may aid practitioners in this effort.

Acculturation

Acculturation is a complex process in which psychological and cultural adaptations must be made to better assimilate into the new environment. Through the acculturation and assimilation process, individuals must learn to cope with the stressors of a new and unknown environment, and in the case of refugees and asylum seekers, learn how to cope with past traumas in an entirely new context. Acculturation plays a fundamental role in the neuropsychological performances of ethnic minorities and/or immigrants who live outside of their country of origin.[61-3]

As the percentage of Arab-speaking individuals living outside of the Arab world continues to grow, there is an increasing need to develop neuropsychological tests that are sensitive to one's native culture but that also take into account the new cultural influences of living in a novel place. When looking at the literature related to neuropsychological performance of healthy Arab adults living outside their country,[64,65] it would be safe to assume that tests that have not yet been culturally adapted could potentially erroneously diagnose Arab individuals as having neuropsychological sequelae consistent with brain damage. For this reason, it is important to administrate validated and adapted tests in the assessment process. Even if the practitioner discerns that the patient has a good level of the language spoken in the host country, he/she cannot assume that the help of a translator will solve this problem. Language is not the sole measure for level of acculturation, and the practitioner must be aware of a variety of cultural biases that could influence one's performance. In a meta-analysis regarding acculturation and its impact on cognitive testing, a series of acculturation factors are highlighted as relevant to neuropsychological testing.[66] Acculturation can be seen as a multidimensional process that occurs in different "domains" and can vary depending on one's life situation and developmental stage. Typically, these "domains" include variables such as language proficiency, ethnic identity, media preferences, and eating habits.[67] Beyond these variables, others highlight *proxies* of acculturation (e.g., years of residency), which oftentimes branches into other sociocultural constructs (such as SES).[66] Practitioners may include an analysis of these domains in the clinical interview and through questionnaires to consider their level of acculturation and how it could influence performance when interpreting test results.

Ideally, practitioners would also be able to use validated tests and norms for the individual's dominant culture. Yet despite growing efforts, there remains an urgent need to create construct-relevant neuropsychological tests as well as appropriate norms for each cultural group. In the absence of these tools, practitioners and researchers alike should consider the level of acculturation through qualitative interviews and how that may influence their performance on traditional cognitive testing.

Educational Level and Quality of Education

Educational level is traditionally one of the central variables to control in neuropsychology and cultural neuropsychology. However, educational levels (as counted by years of education) could be affected by the differences in educational systems around the world. For example, in some countries, preschool education is obligatory and in others it is not.

The central clinical implications of not attending preschool are two-fold: (1) accuracy in measuring abnormalities in learning abilities and (2) difficulties in comparing performance with normative scores. If children do not receive preschool training, they may not develop the skills needed to perform well on neuropsychological tests commonly used to assess for learning disabilities and writing skills. Thus, poor scores may be interpreted as delays or abnormalities, when in reality they simply may not have received specific training. With regard to the latter, it may be difficult to compare their results to normative scores, which are typically based on educational level. Without a proper comparison group, practitioners may face important barriers when making a clinical interpretation of their performance.

In addition, the quality of education plays an important role in neuropsychological functioning and performance. Reading ability is widely used to evaluate quality of education among English speakers. However, calculation skills could be an alternative approach to evaluate the quality of education among Arab individuals. It has been suggested to use non-verbal tests to assess cognitive performance in culturally diverse individuals due to the supposition that they depend less on language capacity.[68] In a previous study, we found that even after controlling for the traditional confounding variables of acculturation, occupational social class, and IQ, non-verbal abilities (such as calculation skills) remained a significant predictor of neuropsychological performance between different cultural groups[69] however, these differences disappeared after controlling for calculation skills. Therefore, we think that calculation as measured by an adequately adapted calculation test skills could be used to evaluate the quality of education among non-English speakers as they may differ depending on the educational system of each country.

In our cross-cultural research on verbal memory, we found differences in performance between Spanish-speaking children from Ecuador and Moroccan children.[70] When conducting a deeper analysis of these differences, we came across important uniquities in the educational system and teaching methodology that may have influenced the discrepancies we found. In Morocco, children are taught to repeat aloud everything they have learned in class, which may in turn contribute to strengthening their verbal memory capacity. It is possible that this teaching method, which emphasizes the communication of memorized material, strengthens verbal memory capacities over other cognitive abilities (such as reasoning and planning) that may be fomented more by other didactic methodologies that focus on critical analysis and synthesis of information.

Socio-Economic Status

As we have alluded to before, SES is an important variable to be considered in neuropsychological test performance. Considering the vast differences found in SES between the 22 countries making up the Arab world, it is especially relevant for practitioners evaluating Arab populations to use normative scores that are representative of their historical context. In a recent study conducted by Lozano et al.,[71] researchers found differences in non-verbal IQ tests between normative scores of children from different Arabic-speaking countries (Morocco and Oman). Critically, about 8% of the healthy Morrocan sample of children were misclassified as intellectually impaired when applying the Omani norms of the Raven Test. These findings highlight not only the urgent need to develop culturally sensitive normative scores but also the need for practitioners to apply scores that best reflect their patient's background.

In light of a trend toward a more globalized world and growth in Arab immigration, clinicians will have to take on more patients from different cultures, likely outnumbering the amount of culturally representative tests and normative scores. While these demographic fluctuations can be expected to happen at a much quicker pace than appropriate test development, practitioners can take into account the variables highlighted throughout this chapter (bilingualism, acculturation, quality and level of education, SES) in order to make cultural adaptations to testing protocol and interpretation.

Conclusion

In Arabic countries, few neuropsychological studies have been conducted, and the number of available neuropsychological tests that are culturally adequate is small. To further compound this issue, cultural differences in neuropsychological test performance exist (both in adults and in children) within Arabic countries as well as between individuals from different Arab countries.

In this chapter, we have highlighted some of the important cultural differences that may influence test performance, such as teaching methodologies and the perception of time. Teaching methodologies have been found to impact the types of cognitive domains that are reinforced, while time perception has been associated with performance on timed neuropsychological tests. Further, research has shown that Arabic individuals may use different cognitive abilities to complete the same task on a neuropsychological test.[40] As such, construct relevance must be considered by all practitioners and researchers working with Arabic individuals. In addition to selecting validated and adapted neuropsychological tests during the assessment, it may be helpful to employ subtests for IQ that have demonstrated adequate construct validity. For example, the Stanford Binet and WAIS have been validated in different Arab countries such as Egypt, Jordan, and Saudi Arabia, and the subtests of these instruments could be used in neuropsychological testing for Arab individuals (see Refs. 30, 31 for more detail on available validated tests).

An additional central finding is that verbal tests and non-verbal tests are not "culture-free," and using these types of tests can lead to diagnostic errors in Arab children and adults. Therefore, tests must undergo an extensive and detailed adaptation before they can be used properly. Due to these cultural biases, practitioners may consider employing a few different strategies. On the one hand, practitioners may use various tests to evaluate the same function and analyze results both qualitatively and quantitatively. Ideally, practitioners will be able to use a mixed-method approach in which he or she combines both objective quantitative data from standardized neuropsychological tests (in the best case, adapted, and validated with representative normative scores) with qualitative information on the patient's history. Qualitative analysis can be done by pulling from external resources, such as by collecting information from the family or school teachers. Finally, we consider it important for practitioners to mention the challenges and limitations of testing in the neuropsychological report so that interpretations are made with precaution.

Despite the challenges mentioned in this chapter for Arab neuropsychologists working in the Arab world as well other Arab neuropsychologists working with Arab patients around the world, the field of neuropsychology in the Arab world has been emerging. In the last 20 years, a number of neuropsychological studies and initiatives, projects, and programs have been implemented with the objective of improving the field of neuropsychology in the Arab world. Notably, among these initiatives is the NeuCare project, which is an international collaborative effort centered on the development of a graduate program about neurodevelopment. This project will help qualify Arabic-speaking clinical neuropsychologists as well as formalize a standardized training for professionals in the Arab world.

Many of these challenges can be addressed by the need for an international Arabic board that can establish standardized cross-cultural training for neuropsychologists in the Arab world as well as develop testing protocols and guidelines for the Arabic population. The APA guidelines for working with people of different cultures may serve as a reference point in this initiative. The creation of such a body may also be useful in connecting professionals across the Arab world to discuss central issues in evaluation and treatment and to develop new neuropsychological programs for researchers and practitioners. The aforementioned national and international efforts are leading the field of neuropsychology in this direction toward a more culturally representative and conscientious science and practice.

References

1. Barakat H. Al-mujtam'al-arabi al-mu'asir: Bahth fi taghayyor alahual waa'al'alaqat [The modern Arab society: Research on changing situations and relations]. Beirut: Center for Arab Unity Studies; 2008.
2. Hammad A, Kysia, R, Rabah, R, Hassoun, R, Connelly M. Guide to Arab culture: health care delivery to the Arab American community. Dearborn (MI): Arab Community Center for Economic and Social Services (ACCESS); 1999.
3. Harb C. The Arab region: cultures, values, and identities. In: Amer MM, Awad, GH. Handbook of Arab American psychology. New York (NY): Routledge; 2015. p. 23–38.
4. World Bank. Population Total—Arab World. The World Bank Data [Internet]. 2019. Retrieved April 8, 2021 from: https://data.worldbank.org/indicator/SP.POP.TOTL?locations=1A
5. UNICEF. MENA Generation 2030 [Internet]. Division of Data, Research and Policy: United Nations Children's Fund; 2019 April. Retrieved from: https://www.unicef.org/mena/reports/mena-generation-2030
6. United Nations Relief and Works Agency for Palestine Refugees in the Near East (UNRWA). 2019 December. Retrieved from: https://www.unrwa.org/where-we-work/lebanon
7. Bogic M, Njoku A, Priebe, S. Long-term mental health of war-refugees: a systematic literature review. BMC Int Health Hum Rights. 2015;15(1):1–41.
8. Munyandamutsa N, Nkubamugisha PM, Gex-Fabry, M, Eytan, A. Mental and physical health in Rwanda 14 years after the genocide. Soc Psychiatry Psychiatr Epidemiol. 2012;47(11):1753–61.
9. Abdullahi I, Leonard H, Cherian S, Mutch R, Glasson EJ, de Klerk N, et al. The risk of neurodevelopmental disabilities in children of immigrant and refugee parents: current knowledge and directions for future research. Rev J Autism Dev Disord. 2018;5(1);29–42.
10. Turley, MR, Obrzut JE. Neuropsychological effects of posttraumatic stress disorder in children and adolescents. Can J Sch Psychol. 2012;27(2):166–82.
11. Arab American Institute. Where do Arab American live? [Internet]. 2017. Available from: https://www.aaiusa.org/demographics
12. Buckwalter T, Parkinson D. A frequency dictionary of Arabic: core vocabulary for learners. New York (NY): Routledge; 2010.
13. Ibrahim R, Eviatar Z, Aharon-Peretz J. The characteristics of Arabic orthography slow its processing. Neuropsychology. 2002;16(3):322–6.
14. Zaborowski JR. From Coptic to Arabic in medieval Egypt. Mediev Encount. 2007;14(1);15–40.
15. Aabi M. The syntax of Arabic and French code switching in Morocco. Cham, Switzerland: Palgrave Macmillan; 2020.
16. Amazouz D, Adda-Decker M, Lamel L. Addressing code-switching in French/Algerian Arabic speech. In Annual Conference of the International Speech Communication Association, ISCA. Stockholm, Sweden. 2017. pp. 62–6.
17. Abu-Rabia S. Effects of exposure to literary Arabic on reading comprehension in a diglossic situation. Reading and Writing. 2000;13:147–57.
18. Assaf AS. Palestinian students' attitudes towards modern standard Arabic and Palestinian City Arabic. RELC. 2001;32(2):45–62.
19. Mahmoud OM. Neuropsychological assessment in the Arab World: Observations and challenges. International Neuropsychological Society Liaison Committee Bulletin. 2015;35(1):4–6.
20. World Bank. Literacy Rates, Youth Female (% of Females Ages 15–24)—Arab World. World Bank Data. 2020; Retrieved April 9, 2021 from https://data.worldbank.org/indicator/SE.ADT.1524.LT.FE.ZS?locations=1A

21. World Bank. Literacy Rates, Youth Male (% of Males Ages 15–24)—Arab World. World Bank Data. 2020; Retrieved April 9, 2021 from https://data.worldbank.org/indicator/SE.ADT.1524.LT.MA. ZS?locations=1A

22. Lezak MD, Howieson DB, Loring DW. Neuropsychological assessment. 4th ed. New York (NY): Oxford University Press; 2004.

23. Puente AE, Pérez-García M, Vilar-Lopez R, Hidalgo-Ruzzante N, Fasfous AF. Neuropsychological assessment of culturally and educationally dissimilar individuals. In: Paniagua F, Yamada AM, editors. Handbook of multicultural mental health: assessment and treatment of diverse population. 2nd ed. New York (NY): Elsevier; 2013. pp. 225–41.

24. Maoz Z, Henderso EA. The world religion dataset, 1945–2010: logic, estimates, and trends. Int Interact. 2013;39(3):265–91.

25. Zolezzi M, Alamri M, Shaar S, Rainkie D. Stigma associated with mental illness and its treatment in the Arab culture: A systematic review. Int J Soc Psychiatry. 2018;64(6):597–609.

26. Al-Krenawi A. Mental health practice in Arab countries. Curr Opin Psychiatry. 2005;18(5):560–4.

27. Chiao JY. Cultural neuroscience: a once and future discipline. Prog Brain Res. 2009;178:287–304.

28. Puente AE, Pérez-García M. Handbook of multicultural mental health. In: Cuellar I, Paniagua FA, editors. Neuropsychological assessment of ethnic minorities: clinical issues. New York (NY): Academic Press; 2000. pp. 419–35.

29. Arnett JJ. The neglected 95%: why American psychology needs to become less American. Am Psychol. 2008;63(7):602–14.

30. Fasfous AF, Al-Joudi HF, Puente AE, Pérez-García M. Neuropsychological measures in the Arab world: a systematic review. Neuropsychol Rev. 2017;27(2):158–73.

31. Zeinoun P, Iliescu D, El Hakim R. Psychological tests in Arabic: a review of methodological practices and recommendations for future use. Neuropsychol Rev. 2021; 1–19. doi: 10.1007/s11065-021-09476-6

32. Grégoire J. International Test Commission. Corsini Encycl Psychol. 2010. doi: 10.1002/9780470479216.corpsy0460

33. Echemendia RJ, Harris JG. (2004). Neuropsychological test use with Hispanic/Latin populations in the United States: part II of a national survey. Appl Neuropsychol. 2004;11(1):4–12.

34. Bellaj T, Ben Jemaa S, Attia-Romdhane N, Dhiffallah M, Ben Ali N, Bouaziz M, Mrabet A. Version Arabe du Mini Mental State Examination (A-MMSE): Fidélité, validité et données normatives [Mini Mental State Examination Arabic version (A-MMSE): reliability, validity and normative data]. La Tunisie Medicale. 2008;86(7):768–76. Retrieved from http://www.latunisiemedicale.com

35. Abou-Mrad F, Tarabey L, Zamrini E, Pasquier F, Chelune G, Fadel P, Hayek M. Sociolinguistic reflection on neuropsychological assessment: an insight into selected culturally adapted battery of Lebanese Arabic cognitive testing. Neurol Sci. 2015;36(10):1813–22.

36. Zamrini E, Abou-Mrad F, Duff K, Pasquier F, Kawas C, Chelune, G et al. Normative data on dementia screening tests in an elderly Lebanese sample. Alzheimers Dement. 2014;10(4): 723. doi:10.1016/j.jalz.2014.05.1341

37. van de Vijver F, Hambleton RK. Translating tests: some practical guidelines. Eur Psychol. 1996;1(2):89–99.

38. AERA, NCME [American Educational Research Association, American Psychological Association ve National Council on Measurement in Education]. Standards for Educational and Psychological Testing. Washington, DC: American Educational Research Association; 1999.

39. American Psychological Association. APA Task Force on Psychological Assessment and Evaluation Guidelines. APA Guidelines for Psychological Assessment and Evaluation. APA; 2020. Retrieved from: https://www.apa.org/about/policy/guidelines-psychological-assessment-evaluation.pdf

40. Fasfous AF, Hidalgo-Ruzzante N, Vilar-López R, Catena-Martínez A, Pérez-García M. Cultural differences in neuropsychological abilities required to perform intelligence tasks. Arch Clin Neuropsychol. 2013;28(8):784–90.

41. American Educational Research Association, American Psychological Association, National Council on Measurement in Education, editors. Standards for educational and psychological testing. Lanham, MD; 2014.

42. Merrell KW. Assessment of children's social skills: recent developments, best practices, and new directions. Exceptionality. 2001;9(1–2):3–18.

43. Ardila A. Cultural values underlying psychometric cognitive testing. Neuropsychol Rev. 2005; 15(4):185–95.

44. Díaz A, Sellami K, Infanzón E, Lanzón T, Lynn R. A comparative study of general intelligence in Spanish and Moroccan samples. Span J Psychol. 2012;15(2):526–32.

45. Barcelo F, Escera C, Corral MJ, Periáñez, JA. Task switching and novelty processing activate a common neural network for cognitive control. J Cogn Neurosci. 2006;18(10):1734–48.

46. Kishiyama MM, Yonelinas AP, Knight RT. Novelty enhancements in memory are dependent on lateral prefrontal cortex. J Neurosci. 2009;29(25):8114–8.

47. Løvstad M, Funderud I, Lindgren M, Endestad T, Due-Tønnessen P, Meling T et al. Contribution of subregions of human frontal cortex to novelty processing. J Cogn Neurosci. 2011;24(2):378–95.

48. Abu Zaydeh H, Zalina I, Wan A, Aljeesh Y. Visual spatial and executive functions disorders among Palestinian children living under chronic stress in Gaza. IUG J Nat Eng Stud. 2012;20(2):55–71. Available from: http://www.iugaza.edu.ps/ar/periodical/

49. El Hioui M, Azzaoui FZ, Touhami Ahami AO, Rusinek S, Aboussaleh Y. Iron deficiency and cognitive function among Moroccan school children. Nutr Ther Metab. 2012;30(2):84–9.

50. Shonkoff JP. Building a new biodevelopmental framework to guide the future of early childhood policy. Child Dev. 2010;81(1):357–67.

51. Maass A, Russo A. Directional bias in the mental representation of spatial events: nature or culture?. Psychol Sci. 2003;14(4):296–301.

52. Ouellet M, Santiago J, Israeli Z, Gabay S. Is the future the right time?. Exp Psychol. 2010;57(4):308–14. doi:10.1027/1618-3169/a000036.

53. Khalil MS. Preliminary Arabic normative data of neuropsychological tests: the verbal and design fluency. J Clin Exp Neuropsychol. 2010;32(9):1028–35.

54. Gollan TH, Fennema-Notestine C, Montoya RI, Jernigan TL. The bilingual effect on Boston Naming Test performance. J Int Neuropsychol Soc. 2007;13(2):197–208.

55. Puente AE, Zink DN, Hernandez M, Jackman Venanzi T, Ardila A. Bilingualism and its impact on psychological assessment. In: Benuto L, editor. Guide to psychological assessment with Hispanics. New York (NY): Springer; 2013. pp. 15–31.

56. Ardila A. Language representation and working memory with bilinguals. J Commun Disord. 2003;36(3):233–40.

57. Shebani, MF, van de Vijver FJ, Poortinga YH. Memory development in Libyan and Dutch school children. Eur J Dev Psychol. 2008;5(4):419–38. doi:10.1080/17405620701343204.

58. Fasfous AF, Puente AE, Pérez-Marfil MN, Cruz-Quintana F, Peralta-Ramírez MI, Pérez-García M. Is the color trails culture free? Arch Clin Neuropsychol. 2013;28(7):743–9.

59. Agranovich AV, Puente AE. Do Russian and American normal adults perform similarly on neuropsychological tests? Preliminary findings on the relationship between culture and test performance. Arch Clin Neuropsych. 2007;22(3):273–82.

60. Agranovich AV, Panter AT, Puente AE, Touradji P. The culture of time in neuropsychological assessment: exploring the effects of culture-specific time attitudes on timed test performance in Russian and American samples. J Int Neuropsychol Soc. 2011;17(4):692–701.

61. Boone KB, Victor TL, Wen J, Razani J, Pontón M. The association between neuropsychological scores and ethnicity, language, and acculturation variables in a large patient population. Arch Clin Neuropsychol. 2007;22(3):355–65.

62. Coffey DM, Marmol L, Schock L, Adams W. The influence of acculturation on the Winconsin Card Sorting Test by Mexican Americans. Arch Clin Neuropsychol. 2005;20(6):795–803.

63. Saez PA, Bender HA, Barr WB, Mindt MR, Morrison CE, Hassenstab J et al. The impact of education and acculturation on nonverbal neuropsychological test performance among Latino/a patients with epilepsy. Appl Neuropsychol Adult. 2014;21(2):108–19.

64. Daugherty JC, Puente AE, Fasfous AF, Hidalgo-Ruzzante N, Pérez-Garcia M. Diagnostic mistakes of culturally diverse individuals when using North American neuropsychological tests. Appl Neuropsychol Adult. 2017;24(1):16–22.

65. Stanczak DE, Stanczak EM, Awadalla AW. Development and initial validation of an Arabic version of the Expanded Trail Making Test: implications for cross-cultural assessment. Arch Clin Neuropsychol. 2001;16(2):141–9.

66. Tan YW, Burgess GH, Green RJ. The effects of acculturation on neuropsychological test performance: a systematic literature review. Clin Neuropsychol. 2020;5(3):541–71.

67. Celenk O, Van de Vijver FJ. Assessment of acculturation: issues and overview of measures. ORPC. 2011;8(1):1–22.

68. Kellogg CE, Morton NW. Revisited beta examinationThird edition. San Antonio, TX: Psychological Corporation; 1999.

69. Fasfous AF, Hidalgo-Ruzzante N, Vilar-López R, Gálvez-Lara M, Pérez-García, M. Mathematical achievement as a proxy for measuring quality of education among non-Native English speakers. Bethlehem Univ. J. 2017;34:113–28.

70. Fasfous A. Neuropsicología cultural en población árabe: evaluación en adultos y niños [Dissertation]. Granada: Universidad de Granada; 2014.

71. Lozano-Ruiz A, Fasfous AF, Ibanez-Casas I, Cruz-Quintana, F, Perez-Garcia M, Pérez-Marfil, MN. Cultural bias in intelligence assessment using a culture-free test in Moroccan children. Arch Clin Neuropsychol. 2021; acab005. doi:10.1093/arclin/acab005

Lebanese

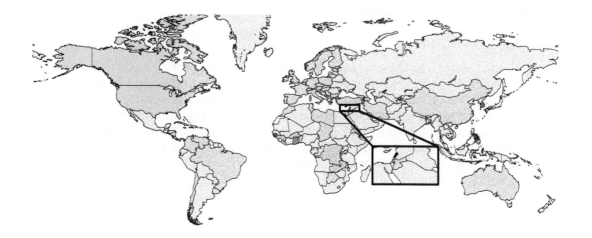

10 Neuropsychological Evaluation of the Lebanese Examinee

Considerations for Multiple Cultures, Multiple Languages, and Multiple Religions

Karim Yamout

Section I: Background Information

Terminology and Perspective

People of Lebanon are referred to as Lebanese and belong to the broader Middle Eastern heritage. My perspective about Lebanon and Lebanese patients comes from being a bilingual (Arabic and English) speaking Lebanese immigrant who traveled to the United States as an adult after completing undergraduate studies and two years of research and clinical training in Psychology in Lebanon. My clinical practice with Lebanese examinees is informed by my clinical and personal experience in Lebanon as well as by my graduate training in Clinical Psychology and Neuropsychology in the United States. I currently provide forensic and clinical services in a private outpatient setting in the Southeastern United States.

Geography

Lebanon is a country in the Middle East.[1] The Mediterranean Sea borders it on the West and it is engulfed otherwise by land. According to Lebanon's Ministry of Tourism website, Lebanon measures about 4,000 square miles with a population of 4.4 million.

History

Lebanon was under a French Mandate until its official independence in November of 1943. As such, there is much French influence. For example, while Arabic is the official language of Lebanon, French continues to be a form of second official language. Political turmoil plagues the history of Lebanon. An accounting of the wars and political tensions is beyond the scope of this chapter. However, it is valuable to note that the Lebanese population has experienced a variety of potentially individual and inter-generational trauma from war and political tensions.

People

In addition to Lebanese nationals, about 4% of the Lebanese population is of Armenian heritage.[2] Further, there is a sizeable Syrian and Palestinian refugee population.[3]

Immigration and Relocation

Lebanese migration is a common occurrence and a topic of both humor (e.g., jokes, humorous experiences of ex-patriates) and lamentation (e.g., about "brain drain," distant family relations,

DOI: 10.4324/9781003051862-21

and other immigration stressors) among the Lebanese people. Immigration to the United States is documented as far back as 1880.[4] Since the 1970s, many emigrated to escape the civil war. More recent migration patterns have been in pursuit of education and work opportunities.

Within Lebanon there is also much relocation. Lebanon is a mountainous country, and commonly individuals who are natives to villages in the mountains typically commute or relocate to cities for work and other opportunities.

Language

Arabic is the official language of Lebanon. However, since Lebanon was under a French mandate, French remains a common second language. It is common in Lebanese culture to code-switch seamlessly between Arabic and one or both of English and French. In fact, it is not uncommon for Lebanese nationals to speak among each other in mostly French or English and to interject Arabic words occasionally. It is also conceivable for Lebanese patients to prefer being tested in English or French rather than in Arabic.

About 4% of the Lebanese population consists of individuals of Armenian heritage. As such, some Armenian Lebanese nationals may be monolingual in Armenian, or multilingual in Arabic and Armenian, in addition to English and/or French.

Arabic itself is a complex language. This has been elaborated on in the Arabic overview chapter of this book. Suffice to mention here that spoken Arabic ("mahkiyeh") even differs between Arabic regions sometimes to the point that an Arabic speaker from one Arab country may not understand an Arabic speaker from another Arab country. The unifying language is Classic Arabic ("fus-ha"), an old version of Arabic that is used mostly in writing but which is archaic and therefore not very familiar to all Arabic speakers. A more accessible version of a unifying Arabic dialect is the Modern Standard Arabic (MSA), which was created as an attempt to provide a common dialect with which different Arabic speakers can communicate. MSA is commonly used in professional settings including newscasts, speeches, psychological tests, and other writings.

Communication

The most observable characteristic of Lebanese communication is that Lebanese individuals are often bilingual or multilingual, as discussed above. Lebanese individuals also typically use emphatic and animated gestures and intonations. Further, it is not unusual in a group discussion for individuals to talk over each other or to speak simultaneously. An individual not familiar with such communication patterns may misinterpret them as hostile or impolite, when in fact they are culturally acceptable.

Education

The Lebanese education system has three main streams or curricula into which students enter as early as Kindergarten. The English stream/curriculum is where students are entered into schools where English is taught alongside Arabic. For example, in middle school Math and Sciences may be taught from English texts printed in the United States. The French stream/curriculum is where students are entered into schools where French is taught alongside Arabic. Finally, the Arabic stream/curriculum is where students are primarily taught in Arabic but with some subjects taught in English or French. In all cases, there is typically a "second" language (actually, a third language for the English and the French curricula) introduced usually in middle school. As such, it is very common for Lebanese nationals to be bilingual. It is also conceivable for Lebanese patients to prefer being tested in English or French rather than in Arabic.

Literacy

According to the CIA Factbook, Lebanon's literacy rate is 96.9% for males and 93.3% for females.[2]

Values and Customs

Lebanese individuals have a wide variety of values and customs. For expatriates and immigrants, these can be influenced by countries of origin as well as country of residence. Even within Lebanon, the intra-cultural differences are varied. As such, while the psychologist may be prepared with knowledge about possible cultural scenarios to be aware of (e.g., being aware of patriarchal influences), the examiner cannot predict ahead of time (prejudge) what the patient's cultural values and customs will be. Further, as is the case with immigrants from any country, one can find different levels of acculturation, and therefore different levels of American values and customs, among the Lebanese immigrants and their subsequent generations.

Lebanon is a diverse culture, influenced by Arab as well as European values and customs, and by Muslim as well as Christian beliefs and practices. This makes it difficult for the clinician to predict the level of conservatism of a Lebanese patient's values ahead of time.

Some values and customs that may sometimes, but not always, exist with Lebanese patients fall under themes of patriarchy, interaction between individuals of the opposite sex, mental/cognitive illness taboos, family unity, and filial piety.

Regarding patriarchy, in some families and cultures, men may take the lead in speaking. Therefore, if the patient is a female, a male in the room such as a spouse or a son may interrupt her, respond before she has the time to respond, or even speak on her behalf. It would behoove the psychologist to find ways of obtaining the female patient's report in a safe and culturally sensitive manner (for example, during face-to-face testing in private).

Regarding interaction with the opposite sex, in some families and cultures, interactions between non-family members of differing sex must adhere to some rules. For example, some individuals avoid shaking hands with members of a different sex. Therefore, a safe way to interact with a patient of a different sex whom you are meeting for the first time would be to not extend your hand for shaking unless the patient extends theirs first. In some families, it is taboo for two individuals of differing sexes to be alone in a closed room. The clinician may want to check with the patient, if the patient and the clinician are of differing sexes and are to be in an office space alone, if the patient is comfortable with the door being closed.

In Lebanon and the Arab world as a whole, there is significant taboo associated with mental illness or any perception of mental infirmity. Often, matters of mental illness are discussed in terms of blood pressure ("daghet"), risk of a stroke ("jalta"), or of a heart attack ("bil alib"), or other supposed health sequelae of stress and low mood. Typically, Lebanese individuals are more comfortable, or less embarrassed, to suffer from physical ailment than mental illness.

Regarding family unity, family is regarded with high respect in the Lebanese culture. Family usually includes extended members, typically parents, grandparents, uncles, aunts, cousins, and beyond. Family ties are to be maintained and protected, and family members are to support and stand behind each other before other affiliations. Further, it is frowned upon to speak ill of one's family members in public. This level of affiliation can impede access to mental health care, as individual and family struggles are expected to be kept in the family.

Finally, filial piety, the practice of "being good to one's elders" including caring for one's elders, is a common cultural norm. This coincides with deference and respect toward one's elders such that caring for a parent is generally considered a sign of respect and virtuous duty, and not condescension.

A note of caution is warranted here. The above cultural considerations are just that, considerations. They are not always relevant or applicable to every Lebanese patient. As such, a prudent approach would be that prejudgment is not advised, but awareness is.

Spirituality and Religion

There are 18 religious sects recognized in Lebanon, primarily of Muslim and Christian origin. There is a significant minority of Druze (about 5%[2]), a religious affiliation present primarily in Lebanon and Syria. As such, the Lebanese culture is influenced by a wide variety of religious and spiritual beliefs and customs. Further, any individual identifying with a specific religious sect may or may not be observant of that sect's customs and values. Again, prejudgment is not advised but awareness is.

Health Status

According to a WHO 2019–2023 Country Cooperation Strategy report, more than 85% of the healthcare services in Lebanon are provided in the private sector, and good high-quality services are available in the major cities, but rural areas are underserved.[5] According to this WHO report, two-thirds of the Lebanese population suffer from overweight/obesity, half lack low physical activity, and one-third smoke. As such, one can imagine that the burden of vascular risk factors, such as vascular cognitive impairment, can present as a real risk among the Lebanese population.

Mental Health Views

In a 2015 report, The World Health Organization (WHO[6]) indicated that there were 42 mental health outpatient facilities and five mental health hospitals and eight community-based psychiatric inpatient units in Lebanon. According to the WHO (2015) report, the most commonly assigned diagnosis in mental hospitals was schizophrenia, and the most commonly assigned diagnosis in outpatient facilities and inpatient units was mood disorders. One epidemiological study[7] showed the lifetime prevalence rate of a DSM-IV mental disorder in Lebanon was 25.8%, with the highest prevalence for anxiety disorders (16.7%) followed by mood disorders (12.6%). According to a WHO 2019–2023 Country Cooperation Strategy—At A Glance 2018 report, mental health conditions, especially post-traumatic stress disorder, depression, and anxiety, were on the rise.[5] This is not surprising since the history of Lebanon is characterized by decades of political turmoil, raising the risks for individual and inter-generational trauma.

There is no specific allocation in the public/governmental health expenditure for mental health services. The WHO estimated that 78% of the Lebanese population had free access to essential psychotropic medications but that psychotherapy interventions were not covered by social insurance plans and majority of private insurances did not cover mental health care.[5] As such, due to limited mental health coverage by insurance plans, lack of affordability can present an obstacle to mental health access in Lebanon.

Other factors also compromise access to mental health care. Mental illness has a significant taboo attached to it in Lebanon. As Hilal and Soufia[8] noted, "(t)he effect of stigma on people with mental illness is more burdening than the disease itself" and concluded that "the lack of effective mental health awareness is the main reason that leads to negative attitudes" (p.70) in their sample of respondents. Further, according to the WHO 2019–2023 report, there is a lack of mental health training among primary care workers, and "interactions between the primary care and mental health systems are rare."[5] However, anecdotally, there are efforts by mental health providers, through social media and other campaigns, to provide education about mental illness, provide resources for help, and de-stigmatize mental illness.

Approach to Neuropsychological Evaluations

One of the early considerations before identifying a test list for the Lebanese (and in general, Arabic-speaking) examinee is to consider the examinee's proficiency with, and preference for, non-Arabic languages. As mentioned earlier, in several Arab countries, a second language, typically English or French, is taught and emphasized at home and in school from a very early age. It is common practice in Lebanon for examinees to be examined in a second language (typically English or French) in addition to, or instead of, in Arabic.

There exist Lebanese institutions, such as universities (e.g., American University of Beirut, Lebanese University) and medical clinics (e.g., Medical Institute for Neuropsychological Disorders) where clinical neuropsychology is practiced and where neuropsychological research is burgeoning. In those clinics, it is typical practice to test in more than one language. One particular example stands out for the test of Trail Making. Some Arab individuals are much more familiar with the alphabet sequence in English or French (same sequence in both languages) than the alphabet sequence in Arabic. As such, an Arabic-speaking examinee may have an easier time completing the Trails B test in English than in Arabic.

Beyond multilingualism, as noted, the Arabic language itself comes in different dialects. As such, test instructions written in one Arabic dialect may not be well understood by speakers of a different Arabic dialect. Further, a stimulus word (e.g., on a word-list learning test) in one Arabic dialect may be understood but still not carry the same level of familiarity for an examinee who speaks a different Arabic dialect. Therefore, even a verbal test translated to one Arabic dialect may not be applicable to an examinee of a different Arabic dialect.

Another consideration is the use of non-Arabic terms in the Arabic language. For example, the word for "computer" in Arabic is transliterated to "hasoub." The word "hasoub" can be used, and technically is used, to refer to a computer. However, most Arabic speakers, even when speaking Arabic, would not refer to a computer as "hasoub" but would instead simply use the word "computer." As such, when developing instructions and test materials (e.g., word-list for memorization, object-naming test, vocabulary test), one needs to consider which word would be most appropriate.

Broadly speaking, there is not one Arabic language, and there is not one Arabic culture. As such, when consulting with examiners evaluating Arabic-speaking examinees, I often caution them that they would want to ensure that the examinee's Arabic dialect and culture is consistent with the dialect and culture of the Arabic tests they are using (or, alternatively, of the interpreter upon whom they are relying).

As a consequence of these obstacles, there is a significant paucity of Arabic neuropsychological tests available for clinical use. The reader is referred to the review article by Zeinoun, Iliescu, and El Hakim (2021) for a listing of available tests.[9]

Given the many levels of considerations that neuropsychologists would have to attend to before even getting to the point of choosing a testing battery for their Arab examinee, it would behoove the neuropsychologists to recognize that they are a clinician with several clinical tools and that the neuropsychological tests represent only one of those tools. When examining an Arabic-speaking examinee, reliance on a detailed clinical history, collateral information, mental status examination, behavioral observations, review of records, and an understanding of functional neuroanatomy and neuropsychological manifestations of different medical and mental health conditions becomes particularly invaluable.

In the case study presented here, a case of dementia in a Lebanese examinee is presented. The case was chosen purposefully predating the publication of normative data for a Lebanese dementia screening battery.[10] The purpose for that choice was to keep in line with the goal of walking through the more typical scenario of having an Arabic-speaking examinee while the examiner has a very limited choice of Arabic tests to administer.

Section II: Case Study — "No Test in Sight, and One Language Won't Suffice"

Note: Possible identifying information and several aspects of history and presentation have been changed to protect patient identity and privacy.

Reason for Referral

Ms. A is a 78-year-old female who was referred to this examiner for a dementia evaluation. She reported that Arabic was her primary language, and she was fluent in French but spoke very little English.

History of Presenting Illness

Ms. A did not believe that she had any cognitive problems and felt indignant that her family was suggesting that she was "kharfaneh" (senile) by asking her to have her mental skills evaluated. Ms. A had been living with her husband, who passed away two years prior to the evaluation. After her husband passed away, Ms. A continued to live on her own. Due to language barriers, however, her son and her daughter-in-law (who lived nearby) helped her out with more complex tasks such as filling out paperwork or paying bills. In the past year, Ms. A's family members started noticing her forgetting things. For example, they would alert her to an upcoming doctor's appointment, and when they showed up to pick her up she was oblivious to having any appointments. They reported that she would repeat her questions to them sometimes. Her family members denied any decline in Ms. A's judgment, reasoning, problem-solving, or visual-spatial perception. They noted that she sometimes paused for words but denied that this interfered with her ability to communicate. She was able to take her medications accurately every morning. She was able to drive to her already restricted routes, mostly to the grocery store and to her son's home nearby. She was described as having been a "phenomenal" cook, but recently her cooking had declined in quality.

The family had brought up the concern about Ms. A's forgetfulness to her primary care physician, who in turn ordered a brain MRI scan and referred her for neuropsychological testing with this examiner. The brain MRI was interpreted by the radiologist to show mild volume loss that was believed to be consistent with her age. There was mention of white matter degradation, but no opinion was given about the level of severity/abnormality of this degradation.

At this point, her son and daughter-in-law were considering having Ms. A move in with them, but they had not broached the subject with her.

Other Pertinent History

Ms. A was born, raised, and educated in Beirut, the cosmopolitan capital of Lebanon. She immigrated to the United States from Lebanon at the age of 64, on the behest of her three children, who all lived in the United States. In Lebanon, she graduated high school and later married at the age of 21. She denied any difficulty learning in school. She was a full-time homemaker and mother of three children. While she picked up some English during her almost 14 years living in the United States, for the most part she spoke Arabic and French in her community.

Ms. A's health history was significant for high cholesterol, high blood pressure, and osteoporosis, all of which were kept under control with medications. Her medication list consisted of atorvastatin, alendronate, losartan, and over-the-counter pain medications. A blood workup from three months prior did not reveal any abnormal findings pertinent to the cognitive complaints (e.g., vitamin deficiency, thyroid dysfunction).

There were no complaints about sleep, appetite, or eating habits in general. However, Ms. A lived alone, and so no one observed her sleeping. There was no chronic history of depression or anxiety or any other mental health complaints. While Ms. A reported that she missed her deceased husband, she reported generally being in good spirits and feeling happy to have her family and grandchildren around her. She reported feeling satisfied with her life and ready to join with her husband in the afterlife; however, she vehemently denied any suicidal thoughts.

Ms. A did not have much of a social circle except for her family and a very small and dwindling circle of Arabic-speaking friends. She did not engage in any formal exercise. She enjoyed reading and knitting and watching television. She denied using any alcohol or drugs. She used to smoke about one pack of cigarettes per day between the age of 17 and 24 (she quit smoking when she first became pregnant).

Regarding family history, Ms. A's father passed away in his 50's from heart problems, and her mother passed away at age 74 from "old age." She and her children did not know of any history of dementia or cognitive decline in the family.

Cultural Notes

Ms. A came from an affluent family that stressed academic achievement. Her father was a politician, and her mother was a housewife whom Ms. A described as a socialite. Ms. A's son reported that his grandmother (Ms. A's mother) was a "formidable" "matriarch." He described his mother as being the same. Ms. A's son described that even though in Lebanese culture the children are expected to care for their parents, he described his mother as "prideful," "secretive," and "stubborn," and she refused help. This was valuable information that prompted me to decide to interview Ms. A in private, in order to provide her a more confidential space and hopefully provide her a safer space to be vulnerable.

Ms. A's son also reported that his mother adhered to certain rules of conduct, such as wearing a headscarf ("hijab") in public and not shaking men's hands. This was valuable to know as a male examiner so that during my examination of Ms. A, I made sure not to accidentally make physical contact with her (e.g., when passing papers or other materials back and forth with her).

Ms. A expressed being comfortable with meeting with me, in a private room, alone, with the door shut.

Mental Status Examination

Ms. A presented as alert and aware of the reason for her examination today. Since she had to travel from her hometown about 150 miles away from this examiner's office location, Ms. A did not know exactly what city we were in. However, she was able to provide her address, and she knew that she was still in the same state as where she resided, and she knew the present month and year but not the date. She happily provided detailed information about her distant past. However, when asked about more recent events in her life she hesitated and generally gave vague information. With Ms. A's permission, I interviewed her son and daughter-in-law to obtain a more detailed recent history. Ms. A was able to express herself fluently and did not evidence any significant problems with word finding. There were no deficits noted in her comprehension. She occasionally interjected some French words but mostly spoke in Arabic. She was able to attend to conversations. Her thought process was clear and coherent and logical. Her mood was euthymic. Her affect ranged appropriately. While she was quite respectful and pleasant, it was clear that she was not happy to have her mental skills evaluated. She was nevertheless able to build rapport easily, and she enjoyed reminiscing about her home country. There were no signs of psychosis. There were no signs of disinhibition or impulsivity.

Neuropsychological Testing

At the time of the present evaluation, the examiner was only aware of two neuropsychological screening instruments that were validated with Arabic-speaking populations, the modified version of the Mini-Mental Status Examination (3MS[11]) and the Montreal Cognitive Assessment (MoCA[12]). I administered the Arabic version of the MoCA to Ms. A.

The following tests were then used. The tests were chosen for the cognitive domain they survey and for the ease of their translation. Unless noted otherwise, the test instructions were provided in Arabic and with test stimuli translated to Arabic when needed:

- Wechsler Adult Intelligence Scale-4th Edition (WAIS-IV) Digit Span[13]
- Arabic version of the Rey Auditory Verbal Learning Test-Revised.[14] This Arabic version of the AVLT already exists but has only been validated with younger adults.
- Brief Visuospatial Memory Test-Revised.[15] Norms only available for young adult Arabic speakers.
- Benton Judgment of Line Orientation.[16] No norms for Arabic speakers.
- Rey-O Complex Figure Test.[17] Norms only available for young adult Arabic speakers.
- Trail Making Test, original English version.[18] Ms. A reported that she was more fluent with the sequence of the alphabet in French (same as English) than she was with the alphabet sequence in Arabic. As such, the original English version of the Trail Making Test was administered.
- Arabic version of Phonemic Fluency and Semantic Fluency tests.[19] Ms. A verbalized a preference for performing this test in Arabic rather than in French. Arabic norms were only available for young adult Arabic speakers.
- Arabic version of the Beck Depression Inventory-II.[20] *Out of cultural sensitivity, I typically exclude the question about sexual interest, particularly with female examinees.*

Test results were as follows.

Montreal Cognitive Assessment (MoCA)

- Trails: 1/1
- Cube: 0/1
- Clock: 2/3
- Naming: 2/3
- List Learning: –
- Digit Span: 2/2
- Letter Vigilance: 1/1
- Serial Subtraction: 2/3
- Sentence Repetition: 1/2
- Abstraction: 2/2
- Delayed Recall: 1/5
- Orientation: 3/5
- Total: 17/30 (Education-Corrected score = 18/30)

Overall, a total score of 18/30 was interpreted as a "red flag" signaling possible cognitive impairment. There are no norms for Arabic-speaking examinees on the MoCA. Further, score equivalencies from English examiners cannot be assumed. However, a qualitative examination of her performances suggested memory problems. For example, she learned four words but recalled only one and recognized only two, and her orientation was inaccurate. There were equivocal signs of executive functioning problems as well, on clock drawing and serial subtraction. Her language scores were less relevant as I tend to take a conservative approach to minimize false-positive errors when interpreting performance on Arabic translated language tests that are not robustly validated and normed.

Attention/Executive

Table 10.1 outlines Ms. A's attention/executive functioning test raw scores.

Ms. A's attention span score on the Digit Span forward appeared good, compared to English-speaking samples (age-matched manual-based norms). Her backward span, again compared to English-speaking samples, based on the manual norms, was significantly lower. In isolation, her backward span performance may not necessarily be interpreted to reflect a deficit. However, when one considers the difference between her forward and her backward span, it would not be unreasonable to propose that there is a red flag signaling possible impairment in the cognitive domain measured by the backward span subtest.

On Trails A, Ms. A again scored favorably against similarly aged American normative samples (e.g., Mayo Older American Normative Study (MOANS), 63rd percentile).

On Trails B, Ms. A's speed, again compared against the MOANS sample, fell at the 5th percentile. Considering how quickly she completed the Trails A test, this score reflects a possible decline in the cognitive domain measured by Trails B. Further, she made 2 errors (lost set) on the test but was able to recover and get back on track.

On clock drawing from the MoCA, Ms. A was able to draw the contour of the cock, set the numbers appropriately, set the hour hand appropriately, but she set the minutes hands inaccurately (pointing to the number 10).

Overall, for each individual task above, and in the absence of validated norms, Ms. A's performance on each test cannot be interpreted in isolation. However, when all the tests are taken into consideration, in light of her intact performances on simpler tasks such as Forward Digit Span and Trails A, one sees that a trend emerges whereby Ms. A struggled with tasks that required higher levels of set-shifting, longer duration of focus and self-tracking, and complex amounts of multi-processing. A conclusion, in this clinical context, may be made that Ms. A exhibited likely declines in executive functioning.

Table 10.1 Attention/executive functioning test results

Test	Raw score
WAIS-IV Digit Span Forward	11
WAIS-IV Digit Span Backward	6
Trails A	39 seconds
Trails B	238 seconds, 2 errors
MoCA Trails	1/1
MoCA Clock	2/3 set the minute hand incorrectly

Visual/Spatial

Table 10.2 outlines Ms. A's visual/spatial test raw scores.

Table 10.2 Visual/spatial test results

Test	Raw score
BVMT-R Copy	12/12
Benton Judgment of Line Orientation	20/30
Rey-O Complex Figure Test	12/36
MoCA Cube Copy	0

Ms. A was able to copy the relatively simple diagrams on the BVMT-R without error. Her judgment of line angulation score, when compared against similarly aged American samples (MOANS sample), did not raise significant concern about a problem with her visual-spatial perception. However, her copy of more complex diagrams, such as a cube and the Rey-O Complex Figure, were comparatively problematic. In light of her executive functioning findings so far, this examiner believes that her difficulties with the cube and with the complex figure further point to the hypothesis that Ms. A likely has executive functioning declines (e.g., organization, planning).

Language

Table 10.3 outlines Ms. A's language test raw scores.

Table 10.3 Language test results

Test	Raw Score
Letter fluency (3 letters total)	24
Animal fluency	11

This examiner found that Ms. A's scores on word generation exercises were too equivocal and borderline to be interpreted clinically as either reflecting normal functioning or reflecting abnormal functioning.

Learning/Memory

Table 10.4 outlines Ms. A's learning/memory test raw scores.

Compared against original American samples, Ms. A's learning of the drawings on the BVMT-R and of the words on the R-AVLT showed a consistent pattern of suboptimal initial memorization

Table 10.4 Learning/memory test results

Test	Raw score
BVMT-R Trials 1–3	1,4,5 = 10
BVMT-R Learning	4
BVMT-R Delayed Recall	0
BVMT-R Recognition Discrimination	3
Rey AVLT Trials 1–5	2,5,6,6,5 (LOT:14)
Rey AVLT Trial B	1
Rey AVLT Trial 6	1
Rey AVLT Delayed Recall	0
Rey AVLT Recognition Hits	7
Rey AVLT Recognition False Positive Errors	0

but an apparent fair ability to memorize over repetition. Her learning curves (BVMT-R Learning and AVLT Learning Over Trials) when compared against similarly aged American normative samples were in the average range (both 50th percentile).

However, after delays with distractions, Ms. A recalled little to none of the information she had originally memorized from the drawings (made a guess that landed her 1 point) or from the list (no words recalled). When asked to recognize the material, she again struggled and made minimal improvements over her recall.

In the absence of relevant normative data, given the qualitative nature of her learning and memory performances detailed here, the examiner made the clinical conclusion that Ms. A exhibited impairment in her ability to retain new information over time.

Mood

On the Beck Depression Inventory-Second Edition (Arabic translation[21]), Ms. A scored a total of 3 points, providing 1-point responses to each of the symptoms of decreased energy, increased appetite, and fatigue.

Case Discussion

In the absence of culturally relevant normative test data on which to rely for neuropsychological evaluations, the examiner evaluating an Arabic-speaking examinee is not devoid of options. Under certain circumstances, and with the help of a thorough clinical interview and a mental status examination, review of medical records, and reliance on as much reliable data as possible, a clinician may still opt to administer neuropsychological testing in search of quantitative and qualitative data to inform the evaluation. The test results can be interpreted using intra-individual norms (looking at patterns of strengths and weaknesses, comparing analogous tests to each other) and can also be used to establish the individual's baseline for future evaluations. Ideally, the examiner would first gather as many tests as possible that have been adapted, validated, and normed on Arabic samples similar to the examinee. In the absence of this ideal, the examiner may choose tests that have been adapted and validated for Arabic speakers but that do not provide relevant norms. In addition, the examiner may choose tests that have not necessarily been validated and adapted to Arabic speakers but that have demonstrated minimal cultural and linguistic influence. Finally, the examiner may choose tests that have not been adapted or validated on Arabic examinees but with which the examiner is well familiar and which provide an adequate sampling of the function being tested.

With regards to test selection in the case of Ms. A, In the absence of tests that had been adapted, validated, and normed on older adult Arabic-speaking samples, I still had access to one common test adapted to the Arabic population (MoCA) and several other tests that were easily available, translatable without complexity, and with which the examiner had close familiarity.

With regards to data integration and interpretation in the case of Ms. A, her children's reports, her medical records (ruling out medical and metabolic causes of subjective cognitive decline), the ruling out of psychological factors contributing to subjective cognitive and functional decline, all raised a significant consideration for the presence of progressive cognitive decline.

After completing her neuropsychological testing, I relied on multiple levels of interpretation of Ms. A's test performance scores:

1. Deferring conclusions. Where I did not feel comfortable interpreting a test score as either normal or abnormal (for example, scores were equivocal, there was no clear overall pattern), I deferred interpretation of those specific test results.
2. Conclusions based on neuropsychological principles, where test performances followed a convincing neuropsychological pattern. For example, Ms. A's learning of new information

was adequate, but her delayed recall and recognition were clearly low, thus suggested abnormal forgetting.

3. Conclusions based on normal scores compared against the original English-speaking normative sample. Normative data typically show that interpreting abnormal scores (compared to standard normative samples) in an examinee that is very different from the original normative sample runs the risk of over-pathologizing (false-positive errors) the examinee's performance. On the other hand, there is no clear indication that normal scores (compared to standard normative samples) lead to under-pathologizing and false negatives. In other words, if the Arabic examinee's score on an American normed test falls in the normal range when compared to the American normative sample, particularly when there is no reason to suspect that the examinee is impaired in the domain measured by this test, then I typically interpret the Arabic examinee's score as normal.

After considering the above, I diagnosed Ms. A with Amnestic Mild Cognitive Impairment, with deficits in memory and equivocal deficits in executive functioning.

In terms of recommendations, I discussed the testing results with the family. Ms. A elected to allow her son and daughter-in-law to be present. Her daughter who resided out of state was present via telephone (again, with Ms. A's permission). Awareness of cultural sensitivities, such as discomfort with mental infirmity (e.g., forgetfulness) and cognitive labels (e.g., "kharaf"—senility or dementia), dictated my choice of language and choice of how to present Ms. A's symptoms. I was able to invoke cultural practices, such as family unity and filial piety, as permission to engage the family in conversation about the mother's living arrangements and future planning. Using Arabic as our language of communication hopefully placed Ms. A at some level of ease as she was quite open and engaged in our discussions. The family, as a whole, felt like they had the information they needed to make decisions about support and living arrangements. The referring physician was provided with the test results for treatment planning.

Section III: Lessons Learned

- Conducting evaluations with less-than-adequate tools requires clinical judgment, which in turn requires the acceptance of liberties in interpretation. The context of an examination will likely influence the examiner to determine to what extent clinical judgments and liberties are acceptable or not. For example, a high-stakes evaluation where findings lead to very consequential outcomes may not tolerate as much clinical judgment as lower stakes evaluations.

  Every case has different parameters. A clinician's options when faced with an examination of an Arabic-speaking individual can be to decline the examination, refer out to another examiner, or undertake the examination using the best clinical tools available.

  The specific information presented in the overview chapter relating to examining Arabic-speaking examinees, combined with principles of cross-cultural examination and considerations for neuropsychological principles of examinations in general can help the clinician make decisions most appropriate to each individual case, to the examinee, and to the clinician.

- I would state an obvious caveat, which is that the above case presentation was used to demonstrate one examiner's (myself) approach, at one point in the examiner's cultural growth, for one particular case (dementia, clinical non-forensic examination). The above presentation is not made as an example of all examiners or all Arab examinees. It is simply a tool to contribute to discussions about some considerations to keep in mind when evaluating an Arab examinee.

References

1. Khalaf SG, Ochsenwald WL, Barnett RD, Maksoud CF, Kingston P, Bugh GR. Lebanon. Encyclopedia Britannica [Internet]. 2021. Available from: https://www.britannica.com/place/Lebanon
2. CIA World Factbook—Lebanon. Available from: https://www.cia.gov/the-world-factbook/countries/lebanon; 2021.
3. United Nations High Commissioner for Refugees. 2021. Available from: www.unhcr.org/lb
4. Khayrallah Center for Lebanese Diaspora, North Carolina State University. 2021. Available from: https://lebanesestudies.ncsu.edu/
5. World Health Organization Lebanon. Country Cooperation Strategy 2019–2023 [Internet]. 2018. Available from: https://apps.who.int/iris/rest/bitstreams/1172324/retrieve
6. Health W, Organization. A report of the assessment of the mental health system in Lebanon using the World Health Organization-Assessment Instrument for Mental Health Systems (WHO-AIMS). Beirut, Lebanon; 2015.
7. Karam EG, Mneimneh ZN, Dimassi H, Fayyad JA, Karam AN, Nasser SC, et al. Lifetime prevalence of mental disorders in Lebanon: first onset, treatment, and exposure to war. PLOS Medicine. 2008;5(4):e61.
8. Hilal N, Soufia M, editors. Perception of mental illness in the Lebanese society. 27th International Conference on Psychiatry & Psychology Health; 2018; Paris, France.
9. Zeinoun P, Iliescu D, El Hakim R. Psychological tests in Arabic: a review of methodological practices and recommendations for future use. Neuropsychol Rev. 2021. doi:10.1007/s11065-021-09476-6
10. Abou-Mrad F, Chelune G, Zamrini E, Tarabey L, Hayek M, Fadel P. Screening for dementia in Arabic: normative data from an elderly Lebanese sample. Clin Neuropsychol. 2017;31(supl):1–19.
11. El Tallawy HN, Farghly WM, Badry R, Rageh TA, Shehata GA, Hakeem MNA, et al. Prevalence of dementia in Al-Quseir city, Red Sea Governorate, Egypt. Clin Interv Aging. 2014;9:9–14.
12. Rahman TT, El Gaafary MM. Montreal Cognitive Assessment Arabic version: reliability and validity prevalence of mild cognitive impairment among elderly attending geriatric clubs in Cairo. Geriatr Gerontol Int. 2009;9(1):54–61.
13. Wechsler D. WAIS-IV. Wechsler Adult Intelligence Scale—Fourth Edition. San Antonio (TX): Psychological Corporation; 2008.
14. Poreh A, Sultan A, Levin J. The Rey Auditory Verbal Learning Test: normative data for the Arabic-speaking population and analysis of the differential influence of demographic variables. Psychol Neurosci. 2012;5:57–61.
15. Benedict RH. Brief visuospatial memory test-revised. Lutz (FL): Psychological Assessment Resources; 1997.
16. Benton AL. Judgment of line orientation. New York (NY): Oxford University Press; 1983.
17. Osterrieth P. Le test de copie d'une figure complex: Contribution a l'etude de la perception et de la memoire. Archives de Psychologic. 1944;30:206–353.
18. Reitan RM. Validity of the Trail Making test as an indicator of organic brain damage. Percept Mot Skills. 1958;8(3):271–6.
19. Khalil MS. Preliminary Arabic normative data of neuropsychological tests: the verbal and design fluency. J Clin Exp Neuropsychol. 2010;32(9):1028–35.
20. Abdel-Khalek AM. Internal consistency of an Arabic Adaptation of the Beck Depression Inventory in four Arab countries. Psychol Rep. 1998;82(1):264–6.
21. Abdelfattah G. Beck Depression Inventory-II. Cairo, Egypt: Al-Anglo Library Publishing; 2000.

C. Asia
Overview

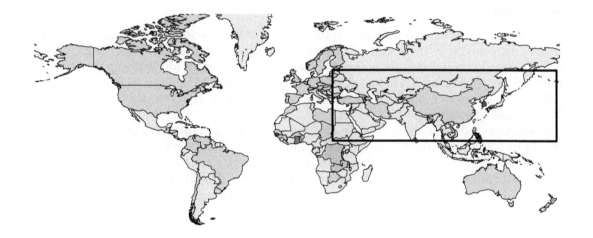

11 General Issues in the Neuropsychological Assessment of Asian Americans

Daryl Fujii

Introduction

Asians, which for the purposes of this chapter will refer to East, South, and Southeast Asians, are the most populous "race" in the world. People from 28 Asian countries make up about 55% (4.28 billion) of the world's population (7.8 billion) as Asia accounts for 8 of the top 20 most populous countries: (1) China—1.4 billion, (2) India—1.38 billion, (5) Pakistan—221 million, (8) Bangladesh—164 million, (11) Japan—126 million, (13) Philippines—109 million, (15) Vietnam—97 million, and (20) Thailand—69 million.[1]

In addition, there are about 52 million people of Asian descent living in other countries, with India (18 million) and China (11 million) ranking first and third, respectively, for country of origin for migrants.[2] Countries with the largest Asian populations include the United States (20.4 million), Canada (6.09 million), Saudi Arabia (6.02 million), United Arab Emirates (5.82 million), Great Britain (4.37 million), France (3.75 million), Australia (3.55 million), and Germany (1.89 million).[3]

The timelines, circumstances for, and locations of diasporas for each Asian country vary, although the primary reasons for migration are labor, family reunification, and asylum. For example in China, out-migration accelerated in the mid-nineteenth century, which was a time of political and economic upheaval with the Opium Wars and Taiping Rebellion, natural disasters, and population growth. In Vietnam, migration occurred after the end of the war in the 1970s as people fled the communist government and abusive refugee camps. More recently is the massive, government-sponsored, and directed out-migration of Filipino workers who drive the country's economy by routinely sending money back to family in the Philippines.[4]

The sheer population numbers would implicate a significant need for neuropsychological services for Asians, with each country facing specific challenges. Indeed, common neurological diseases in Asia include cerebrovascular diseases, headaches, seizure disorder, and Alzheimer's disease and Parkinson's disease in geriatric populations, which is very similar to Western countries. Diseases specific to Asian countries include a high number of strokes in younger adults secondary to premature atherosclerosis, relative commonality of neuromyelitis optica and the optic-spinal variant of multiple sclerosis, and a high incidence of sex-linked dystonia-Parkinsonism in the Philippines. Japanese encephalitis, tuberculous meningitis, cysticercosis, rabies, and tetanus are common infectious diseases, while enterovirus-71 encephalitis, dengue, sarcocystosis, and Nipah encephalitis are emerging infections with neurologic involvement.[5]

Unfortunately, not all Asian countries have neuropsychological services, and there is significant variability in the availability and standards of practice in countries where services exist. For example, neuropsychology is much more developed in countries such as China, Korea, and India,

DOI: 10.4324/9781003051862-23

where there is specific training to become a neuropsychologist, as well as more translations and validation of cognitive tests than in countries such as Vietnam and Thailand where the discipline of psychology is still developing. In China, Korea, India, and the Philippines, neurocognitive assessments are performed by neuropsychologists, whereas in Japan, neuropsychologists are typically psychometrists for physicians who are the only professionals who can legally interpret neuropsychological test results.[6] Thus the state of neuropsychology for Asians would indicate a need for a general framework for understanding Asian culture to provide guidance for approaching a neuropsychological assessment with this population and knowledge of specific cultures.

This section overview chapter is a primer for neuropsychologists when working with Asians with a focus on Asian American (AA) patients. It describes general issues and dispels inaccurate preconceptions of AA as a relatively homogenous group. Issues will be organized according to the ECLECTIC framework.[7] General implications will be provided for each issue which will provide a context for the sectional chapters on specific AA groups.

Asian Americans

Asian Americans (AAs) are a highly heterogeneous racial group of 20.4 million people that account for about 5.4% of the US population. The US census reports 19 unique ethnicities with the largest 6 groups, Chinese (4,948,000), Indian (3,982,000), Filipino (1,980,000), Korean (1,822,000), and Japanese (1,411,000) accounting for 85% of the population. Other AA ethnic groups include: Pakistani (519,000), Cambodian (330,000), Hmong (299,000), Thai (295,000), Laotian (271,000), Bangladeshi (180,000), Burmese (168,000), Nepalese (140,000), Indonesian (113,000), Sri Lankan (60,000), Malaysian (30,000), Bhutanese (24,000), and Mongolian (21,000).[8] Given the numerous countries of origin, it is not surprising that AAs are culturally and linguistically diverse. AAs are also significantly diverse in key demographic variables such as level of education, socio-economic status, percentage foreign-born, and English proficiency.[9] Despite the diversity, scholars have argued for a pan-Asian culture and experiences.[10]

Education/Literacy

Asian countries vary considerably in quantity and quality of education and literacy. Expected years of education range from a high of 16.4 years for South Koreans to a low of 8.5 years for Pakistanis.[11] Similar discrepancies are demonstrated on international test scores, such as the Programme for International Student Assessment (PISA), which could be considered a measure of education quality. In 2018, China, South Korea, and Singapore were among the highest-performing countries, while students from Malaysia, Thailand, and the Philippines scored in the bottom third.[12] Ranges in literacy rates are also considerable, with Japan (99%) and South Korea (98%) approaching 100%, while India (69%), Bhutan (53%), and Pakistan (55%) fall in the lowest 20% of countries for literacy.[13]

Although AAs are the highest educated ethnic group within the United States, with 51% having a bachelor's degree or higher, educational attainment for specific Asian ethnic groups varies considerably. The most educated ethnicities of Indian (72%) and Malaysian (60%) have twice the national average (30%), while the least educated ethnicities are about two times below the national average (Laotian 16%; Bhutanese 9%).[9]

Implications: (1) As education is one of the strongest predictors of neuropsychological test performance, it is imperative that the neuropsychologist is aware of the AA patient's educational background, including the quality of education. This understanding is particularly important for first-generation AAs who were educated in their home country. Scores on international standard tests such as PISA,[12] Trends in Mathematics and Science Study (TIMSS), and Progress in Reading and Literacy Study (PIRLS)[14] can be a proxy for education quality for a country, although not every Asian country participates in testing. For first-generation AAs who are educated in the United States, it is also imperative that the neuropsychologist is aware of school's services for foreign students, such as the English as a Second Language (ESL) Program. (2) It is essential to procure demographically matched norms for test interpretation, as education levels can significantly vary between and within a country. For example, Asian Indians in the United States are highly educated, yet continental India has among the highest illiteracy rate in the world. If these norms are not available, it is recommended that neuropsychologists use the individual comparison method,[15] which uses premorbid estimates of cognitive functioning as a benchmark to interpret current test scores (for a general strategy to determine premorbid functioning see Fujii[16]).

Culture/Acculturation

In America, the majority of AAs are foreign born (59%), although percentages vary by ethnicity. For example, the vast majority of Bhutanese (92%) and Nepalese (88%) are first-generation American, while only 27% of Japanese and 39% Hmong are foreign born.[9] Thus it is essential that a neuropsychologist understand the specific culture of an AA's country of origin and their acculturation to Western society to provide competent and meaningful services. Specifically, macrosocietal structures such as a country's geography, sociopolitical-economic history, population demographics, government, and educational system can provide important clues to determine language(s) spoken, English proficiency or bilingualism, educational opportunities, intellectual functioning on Western tests, and historical events that may impact the relationship between the neuropsychologist and AA patient.[16] Values, beliefs, worldviews, religions, family structures, and norms for social interactions[17] can guide approaches for developing rapport, optimizing communication, understanding conceptions of intelligent behavior, and generating meaningful recommendations. Common medical conditions and neurological disorders, attitudes and beliefs regarding health and illness, and common treatments for illnesses[17] are useful for generating hypotheses about diagnoses and making useful treatment recommendations.

Despite unique differences between Asian countries, there is a general collectivist pan-Asian culture emphasizing interdependency that manifests itself in norms of social conformity and restraint, strongly defined roles, suppression of emotional expression, indirect communication, and family loyalty with a fierce obligation to avoid bringing shame to one's family. These values are influenced by Eastern philosophical traditions such as Hinduism, Buddhism, Taoism, and Confucianism, which stress interdependency of the person with the universe.[10,18]

Although cultural knowledge is important for developing a contextual understanding of AA patients, level of acculturation defined for neuropsychological purposes as "the similarity of a patient's culture and experiences to, and adoption of, mainstream culture"[16] (p. 67) is essential to individualize conceptualization of the patient. Knowledge of a patient's acculturation will help neuropsychologists titrate the impact of an AA patient's home culture on presentation and functioning. This information can then guide the evaluation process. Acculturation can be determined through formal assessment such as the Asian American Multidimensional Acculturation Scale,[19] or clinically based upon characteristics such as age at immigration or generation in the United States, exposure to mainstream culture, or cultural identity.[20]

Implications: (1) Neuropsychologists need to research an AA patient's culture and at a minimum informally assess for acculturation prior to the assessment to develop plans for the assessment. To reduce testing biases, neuropsychologists should refer to the American Education Research Association (AERA) Standards for Educational and Psychological Testing (2nd ed.)[21]

and determine how culture can impact the four pillars for fairness in testing: (a) comfort with the testing situation, (b) test bias, (c) accessibility, and (d) validity.[7] A cultural conceptualization can then assist in developing useful recommendations. (2) Asians' collectivist culture has implications for cognition and underlying brain functioning. For example, in comparison to Westerners, Asians engage in more holistic versus detail visual processing focusing on both object and foreground, formulate memories within contexts versus discrete details, and classify objects through experiential relationship-oriented categories.[22]

Language

Unlike ethnically diverse Latinos who generally speak a form of Spanish, each Asian country has its own language. In some countries, such as India and the Philippines, several major languages are spoken with even more regional dialects. For example, India has 22 official languages and over 1599 other languages. Given that 59% of AAs are foreign born, and 68% of AA speak a language other than English at home, language and English proficiency are salient issues for the neuropsychological evaluation process. English proficiency varies widely across Asian ethnic groups with large majorities of Japanese (84%), Filipinos (82%), and Indians (80%) being proficient in English, while ethnicities with large populations of recently arrived immigrants such as Bhutanese (27%) and Burmese (28%) are less proficient.[8] An important factor affecting English proficiency is generation in the United States, as 94% of native-born AAs speak English well versus 55% of foreign-born AAs. Other factors include age at immigration, number of years educated in the U.S., and exposure to English in country of origin.[23] For example, English is considered one of the national languages in India, Singapore, Hong Kong, and the Philippines; thus AAs from these countries are generally proficient in English. In countries such as China, Japan, and South Korea, English reading and writing is emphasized versus speaking, resulting in stronger reading versus expressive language and comprehension skills. Another consideration is that many Asian languages are very different than English; thus learning English for Asians may be more challenging than someone who is a native speaker of a European language.[24]

Implications: (1) Neuropsychologists need to determine the need for interpreter services and test translations prior to assessment. Clinicians should be mindful that not all AA patients will require these services, and conducting the evaluation in English may be appropriate for AAs born in the United States, immigrated at a young age and educated in the United States, or those immigrating from countries where English is a primary language.[23] (2) If it is determined that an interpreter is needed, neuropsychologists need to find trained interpreters and procure appropriately translated tests. Clinicians should be aware of best practices in working with interpreters,[25] and translating tests if none are available.[26] (3) Neuropsychologists should also be versed in the bilingualism literature.[27]

Economics

Another area of high variability is economics. World economic rankings indicate that Asian countries are among both the strongest (Singapore, China, Japan, South Korea) and weakest (Bhutan, Nepal) economies in the world. Even in countries with strong economies, there can be significant discrepancies in income among the people with areas of high poverty, particularly in rural areas. This pattern of significant economic inequality is also present in the United States, where several Asian ethnicities rank among the highest median household incomes (Indians $100,000, Filipinos $80,000, Japanese $74,000), while other ethnic groups such as the Bhutanese (33.3%) and Burmese (35%) have poverty rates that are twice the national average (12.1%).[9]

Implications: (1) Economics has significant implications for understanding the cognitive functioning and test performance of AA patients. On a global level, countries with stronger economies have better educational systems and network infrastructure for access to information.[28-30] Thus it is not surprising that a country's economy is correlated (0.59) with performance on academic and Western intelligence tests.[31] One implication is that a country's economy can be used as a rough indicator to adjust expected performance on neuropsychological tests for patients from AA ethnicities where there are no normative data.[16] (2) On an individual level, poverty has been associated with less stimulating reading environments[32] and stressful, chaotic, traumatic environments, which have been associated with smaller frontal and hippocampal areas that modulate memory and executive functioning.[33]

Communication Style

Communication style refers to the manner in which information is transmitted between people. It not only involves how information is imparted but also what information is appropriate to disclose and to whom. Incongruence in communication style between a neuropsychologist and patient can result in miscommunication, negative perception of the other, and impact rapport.[33] Due to contrasting styles between individualist and collectivist cultures, it is important for neuropsychologists to be familiar with communication styles of AAs. Individualistic cultures communicate more directly with meaning primarily contained in the content of what is said. Thus the onus for communication is on the speaker. By contrast collectivist cultures emphasize relationships, thus communicate more indirectly with a greater emphasis on nonverbals and the absence of content to avoid conflict or offending. The onus for communication is on the listener.[34]

Another significant difference is the meaning of head nodding. For Westerners, nodding one's head signifies agreement. However, for many Asian societies, head nodding in response to an authority figure, such as a neuropsychologist, means "I am listening to you." Thus AAs may nod even if disagreeing with or not understanding the clinician. This behavior results from respect, as disagreeing with an authority figure is considered rude.[35]

Another pertinent aspect of communication is idioms of distress, which is the manner that people of a culture express emotional distress. This expression reflects a shared way of experiencing or communicating emotional concerns and may or may not involve specific symptoms or syndromes.[36] Understanding an AA patient's idiom of distress is not only important for diagnostic purposes but can also facilitate rapport.[37] For Asians, emotional problems are typically demonstrated through somatic symptoms.[38] In addition, due to the stigma of mental illness, Asians tend to delay seeking assistance for mental health or neurological issues until symptoms are severe.[39] Awareness of this tendency is crucial as neuropsychologists can easily underestimate distress from the patient's self-report due to somatization of emotional problems and low emotional expressiveness.

Implications: (1) Neuropsychologists should be cognizant of AAs' communication style and be vigilant for indirect or subtle signs of discomfort or distress. (2) AA patients should be given permission to ask questions if they do not understand test instructions or any aspect of the assessment. Check-ins throughout the assessment can reinforce this behavior as some AA cultures acquiesce only after several offers to avoid appearing rude. (3) AAs' indirect communication style is moderated by generation and acculturation.

Testing Situation: Perception and Goals

According to Greenfield,[40] neuropsychological testing is a Western technology with its values and cultural assumptions inherent in the process. Due to the Western cultural bias, the process can be unfair for people from cultures who are unfamiliar and/or uncomfortable with the testing situation, or whose behaviors, values, and worldviews are dissimilar to the west. Specifically, biases can impact motivation and test performances.[41] For many AAs who come from countries with good educational systems or are educated in the United States, the testing situation is a familiar one. These AAs are typically motivated to perform well as education is highly valued, and there is pressure to perform well in testing situations. However, AAs are a highly heterogeneous group, and not everyone fits into this stereotypical category. Testing situations can be perceived as stressful and uncomfortable for AAs who have low levels of education or do not speak English well, for example, elderly who were born in countries with poor educational systems. AAs who have historically performed poorly on tests may also experience more discomfort. It can also be stressful if the patient feels the neuropsychologist is asking intrusive questions about their family, or if the evaluation is perceived to be associated with psychiatric issues due to the stigma of mental illness. In addition, perceived microaggressions by the neuropsychologists can negatively impact rapport and test performance.[42]

Implications: (1) Neuropsychologists should be aware of the AA patient's culture and level of acculturation to develop hypotheses of how they will perceive the testing situation and adapt approaches to address issues and maximize comfort. For example, engaging in small talk, framing the evaluation as a medical versus psychological assessment, or mirroring the less direct eye contact of the AA patient may reduce discomfort. (2) Neuropsychologists can maximize engagement in the assessment by determining the AA's concerns or goals for the evaluation and then tailoring recommendations toward these goals. To determine what is useful for the patient, the neuropsychologist should (a) probe what is most bothering the patient or how the patient's purported neurological condition is causing him/her distress, (b) provide a general description of the neuropsychological evaluation, including purpose and types of information it can provide, (c) inform the patient how this information can be useful to understand his/her concerns, and (d) describe how this information can guide recommendations to address the patient's concerns.

Intelligence: Conception

Estimates of premorbid intelligence are integral for the neuropsychological assessment as it serves as a benchmark for interpreting test scores and comparing current abilities.[15] Despite its anchoring role, the construct is somewhat amorphous as psychologists have not agreed upon a standard definition.[43] Concepts of intelligence become more complicated when examining different cultures. Numerous theorists purport that intelligence is intimately tied to survival and advancement within one's social and physical environment.[44,45] Thus, intelligence across cultures will differ contingent upon unique challenges faced in adapting to and problem solving within environments.[46]

For many AAs, intelligent behavior is associated with high academic achievement. Although performance differs by country of origin, as a whole AAs demonstrate stronger academic achievement and score higher on standardized tests than Whites, particularly in science, technology, engineering, and mathematics (STEM).[12,47] The academic achievement of AAs has been attributed to several social and cultural factors. AAs are more inclined to believe that academic achievement is something that can be developed versus Western beliefs in innate abilities. East Asians are influenced by Confucian ideals of the perfectibility of humans through learning and self-cultivation. Immigration status is another influence as immigrants leave their home country in search of a better life. For many AAs, educational attainment is perceived to be associated with social prestige and upward mobility, particularly for STEM fields. Parents have higher expectations and are highly influential on children due to parenting styles that engender interdependence and collectivism.[48] The importance of motivational factors is illustrated by weak correlations for socio-economic status and academic achievement, particularly for Southeast Asians.[49]

Academic differences are also demonstrated in the school systems of many Asian countries and the United States. In Asian schools, the teacher is a respected authority who is not questioned. Emphasis is on rote learning and mastering a breadth of knowledge that facilitates high achievement on tests. By contrast, in the US, teachers are viewed more as facilitators of learning. Although course attainment is an aspect of learning, there is more emphasis on discussion and cultivation of critical thinking versus knowledge acquisition.[50]

Implications: (1) When interpreting test data, neuropsychologists should be aware of the general pattern for higher math versus verbal abilities, as well as weaker association between socio-economic status of AA immigrants and academic achievement.

Context of Immigration

Not everyone from a given country who wants to emigrate to the United States is successful. The person must meet eligibility criteria for one of the immigration categories, which includes family reunification, employment, political, and lottery. Access to resources to travel to the United States is also needed. Thus, there is a selection bias of who emigrates. Biases differ per country as each has its own economic, political, and geographic realities. For example, despite being in the bottom third of the world countries for total literacy rate (71.2%),[51] Indians who successfully emigrate are the most highly educated (72% bachelor's degree) and have the highest household median income ($100,000) in the United States.[8] A related issue is when a person immigrates in relation to the country's immigration history, as there can be several "waves" of immigration associated with different sectors of society. For example, the first wave of Vietnamese immigrants, who arrived shortly prior to the fall of Saigon in 1975, were primarily urban, well-educated business owners or those with ties to the US military personnel. The second wave, known as "the boat people," were largely less-educated rural farmers or fishermen, who fled to refugee camps to escape worsening political and economic conditions before relocating to a host country during the late 1970s to late 1980s. The third wave are those seeking family reunification.[52]

Although people of a country generally share the same culture and experiences, there is often significant heterogeneity which can include demographics that are salient for neuropsychologists such as language spoken, education level and quality, occupation, and socio-economic status. Thus, the selection biases of immigration can provide important clues for understanding how the AA patient fits within their own culture of origin. Determining a person's status within her country is a key issue when attempting to estimate premorbid functioning on Western tests when no relevant norms exist for that country.[16] A contextual understanding is especially important for AAs who may not present as the prototypical person for that country.

Another important aspect of immigration is the process or journey for the patient. This issue is particularly salient for refugees as many have experienced physical and psychosocial traumas during the immigration process. Experiences can be associated with psychiatric conditions and also neurological considerations for differential diagnoses.[52]

Implications: Immigration is a salient issue for many AAs as 59% are foreign born, and many more are second generation, thus children of immigrants. Although third-generation citizens are typically English-speaking and acculturated, understanding a family's immigration history can still provide important contextual information for understanding them.

Summary

In summary, AAs are highly diverse people originating from 19 different countries. Each country has a unique culture associated with specific sociopolitical economic histories, and most speak at least one unique language. This chapter provided a cultural framework for appreciating how culture interfaces with neuropsychological assessment. Due to the heterogeneity in AAs, neuropsychologists should be knowledgeable of the Asian patient's specific culture to guide approaches for collecting accurate data, provide a context for interpreting data, and generate useful recommendations. The following chapters in this section will describe cultural specifics for Asian Indian, Chinese, Filipino, Japanese, Lhotshampa (Nepali Bhutanese), Pakistani, South Korean, Taiwanese, and Vietnamese Americans.

References

1. Worldometer. Current world population [Internet]. [Place unknown: Worldometer]; n.d. [cited 2020 Jul 30]. Available from: https://www.worldometers.info/world-population/
2. United Nations. The number of international migrants reaches 272 million, continuing an upward trend in all world regions, says UN [Internet]. [New York (NY): United Nations]; 2019 Sep 17 [cited 2020 Mar 6]. Available from: https://www.un.org/development/desa/en/news/population/international-migrant-stock-2019.html
3. Wikipedia: The Free Encyclopedia. Category: Asian diasporas [Internet]. [Place unknown]: Wikimedia Foundation, Inc; n.d. [Updated 2020 Apr 26, cited 2020 Jul 30]. Available from: https://en.wikipedia.org/wiki/Category:Asian_diasporas
4. Hu-DeHart E. Diaspora. In: Schlund-Vials, CJ, Võ LT, Wong KS, editors. Keywords for Asian Amer. Studies [Internet]. New York (NY): New York University Press; 2015 [cited 2020 Jul 31]. Available from: https://keywords.nyupress.org/asian-american-studies/essay/diaspora/
5. Tan CT. Neurology in Asia. Neurology. 2015 Feb 10;84(6):623–5.
6. Lee TMC, Kai W, Collinson SL. History of neuropsychology in Asia. In: Barr WB, Bieliauskas LA, editors. Oxford handbook of history of clinical neuropsychology [Internet]. New York (NY): Oxford University Press; 2016 Oct [cited 2020 Mar 6]. Available from: https://www.oxfordhandbooks.com/view/10.1093/oxfordhb/9780199765683.001.0001/oxfordhb-9780199765683-e-36
7. Fujii D. Developing a cultural context for conducting a neuropsychological evaluation with a culturally diverse client: the ECLECTIC framework. Clin. Neuropsych. 2018;32(8):1356–92.
8. Lopez G, Ruiz NG, Patten E. Key facts about Asian Americans, a diverse and growing population [Internet]. Washington (DC): Pew Research Center; 2017 [cited 2020 March 6]. Available from: https://www.pewresearch.org/fact-tank/2017/09/08/key-facts-about-asian-americans
9. Budiman A, Cilluffo A, Ruiz NG. Key facts about Asian origin groups in the U.S. [Internet]. Washington (DC): Pew Research Center; 2019 [cited 2020 Mar 6]. Available from: https://www.pewresearch.org/fact-tank/2019/05/22/key-facts-about-asian-origin-groups-in-the-u-s/
10. Guo T, Uhm SY. Society and acculturation in Asian American communities. In: Davis, J, D'Amato, editors. Neuropsychology of Asians and Asian-Americans. New York (NY): Springer; 2014. p. 55–76.
11. United Nations Development Programme. Human Development Reports Pakistan [Internet]. Place unknown: Human Development Report Office; n.d. [cited 2020 Mar 6]. Available from: http://hdr.undp.org/en/countries/profiles/PAK
12. OECD Programme for International Student Assessment. PISA 2018 results [Internet]. Place unknown: Organisation for Economic Co-operation and Development (OECD); 2019 [cited 2020 Mar 6]. Available from: https://www.oecd.org/pisa/PISA-results_ENGLISH.png
13. Burton J. List of countries by literacy rate [Internet]. Place unknown: WorldAtlas; 2020 Aug 12 [cited 2020 Mar 6]. Available from: https://www.worldatlas.com/articles/the-highest-literacy-rates-in-the-world.html
14. International Association for the Evaluation of Educational Achievement. About IEA [Internet]. Place unknown: TIMSS & PIRLS International Study Center, Lynch School of Education, Boston College; 2009 [cited 2020 Mar 22]. Available from: https://www.iea.nl/
15. Gasquoine PG. Race-norming of neuropsychological tests. Neuropsych. Rev. 2009 Jun 1;19(2):250.
16. Fujii D. Conducting a culturally informed neuropsychological evaluation. Washington (DC): American Psychological Association; 2016.
17. Judd T, Beggs B. Cross-cultural forensic neuropsychological assessment. In: Barrett K, George WH, editors. Race, culture, psychology, and law. Thousand Oaks (CA): Sage Publications, Inc; 2005. p. 141–62.

18. Lau EY. Clinical interviewing and qualitative assessment with Asian heritage clients. In: Davis J, D'Amato R, editors. Neuropsychology of Asians and Asian-Americans. New York (NY): Springer; 2014. p. 135–50.

19. Gim-Chung RH, Kim BS, Abreu JM. Asian American multidimensional acculturation scale: development, factor analysis, reliability, and validity. Cultur Divers Ethnic Minor Psychol. 2004 Feb;10(1):66.

20. Birman D, Simon CD. Acculturation research: challenges, complexities, and possibilities. In: Leong, FTL, editor. APA handbook of multicultural psychology, Vol 1: Theory and research. Washington (DC): American Psychological Association; 2013. p. 207–30.

21. American Education Research Association; American Psychological Association; National Council on Measurement in Education (US). Standards for educational and psychological testing. 2nd ed. Washington (DC): American Education Research Association; 2014.

22. Yang L, Wong B, Li LQ. Culture and memory. In: Pedraza O, editor. Clinical cultural neuroscience: foundation and assessment. New York (NY): Oxford University Press; 2020. p. 169–99.

23. Artiola i Fortuny L. Research and practice: ethical issues with immigrant adults and children. In: Morgan JE, Ricker JH, editors. Textbook of clinical neuropsychology. New York (NY): Taylor & Francis; 2008. p. 960–81.

24. National Virtual Translation Center. Learning language difficulty for English speakers [Internet]. Place unknown: NVTC; 2007 [cited 2020 Mar 7]. Available from: http://web.archive.org/web/20071014005901/http://www.nvtc.gov/lotw/months/november/learningExpectations.html

25. Santos O, Fujii D, Pedraza O. Neuropsychological assessment of non-English speakers. In: Pedraza O, editor. Clinical cultural neuroscience: foundations and assessment. New York (NY): Oxford University Press; 2020. p. 169–99.

26. International Test Commission (ITC). ITC Guidelines for translating and adapting tests [Internet]. Lincoln (NE): International Test Commission; 2017 [cited 2020 Mar 22]. Available from: https://www.intestcom.org/page/16

27. Freeman MR, Shook A, Marian V. Cognitive and emotional effects of bilingualism in adulthood. In: Nicoladis E, Montanari, S, editors. Bilingualism across the lifespan: factors moderating language proficiency. Washington (DC): American Psychological Association; 2016. p. 285–303.

28. McPhillips D. Best countries for education: from primary school to university, a look at how countries invest in the world's future leaders [Internet]. Place unknown: US News & World Report LP; 2017 [cited 2017 May 20]. Available from: https://www.usnews.com/news/best-countries

29. Organisation for Economic Co-operation and Development (OECD). Broadband statistics update [Internet]. Place unknown: OECD; 2020 Jul 22 [cited 2017 May 20]. Available from: https://www.oecd.org/sti/broadband/broadband-statistics-update.htm

30. World Bank. 2019. GDP World [Internet]. Retrieved on October 24, 2020 from https://data.worldbank.org/indicator/NY.GDP.MKTP.CD?locations=1W

31. Lynn R, Meisenberg G. National IQs calculated and validated for 108 nations. Intelligence. 2010 Jul 1;38(4):353–60.

32. Sénéchal M, LeFevre JA. Parental involvement in the development of children's reading skill: a five-year longitudinal study. Child Dev. 2002 Mar–Apr;73(2):445–60.

33. Ursache A, Noble KG. Neurocognitive development in socioeconomic context: multiple mechanisms and implications for measuring socioeconomic status. Psychophysiology. 2016 Jan;53(1):71–82.

34. Tannen D. The pragmatics of cross-cultural communication. Appl Ling. 1984 Sep;5(3):189–95.

35. Fujii D, editor. The neuropsychology of Asian Americans. New York (NY): Psychology Press; 2011 Jan 11. p. 324.

36. American Psychiatric Association. American psychiatric association: diagnostic and statistical manual of mental disorders. 5th ed. Arlington (VA): American Psychiatric Association; 2013. p. 947.

37. Nichter M. Idioms of distress revisited. Cult Med Psychiatry. 2010 Jun;34(2):401–16.

38. Maffini CS, Wong YJ. Assessing somatization with Asian American clients. In: Benuto, L. T., Thaler, N. S., & Leany, B. D. (Eds.). (2014). Guide to psychological assessment with Asians. New York (NY): Springer; 2014. p. 347–60.

39. Kim JE, Saw A, Zane NW, Murphy BL. Patterns of utilization and outcomes of inpatient psychiatric treatment in Asian Americans. Asian Am J Psychol. 2014 Mar;5(1):35.

40. Greenfield PM. You can't take it with you: why ability assessments don't cross cultures. Am Psych. 1997;52(10):1115–24.

41. American Education Research Association, American Psychological Association, and The National Council on Measurement in Education. Standards for educational and psychological testing. 2nd ed. Washington (DC): American Education Research Association; 2014.

42. Thames AD, Hinkin CH, Byrd DA, Bilder RM, Duff KJ, Mindt MR, et al. Effects of stereotype threat, perceived discrimination, and examiner race on neuropsychological performance: simple as black and white?. J Int Neuropsychol Soc. 2013 May;19(5):583.

43. Sternberg RJ, Kaufman SB, editors. Cambridge handbook of intelligence. New York (NY): Cambridge University Press; 2011.

44. Sternberg RJ. Teaching about the nature of intelligence. Intelligence. 2014 Jan 1;42:176–9.

45. Vygotsky LS, Cole M, John-Steiner V, Scribner S, Souberman E. The development of higher psychological processes. Mind Soc. 1978:1–91.

46. Laboratory of Comparative Human Cognition. Culture and intelligence. In: Sternberg RJ, editor. Handbook of human intelligence. Cambridge: Cambridge University Press; 1982. p. 642–719.

47. FairTest (US). 2019 SAT Scores: gaps between demographic groups grows larger [Internet]. Place unknown: publisher unknown; 2019 Sep 24 [cited 2020 Mar 20]. Available from: https://www.fairtest.org/2019-sat-scores-gaps-between-demographic-groups-gr

48. Hsin A, Xie Y. Explaining Asian Americans' academic advantage over whites. Proc Nat Acad Sci. 2014 Jun 10;111(23):8416–21.

49. Kim SW, Cho H, Song M. Revisiting the explanations for Asian American scholastic success: a meta-analytic and critical review. Educ Rev. 2019 Nov 2;71(6):691–711.

50. Clegg, DS. Why Asian education is better, and why It Is Not [Internet]. Place unknown: Verizon Media; 2014 Sept 5 [updated 2017 Dec 6; cited 2020 Mar 6]. Available from: https://www.huffpost.com/entry/why-asian-education-is-be_b_5695418

51. Central Intelligence Agency. World Factbook 2020 India [Internet]. Washington DC: Central Intelligence Agency; 2021 Sept 3 [updated 2020 Oct 5; cited 2017 Jul 15]. Available from: https://www.cia.gov/the-world-factbook/countries/india/

52. Ngo D, Le M, Le PD. Neuropsychology of Vietnamese Americans. In: Fujii D, editor. The neuropsychology of Asian Americans. New York (NY): Psychology Press; 2011 Jan 11. p. 181–200.

Asian Indian

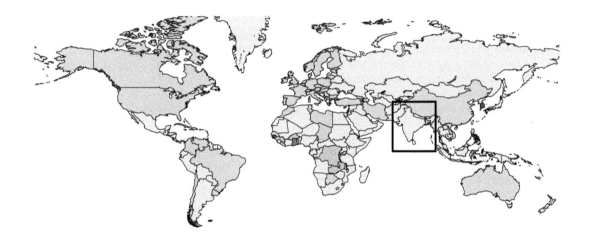

12 Neuropsychological Assessments with Asian Indians

One Size Does Not Fit All

Farzin Irani

Section I: Background Information

Terminology and Perspective

People descended from India are referred to as Indians, Asian Indians, "desi", East Indians, or Indian American/Canadian, etc. My preferred terminology is Indian for those living in India and Asian Indian for those residing in the United States.

One aspect of my identity that frames my perspective for this chapter is of a Gujarati- and Hindi-speaking naturalized American citizen who immigrated to the West as an adolescent. I was professionally trained in the northeastern United States, where I currently teach and practice neuropsychology in a private setting. As reflective of my own transnational bicultural identity, this chapter straddles information about Indians and Asian Indians. I do not claim to speak for the entire community and cannot offer all background information about India.

Geography

India is the 7th largest country in the world, spanning 29 states and 7 union territories. It is located in South Asia and is bound by the Indian Ocean, Arabian Sea, and the Bay of Bengal. It shares land borders with Pakistan, China, Nepal, Bhutan, Bangladesh, and Myanmar.

History

Humans likely first arrived on the Indian subcontinent from Africa between 73,000 and 55,000 years ago.[1] The Indus valley civilization began 4,500 years ago. The ancient cities of Mohenjo-Daro and Harappa were the most advanced of their time. Alas, the region has been invaded many times, starting with Indo-Aryan tribes in 1500 BC. After rule by **Hindu** dynasties, from the 8th century onwards, India faced conquests by Arab, Turkish, and Persian Moghuls. European colonization began with Portuguese traders in the 1500s and the British East India Company's **raj** from 1858 until India's independence on August 15, 1947. The region was subsequently partitioned into primarily Hindu India and mostly Muslim Pakistan, with ongoing ethnic tensions. Almost a century of imperial rule impacted India's global economic and social position[2] and the psychology of its people.[3] Yet, subsequent Indian nationalism engenders pride in cultural and historical accomplishments, such as being the birthplace of early modern language (Sanskrit), alternative medicine (Ayurveda), brain surgeries, yoga, mathematics, chess, the world's first university (Nalanda University in 4th century BC) and several ancient religions.

DOI: 10.4324/9781003051862-25

People

India is the world's largest democracy, with a population of over 1.3 billion people and the largest youth population in the world. I was born in the Indian city of Mumbai, where I spent the first nine years of my life. India has a surface culture of vibrant colors, intoxicating fragrances, melodious music, energetic dances, fun festivals, spicy foods, and lively clothing. I remember people who are hard-working, passionate, humble, generous, caring, respectful, and full of laughter and life despite hardships and sorrows. Yet, the deep culture of people from modern Mumbai is as different from other metropolitan and rural communities as the unique languages, educational backgrounds, socio-economics, values and customs, that exist throughout the country. Indians are by no means a "one size fits all" people. Within-group ethnic diversity and cultural pluralism is the norm.

Immigration and Relocation

India has the world's largest transnational community, with 18 million of its citizens living in the United Arab Emirates, United States, Saudi Arabia, or other places throughout the globe.[4] Common reasons to leave India include economic opportunities, family reunification, or temporary school or work-related relocation.

In the United States, Asian Indians make up 1% of the population and the third-largest foreign-born resident population.[5] In addition to US-born and naturalized citizens, Asian Indians include legal permanent residents, students, workers, and spousal visa holders, refugees, and undocumented immigrants.

Historically, before the 1800s the British East India Company brought indentured Indian servants to the American colonies. The first recorded immigration wave (1899–1908) included ˜6,800 Punjabi Sikhs arriving in California from primarily semiliterate, agricultural, or military backgrounds.[6,7] The 1917 Immigration Act barred migration from India ("Asiatic barred zone") with warnings of a "tide of turbans." After the Immigration and Naturalization Act of 1965 the second phase allowed wealthier, more educated Punjabi and Gujarati speaking professionals to enter and pursue the American dream. The 1990 Family Reunification Act allowed migration under family sponsorship visas. This group was less educated, sought service sector jobs, and faced more challenges for access to services and social networks. More recent employment-based relocation has included an influx of skilled professionals, particularly in technology and medicine, mainly from southern states of India.[6,7] These immigration trends help understand differences in linguistic, educational, occupational, and socio-economics depending on when an Indian came to the United States.

Acculturation and Systemic Barriers

The cultural psychology of immigration[8] is worth considering since sometimes cognitive complaints may reflect emotional distress due to acculturation stress or racism. Migrating to a foreign land can involve culture shock when learning new social rules, managing stressors of coping with unfamiliar environments, and changing cultural identities.[9] Patients may be struggling with pre-immigration traumas, stressors related to green card or visa, changes in cultural identity or socio-economic status, and racism or stereotype threat.[10] Those born to Indian immigrants may live vicariously through their family's immigration stressors, while others may prefer to eschew their ancestral homeland and maintain an "American" identity.[11] Some Indians effectively navigate immigration stress using **Berry's acculturation model's**[12] strategy of integration, while separation, marginalization, or assimilation is less effective for Asian Indians.[13]

Integration to mainstream culture becomes more challenging when Asian Indians are faced with racism due to skin tone, "accents", "body odor", choice of clothing, food preferences, religious beliefs, or oppression due to other aspects of intersectionality. Complaints of glass ceiling effects are rampant in workplaces. Racial injustices include increased hate crimes against Sikh men who wore turbans after 9/11, increased government scrutiny (e.g., FBI surveillance of Muslim communities, greater profiling in immigration policies), and increased "communities on fire" with violence and xenophobic political rhetoric, often motivated by anti-Muslim sentiment.[14,15] In a recent survey, 1 in 2 South Asians in the United States report regularly encountering discrimination.[11] Yet, along with other Asian American communities Asian Indians grapple with the "model minority myth" based on stereotypes of achieving socio-economic success due to higher education, work ethic, low criminality, and family/marital stability. However, this myth has been used historically to create racial wedges and exclude those with genuine economic need from receiving social assistance.

Understanding these systemic barriers within the context of personal biases is important since stereotype threat and perceived discrimination impacts examiner-examinee racial discordance during neuropsychological testing[16] and is linked to neuropsychological test performance for Asian Indians in the United States.[17]

Language

Accurate evaluation of language proficiency ensures that evaluations assess cognitive ability and not English language proficiency. India is one of the most linguistically diverse nations in the world. Multilingualism is the norm, with 22 official languages with their own written scripts. These languages are of Indo-Aryan, Dravidian, Austroasiatic, and Sino-Tibetan origin.[18] Hindi, Bengali, Marathi, Telugu, Tamil, Gujarati, Urdu, Kannada, Odia, Malayalam, and Punjabi are commonly spoken, but there are over 19,000 spoken dialects, many without writing systems. Most Indian languages have significant linguistic and cultural differences from English.

In the United States, 82% of Asian Indians are proficient in English.[19] In India, 11% of the population speaks English, 26% are bilingual, and 7% are trilingual.[20] English and Hindi are commonly spoken in India, but depending on the context, different languages can be used for ethnic identity, business transactions, official dealings, or entertainment.[21] Use of language mixed and borrowed words are frequent in daily communication. While there may be overlap among some languages, knowledge of one language does not imply knowledge of another regional language. This is important to keep in mind when working with interpreters and translators, or decisions to refer to another provider.

Recommendations for testing bilingual speakers in the Indian context include evaluating the linguistic proficiency of the patient and examiner, considering language interference from borrowed/language-mixed words when interpreting responses, and not separating monolingual and bilingual norms for select cognitive batteries.[22] It is practically impossible to develop/adapt tests in all Indian languages and dialects, but some tests and normative data are currently available and others are emerging (see Appendix and Porrselvi & Shankar (2007)[23] for a review).

Communication

Understanding communication preferences helps establish rapport, gather accurate history, ensure testing fairness, and deliver effective feedbacks. While private communication patterns among family or friends can vary, public communication for most Indians tends to be polite, respectful, and indirect. Even before COVID-19 social distancing, many Indian Hindus traditionally preferred to formally join hands (namaste) or touch an elder's feet in greeting instead of shaking hands. For some, initiating a conversation without being asked could be considered disrespectful, since Indian schools teach students not to speak unless spoken to. So, patients may not volunteer information unless explicitly asked.

Age, seniority, and educational achievements are highly regarded. Formal language tends to be preferred for authority figures (e.g., Dr., Sir/Madam, Mr/.Mrs, uncle/aunty) rather than first names. Doctors tend to be revered, so in interactions with neuropsychologists, verbal responses could be incongruent. For example, patients may blindly follow recommendations without questions or criticism, despite internal conflict. On the other hand, they may also verbally agree with recommendations but not act on them because direct verbal refusals such as saying 'no' to a doctor could be perceived as harsh. More evasive communication styles such as hand or head gestures, vague responses (e.g., "I'll try"), or silence may be used instead. However, this isn't true for all Indians. Global exchanges through social media have brought Westernized influences, with many preferring direct communications.

For Indian immigrants, nonverbal gestures and Indian English vernacular can challenge communication in clinical encounters. Gender boundaries may be communicated nonverbally. For example, some may avert eye and physical contact with the opposite gender. It may be challenging for some to work with a different gendered person in a small testing room for extended periods of time.

I recall a funny incident with an older Indian immigrant who was not fluent in English. He was asked by our receptionist whether he wanted coffee. He responded with an "Indian head shake", which looks like a mix between a nod and a head shake. Our receptionist was utterly puzzled about whether he meant "yes", "no", or "maybe." After unsuccessful attempts to clarify, she brought coffee that he politely accepted. She left pleased that she had deciphered the cryptic gesture. Once the doors to my office closed, he laughed and offered the full cup of coffee to me. He told me in Hindi that he doesn't drink coffee and was trying to express that he understood what she was asking but didn't want her to feel bad by refusing. This was his way of not making a firm commitment without being offensive. So, guess who then drank the coffee to not offend our receptionist? And even I don't like coffee!

Education

Accurate assessment of education quality and quantity is important for neuropsychological test interpretation.[24] In the United States, many Asian Indians are well-educated, with 85% having at least some college education.[19] Yet, in India, while 95% complete primary school (class 1–8), subsequent dropouts lead to 69% completing secondary (class 9–12) and only 25% completing post-secondary school.[25]

There are also vast disparities in the quality of educational experiences in India. Schools can be funded by government, private, or international sources with different resources and "mediums" of instruction (i.e., local language emersion versus English-based instruction). Schooling can range from village leaders teaching children under a tree to urban classrooms bulging with 65+ children to some of the most elite private and technical schools in the world. Therefore, it is important to ask about the quality of educational experiences, beliefs about education, and mediums of instruction during school.

The mindset around learning is also worth understanding since it can affect test-taking style. In Indian schools, focus is frequently on rote memorization rather than application. Standardized examinations occur at transition points and are stressful for students and families since they determine financial and social success. This contributes to an environment that values academic and occupational achievement, particularly in science, technology, engineering, and mathematics (STEM) fields. Achievement is often viewed as something that can be developed through hard work versus innate intelligence.

There is significant outbound student mobility from India, which has the second-largest international student population worldwide.[26] Unfortunately, there are many Indian migrants with advanced degrees whose training is not recognized after immigrating to the West. I evaluated a pediatrician from India who accepted a research assistant position to support his family. Over time, this eroded his self-esteem, impacted mood and chronic pain, and took him down a slippery slope of prescription drug abuse with associated cognitive deficits. Uncovering this core issue during the assessment helped accurately determine his treatment needs.

Literacy

India has one of the largest illiterate populations in the world (~1 in 4 people). Literacy rates are higher in urban areas (87%) compared to rural (73%), with gender disparities between men (84%) and women (70%).[20] In rural areas, contributors to these disparities include shortage of classrooms, lack of sanitation or drinking water, **caste** disparities, and gender role expectations.[27]

Formal and informal ways of learning to read and write in multiple languages at various ages are common in India. Most Indian schools formally teach three languages such as English, Hindi, and a regional language. In some schools, a foreign language such as French or German may be an option. Interpreters should be asked about their multilingual literacy in all the patient's preferred languages due to high likelihood of language code-switching during evaluations. Asking about the nature and type of formal and informal educational experience also helps understand how patients create and communicate using written materials in multiple languages.

I was referred to a Gujarati-speaking patient due to dementia concerns. The neurologist observed difficulty recalling words during a cognitive screener administered in English. The patient also worked very slowly when completing a simple written alphanumeric sequencing task. In gathering history, I learned that he had briefly attended a rural school in his village in India where he was taught to speak, read, and write in basic Gujarati for "a couple" of years. After immigrating to America over 40 years ago, he picked up basic conversational English, but with limited reading or writing ability in English. As a cashier, he was able to calculate change for his customers. He could also recite numbers and the Gujarati alphabet aloud during his neuropsychology appointment. Yet, his performance was much slower on written tasks. He explained that in school, they used small, hand-held chalkboards rather than paper and pencil to write. He was taught to take his time when writing to ensure accuracy. Thus, he was forming each number in his mind on his mental chalkboard first before transferring it to the paper. He did not have processing speed concerns - he just had a different test-taking approach. When presented with simple words to remember in Gujarati rather than English, he could learn and recall the words, highlighting intact memory abilities. This patient could have been misdiagnosed with dementia, which may have robbed him of driving or led to unnecessary treatments and costs.

Socio-Economic Status

While Asian Indians in the United States have high annual household incomes compared to the general population, there is a bimodal distribution for wealth, with many living in poverty.[19,28,29] India has a developing market economy with positive long-term growth projections due to its young population (more than 80% are younger than 44 years old) and integration into the global economy.[30] India struggles with paradoxical disparities between rich and poor. Mansion gates open onto shanty-towns where young children hold even younger siblings on their hips and beg for money. Tasty and nutritious food is abundant yet inaccessible to children who can be found picking food from garbage. Poor communities also don't have resources to afford medical or mental health care. Urban areas have access to bottled or public water, but in remote villages, girls and women walk for miles carrying water from rivers or lakes. Sanitation levels vary greatly, with some of Asia's biggest slums riddled with extremely poor living and toileting facilities. Air pollution is common in over-populated urban cities with detrimental effects on pulmonary and other health conditions, yet rural communities enjoy open fields and fresh air. These socio-economic disparities and lack of access to nutritional and environmental resources impact Indian children's physical, cognitive, and brain development.[31,32] Most recently, the COVID-19 pandemic adversely impacted mortality for Indians from poor and illiterate backgrounds due to comorbidities associated with socio-economic inequities.[33]

I evaluated a middle-aged Indian immigrant for attentional concerns. In relaying history, he shared that during adolescence he was an "awful" student who was easily distracted, got into trouble with his teachers, and failed his classes. This could have been attributed to an attention-deficit/hyperactivity disorder. Yet, after becoming more comfortable, he disclosed that these academic difficulties occurred during a time of stress and family disruption. His father had unexpectedly abandoned the family, and his mother had to make ends meet as a maid. He described a situation where they lived meagerly with poor nutrition and unhygienic living conditions. He frequently became sick with illnesses that went uninvestigated. He couldn't attend to his health and education because of increasing financial responsibilities to support his mother and sister. There were no social support services that came to his rescue, and the new family unit struggled. These economic and social circumstances likely impacted brain-behavior development, with downstream influences on his ability to make educational and occupational gains.

Values and Customs

Awareness about commonly held values and customs in Indian communities can support rapport, thoughtful interviews, and successful feedback sessions. Yet, it's important to recognize that individual values vary greatly, and patients are always the best source of their unique world views.

In general, traditional Indian views value hospitality, respect, humility, selflessness, inter-dependence, family-centrism, and collectivism. These values manifest in an amalgam of perspectives and behaviors. For example, gifts or food items can be offered to doctors to show gratitude and respect, and rejection of these gifts may be hurtful. In accord with values of collectivism and belongingness, children may be taught from a young age that individual decisions need to be in harmony with family and social structures. In my practice, some Indian patients have chosen to reject treatment recommendations that involved allocating limited financial resources on themselves instead of their families.

Though contemporary Indian culture is trending away from traditional, arranged marriages and joint family structures, many Indians continue to make family decisions cooperatively. I once completed a feedback session with a frightened woman recently diagnosed with multiple sclerosis. During the session, she brought both her in-laws, husband, sisters-in-law, and teenage children. My office no longer had any place to move. Yet, we knew that the treatment plan we had come up with jointly was well understood and likely to be successfully implemented with the support and commitment she received from her entire concerned family that day.

Those who immigrate at young ages or were born in the West are more likely to be integrated into mainstream culture, so they may think or behave differently from their parents, which can be a source of intergenerational conflict. Youth born in the United States who have Indian immigrant parents may be secretive about dating, clothing, smoking, drug or alcohol use. This can impact accurate assessment of the influence of factors such as substance abuse on an evaluation.

It is also worth noting that time is valued differently between Indians and the West. Many Indians prefer to function at a relaxed pace rather than feeling confined to inflexible routines or structures. This may translate into arriving late to appointments, impromptu meetings, and rescheduling appointments. The time pressure of neuropsychological assessments has not always been appreciated by some of my less test-wise Indian immigrant patients. Notably, Asian Indians accustomed to competitive academic environments in India have been ready to go before the stopwatch is even pulled out!

Gender and Sexuality

In India there are gender disparities in cognitive functioning for women moderated by region (e.g. southern versus northern India), educational attainment, health, and socio-economics.[34] Paradoxically, while Hindu scriptures revere women as Goddesses, there are gender inequalities with low female to male sex ratios in certain regions due to "missing women" who perish due to socially determined excess female mortality.[34] In traditional male-dominated patriarchal homes, women are viewed as mother figures and homemakers who don't pursue higher education or work outside the home. Understanding these values helps avoid Westernized assumptions and supports culturally consistent treatment planning. For example, some of my traditional female patients have not wanted to make health decisions without their husband or family's involvement. In situations of financial dependence, this has guided referrals to free or low-cost clinics.

Indians tend to be conservative sexually. Discussions about sexual functioning relevant in some neuropsychological contexts have not spontaneously emerged with my Indian patients. In addition, despite historical literary evidence of a spectrum of sexual and gender identities in ancient texts (e.g., Kama Sutra), discrimination toward the LGBTQ+ community is common. A colonial-era law that made gay sex punishable with up to ten years in prison was only recently struck down in 2018 by the Supreme Court of India. It was only a few years prior in 2014 that the Supreme Court of India officially recognized hijras or a third gender of people in India.

The intersection of social challenges in LGBTQ+ communities with those of the Indian culture can create unique systems of disadvantage. A young Asian Indian gay patient presented for an ADHD evaluation, but was instead clearly depressed and struggling to come out to traditional Indian parents who were cluelessly planning an arranged marriage. Creating an affirming space can allow neuropsychologists to appreciate the influence of extrinsic and intrinsic contextual factors on cognitive complaints.

Spirituality and Religion

In India, the majority religion of Hinduism co-exists with Islam, the largest minority religion. Other faiths include Sikhism, Christianity, Buddhism, Jainism, Zoroastrianism, Judaism, and the Baha'i Faith. People of different religions, castes, and cultures generally live in harmony and celebrate each other's festivals (e.g., Holi, Diwali, Eid, Navroz, Christmas). Yet, there are painful religious and caste-based conflicts historically rooted in colonial influences that lead to violence that has impacted the physical and psychological health of millions of Indians. Islamophobia and Hindu-Muslim conflicts are rampant, including current escalations. Caste-system politics and societal stratifications have created injustice, socio-economic inequalities, and violence within and outside the caste group structure. The oppression of **Dalit** and indigenous peoples of South Asia is also present in the United States.[35] As a religious minority, I listen closely when caste-oppressed South Asians share workplace discrimination experiences[35] so that I can affirm the presence of these within-group injustices and their potential impact on emotional and cognitive health.

Health Status

Our recent review on biopsychosocial and health characteristics in the Asian Indian population in the United States highlights concerns about health data aggregation with Asians broadly and the marginalization of the Asian Indian community in the neuropsychology literature.[36] This is despite disproportionally high rates of salient health conditions with increased cognitive burden. This includes metabolic and cardiovascular disorders (e.g., coronary artery disease, hypertension, type 2 diabetes) with associated mortality burden, particularly for younger Asian Indian males. Stroke and dementia although prevalent are poorly understood in the community. Other primary health conditions also prevalent in the community include cancer (prostate, colorectal, lung, breast, ovarian, uterine), tuberculosis, and HIV/AIDS, although one in five South Asian Americans lacks health insurance to treat these conditions.[37] There has also been a disparate impact of COVID-19 across South Asian communities in the United States,[38] with the neuropsychological impacts of these health conditions in the community neglected in the literature so far.

Mental Health Views

Asian Indians have elevated depression, stress, suicide, smokeless tobacco use, and domestic trauma rates, yet understanding of the culturally relevant treatment needs for the community is limited.[36] In India too, there are barriers to accessing services due to stigma and discrimination against people with mental disorders.[39] It is common to go to a medical doctor for physical ailments, yet seeking help from an "outsider" about personal issues could be viewed shamefully. There may be a tendency to rely on alternative coping systems involving elders or extended family/friends who drop by uninvited to converse about each other's problems. Consultation with religious leaders such as yogis, pandits, imams or priests may be more acceptable for some than seeking out help from a psychologist. Mental health services may be a luxury few can afford. Holistic options may be used as alternatives. Some may believe that cognitive or emotional issues can be cured by trying harder. Some Hindus may view their problems as "karma" due to a pre-destined fate for which nothing can be done. However, influences of age, education, family dynamics, geographic location, and acculturation status all moderate such beliefs.

Approach to Neuropsychological Evaluations

Despite a long immigration history and increasing US census representation, neuropsychological considerations for Asian Indians as a distinct group have been absent. In the absence of neuropsychological tools adapted to the Asian Indian immigrant context, a one size fits all approach cannot be used. Each case needs careful consideration for whether it is more appropriate to use existing measures and norms developed in a Western context or whether tools from India are a better fit. There are some linguistically diverse global and domain-specific tests that have been adapted/translated in various Indian languages, and specific test batteries have recently been developed, standardized, and normed in multiple languages at a larger scale using Indian epidemiological samples (see Appendix for list).

Neuropsychology in India started over 40 years ago from Western influence but has faced challenges related to growing training pathways, infrastructure, lack of awareness, linguistic, educational and literacy-related diversity, and access/affordability concerns.[40] There are very few doctoral-level neuropsychologists in India, most of whom work at the National Institute of Mental Health and Neurosciences or practice as clinical psychologists in neurological or psychiatric settings. Thus, many Indians immigrants are unlikely to be familiar with neuropsychological services.

Often, when Asian Indians present for services, it is under the guise of physical or somatic complaints since body concerns are more culturally acceptable.[41],[42] In my practice with Asian Indians, clinical referrals come from trusted primary care physicians, with rare self-referrals or referrals from mental health providers. I believe this is in part because neuropsychologists serve as a bridge from the medical/neurological to psychological world. We act as a gateway to engage in discussions about emotional and social concerns along with neurological considerations. Physical or cognitive complaints can uncover psychological or social issues. During clinical interviews, paying close attention to unspoken and indirect messages can help identify true cognitive, emotional, or social needs.

When Indian immigrants present for an evaluation, they may be unsure about what to expect or why they were referred. A preliminary orientation to the nature and purpose of assessment can increase comfort. Providing clear explanations about the focus on the body and brain may ease fears about stigmatization. For example, explaining that sadness or nervousness can affect chemicals released in the brain and body has allowed patients to feel more invested. I also prepare patients for the nature of the clinical interview by indicating that my questions about history are not meant to be inquisitive but to understand them better and be helpful. Family members may prefer to share concerns privately out of respect for their loved one. The idea of confidentiality (with its limits) may be new, so patients may welcome assurance that private information will not be disclosed to anyone not authorized.

If testing is indicated and appropriate, even though I understand multiple Indian languages, I can't read or write in all those languages, so I consider whether a regional language-specific interpreter or referral to another Indian provider is more appropriate. During testing, it's important to minimize measurement bias by evaluating whether available tools are psychometrically, linguistically, and regionally appropriate for each Indian patient. I also try to assess test wiseness to ensure physical/emotional comfort, understanding of the test setting, and/or computer savviness. For some patients from illiterate or rural backgrounds, psychometric testing may not be appropriate.

In feedback sessions, due to the reverence given to doctors and preference for directive stances, Indian patients and families often expect advice and clear directions on what to do next. For patients with language barriers or those less familiar with how to implement treatment recommendations, I often pick up the phone during the session to provide connections to culturally or linguistically appropriate referrals. Occasionally, Indian patients feel insecure about terminating the assessment relationship after establishing trust, so extra steps need to be taken to support smooth transfer of care.

If referring for psychotherapy or cognitive remediation, allaying patients' concerns about the unknown by orienting them to what to expect can be helpful. Culturally aware interventions in the hands of a multiculturally competent provider are most likely to be effective and reduce risks for premature termination of care. Recommendations for family-based therapy can be helpful for some patients who do not view their own well-being as different from that of the family unit. Some of my Indian patients have not welcomed groups, which they considered publicly humiliating or unnecessarily intrusive. Yet, some of their children and extended family have been quite ready to hear about much-needed respite and supportive resources.

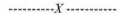

----------*X* -----------

Overall, these personal and professional experiences, as well as my knowledge about India and awareness of my own skills and limitations helped prepare me to meet Mrs. Rama and see her as more than a "40-year-old, right-handed, Asian Indian woman with twelve years of formal education referred by her family doctor due to concerns about her cognition." Despite some common aspects of our cultural heritage, I knew that Mrs. Rama had her own story to tell that I needed to carefully hear and learn from in order to be helpful to her.

Section II: Case Study — "I'd Rather Have a Stroke than Be Depressed"

Note: Possible identifying information and aspects of history and presentation have been changed to protect patient identity and privacy.

Behavioral Observations

Mrs. Rama came to her neuropsychology appointment alone after being dropped off by her husband who left for work. She was 20 minutes late, which we later joked about being "Indian Standard Time." She brought intake paperwork which she completed with the help of her husband. She was alert, fully oriented, polite, and pleasant. She wore the top of a traditional Indian outfit and had red powder sprinkled in the middle part of her hair to indicate she was a traditional married Hindu woman. She was conversational in Indian English. She expressed a preference for the evaluation to be conducted in her first language, Hindi. The rest of her informed consent process and mental status exam was unremarkable. There were no difficulties noted in her vision, hearing, movements, speech, language, social or sensory-motor functions. While she was politely responsive to humor, her facial expressions were generally restricted, and she cried at various points when discussing her history. She appeared nervous at the outset and initially expressed uncertainty about what to expect. She visibly relaxed as the interview progressed and after receiving clarifying explanations about the process in assessing brain-behavior relationships. Prior to gathering history, I prefaced my questioning by clarifying that I was not trying to be inquisitive but wanted to understand her experiences. She was occasionally evasive, and I did not press her directly for information during those moments. We built a good rapport. During the testing session, she indicated she was used to standardized testing from her schooling days in India, yet I took care to ensure that she was comfortable in our testing environment. She remained focused and eager to do well and gave good effort throughout the session. We started our conversation with her reasons for seeking the current evaluation.

Presenting Concerns

Mrs. Rama shared that she became concerned about something being "wrong" with her after seeing her father and a family friend have a stroke. She approached her family doctor for concerns about forgetfulness about names of acquaintances at her place of worship and absent-mindedness (e.g., walked away with groceries without paying, misplacing her purse). She sometimes found it hard to understand what people were saying to her; however, this didn't occur when speaking in Hindi. She denied any expressed concerns from her husband or others. She denied acute medical events and stated these cognitive difficulties had been there "on and off" for a few years. She denied problems with balance, falls, head injuries, vision, or changes in her reading or writing.

Daily Functioning

Mrs. Rama had never worked outside her home. She spent her days cooking, cleaning, and half-heartedly watching Hindi television serials or movies. She had been getting tired easily for the past few years and didn't feel motivated. She had never driven and relied on her husband for transportation. Her husband also managed finances, but she managed her own medical appointments on a calendar. She had friends from the Hindu temple where she worshiped but had been avoiding socialization. She also rarely made long-distance calls to her friends in India anymore.

Health History

Mrs. Rama denied problems with her birth or early development. She was medically healthy and only took medication to control type II diabetes. She struggled with obesity after dietary changes since moving to the United States. She reported occasional headaches treated with over-the-counter medications. Her most recent blood work was unremarkable, with normal thyroid function, vitamin D and B12 levels. Neuroimaging was not available at the time of her initial appointment. She had no history of smoking, drinking, or abusing drugs. She was a strict vegetarian based on her religion. She slept well at night and napped during the day. She denied night-time awakenings, a history of snoring, gasping, or morning headaches. There was no known family history of dementia. Her father died of a stroke, and her mother had a history of psychosis. She did not have siblings or children.

Educational History

In India, Mrs. Rama was taught in a rural setting in Hindi-medium schools, which included some instruction in English. She passed nationally administered 12th grade Indian School Certificate Examinations in English. She was enrolled in college in the Humanities before discontinuing her education in less than a year. She denied history of distractibility, being held back, or struggling academically in any particular subject. She described herself as an average student. She had not completed any formal classes in English as a Second Language or schooling after migrating to the United States.

Language Proficiency

Using a language experience and proficiency questionnaire,[43] I determined that Mrs. Rama's dominant language was Hindi. She acquired Hindi first since it was spoken at home by her family. She currently had 80% exposure to Hindi, 15% English, and 5% Punjabi. She described herself as having "excellent, 9/10" ability to speak, understand, read and write in Hindi, which was taught formally throughout her schooling. Internalized language involving thinking or dreaming was also in Hindi. Mrs. Rama's English language proficiency was "adequate, 5/10" for speaking, reading, and writing. She described herself as "very good" at understanding Punjabi but had "low" capacity to read and write in Punjabi.

It was clear that Mrs. Rama's dominant language was Hindi, followed by English, and then Punjabi. Her degree of English language proficiency was not sufficient to match age-based expectations of available English-based neuropsychological test measures. She expressed a preference for testing in Hindi. An evaluation in her native language was the most accurate way to ensure that the testing captured her current cognitive status rather than English language proficiency. I am able to speak, read and write in Hindi and felt comfortable proceeding with a Hindi evaluation.

Cultural History

Mrs. Rama was an only child born into a traditional, religious Hindu family in India. Her parents lived jointly with her paternal grandparents, uncles and aunts, and their children. When Mrs. Rama was born her parents were thrilled despite initial disappointment expressed by her grandparents that she wasn't a boy. She was aware of her "burden" to her family as a female since childhood.

Mrs. Rama's father worked at a local clothing shop, and her mother did not work outside the home. Her family lived modestly in a clean, hygienic environment with good access to nutritious food and clean water. She denied history of abuse stating she was a "good girl" who escaped the occasional corporal punishment inflicted on her male cousins. Expectations in her family were that, like her older cousins, when she reached a marriageable age, she would have an arranged marriage with someone selected by her family from her religion and caste. Yet, Mrs. Rama would often worry about not getting an acceptable marriage proposal due to her mother's mental health.

Mrs. Rama shared that her mother was known as the "pagal" (crazy) lady in her town after several public psychotic episodes. Early on, her mother was kept locked in her home during these episodes, and her family would pray for her to get better. She eventually received psychiatric treatment, but this was a source of shame for the family. A marriage proposal for her older cousin was broken due to this situation. Mrs. Rama learned early to be ashamed and secretive about mental health.

In college, she fell in love with a Muslim man and knowing that their inter-faith relationship would not be accepted by their families, they ran away to a big city together. They became estranged from both families. Mrs. Rama shared that her family considered her to be selfish since she had ignored the family's honor. Yet, the couple was in love and happily settled in the big city. Mrs. Rama described feeling at peace and happy during those days. They successfully built a circle of friends, and she was active in social circles. She enjoyed reading, yoga, cooking, shopping, exercising, watching television/movies, and attending community and spiritual gatherings. Over the years, Mrs. Rama and her husband were unable to conceive children, which became a source of shame. She viewed this as being her "karma" (action) based on her inability to fulfill her "dharma" (duty) to her family and religion.

Eventually her husband's company transferred his job to the northeastern United States, and they left India with trepidation yet excitement about new opportunities. Mrs. Rama shared that when she reached America at the age of 32, she experienced culture shock. She initially enjoyed the luxuries of the West including abundance of food, living space, entertainment, places to see, and things to buy. Yet, after a few months she began to feel anxious about communication barriers and trying to learn entirely different ways of doing things. She was on a spousal visa and could not work. Her husband traveled frequently for his job, and they lived in a suburban area without easy access to transportation. Her neighbors did not reach out to her socially. This was in stark contrast to her lifestyle in India, where neighbors would drop by uninvited to socialize over tea. She began to miss the communal and familiar aspects of her life in India, including the subtropical climate of her home when faced with harsh winters. She isolated herself within the safety of her home, which compounded her loneliness.

Privately, Mrs. Rama became guilt ridden about past decisions to abandon her family and home and became resentful about leaving India. As time went on, she became more spiritual and immersed in her own cultural identity as a Hindu woman. Over time, even her faith became a solitary act in her *puja* room at home, compared to communal prayer and chanting sessions.

Mrs. Rama experienced racist encounters that impacted her acculturation. She became scared about interacting with "Americans" after being yelled at during communication barriers where she was told "go back to where you came from" or "learn English if you want to live in my country." Her husband and main confidant was supportive but did not know what to do about these situations and so suggested she "walk away and forget them."

Emotional Functioning

Mrs. Rama expressed feeling lonely, sad, and crying frequently. She shared thoughts about wishing she had never been born but denied active suicidal ideation due to her faith. She became preoccupied with excessive guilt about not having resolved her relationship with her father before he died of a stroke a few years ago. While she regularly sent money to India for her mother's psychiatric care, she also felt ashamed about abandoning her and did not want to face her family and "bring them more shame." She worried about "catching" her mother's "bimari" or illness, yet there was no evidence of any history of psychosis for Mrs. Rama. She had decreased interest in doing things, was sleeping a lot, felt fatigued, and had trouble concentrating due to her thoughts and worries.

Preliminary Formulation

At the end of the interview, it was clear to me that Mrs. Rama was clinically depressed and anxious but did not recognize or want to acknowledge it. In addition to personal and historical family of origin-related contributions, acculturation and immigration-related stressors were clearly at play.

Mrs. Rama had experienced culture shock after losing familiar cues, breakdown of interpersonal communication, and an identity crisis. Her physical and social isolation reflected a *separation* stage of acculturation where she deeply valued her own cultural identity but was unable to develop a satisfying relationship with her new home. Additional barriers included racist experiences, problems with communication, and lack of access to knowledge about majority culture.

While the referral question involved evaluation for memory loss, psychological and cultural factors were much more salient. However, I did not want to make premature conclusions. She had been referred to a neuropsychologist, had increased cardiovascular and stroke risks (diabetes, obesity, family history, sleep and mood disturbance, unhealthy lifestyle with lack of exercise and poor diet), and was seeking physical explanations for her attention/"forgetfulness" and language comprehension type complaints. While it was unlikely that Mrs. Rama had a stroke, the possibility of early metabolic or vascular-related cognitive dysfunction was worth exploring given increased burden in the Asian Indian population.

Throughout my work with Mrs. Rama, I tried to remain aware of my soft spots for her as an Indian woman and also reflected on hot spots related to the injustices she experienced. I then proceeded to select and administer a brief neuropsychological test battery that could assess her cognitive functioning in a culturally fair manner to rule out possible brain dysfunction and establish a baseline for the future.

Test and Norm Selection

There are limited tests available in Hindi, and unfortunately no comprehensive demographically corrected normative data for Indians immigrants living in the United States at the time I saw her. While Mrs. Rama lived in the United States, based on her acculturation and language proficiency in Hindi, Indian norms were a better fit. I used a neuropsychological test battery adapted to the Indian context with available age and education adjusted normative data from healthy Hindi-speaking individuals in northern India.[44] This population was a good match for Mrs. Rama's background. This test battery has been modified[44] as described below:

1 Hopkins Verbal Learning Test-Revised[45] with adaptations involving items representing gemstones opal and ruby which are unfamiliar in the northern Indian context, and replaced with Hindi gemstone names (e.g., moonga and pukhraj).
2 Brief Visuospatial Memory Test-Revised.[46]
3 Digit Symbol-Coding and Symbol Search subtests from Wechsler Adult Intelligence Scale-III.[47]
4 Grooved Pegboard Test.[48]
5 Color Trails Test 1 and 2.[49]
6 Spatial Span subtest from Wechsler Memory Scale III.[47]
7 Controlled Oral Word Association Test[50] with modifications of changing letters F, A, and S to P, A, and R to match rate of occurrence of letters in Hindi.
8 Category Fluency Test.[50]
9 Stroop Color and Word Test.[51]
10 Wisconsin Card Sort Test 64.[52]

For emotional functioning, I complemented my clinical interview with brief depression (Patient Health Questionnaire-9) and generalized anxiety disorder (GAD-7) screeners that have been translated into Hindi.

Test Results and Impressions

After adjusting for age and education, Mrs. Rama performed in the average range across all cognitive tests administered. She slowed down slightly on one processing speed measure (symbol search, $z = -0.75$, 21st percentile), but this was not consistent with average range speed demonstrated on other measures. She had a deliberate approach during this task that accounted for her slowing. Learning and memory showed subtle initial dips in encoding of new verbal and visual information during the first trial, but her total learning and recall of previously learned information was intact, and there were no problems with delayed recall. Language and problem-solving skills were adequate. Overall, her neurocognitive profile was intact.

Emotionally, she endorsed moderate levels of depression (PHQ-9 = 13) with daily loss of interest/pleasure, feeling down/hopeless, feelings of failure, excessive sleeping, fatigue, poor appetite, and trouble concentrating. These symptoms made it difficult for her to take care of things at home and get along with others. Mrs. Rama also reported moderate levels of anxiety (GAD-7 = 12) with daily worries, trouble relaxing, and feeling afraid about something awful happening. She reported several days when she feels nervous, has trouble relaxing, and feels irritable.

Overall, Mrs. Rama was diagnosed with a major depressive disorder, single episode, moderate, with anxious distress (F32.1). I also acknowledged problems related to her social environment including acculturation difficulties (Z60.3) and exclusion and isolation (Z60.4).

Feedback Session and Follow-Up

For her feedback session, Mrs. Rama brought her husband to the appointment. Her first direct question was whether she had a stroke. I shared my impression that she had not had a stroke based on her neuropsychological test data and the normal neuroimaging results subsequently received. I provided education about stroke signs and symptoms, and we discussed her fears about having a stroke like her father and friend. I also helped her understand her cognitive struggles from an attentional and motivational framework rather than one involving brain damage from stroke. She became visibly relieved.

I then gently proceeded to engage her and her husband in a discussion that validated her feelings and historical conflicts with her family of origin. I normalized her immigration-, acculturation-, and racism-related stress, and we spoke about her worries about losing her cultural identity. We discussed her social isolation and psychosocial influences on her mood. She expressed an interest in finding a balance between her relational and individual needs.

When I shared my impressions regarding depression and anxiety, she acknowledged it but noted that she was secretly hoping I would tell her that she had a stroke. She cried and shared that a mental health diagnosis was stigmatizing given her mother's history, and she didn't want to be considered "pagal." It would be much easier for her to accept that she had a medical problem. I was glad that she asserted her thoughts and did not just agree with me, given my position as an authority figure for her. I expressed understanding of the influence of her beliefs and her struggle with her diagnosis. I provided education about psychotic disorders and reassured her regarding the absence of evidence for psychosis. I then explained the neurobiology of depression and anxiety so that she could view them as common medical conditions that many people struggle with.

To improve her mood and health behaviors, we discussed behavioral activation by returning to attend the Hindu temple regularly, calling her friends in India, taking daily walks with her husband, exploring local hobbies (e.g., floral arrangement, cooking or yoga classes) or reaching out to a neighbor by taking over home-made food. We spoke about using Uber/Lyft for transportation so that she could have access to community resources without relying on her husband. We also discussed additional prevention strategies for brain health (e.g., regular health care, diet for brain/ heart health, mindfulness, cognitive engagement).

We then discussed options of seeing a psychiatrist for medication management and a psychologist/counselor for talk therapy. She preferred to start with a bilingual, Hindi-speaking psychiatrist to get medications to help her feel better. Based on her acculturation (*separation*) and traditional loyalties, it was not surprising that she selected this concrete and time-limited medical option with someone who shared her cultural background.

She needed psychotherapeutic support too. Her husband had integrated more into majority culture and was eager to hear how to support his wife. I presented the option of couples' therapy. To allay their concerns about the unknown, I explained what therapy can involve and how they could communicate about current and past stressors. They agreed, and Mrs. Rama was particularly pleased about the prospect of having a weekly hour with her husband's full attention. I referred them to a culturally sensitive couples' therapist who was likely to validate their experiences without pathologizing their cultural experiences. I asked Mrs. Rama to reach out to me again if she needed referrals in the future for a culturally aware individual therapist. She left smiling.

Upon her request and with her written permission, I reached out to her new psychiatrist and couples' therapist to share my impressions and suggestions for her treatment plan. After more than a year, I received a call from Mrs. Rama inquiring about individual therapist referrals. She shared that she was doing well, her mood had lifted, and she was more socially engaged and healthier. The couple had been discharged from counseling, and Mrs. Rama was now planning to enter the workforce! Her couple's therapist suggested that she gain individual support through this new endeavor in her life. When Mrs. Rama asked for referrals this time she was open to working with a non-Indian therapist. Her new help-seeking behavior suggested more positive attitudes toward mental health and greater integration.

Overall, I was glad that Mrs. Rama's neuropsychological evaluation helped provide a bridge to the psychological supports she needed to treat her emotional symptoms and put her on a path of improved well-being.

Section III: Lessons Learned

- India is rich in historical, linguistic, educational, socio-economic, religious, and cultural heterogeneity.
- Knowledge about deeper aspects of Indian culture (e.g., communication preferences, values/ customs) can help establish trust and rapport in a community that is guarded about seeking psychological/neuropsychological services. This can support gathering accurate biopsychosociocultural histories, ensuring test fairness, making accurate clinical impressions, and delivering effective feedback that is likely to be implemented.
- Orientation to the assessment process, brain and body-based explanations, and clearly setting expectations about the clinical interview and confidentiality can help ease patients into an unfamiliar experience.
- Consideration of the psychology of immigration and systemic barriers faced by Asian Indians can reveal acculturation-, racism-, casteism-, sexism-, classism-, or heterosexism-related stress masked as cognitive or physical complaints.
- Linguistic, educational, and literacy-based diversity in India deserves inquiry into the nature and quality of these experiences to ensure that evaluations assess cognitive ability and not English language proficiency, test wiseness, or different ways of communicating in oral or written materials.
- Multilingualism is the norm and providers/interpreters need to consider language interference from borrowed/language-mixed words when interpreting responses.

- Despite being the largest transnational community in the world, having a long immigration history in the United States and increasing census representation, the Asian Indian population has been invisible in the Western neuropsychology literature. More attention is needed to uncover cognitive sequelae of health disparities in Asian Indians.
- In the absence of comprehensive neuropsychological tools adapted to the Asian Indian immigrant context, a one size fits all approach cannot be used. Each case needs consideration for appropriateness of using existing measures developed in Western contexts or available tools from India.
- Neuropsychologists can serve as a bridge between the medical and psychological worlds by engaging Indian patients in discussions and treatment plans that address emotional and social concerns along with neurological concerns.

Acknowledgments

Thank you to my desi colleagues who read drafts of this chapter and provided helpful cultural expertise—Drs. Preeti Sunderaraman, Vidya Kamath, Narinder Kapur, and Aparna Dutt. Dr. Tedd Judd's early comments also allowed this chapter to evolve. Sana Arastu's editorial assistance and thoughtful comments have been invaluable. The South Asian Special Interest Group of the Asian Neuropsychology Association, especially the core group of Drs. Jasdeep Hundal, Kamini Krishnan, and Preeti Sunderaraman, have provided peer support and collaboration throughout. This case presentation would not have been possible without "Mrs. Rama" and other Indian patients who entrust us with their stories. Thank you!

Glossary

Berry's (1992) acculturation model[12]. This model categorizes adaptation strategies along two dimensions of retention or rejection of one's native culture and host culture:

		Is it considered of value to maintain identity of culture of origin?	
		Yes	No
Is it considered of value to develop	Yes	Integration	Assimilation
relationships with the host culture?	No	Segregation	Marginalization

Caste. A system of religiously sanctioned social division in India by which people are ranked in a hierarchy based on birth, with position within the hierarchy determining social and economic outcomes (www.equalitylabs.org).

Dalits. Formerly known as "untouchables," this group was excluded from traditional Hindu caste hierarchy due to being considered spiritually and physically polluting to caste-ed Hindus. The community has been subjected to extreme violence and discrimination (www.equalitylabs.org).

Hindu. A person who follows the religion of Hinduism. It is not the same as Hindi, which is a language.

Raj. A term used to indicate British reign of the Indian subcontinent from 1858 to 1947.

References

1. Petraglia MD, Allchin B. The evolution and history of human populations in South Asia: Interdisciplinary studies in archaeology, biological anthropology, linguistics, and genetics. Dordrecht: Springer; 2007. xiii, p. 464.
2. Carey S. The legacy of British colonialism in India post 1947. New Zealand Rev Econ Finance. 2012;2:37–47.

3. Bhatia S, Priya KR. Decolonizing culture: Euro-American psychology and the shaping of neoliberal selves in India. Theory & Psychology. 2018;28(5):645–68.

4. United Nations Department of Economic and Social Affairs PD. International Migration 2020 Highlights (ST/ESA/SER.A/452). 2020.

5. US Census Bureau. Asian alone or in combination with one or more other races: 2015 American Community Survey 1-Year Estimates. 2017.

6. Chakravorty S, Kapur D, Singh N. The other one percent: Indians in America. Oxford University Press [Internet]; 2016.

7. Pillari V. Indian Hindu families. In M. McGoldrick, J. Giordano, & N. Garcia-Preto (Eds.), Ethnicity and family therapy (pp. 395–406). 3rd ed. New York (NY): Guilford Press; 2005.

8. Mahalingam R, editor. Cultural psychology of immigrants. Mahwah (NJ): Lawrence Erlbaum Associates Publishers; 2006. New Jersey, US.

9. Ward C, Bochner S, Furnham A. The psychology of culture shock. Hove, East Sussex: Routledge; 2001.

10. Díaz -Santos M, Hough S. Cultural competence guidelines for neuropsychology trainees and professionals: Working with ethnically diverse individuals. In: Ferraro FR, editor. Minority and cross-cultural aspects of neuropsychological assessment: Enduring and emerging trends. 2nd ed. Philadelphia (PA): Taylor & Francis; 2016. p. 11–33.

11. Badrinathan S, Kapur D, Kay J, Vaishnav M. Social realities of Indian Americans: Results from the 2020 Indian American Attitudes Survey. Washington, DC: Carnegie Endowment for International Peace; 2021.

12. Berry JW. Immigration, acculturation, and adaptation. Appl Psychol. 1997;46(1):5–34.

13. Krishnan A, Berry JW. Acculturative stress and acculturation attitudes among Indian immigrants to the United States. Psychol Dev Soc. 1992;4(2):187–212.

14. Asian Americans Leading Together (SAALT). Racial Justice.: SAALT [Internet]. 2021. Available from: https://saalt.org/policy-change/racial-justice/

15. South Asian Americans Leading Together (SAALT). Communities on Fire: Confronting Hate Violence and Xenophobic Political Rhetoric [Internet]. 2018. Available from: https://saalt.org/wp-content/uploads/2018/01/Communities-on-Fire.pdf

16. Thames AD, Hinkin CH, Byrd DA, Bilder RM, Duff KJ, Mindt MR, et al. Effects of stereotype threat, perceived discrimination, and examiner race on neuropsychological performance: Simple as black and white? J Int Neuropsychol Soc. 2013;19(5):583–93.

17. Nagra A, Skeel RL, Sbraga TP. A pilot investigation of the effects of stress on neuropsychological performance in Asian-Indians in the United States. Cultur Diver Ethn Minor Psychol. 2007;13(1):54–63.

18. Asher RE, Moseley C, Darkes G. Atlas of the world's languages. Milton Park, Abingdon: Routledge; 2007.

19. Budiman A. Indians in the U.S. Fact Sheet. Washington (DC): Pew Research Center; 2021.

20. India Co. Language: India, States and Union territories. New Delhi, India: Office of the Registrar General; 2011.

21. Vasanta D, Suvarna A, Sireesha J, Raju SB. Language choice and language use patterns among Telugu-Hindi/Urdu-English speakers in Hyderabad, India. International Conference on Language, Society, and Culture in Asian Contexts (LSCAC) Proceedings; 2010. pp. 57–67.

22. Paplikar A, Alladi S, Varghese F, Mekala S, Arshad F, Sharma M, et al. Bilingualism and its implications for neuropsychological evaluation. Arch Clin Neuropsychol. 2021.

23. Porrselvi A, Shankar V. Status of cognitive testing of adults in India. Ann Indian Acad Neurol. 2017;20(4):334–40.

24. Manly JJ. Deconstructing race and ethnicity: implications for measurement of health outcomes. Med Care. 2006;44(11 Suppl 3):S10–6.

25. India Go. Educational Statistics at a Glance New Delhi [Internet]. 2016. Available from: https://www.education.gov.in/sites/upload_files/mhrd/files/statistics-new/ESG2016.pdf

26. Trines S. Education in India: World Education News and Reviews [Internet]. 2018. Available from: https://wenr.wes.org/2018/09/education-in-india

27. The Challenges for India's Educational System. 2005 https://www.chathamhouse.org/sites/default/files/public/Research/Asia/bpindiaeducation.pdf

28. Chen Jr MS, Hawks BL. A debunking of the myth of healthy Asian Americans and Pacific Islanders. Am J Health Promot. 1995;9(4):261–8.

29. Tanjasiri SP, Wallace SP, Shibata K. Picture imperfect: hidden problems among Asian Pacific Islander elderly. Gerontologist. 1995;35(6):753–60.

30. Wikipedia. Economy of India [Internet]; n.d.. Available from: https://en.wikipedia.org/wiki/Economy_of_India

31. Ghosh S, Chowdhury SD, Chandra AM, Ghosh T. Grades of undernutrition and socioeconomic status influence cognitive development in school children of Kolkata. Am J Phys Anthropol. 2015;156(2):274–85.

32. Fernald LCH, Kariger P, Hidrobo M, Gertler PJ. Socioeconomic gradients in child development in very young children: evidence from India, Indonesia, Peru, and Senegal. Proc Natl Acad Sci. 2012;109(Supplement 2):17273.

33. Sharma AK, Gupta R, Baig VN, Singh TV, Chakraborty S, Sunda JP, et al. Socioeconomic status and COVID-19 related outcomes in India: hospital based study. medRxiv. 2021.

34. Lee J, Shih R, Feeney K, Langa KM. Gender disparity in late-life cognitive functioning in India: findings from the longitudinal aging study in India. J Gerontol B. 2014;69(4):603–11.

35. Zwick-Maitreyi M, Soundararajan T, Dar N, Bheel RF, Balakrishnan P. Caste in the United States: A survey of caste among South Asian Americans. Equality Labs, USA; 2018.

36. Sunderaraman P, Irani F, Krishnan K, Hundal J. A narrative review of the biopsychosocial and health characteristics of Asian Indians in the United States: Clinical and research implications for neuropsychological functioning. Clin Neuropsychol. 2021 Nov 25:1–19.

37. SAALT. Health Care Issues Affecting South Asians in the United States. 2009.

38. SAALT. Unequal Consequences: The Disparate Impact of COVID-19 Across South Asian American Communities. 2020.

39. Shidhaye R, Kermode M. Stigma and discrimination as a barrier to mental health service utilization in India. Int Health. 2013;5(1):6–8.

40. Kumar JK, Sadasivan A. Neuropsychology in India. Clin Neuropsychol. 2016;30(8):1252–66.

41. Leung P, Cheung M, Cheung A. Developing help-seeking strategies for Pakistani clients with depressive symptoms. Asia Pac J Soc Work Dev. 2011;21(2):21–33.

42. Conrad MM, Pacquiao DF. Manifestation, attribution, and coping with depression among Asian Indians from the perspectives of health care practitioners. J Transcult Nurs. 2005;16(1):32–40. doi:10.1177/1043659604271239

43. Marian V, Blumenfeld HK, Kaushanskaya M. The Language Experience and Proficiency Questionnaire (LEAP-Q): assessing language profiles in bilinguals and multilinguals. J Speech Lang Hear Res. 2007;50(4):940–67.

44. Waldrop-Valverde D, Ownby RL, Jones DL, Sharma S, Nehra R, Kumar AM, et al. Neuropsychological test performance among healthy persons in northern India: development of normative data. J Neurovirol. 2015;21(4):433–8.

45. Benedict RHB, Schretlen D, Groninger L, Brandt J. Hopkins Verbal Learning Test—Revised: normative data and analysis of inter-form and test-retest reliability. Clin Neuropsychol. 1998;12(1):43–55.

46. Benedict RH. Brief visuospatial memory test-revised. Lutz (FL): Psychological Assessment Resources; 1997.

47. Wechsler D. Wechsler Adult Intelligence Scale. 3rd ed. Pearson; 1997.

48. Grooved Pegboard User's Manual. Lafayette (IN): Lafayette Instruments; 2015.

49. D'Elia L, Satz P, Lyons Uchiyama C, White T. Color Trails Test. PAR; 1989.

50. Borkowski JG, Benton AL, Spreen O. Word fluency and brain damage. Neuropsychologia. 1967;5(2):135–40.

51. Golden CJ, Freshwater SM. Stroop color and word test. 1978.

52. Kongs SK, Thompson LL, Iverson GL, Heaton RK. WCST-64: Wisconsin Card Sorting Test-64 card version, professional manual. PAR; 2000.

Chinese

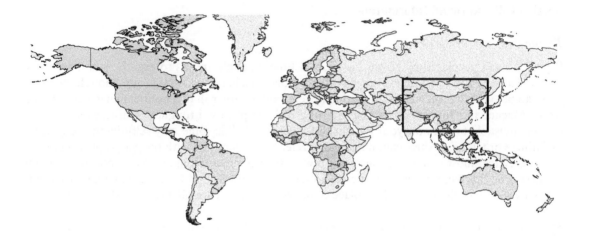

13   Considerations in Neuropsychological Evaluations with Chinese Individuals

Mimi K.W. Wong, Esther Chin, and Yue Hong

Section I: Background Information

Terminology and Perspective

If you ever felt perplexed by whom the term "Chinese people" refers to exactly, you have every right to feel so. People of Chinese descent are members of a heterogeneous group, though their origins can be typically traced back to China (a geographic rather than a political term here), Hong Kong, Macau, and Taiwan. Given the sociopolitical complexity throughout Chinese history, it is always advisable to ask how your patient self-identifies. While some may self-identify in general as Chinese or Chinese American, many may prefer to be identified with the geographic region to which they feel most connected, such as Taiwanese American, Hongkongers, and Singaporean Chinese. For this chapter, though, the broad terms of Chinese and Chinese American are used, we focus on those who identify their place of origin as China, Hong Kong, and Macau.

AUTHOR'S NOTE [MIMI K.W. WONG]: My perspective is that of a bilingual (Cantonese/English) Chinese American neuropsychologist who was born in Guangzhou, China, and immigrated to the United States as a young child. I trained in neuropsychology on the West Coast of the United States, where I currently practice in a teaching hospital inpatient/outpatient setting.

AUTHOR'S NOTE [ESTHER CHIN]: I identify myself as a "Hongkonger" who was born in Hong Kong and completed my college degree there. I then received my master's degree in London and subsequently practiced psychology in both Hong Kong and Boston. My doctoral/post-doctoral training in clinical psychology with specialty in pediatric neuropsychology was mainly in California and later in the Midwest. I currently practice in a neurosciences institute of a teaching hospital in an outpatient setting in the suburb of Chicago.

AUTHOR'S NOTE [YUE HONG]: I identify as a first-generation Chinese in the United States. I grew up in Chengdu, China, completed my undergraduate education in Hong Kong, and received subsequent training in clinical psychology and neuropsychology on the East Coast of the United States. I currently practice in a hospital in Massachusetts.

Geography

The total area of China is estimated to be around 3.7 million square miles and is similar to that of the United States. The term "mainland China" commonly refers to the 32 first-level administrative divisions (i.e., provinces, autonomous regions, and municipalities) that are under the direct jurisdiction of the People's Republic of China (PRC). This term typically excludes the Special Administrative Regions (SARs) of Hong Kong and Macau, which are former colonies of the

DOI: 10.4324/9781003051862-27

Britain and Portuguese Empires, respectively, and were returned to Chinese rule in 1997 and 1999, respectively. Although the PRC considers Taiwan to be its 23rd province, Taiwan has identified itself as the Republic of China since 1949 and rejected the PRC's claim of sovereignty.

History and Society

China has the longest continuous history in the world of over 5,000 years and is considered one of the four cradles of civilization. It is impossible to summarize Chinese history in any meaningful way in a few paragraphs; instead, we focus on significant events over the past century that may help create a broad context to understand the drastic changes the Chinese population has witnessed. To make things easier to follow, we invite the readers to join us for a walk-through of the life of a centenarian, S, who was born in 1920.

Eight years before S was born (1912), the last imperial dynasty of China had collapsed. It was during this tumultuous dynasty that Hong Kong and Macau were ceded, and they have since been under Western administrations until the late 1990s. S was born into the Republic of China founded in 1912. S's early life was filled with political and military instability. He witnessed two civil wars (1927–1937; 1945–1949) between the two major parties in the Republic of China, as well as the Second Sino-Japanese War (1937–1945) between China and Japan. At age 29 (1949), S and his family finally saw an end to the wars, marked by the establishment of the PRC by the Communist Party and the evacuation of the Nationalist Party to the island of Taiwan.

The first three decades of the newly founded PRC were marked by a series of highly controversial reforms and movements. The country endured extreme economic difficulties marked by a nationwide famine between 1959 and 1961, right around the time when S's children were born. A few years later came the Great Proletarian **Cultural Revolution** (1966–1976), during which S and many of his friends and colleagues were politically persecuted. It was an extremely difficult time for S and his family, but these memories were such a taboo that he rarely talked about even to his grandchildren.

Since the late 1970s, leadership of the PRC has implemented significant economic reforms that were proven successful. The Chinese society has since undergone drastic changes due to rapid economic growth and globalization that at times overwhelmed S. Fifty years ago, he was struggling to feed his family; by comparison, present-day China has had the world's second-largest economy. Had S left the country during different times, his memory of China would depict a different world. S has his concerns about the current society. The rapid economic growth is accompanied by a high degree of economic inequality, resulting in a significant urban-rural disparity in terms of accessibility to resources in education, healthcare, and employment opportunities. The younger generations seem to be struggling with their traditional value and beliefs challenged by the swirling globalization. For S, at age 100, he is ready to hand over the challenges to the next generation.

People

According to the national census of 2010, the population of the PRC is approximately 1.37 billion.[1] Since the 1950s, China has established a series of family planning policies to address the concerns of overpopulation. These policies reached their most strict form, the one-child restriction, in the late 1970s and have gradually loosened up over the past two decades. These policies, though effective in controlling population size, created many unintended consequences on the composition of the population.[2] For instance, there is a huge gender imbalance in China, with the male population exceeding the female population by more than 30 million, underlined by a patriarchal preference for sons over daughters. Girls, particularly those who are less socio-economically resourceful, often struggle with issues surrounding self-worth. Additionally, with the decreasing birth rate, China is now faced with an aging society that will challenge the system's ability to care for its people. On the family level, one sees a typical 4:2:1 (4 grandparents, 2 parents, 1 child) structure that funnels all resources and attention to this one child, who eventually becomes the sole caregiver for their entire aging family.

It is also important to note the ethnic and religious composition of the Chinese population. Besides the largest ethnic group of the Han people (approximately 92% of the population[1]), China recognizes other 55 ethnic minority groups, most of which reside in areas bordering other countries. Whereas in Hong Kong and Macau, though the majority (92%–95%) of the population are ethnic Chinese, the ethnic minorities are often from Southeast Asian countries and descendants of British and Portuguese. In terms of religious affiliation, the majority of the population in mainland China identify as atheists and agnostics. Five religions are currently acknowledged in mainland China, including **Taoism**, Buddhism, Catholicism, Protestantism, and Islam. In Hong Kong and Macau, there is a higher rate of reported religious affiliations with Buddhism, Taoism, and Christianity.

Immigration and Relocation

Depending on the definition of the "Chinese diaspora," population estimates vary between 10 million and 45 million.[3] The number of Chinese individuals residing in the United States is estimated to be around 5.2 million, with California and New York hosting the largest Chinese communities.[4] Immigration of Chinese into the United States mainly consists of two waves: the mid-19th century and the 1970s to the present. In the 1800s, Chinese immigrants were primarily male, low-skilled manual laborers in agriculture, mining, and railroad construction who migrated to the West Coast. As US–China relations improved in 1979, the second wave of Chinese migration to the United States began. From 1980 to 1990, the number of Chinese immigrants nearly doubled and has been growing since. For older generations of immigrants, the principal reason for migration was the search for jobs and/or political asylum, whereas younger generations of immigrants are largely seeking to enhance employability and academic background. The context of immigration can shed light on socio-economic status and immigration-related stressors.

Language

Just like the term "Chinese people," "Chinese language" is also a hugely heterogeneous umbrella term. There are hundreds of dialects spoken in China typically classified into seven groups; many of these dialects are not mutually intelligible from a linguistic perspective.[5] Of the seven groups, a dialect of the Mandarin group became the official language in mainland China in the 1950s (known as Putonghua). Though Mandarin is generally spoken across most of northern China, southern Chinese of older generations or those from rural areas may not be familiar with the official dialect. Of note, another variation of Mandarin (Guoyu) serves as the official language in Taiwan. The Yue group, consisting of at least 14 dialects including Cantonese and Taishanese, is a group of Chinese dialects primarily spoken in the provinces of Guangdong and Guangxi, as well as Hong Kong and Macau. For the Chinese immigrant population in the United States, Mandarin/Putonghua and Cantonese are reported to be the most commonly spoken dialects.[6]

It is also important to differentiate two writing systems of Chinese, the traditional and the simplified Chinese characters. The simplified Chinese characters were introduced in the 1950s and have become the preferred writing system for most mainland Chinese. However, traditional characters continue to be used by Chinese living in Taiwan, Hong Kong, and Macau. For example, a Cantonese-speaking Hongkonger can communicate freely with a Mandarin-speaking Taiwanese by writing since both adopt the traditional characters, whereas a mainlander who uses simplified written Chinese may not understand a Taiwanese's writing as easily even though both are Mandarin-speaking. It is worth noting, though, that both simplified and traditional writing systems of Chinese follow the same vocabulary and grammatical structure of Mandarin. Therefore, while there may be immediate challenges with a mainlander who uses simplified written Chinese not understanding a Taiwanese's writing, this could be overcome with some effort and time, and vice versa. Yet the linguistic differences between different groups of spoken Chinese languages (e.g., Cantonese and Mandarin) are much more difficult to overcome.

In short, "the patient's primary language is Chinese" provides very little information for a culturally informed neuropsychological evaluation. Primary dialect, familiarity with the most commonly used Chinese dialects (Mandarin and Cantonese), preferred writing system (traditional vs. simplified) should be assessed to guide clinical decision-making.

Education

The level of literacy grew substantially over the last half-century in China, from 20% in 1949 to 96% in 2018.[7] Since the 1980s, China has implemented the nine-year compulsory education system, consisting of six years of primary school and three years of junior secondary school, whereas education in Hong Kong is largely modeled after the English system. The average years of schooling in China were estimated to be 7.8 years in 2017, though the education quality likely differs depending on when and where one is educated. Those who went to school before the 1970s in mainland China likely experienced disruptions to their education given the socio-economic upheaval, and those who received education in rural areas are likely at a disadvantage for education quality.

In the United States, over half of the Chinese American population has a bachelor's degree or higher, and the average education attainment of the US-born Chinese is remarkably higher than that of the first-generation immigrants.[8]

Culture

Though Chinese culture is diverse given the enormous temporal and geographic spans, some themes are generalizable given the profound impact of **Confucianism**. Most notably, Confucianism promotes two principles of Li (social rituals) and Ren (humanism). The former is considered more conservative, promoting respect for authorities and conformity to established social roles. The latter is more idealistic and highlights universal values that allow two individuals to coexist in a humane manner. Most germane is how these general principles manifest themselves in the contemporary Chinese society and how they could impact a neuropsychological evaluation. We would like to remind our readers, though, that these summaries are not meant to perpetuate stereotypes and that each individual is unique and should be respected as such.

Harmony and Stability

Harmony is highly valued by Confucianism to maintain the stability of a society and its units. On an individual level, Chinese people are taught to behave in a way that maximizes the interests of the group and obeys those in authority. Should conflicts arise, one is expected to forgo their own personal preferences if they are of a minority/lower status on the social hierarchy. In fact, it is often considered rude and selfish to be vocal about one's own needs without acknowledging the group's preference. On a more societal level, while the sense of belonging is maximized for the majority, deviation from the social norm is discouraged, and the needs of minority groups are often drowned out. In a clinical setting, this can manifest as a particularly agreeable patient who will likely hesitate to ask for clarification or to question a provider in fear of jeopardizing the patient–doctor relationship.

Communal and Familial Orientation

The communal and familial orientation is closely intertwined with the valuation of harmony and stability, as family is considered the basic building unit of a society. Altogether, they enhance commitment to familial/communal relationships because these relational networks are expected to be long-lasting. If used properly, one could find safety and support in a resourceful and nourishing relational network that spans several generations.

However, these relational networks can become entangling and give rise to boundary issues that may appear problematic to someone who is acculturated in an individualistic society. For instance, every single member of these networks is held responsible for the reputation or "face" (**mianzi**) of the group. One's wrongdoing, or deviation from the norm, could be considered a disgrace (loss of face) to the entire group and is, therefore, highly discouraged. Perhaps the other side of the same coin, boundary issues also arise as a way to protect an ingroup member. For instance, it is *very* common for the Chinese to "hide" the diagnosis of a terminal illness from their elder parents, because it is considered insensitive to tell them the diagnosis and unhelpful anyway. Vice versa, it is also common for parents to "hide" their health conditions from their children in fear of creating burden for them. The movie, *Farewell,* did an excellent job depicting these intricacies and is highly recommended for those who are interested.

Shame

Shame is proven to be an effective tool to guide human behavior and is a tool commonly used in child-rearing in traditional Chinese cultures. Lieber et al.[9] define shame in the context of Chinese culture as "a socio-emotional reference and mechanism for fostering the development of children's social sensitivities." In other words, the goal of parenting is to achieve moral socialization in line with the traditional Chinese values through the mechanism of shame. Implanted at a young age, the shame system operates throughout one's life and is easily activated when one is accused of "losing face" by failing to meet expectations from authority. During neuropsychological evaluations, you will likely see the activation of this system when a Chinese examinee becomes highly anxious about their performance and overly apologetic for not knowing an answer. It is critical to note and address these reactions, because one could end up evaluating the power of shame rather than cognitive functioning.

Mental Health Views

Stigma toward individuals with mental illnesses is pervasive in China and is, unfortunately, sustained by many of the traditional Chinese values. People with mental illness are often depicted as dangerous and unpredictable and are considered a threat to a harmonious and stable society. These public stigmas can become internalized, activating the shame system and further prohibiting individuals from seeking help and advocating for themselves. A survey revealed that the number one coping mechanism endorsed by Chinese individuals with severe mental illness is maintaining secrecy about the illness.[10] Moreover, concealing mental illness often becomes a communal act. As previously noted, one's deviation from the norm (in this case, having a mental illness) causes the entire family to lose "face" and, therefore, takes everyone's effort to cover the tracks. The incentive is amplified by common beliefs about the hereditary nature of *all* mental illnesses, implicating the family as pathogenic. Conversely, family members may participate in the deception and "hiding" as a way to protect their loved ones from being discriminated against. In either case, the secrecy often leads to an extreme lack of information and support and, at times, an unbearable burden for the entire family. In addition, individuals with mental illness become increasingly invisible, resulting in biased media coverage that focuses on the most extreme cases, which in turn further fortifies the stereotypes of mental illness being dangerous and unpredictable. The Chinese government passed a new mental health law in 2013 to improve mental health literacy and reduce stigma. However, it will likely take decades before individuals with mental illness become visible in a respectful light.

Health providers are often seen as authorities. A Chinese individual may, thus, conceal mental health history of themselves or family members from medical providers for fear of being sanctioned or discriminated against. A red flag may be raised even higher when one gets introduced to a neuro-*psychologist*. A standard question of "any history of psychiatric illnesses in your family?" will most likely get an answer of "no." It is thus important to build rapport and gain trust before proceeding with those questions, including, but not limited to, clearly explaining the role of a neuropsychologist, proving one's credibility by revealing one's training background, carefully reviewing the confidentiality terms, and explaining the rationale for questions that may feel intrusive or offensive. It is also important to maintain vigilance to reports of somatic symptoms such as chronic pain and general malaise as these are often comorbid with affective symptoms and are considered "safer" options to report.

Health Status

Life expectancy in China has increased steadily over the past half-century, reaching about 76 years and is above the world average.[11] However, significant rural-urban disparity is observed at birth and widens with age. Being a woman and being born during periods of societal instability (e.g., famine cohort (1959–1961), later cultural revolution cohort (1971–1976) are risk factors for worse health outcomes.[12] There is also a rising rate of obesity and high smoking prevalence among Chinese men.

The prevalence of neurodevelopmental disorders in Chinese children is reported to be lower than in highly industrialized countries, which is likely an underestimate. Evidence suggests that, with different methodology for data collection and reporting, the prevalence of Autism Spectrum Disorder (ASD) in China is at least comparable to that of Western societies.[13] Individuals with neurodevelopmental disorders are another "invisibilized" group in China due to similar reasons outlined in the Mental Health section. I (YH) remember having a classmate in primary school who would constantly stand up in the middle of the class, for which he was criticized by teachers and bullied by fellow students. It never occurred to me until many years later that this person may have had attention-deficit/hyperactivity disorder. Similarly, autism, to this day, is still used in a nonchalant way by mass media to refer to social anxiety (e.g., "Nah, I'm gonna skip the party, my autism is flaring up lately"). The reason for sharing these stories is simply to remind our readers that, when you work with a Chinese family, a condition that seems common to you may not be well or accurately understood by the family. It is thus critical to take the time to explain the condition, to go the extra mile to destigmatize it, and to ensure that the family doesn't take the diagnosis as yet another secret to keep.

History of and Approach to Neuropsychological Evaluations

Historically, a Western conceptualization of neuropsychology was introduced to mainland China in the 1980s,[14] followed by various efforts to adapt and validate tests. However, the development of clinical neuropsychology is limited by a lack of systematic training and the healthcare system's capacity to afford such a time-consuming evaluation. In fact, doctoral-level neuropsychologists, who are often trained overseas, work mostly in research settings in China, whereas clinical neurocognitive testing is often performed by physicians and physician assistants, who may possess limited knowledge regarding the background and psychometric properties of testing tools. Clinical neuropsychology witnessed a comparably faster development in Hong Kong, perhaps attributable to a greater degree of Westernization. The Hong Kong Neuropsychological Association was established in 1998 and played an important role in the development of the specialty in the area.[14] A large amount of indigenous test development and test translation/adaptation also took place. Yet, comprehensive neuropsychological evaluation in clinical settings is not readily accessible to everyone for whom it could be a benefit.

One of the biggest barriers for neuropsychologists who are interested in serving the Chinese population is the accessibility of testing instruments. As most neuropsychologists work in research settings, the end goal of test development, adaptation, and validation are often not for clinical application, making the tests difficult to locate. Practical barriers such as the high price of commercialized tests in China and the need to be credentialed through a local professional organization to purchase tests can also impede these local tools/norms from appreciation by a wider audience. A recent systematic review[15] provides detailed information on non-commercialized test validation in mainland China and provides a list of available instruments and normative data that may be of interest to readers of this chapter.

Taken together, providers should bear in mind that a neuropsychological evaluation can be particularly foreign to a Chinese patient. They may find it highly intimidating given the "psychology" root in combination with the testing setting that creates a rather explicit social hierarchy. It is advised that a provider actively seeks ways to enhance rapport and motivation and adopts a communication style that maximizes the patient's comfort level. Extra time is likely required to explain the purpose and procedures of the evaluation. During the evaluation, it is important to watch for signs of when a patient tries to maintain harmonious relationships by not being direct and forthright. In those situations, the patient may instead communicate indirectly with a greater emphasis on nonverbals (e.g., reduced eye contact, closed-off body posture), of which a culturally sensitive neuropsychologist should be mindful.

Section II: Case Studies — "Overcoming Shame in the Family"

Note: Possible identifying information and aspects of history and presentation have been modified to protect patient identity and privacy.

The following two case studies were selected to illustrate some of the cultural considerations mentioned in Section I. Please note that the pediatric case is from Dr. Esther Chin, and the adult case is from Dr. Mimi K.W. Wong.

Pediatric Case

Background

Xiaomin Chan was a 4-year-10-month-old Chinese female with a right-handed preference who immigrated to the United States eight months prior to the evaluation. Her family was referred to me by her social worker at a community center for a neuropsychological evaluation due to concerns with global cognitive delays. In addition to the standard components of a pediatric evaluation, an extensive clinical interview was performed with not only Xiaomin's parents but also her grandparents, homeroom teacher, and school social worker. *[Author's note (EC): In the context of communal culture, both Chinese parents and grandparents are likely to be the main caregivers.*

Her teacher and school social worker provide additional information in order to validate the consistency of information and prevent cultural biases.] Cantonese and Taishanese dialects (referred to as "Cantonese" for the rest of this case study for simplicity) were Xiaomin's primary languages used at home, while English and Cantonese were used at school.

Xiaomin's parents, grandparents, and teachers were concerned about her overall cognitive functioning. According to their report, she demonstrated an inconsistent level of attention, depending on the nature of the activity. With respect to her language functioning, she mainly used physical guidance (e.g., pulling an adult's hand), vocalization (e.g., babbling), and gestures to make requests or express herself. She occasionally communicated with single words and simple phrases in Cantonese. Her ability to follow simple 1-step instructions in Cantonese and English was inconsistent. In terms of her adaptive functioning, she was able to feed herself with utensils and dress herself with assistance. However, she needed help to bathe herself, wash her hair, and button her shirts. She could scribble but couldn't trace lines. She could walk up and down stairs and ride a bike with training wheels. She was also toilet trained. *[Author's note (EC): I was pleasantly surprised by the fact that both her parents and grandparents appeared to have no hesitation to accurately report what she could and could not do. This was a positive sign for me to access their readiness to process any diagnostic information during the feedback.]*

Xiaomin's parents and teachers also reported concerns related to social and emotional difficulties. She struggled to initiate social interactions and maintain social reciprocity, even when the engagement was facilitated in Cantonese. Her eye contact was inconsistent, and affect tended to be flat. Her ability to engage in pretend/imaginative play was limited. Echolalia and behavioral rigidity (e.g., difficulty with transitions) were reported. Excessive interests in specific toys and sensory atypicality (e.g., disliking getting wet, visual examination, looking up at the ceiling lighting) were observed. Emotionally, separation anxiety with her mother was reported. She also easily became frustrated at home, resulting in crying with variable durations. No therapy services had been initiated.

At the time of the evaluation, Xiaomin attended the pre-kindergarten program organized by a Chinese community center. Reportedly, she did not demonstrate knowledge of pre-academic skills (e.g., recognition of color, numbers, or shapes). Of note, she received no formal education prior to her immigration to the United States. Her social worker had been assisting the family in navigating resources provided by their school district in preparation for her attendance to kindergarten in the next academic school year. An Individualized Education Program (IEP) evaluation was initiated; however, she was deemed ineligible as her language delay was attributed to her recent immigration. *[Author's note (EC): Upon record review, her school did not appear to conduct a thorough interview with her family to gather information regarding her development prior to immigrating or involve culturally competent specialists to differentiate between a true language delay and a lack of language proficiency due to recent immigration.]*

Xiaomin's mother reported that she was diagnosed with pre-eclampsia in the last month of her pregnancy. She was otherwise reportedly born full term via cesarean section without postnatal complications. During infancy, she was diagnosed with pulmonary arteriovenous malformation, for which two surgeries were performed at four months and nine months old. The rest of her medical history was unremarkable. Cognitively, her attainment of early gross and language skills was delayed. While she crawled at approximately eight months, she started walking at age two. She started using single words in Cantonese at age two and word phrases at age 4.5. No concerns with her sleep, appetite, functional hearing, or vision were reported.

In May 2018, Xiaomin and her mother immigrated to the United States to reunite with her father, who had been living here. At the time of the evaluation, Xiaomin lived with her parents and paternal grandparents. Her father graduated from high school in China and worked as a busser in a Chinese restaurant. Her mother completed nine years of education in China and was a homemaker. Immediate and extended family medical history was reportedly unremarkable. Of note, the evaluation was performed over three sessions on separate days: 1.5-hour intake, 3-hour testing, and 2-hour feedback.

Behavioral Observations

Xiaomin's mother and grandmother accompanied her to the clinic on the day of testing. Due to her separation anxiety, her mother had to be present in the testing room throughout the evaluation. Xiaomin presented as a pleasant girl, but her social engagement was limited, and eye contact was inconsistent. Her mood was mostly indifferent, but she appeared to show brief moments of pleasure when activities caught her interests (e.g., blowing bubbles). To communicate, she used vocalization, physical guidance/gestures, and simple vocabulary in Cantonese. She wasn't able to follow 1-step instructions consistently and needed frequent redirection and prompting to keep her on task. Despite support, her attention span was short. She struggled to remain seated and tended to walk around in the testing room. She also demonstrated echolalia, visual examination, and repetitive looking up at the ceiling lighting during testing. She was able to walk independently and scribbled with color pencils. Her short attention span and limited social engagement most definitely impacted her testing performance, but these results are likely an accurate representation of her typical functioning.

Tests and Norm Selection

The limitations surrounding availability and accessibility of tests and normative data for Chinese individuals described in previous sections are, unfortunately, prevalent in the pediatric world. The common practice, though not ideal, is to utilize measures developed and normed in the United States with reasonable adaptation, interpret results with caution, and clearly note the limitations in the report. For this case, the following tests and questionnaires were translated and administered in Cantonese.

- Stanford Binet—Fifth Edition (SB-5): Abbreviated battery IQ[16]
- Bayley III—Scales of Infant and Toddler Development: Cognitive composite[17]
- Wide Range Assessment of Visual Motor Abilities (WRAVMA): Drawing and pegboard[18]
- Peabody Picture Vocabulary Test—Fourth Edition (PPVT-4)[19]
- Autism Diagnostic Observation Schedule—Second Edition (ADOS-2): Module 1[20]
- Bracken School Readiness Assessment: School readiness composite[21]
- Adaptive Behavior Assessment System—Third Edition (ABAS-3)[22]
- Social Responsiveness Scale—Second Edition (SRS-2)[23]
- Childhood Autism Rating Scale—Second Edition (CARS-2): Standard form[24]
- Behavior Assessment System for Children—Second Edition (BASC-2): Parent and Teacher Report[25]
- Behavior Rating Inventory of Executive Functioning (BRIEF): Parent and Teacher Report[26]

Cognitive Test Results and Interpretation

Xiaomin's overall cognitive functioning was below age expectation, falling within the moderately impaired range. Her cognitive development was approximately at an age equivalent of 18 months old. She was able to search for missing objects and take blocks out of cups. However, she struggled to engage in relational play (e.g., feeding a baby doll) or match shapes consistently.

Comparably, Xiaomin's other cognitive abilities, including visual-motor integration skills, fine motor dexterity, and language skills, were below age expectation. She particularly struggled with her language skills. In addition to her observed language deficits throughout testing, her performance on a task of receptive language skills was severely impaired, with an age equivalent below two years. A task of pre-academic skills was attempted but was incomplete due to her inattention and limited social engagement.

Autism-Related Measures

The ADOS-2 Module 1 was administered with the presence of her mother in the testing room. Xiaomin demonstrated atypical social communication and interaction, which was evident in Cantonese. For example, she mostly used vocalization but not words in her communication, which was considered as a delay in Chinese language development given her age. She seldom directed her vocalization to her mother/the examiner and used poorly modulated eye contact throughout the evaluation. While she directed some of her facial expressions to her mother, she did not demonstrate a responsive social smile to either her mother or the examiner. Despite her mother's effort, she showed limited engagement in most activities. *[Author's note (EC): Compared to people raised in Western cultures, Chinese people may demonstrate less eye contact, facial expression, and/ or gestures in communication and appear to be relatively reserved with new people or people in higher hierarchy. However, Xiaomin's lack of social communication and interaction even with her mother, with whom she is familiar, was above and beyond what is expected in Chinese culture.]*

In addition, atypical sensory interests (e.g., unusual visual examination, looking up at the ceiling lighting) were observed during the ADOS. She demonstrated an intense and repetitive interest in a particular pop-up toy and often fidgeted and got up out of her seat. Overall, on the ADOS-2 Module 1, her scores showed a moderate level of autism spectrum-related symptoms.

Adaptive Functioning and Emotional/Behavioral Rating Questionnaires

Xiaomin's parents, grandparents, and teachers completed questionnaires assessing her overall adaptive functioning and general emotional/behavioral functioning. Xiaomin's overall adaptive functioning was moderately impaired, mostly functioning at one year and six months to one year and 10 months old. All raters reported similar concerns but with different levels of severity. The concerning areas included lack of inhibition/hyperactivity, emotional dysregulation, atypical behaviors, social problems, and functional communication difficulties. The ratings from her parents and teachers indicated significant concerns, whereas her grandparents endorsed less severe concerns. *[Author's note (EC): As mentioned, based on the observation during intake, both her parents and grandparents appeared to be ready and likely to accept potential diagnoses. Yet, the discrepancy in severity ratings may suggest that her grandparents experience a higher level of "shame" related to the atypical neurodevelopment of their granddaughter. I made a mental note that additional explanation and education for her grandparents may be required during the feedback.]*

Summary

Xiaomin presented as a pleasant girl with a short attention span and limited social engagement. Results of the current evaluation, performed in Xiaomin's first language, revealed overall developmental and intellectual delay. Significant difficulties with socialization/communication, restricted interests, rigidity, and sensory issues were reported by Xiaomin's parents, grandparents, and teachers, consistent with formal testing and clinical observation. Her cognitive delays and language difficulties could not be solely explained by her lack of formal education or English proficiency. Thus, a diagnosis of ASD with accompanying intellectual and language impairment (Level 2) was given.

Feedback and Recommendations

[Author's note (EC): In order to mitigate reactions of shame and help the family focus on strengths and therapeutic options, ongoing psychoeducation and updates on preliminary data were provided throughout the evaluation. This gradual manner was crucial to mentally prepare the family for the possible diagnosis, alleviate the feeling of shame, and cultivate realistic hope to the family by navigating services and resources in the community.] On day one, following the intake, I gently inquired of the family about any "diagnostic" thoughts in their mind and subsequently provided psychoeducation on each possible diagnosis. I also provided education on how the "diagnostic term" was not used to create stigma but to navigate and connect with the appropriate interventions. On the day of testing, I spent the last 15–20 minutes summarizing the preliminary data with Xiaomin's mother and her grandmother. I tied the data to the diagnosis (in this case, autism) and strategically pointed out Xiaomin's relative strengths and areas of potential improvement. With all the mental preparation starting at the intake, the oral feedback provided in the last session became a smooth and constructive discussion with relatively open-minded reception from Xiaomin's family. *[Author's note (EC): Xiaomin's mother and grandmother were both closely involved throughout the evaluation. This was crucial in Xiaomin's case to alleviate her mother's burden to convey the "bad news" and communicate unfamiliar information to members of the higher familial hierarchy. Additionally, having the whole family on board, the strong relational network within the family became an excellent asset to maximize the benefits from appropriate interventions.]*

Based on the results of the current evaluation, a list of recommendations was provided, including therapeutic intervention, special education services, and community resources. Here I highlight the recommendations that are most relevant to this chapter.

1 Xiaomin and her family were recommended to receive applied behavioral analysis (ABA) in-home therapy to address her ASD symptoms. I encouraged participation of the entire family to support her ability to generalize the learned skills across different settings. Given the intricacies of therapy, I recommended arranging a Cantonese-speaking therapist for the family; or, at least, the presence of a medically trained interpreter to assist with communication.

2 Xiaomin's family was recommended to share the report with her school and school district. I made it explicit in the report that her symptoms could not be solely explained by her lack of proficiency in English and/or her history of recent immigration in order to help with the qualification for IEP. In addition to intensive special education services commonly provided to students with ASD, I highlighted the importance for her IEP team to collaborate with bilingual/bicultural providers. Specifically, I recommended collaborating with a qualified bilingual (i.e., English and Cantonese) specialist or teacher to assist with understanding language or cultural factors as they relate to the student's instructional or assistance needs and to design and implement the English as a Second Language (ESL) curriculum. I also recommended consultation with a Chinese-speaking speech/language pathologist in order to maximize her benefit from speech/language therapy at school.

3 Lastly, the following resources for ASD were provided to Xiaomin's family and may be of interest to readers of this chapter.

- Featuring dozens of short files, the website (http://www.interactingwithautism.com) presents the latest evidence-based information on how to understand, treat, and live with people with ASD. Information is available in Chinese.
- Here is a website with autism information packet: https://www.supportforfamilies.org/autism-info-packet

Adult Case

Background Information

"Ms. Chan" was a 55-year-old Chinese female with approximately two years of formal education. Her primary language is Cantonese, which is used with her family and providers. *[Author's note (MW): Given that she came from rural China, it's possible that she speaks other rural dialects such as Taishanese. I would typically ask the patient which language they use at home when communicating with family, which is helpful in determining the language to use in testing].* The patient was referred by her primary care provider for complaints of problems with cognition in general, including memory and comprehension, with a history of possible developmental delay. The provider requested an evaluation of the patient's current neurocognitive status to assist in differential diagnosis and treatment planning.

Ms. Chan appeared to be a poor historian. Records showed contradictory self-reports about her symptoms and history. As a result, I gathered most of her history through available record reviews and collateral information from providers and siblings. Per her providers, Ms. Chan's current cognitive symptoms included problems with memory, attention, and comprehension. She demonstrated difficulties with performing complex activities of daily living, such as shopping, filling out forms, going to unfamiliar places, and following medical directions. Arrangements had to be made for Ms. Chan to visit the primary care clinic daily to ensure medication compliance. Although Ms. Chan reported that she took care of her own finances, Adult Protective Services was involved on two separate occasions due to concerns of possible financial abuse or undue influence. She reportedly had been able to manage her simple daily activities in the past, likely with support from her parents. At the time of the evaluation, Ms. Chan was able to dress, eat, and toilet independently and could use public transportation to get to familiar places. However, records noted poor hygiene in the past. Her sister noted that she usually attempts to present herself in a positive light and was reluctant to acknowledge any cognitive problems.

Ms. Chan was born in Vietnam and raised in rural China. Per Ms. Chan's older sister, she did not meet her developmental milestones for communication. She spoke single words at four years old, spoke two-word phrases and knew a few colors at 8–9, could count at 10, and spoke short sentences at 12. She had a high fever when she was around seven years old, was in a "coma" for three to four days with possible seizures, and was hospitalized for approximately one month in China. Her sister believed that Ms. Chan's functioning further declined after this early illness with tremendous difficulties with communication, memory, and learning. She did not progress through school like her peers and siblings and only completed two years of formal schooling. *[Author's note (MW): Ms. Chan grew up in a rural Chinese family during the Cultural Revolution, which was a time marked by great sociopolitical turmoil. Access to quality education and healthcare was limited. All the family members had limited education and low health literacy, including poor understanding of the impact of mental health and developmental conditions on one's behavior].*

Ms. Chan had been cared for by her family since childhood. She has never worked in gainful employment. Around 25 years ago, she moved to the United States to reunite with her family. She has since lived with and been taken care of by her mother until she passed away around two to three years prior to this assessment. Soon after her mother passed away, Ms. Chan was evicted from the family residence due to increasing conflicts with her siblings, who were concerned by her behavioral problems at home, including refusing to throw away rotting food and being verbally abusive to her brother and sister-in-law. After being evicted, Ms. Chan became homeless. She was living at a shelter and was supported financially by supplemental social security income. She appeared to maintain a somewhat close relationship with her younger brother, whom she called once per week. *[Author's note (MW): Ms. Chan's family may have been aware of her pervasive cognitive deficits to some degree, but shame, in addition to other factors including limited health literacy, may have prevented the family from seeking professional help earlier. Ms. Chan's mother took care of her disabled child's needs into adulthood, which is a common cultural expectation. As mentioned earlier, in traditional Chinese families, the stigma of having a mentally ill family member may lead to overprotection and the phenomenon of being "hidden" from the world. If Ms. Chan was assessed and received appropriate services earlier, she may not have had to endure the hardship of the years of homelessness, abuse, and vulnerability as a result].*

Per records, Ms. Chan has been diagnosed with schizophrenia, psychosis disorder not specified, psychosis unspecified, recurrent major depressive disorder, and severe adjustment disorder.

Approximately two years prior to this assessment, Ms. Chan completed an evaluation with an English-speaking neuropsychologist with the assistance of a Cantonese interpreter for possible cognitive/intellectual disorder. During that evaluation, the family's concerns regarding her problems with behavior and self-management (i.e., difficulties in learning about diabetes management) were confirmed, but no developmental history or other collateral information was gathered from family members. Furthermore, no formal intelligence measures or normative data appropriate for her culture were utilized during that assessment. She was diagnosed with a psychotic disorder not otherwise specified by history and a cognitive disorder NOS, mild, possibly due to a long-standing learning disorder. Following this evaluation, she was referred to the local Regional Center by her primary care provider, but her application was apparently rejected due to insufficient information regarding developmental and educational history and an under-established link between her mental illness and her ongoing symptoms. *[Author's note (MW): It is not entirely clear how the examiner arrived at this diagnosis, given the overall marked impairment demonstrated in test results. It is certainly possible that given the lack of appropriate culturally appropriate measures and normative data available at the time of that evaluation, the examiner took a more conservative stance on conclusions so as not to pathologize the patient].*

Ms. Chan has historically presented conflicting self-reports on symptoms of auditory and visual hallucinations. Providers noted poor, if at all, compliance with her psychotropic medications, yet her symptoms stayed stable. Per Ms. Chan's siblings, they have never observed and heard of any psychotic symptoms such as auditory or visual hallucinations, internal preoccupation, or delusions. They noted disorganized speech and behaviors but noted that they were not a significant change from her baseline post-childhood febrile illness. Recently, a second opinion obtained from a new psychiatrist indicated that although psychotic disorder could not be ruled out, the degree of cognitive impairment appeared to exceed the level that would be expected from psychiatric diagnosis alone. *[Author's note (MW): Gathering detailed collateral information from her siblings was essential for accurately determining the diagnosis and assessing her eligibility for certain programs. Although it was unfortunate that her siblings were unable to be more involved in her care previously, it was my hope that with greater psychoeducation regarding intellectual disability and more support through the RC, they would be more amenable to engage with Ms. Chan. I recall her speaking fondly of her younger brother and how she enjoyed his visits while she was staying at the shelter].*

Behavioral Observations

Ms. Chan came to the appointment alone. She was dressed appropriately but appeared somewhat disheveled with noticeable dirt under fingernails and a report of constant "itchy skin." She looked younger than her stated age. She knew that she was in the hospital to see me but did not know the date or the situation related to this evaluation. She spoke in a loud child-like voice, and her speech felt pressured with mostly short phrases. Enunciation of Chinese words was at times unclear, and

I had to ask her to repeat for me to understand. She also had difficulties with comprehension and following instructions, requiring multiple repetitions on more complex tasks. Reports of her own history appeared questionable after corroboration with her sister and providers. During our inter- action, she had difficulties tracking the conversation and appeared impulsive despite prompting. I noticed that her affect was restricted and was not always congruent with her reported mood. For instance, she did not appear fearful or distressed when talking about her hallucinations, which she stated as distressing.

Ms. Chan reported seeing "ghosts who threaten to harm her with forks and knives." When asked to describe this in greater detail, she stated, "they wear white and it happens both day and night," but could not elaborate further. Other than self-reported visual hallucinations, and circumstantial speech, she did not seem preoccupied with things that were not present in the room or report any beliefs that were detached from reality. Her ability to understand and judge complex situations appeared impaired. During testing, she put forth adequate effort and task engagement, and the test- ing results were considered to be a valid representation of Ms. Chan's current cognitive functioning.

Tests and Norm Selection

Given the limitations surrounding test accessibility as described in previous sections, it is often the practice to use a mix of available tests normed for the Chinese population (when possible) along with tests adapted and translated from measures developed and normed in the United States. In this battery, I used the measures listed below. The instructions for the Beta-4 and the questions for the Independent Living Scales (ILS) subtest: Health and Safety were informally translated into Cantonese. All other tests listed below were normed on neurotypical Chinese individuals. The Beta-4 provides a reliable and valid estimate of non-verbal intellectual functioning, validated on English, ESL, and non-English speaking populations as well as special groups with learning dis- orders and intellectual disabilities. Given Ms. Chan's educational level and unfamiliarity with the testing situation, special attention and arrangements were made in order to optimize her comfort and participation.[27] These included using more simplified explanations on training items in addi- tion to the standard instructions and/or having the examiner read the Chinese word list items if she was unable to read all the words due to low literacy. Deviations from standard administration procedures and cautious interpretation were documented in the report.

- Beta-4[28]
- Brief Visuospatial Memory Test—Revised Form 1 (BVMT-R)[29,30]
- CERAD List Learning Test—Chinese[31,32]
- Category Fluency[33,34]
- Color Trails Test[34,35]
- ILS subtest: Health and Safety[36]
- Wechsler Adult Intelligence Scale—Revised Edition (WAIS-R)[34,37]

    - Selected subtest: Digit Span

Test Results

An estimate of Ms. Chan's non-verbal intellectual functioning based on the Beta-4 suggested strong possibility of intellectual disability (Beta 4 IQ = 52; 0.1 percentile). Her ability to recall a verbal list after ten minutes appeared grossly intact, but her ability to recall visual informa- tion was severely impaired, mostly due to poor comprehension and poor encoding. A teach-back method was used where Ms. Chan was asked to state in her own words what she understood to be the task instructions. She failed this three times with no improvement on prompting. Verbal fluency and visuospatial construction abilities were impaired (Category fluency = mild to moderately impaired; BVMT copy = unable to understand instructions). Simple attention was mildly impaired. Complex attention and executive functioning were severely impaired. She had significant difficulties understanding the instructions for a set-shifting task. Similarly, she was unable to understand how to do digits backward despite repeated teaching and prompting. Understanding of everyday health and safety scenarios assessed using the ILS Health and Safety subtest was impaired, which is typically associated with inability for independent living.

Clinical Impressions

Based on the results of this assessment and reported onset of cognitive and adaptive functional deficits since childhood, it was my impression that Ms. Chan met criteria for Intellectual Disability. She demonstrated significant deficits primarily in comprehension, complex attention, and executive functioning. In spite of the lack of records from Ms. Chan's developmental period, information gleaned from family members and current providers was highly consistent with impaired adaptive functioning prior to age eighteen in the absence of psychiatric disorder, as well as impaired current adaptive functioning. Furthermore, recent questions regarding her self-reported psychotic symptoms had been raised by multiple providers. In fact, providers who have known Ms. Chan for many years have not reported any observable psychotic symptoms other than circumstantial child-like speech.

Recommendations

1 Given repeated concerns regarding possible financial abuse by current payee and prior APS involvement, I recommended that another payee other than the alleged perpetrator be identified to help Ms. Chan manage her SSI income.
2 I encouraged Ms. Chan to continue following up with a psychiatrist within her own health network who can manage her psychiatric treatment.
3 I recommended that Ms. Chan be re-evaluated for eligibility to receive services from Regional Center. Although she was previously found ineligible, it was my hope that Regional Center will reconsider her application given the newly acquired collateral information from siblings, detailed psychiatric records, and updated testing with more culturally appropriate measures and normative data.
4 Ms. Chan is fortunate that her bilingual social worker has been advocating tirelessly to help her obtain the appropriate diagnosis and services. I recommended engaging with other advocacy programs should more support be required.

Follow-Up

Feedback was provided to Ms. Chan's primary care team per her wishes. Ms Chan's application was re-submitted to the Regional Center, which was then evaluated by a separate team of clinicians for eligibility criteria. She underwent another eligibility evaluation, meeting with an intake social worker, and was tested by a new bilingual neuropsychologist, whose report indicated that Ms Chan met criteria for moderate Intellectual Disability and was therefore eligible for Regional Center services. She was assigned a bilingual case manager who met with her regularly and found her appropriate housing, such that she was able to transition from the shelter where she was living.

She later enrolled in a structured day program focusing on helping adults with intellectual disabilities improve both social and daily living skills. According to her social worker, Ms. Chan appeared quite happy with her new living arrangements and daily structure activities, which allowed her to meet new friends and eat "dim sum" together.

Section III: Lessons Learned

- A culture of stigma and shame surrounding mental health and neurodevelopmental diagnoses is prevalent in Chinese communities. Healthcare providers should be mindful of the following.

  - Past experience of internalized and public stigma may impact one's mental health history.
  - Stigma may increase the patient's suspicion about the neuropsychological evaluation. Extra time is likely required to explain the purpose, procedures, and limits of confidentiality and to build rapport and trust.
  - Stigma may prevent patients and families from accepting the diagnosis and following up with recommendations. On-going psychoeducation and destigmatizing efforts are greatly beneficial.

- The following are considered helpful to reach accurate diagnoses and to generate effective recommendations.

  - Language concordant assessment is important. In both cases, having a bilingual/bicultural neuropsychologist who could speak the patients' native language, administer culturally appropriate measures, and navigate nuanced cultural issues, was essential to increasing confidence in diagnostic accuracy.
  - Accuracy of self-reported and collateral information should be considered in light of the possibility that patients or family members may not be fully forthright with disclosure in efforts to "save face," avoid potential conflict, and maintain harmony.
  - Relational network, if used properly, can be a powerful tool to aid effective treatment. Inclusion and/or exclusion of certain family members should be carefully discussed with the patient (and their guardian(s) if applicable). Proper involvement of extended family members can greatly alleviate the patient's pressure to reveal the "bad news" and communicate unfamiliar information to members of the higher familial hierarchy. Conversely, support from the important family members can in return greatly benefit the patient.
  - Better ability to differentiate culturally acceptable/related behaviors from clinical behaviors (e.g., avoidant eye contact due to the presence of elders in the context of Chinese cultural context vs. in the context of ASD) will prevent the possibility of misdiagnosis or underdiagnosis. This is particularly relevant to clinical diagnoses that take the quality of social engagement into consideration (e.g., ASD, social anxiety).

- When working with immigrants, assistance on how to navigate the dominant culture's system of care is often necessary and critical.

  - Inaccurate diagnosis can deprive immigrants who are unfamiliar with the dominant system of the opportunity to access adequate care and services. Providers should assess how past diagnoses/healthcare has or has not made an impact on the patient's daily living.
  - Certain services (for example, the Regional Center, a formulation of an IEP) may require specific and convoluted documentation, which often puts immigrants at a disadvantage.

The process is much easier to navigate when providers working with immigrant populations familiarize themselves with possible barriers and how to overcome them.

- Health providers who are able and willing to engage in advocacy are invaluable. In both cases, the patients were fortunate that many of their providers went above and beyond the call of duty to ensure they received appropriate care and services despite setbacks.

Glossary

Confucianism.   A system of social and ethical philosophy founded by Confucius (孔夫子, 500 B.C.), which promotes Li (礼, social rituals) and Ren (仁, humanism). The philosophy is based on the belief that adherence to ethical social rituals enables one to maximize the fundamental goodness of humans and live a productive and ethical life. Though transformed over time, Confucianism remains one of the most influential philosophies in the Chinese-speaking world.

Cultural Revolution.   A sociopolitical purge movement in mainland China (1966-1976) that began with efforts to rid the population of its "unprogressive values," which resulted in the harassment and persecution of a large body of the country's elderly and intellectuals. Despite the significant short- and long-term effects of this movement, it is commonly considered a taboo to discuss this topic unless a high level of trust has been established.

Mianzi (direct translation of face).   A sociological concept that links the reputation and dignity of an individual, as well as the communal network to which they belong, with one's perceived image in social contexts. Mianzi can be lost or earned and is largely determined by the collective evaluation than by the individual perspective.

Taoism.   One of the five religious' doctrines in mainland China. Taoism is commonly considered both a philosophy and a religion and is connected to the philosophers Laozi (老子, 500 BC) and Zhuangzi (庄子, 400 BC). It is vaguely defined by a belief in cosmic balance maintained and regulated by the Tao ("the Way"). One of the most well-known ideas of Taoism is the belief in balancing forces, or yin and yang. Taoism differs from Confucianism by its lack of emphasis on the rigid rituals and social order.

References

1. Communiqué of the National Bureau of Statistics of People's Republic of China on Major Figures of the 2010 Population Census [Internet]. 2011. [cited 2020 Aug 22]. Available from: https://web.archive.org/web/20131108022004/http://www.stats.gov.cn/english/newsandcomingevents/t20110428_402722244.htm

2. Hesketh T, Lu L, Xing ZW. The effect of China's one-child family policy after 25 years. N Engl J Med. 2005 Sep 15;353(11):1171–6.

3. Goodkind D. The Chinese diaspora: historical legacies and contemporary trends. US Department of Commerce, Economics and Statistics Administration, US Census Bureau; 2019. https://www.census.gov/library/working-papers/2019/demo/chinese-diaspora.html.

4. US Census Bureau. Asian American and Pacific Islander Heritage Month: May 2020 [Internet]. The United States Census Bureau. [cited 2021 Mar 28]. Available from: https://www.census.gov/newsroom/facts-for-features/2021/asian-american-pacific-islander.html

5. Li DCS. Chinese as a lingua franca in Greater China. Annu Rev Appl Linguist. 2006 Jan;26:149–76.

6. US Census Bureau. Language spoken at home for the population 5 years and over [Internet]. 2016. [cited 2021 Mar 28]. Available from: https://data.census.gov/cedsci/table?q=chinese&tid=ACS-DT1Y2018.C16001&hidePreview=false

7. UNESCO Institute for Statistics. Literacy rate, adult total (% of people ages 15 and above)—China | Data [Internet]. 2021. [cited 2021 Mar 28]. Available from: https://data.worldbank.org/indicator/SE.ADT.LITR.ZS?locations=CN

8. Pew Research Center. Chinese population in the U.S., 2000–2015 [Internet]. 2021. Available from: https://www.pewsocialtrends.org/fact-sheet/asian-americans-chinese-in-the-u-s/

9. Lieber E, Fung H, Leung PW-L. Chinese child-rearing beliefs: key dimensions and contributions to the development of culture-appropriate assessment. Asian J Soc Psychol. 2006;9(2):140–7.

10. Chung KF, Wong MC. Experience of stigma among Chinese mental health patients in Hong Kong. Psychiatr Bull. 2004 Dec;28(12):451–4.

11. The World Bank. Life expectancy at birth, total (years)—China [Internet]. 2021. [cited 2021 Mar 28]. Available from: https://data.worldbank.org/indicator/SP.DYN.LE00.IN?locations=CN

12. Jiang J, Wang P. Health status in a transitional society: urban-rural disparities from a dynamic perspective in China. Popul Health Metr. 2018 Dec 27;16(1):22.

13. Sun X, Allison C, Wei L, Matthews FE, Auyeung B, Wu YY, et al. Autism prevalence in China is comparable to Western prevalence. Mol Autism. 2019 Feb 28;10(1):7.

14. Chan AS, Leung WW, Cheung M-C. Clinical neuropsychology in China. In: Bond MH, editor. The Oxford handbook of Chinese psychology. New York (NY): Oxford University Press; 2010. p. 383–97. (Oxford library of psychology).

15. Sun X, Qi WG (Gabriel), Hong Y. Normative data for adult Mandarin speaking populations: a systematic review of performance-based neuropsychological instruments. J Int Neuropsychol Soc. 2021. 1–21. doi:10.1017/S1355617721000667.

16. Roid GH, Pomplun M. The Stanford-Binet intelligence scales, fifth edition. In Flanagan DP, Harrison PL, editors. Contemporary intellectual assessment: theories, tests, and issues. 3rd ed. New York (NY): The Guilford Press; 2012. p. 249–68.

17. Armstrong KH, Agazzi HC. Chapter 2—The Bayley-III Cognitive Scale. In: Weiss LG, Oakland T, Aylward GP, editors. Bayley-III clinical use and interpretation [Internet]. San Diego: Academic Press; 2010 [cited 2021 May 4]. p. 29–45. (Practical Resources for the Mental Health Professional). Available from: https://www.sciencedirect.com/science/article/pii/B9780123741776100029

18. Adams W, Sheslow D. Wide range assessment of visual motor abilities [Internet]. London, England: Pearson Assessment; 1995 [cited 2021 May 4]. Available from: https://www.pearsonassessments.com/store/usassessments/en/Store/Professional-Assessments/Motor-Sensory/Wide-Range-Assessment-of-Visual-Motor-Abilities/p/100001723.html

19. Dunn LM, Dunn DM. Peabody Picture Vocabulary Test. 4th ed. [Internet]. London, England: Pearson Assessment; 2007 [cited 2021 May 4]. Available from: https://www.pearsonassessments.com/store/usassessments/en/Store/Professional-Assessments/Academic-Learning/Brief/Peabody-Picture-Vocabulary-Test-%7C-Fourth-Edition/p/100000501.html

20. Lord C, Rutter M, DiLavore P, Risi S, Gotham K, Bishop S. Autism Diagnostic Observation Schedule, 2nd ed. [Internet].Torrance (CA): Western Psychological Services; 2012 [cited 2021 May 4]. Available from: https://www.wpspublish.com/ados-2-autism-diagnostic-observation-schedule-second-edition

21. Bracken B. Bracken School Readiness Assessment. 3rd ed. [Internet]. London, England: Pearson Assessment; 2007 [cited 2021 May 4]. Available from: https://www.pearsonassessments.com/store/usassessments/en/Store/Professional-Assessments/Developmental-Early-Childhood/Bracken-School-Readiness-Assessment-%7C-Third-Edition/p/100000165.html

22. Harrison P, Oakland T. Adaptive Behavior Assessment System. 3rd ed. [Internet]. Torrance, CA: Western Psychological Services; 2015 [cited 2021 May 4]. Available from: https://www.wpspublish.com/abas-3-adaptive-behavior-assessment-system-third-edition

23. Constantino J. Social Responsiveness Scale. 2nd ed. [Internet].Torrance, CA: Western Psychological Services; 2012 [cited 2021 May 4]. Available from: https://www.wpspublish.com/srs-2-social-responsiveness-scale-second-edition

24. Schopler E, Van Bourgondien M, Wellman G, Love S. Childhood Autism Rating Scale. 2nd ed. [Internet]. Torrance, CA: Western Psychological Services; 2010 [cited 2021 May 4]. Available from: https://www.wpspublish.com/cars-2-childhood-autism-rating-scale-second-edition

25. Reynolds C, Kamphaus R. Behavior Assessment System for Children. 2nd ed. [Internet].London, England: Pearson Assessment; 2004 [cited 2021 May 4]. Available from: https://www.pearsonclinical.co.uk/Psychology/ChildMentalHealth/ChildADDADHDBehaviour/BehaviorAssessmentSystemforChildrenSecondEdition(BASC-2)/BehaviorAssessmentSystemforChildrenSecondEdition(BASC-2).aspx

26. Gioia G, Isquith P, Guy S, Kenworthy L. Behavior Rating Inventory of Executive Function [Internet]. Torrance, CA: Western Psychological Services; 2013 [cited 2021 May 4]. Available from: https://www.wpspublish.com/brief-behavior-rating-inventory-of-executive-function

27. Fujii DEM. Developing a cultural context for conducting a neuropsychological evaluation with a culturally diverse client: the ECLECTIC framework. Clin Neuropsychol. 2018 Nov 17;32(8):1356–92.

28. Kellogg C, Morton N. Beta-4 [Internet]. London, England: Pearson Assessment; 2016 [cited 2021 May 4]. Available from: https://www.pearsonassessments.com/store/usassessments/en/Store/Professional-Assessments/Cognition-%26-Neuro/Non-Verbal-Ability/Beta-4/p/100001642.html

29. Benedict R. Brief Visuospatial Memory Test-Revised [Internet]. Lutz (FL): Psychological Assessment Resources, Inc; 1997 [cited 2021 May 4]. Available from: https://www.parinc.com/Products/Pkey/30

30. Lee CKY, Collinson SL, Feng L, Ng T-P. Preliminary normative neuropsychological data for an elderly Chinese population. Clin Neuropsychol. 2012 Feb 1;26(2):321–34.

31. Welsh KA, Butters N, Mohs RC, Beekly D, Edland S, Fillenbaum G, et al. The Consortium to Establish a Registry for Alzheimer's Disease (CERAD). Part V. A normative study of the neuropsychological battery. Neurology. 1994 Apr;44(4):609–14.

32. Liu K, Kuo M, Tang K, Chau A, Ho I, Chan W, et al. Effects of age, education and gender in the Consortium to Establish a Registry for the Alzheimer's Disease (CERAD)-Neuropsychological Assessment Battery for Cantonese-speaking Chinese elders. Int Psychogeriatr. 2011 Jul 5;23(10):1575–81.

33. Baldo JV, Shimamura AP. Letter and category fluency in patients with frontal lobe lesions. Neuropsychology. 1998;12(2):259–67.

34. Lee T, Wang K. Neuropsychological measures: normative data for Chinese. 2nd revised ed. Hong Kong: Laboratory of Neuropsychology, The University of Hong Kong; 2010.

35. D'Elia LF, Satz P, Uchiyama CL, White T. Color Trails Test Professional Manual [Internet]. Odessa (FL): Psychological Assessment Resources; [cited 2020 Feb 28]. Available from: https://www.parinc.com/Products/Pkey/77

36. Loeb P. Independent Living Scales [Internet]. London, England: Pearson Assessment; 1996 [cited 2021 May 4]. Available from: https://www.pearsonassessments.com/store/usassessments/en/Store/Professional-Assessments/Cognition-%26-Neuro/Independent-Living-Scales/p/100000181.html

37. Wechsler D. Wechsler Adult Intelligence Scale-Revised manual. New York (NY): The Psychological Corporation; 1981.

Filipino

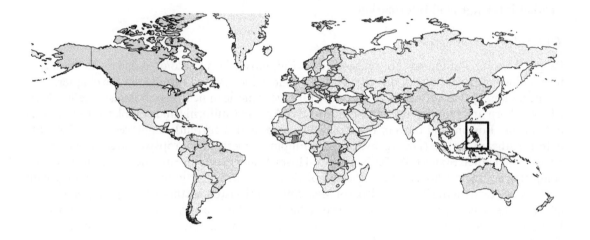

14 Cultural Sensitivity in Neuropsychological Assessment of Filipinos and Filipino Americans

Kristina A. Agbayani, Mario F. Dulay, Jr.,
Regilda Anne A. Romero, and Cherry Ordoñez

Section I: Background Information

Terminology and Perspective

People from the Philippines are referred to as Filipinos, Pinoys, and/or Asians. The preferred terminology of the authors of this chapter is Filipino, which is used throughout the chapter.

The authors' perspectives are that of a (1) Filipino American neuropsychologist (she/her/hers) who was born and raised in the San Francisco Bay Area in California and completed her training in Houston, Boston, and the San Francisco Bay Area, and is currently employed at the VA Palo Alto Healthcare System (Dr. Agbayani); (2) a Filipino American neuropsychologist (he/him/his) born at the United States (US) Balboa Naval Hospital and raised in San Diego, California, who completed graduate school at the University of Cincinnati with post-grad school and employment in Houston, Texas at the Baylor College of Medicine and Houston Methodist Hospital (Dr. Dulay); (3) a Filipino American neuropsychologist (she/her/hers) who was born and raised in Quezon City, Philippines, migrated to California as a young adult, completed her training in Palo Alto, San Francisco, Virginia Beach, and Minneapolis, and is currently employed as a Clinical Assistant Professor at the UF Department of Psychiatry, College of Medicine (Dr. Romero); and (4) a clinical psychology doctoral student (she/her/hers) born in the Philippines and raised in Hawai'i and California with prior training and work in urban planning and finance before returning to school to become a psychologist (Ms. Ordoñez).

Geography

The Philippines is an archipelago consisting of 7,641 islands encompassing almost 300,000 square kilometers in Southeast Asia in the Western Pacific Ocean. It is bordered by the South China Sea in the west and the Philippine Sea in the east. The 2019 population was approximately 108.1 million.[1] The country is divided into three main regions: Luzon (northern), Visayas (central), and Mindanao (southern). The capital city, Manila, is in the Luzon region.

History

The Philippines has a unique historical and cultural background that combines Asian, Spanish, and Western influences. The indigenous peoples were descended from Malaysia. Trade routes with neighboring countries brought Chinese and Indonesian influences. Following the arrival of **Ferdinand Magellan**, the Philippines became a Spanish colony for over 300 years (1521–1898). The lasting Spanish influence is evident in aspects of language (i.e., many Tagalog words are the same or

DOI: 10.4324/9781003051862-29

similar in Spanish), cultural traditions, and the prevalence of Catholicism in the country.[2] Filipino history and culture are also quite similar to those of Latin American countries with Spanish colonial histories.[3] The Philippines was ceded by Spain to the United States with the Treaty of Paris in 1898 and remained a US colony until 1946. American influence is made evident by English being one of the country's national languages, as well as its educational and political system. Currently, the government of the Philippines is a presidential, democratic republic, with power equally divided among the executive, legislative, and judicial branches.[4]

Immigration

Like many immigrants, Filipinos leave their homes in search of freedom, work, and education. Top places of immigration for Filipinos have largely been the United States, followed by Saudi Arabia, Canada, United Arab Emirates, Australia, and Japan.[5] Filipinos arrived in the United States as early as 1587 as indentured servants and slaves on Spanish galleon ships.[6,7] Early 1900s immigration to the United States consisted of Filipino students on American government scholarships, called **pensionados**, to laborers, called **sakadas**, who worked on plantations and canaries.[8]

Post-World War II immigration of Filipinos largely included spouses and children of US military soldiers, healthcare workers, and those seeking refuge from **economic turmoil**. Political repression and human rights violations during the **Ferdinand Marcos** era (1965–1986) pushed many Filipinos to emigrate.[9] After 1965, Filipino immigration to the United States largely consisted of the "brain drain" generation of professionals such as nurses and engineers. Although the post-1965 wave of Filipino immigrants is considered the last official wave of Filipinos immigrating to the United States, there are an invisible group of Filipino undocumented immigrants known as TNTs (tago ng tago/always hiding).[10] Attention to immigration history can shed light on possible pre-immigration traumas, culture shock and acculturation, socio-economic status, and visa documentation stressors that in turn can impact emotional well-being, test performance, and test-taking approach.

Language

Over 170 languages and dialects are spoken in the Philippines that are region-specific. **Filipino** and English are the national languages of the Philippines. Consequently, many Filipinos are able to speak, write, and understand Filipino, English, and their respective regional language/dialect,[11] with varying levels of comfort and fluency among them. Therefore, it is essential for clinicians to obtain detailed information about language education background and preferences as part of a clinical interview to help determine what tests and norms are most appropriate. The effect of testing a patient in their less proficient language can have a detrimental impact on interpretation of neuropsychological test results. English language proficiency can initially be estimated during the clinical interview by gathering information such as age immigrated to the United States, education level, years of education in the United States, language spoken in the home, and language spoken most often. If the person speaks minimal English, an interpreter who speaks the specific Filipino language or dialect may be warranted rather than not completing an evaluation. However, test interpretation when using US tests and norms can reduce validity and require a more qualitative descriptive assessment of the patient's strengths and weaknesses from non-language-based tests and collateral reports.

Education and Literacy

Having a good understanding of a client's literacy, education level, and quality of education is essential to neuropsychological test data interpretation. Asking detailed questions about number of years, quality of and access to education is crucial, as there can be significant variability based on region, socio-economic status, and other factors. The Philippines has high literacy rates, upwards of 94% in adults and 98% in young adults as of 2015.[12] Regional dialects are primarily used for instruction during the initial elementary school years, with English and Filipino instruction starting from grades 4 to 6. Both of the national languages are used exclusively in secondary and higher education. Previously, the basic elementary and secondary education cycle consisted of ten years. The 2011 Kindergarten Education Act and the 2013 Basic Education Act resulted in a mandatory year of kindergarten and extended the elementary and secondary education cycle to 12 years, respectively. Overall, higher education has expanded since the late 1990s.[13] Nevertheless, there continue to be significant disparities in education based on region and socio-economic status. Poverty remains a significant issue in the Philippines compared to other Southeast Asian countries. For example, I (KAA) evaluated an elderly Filipino patient who had minimal formal education. He grew up in a rural area and attended up to the first grade. His attendance in school was very intermittent due to having to help his family in their rice fields. He stated that this practice was typical for children in his community, where many did not complete school because there were more important priorities, such as tending to and harvesting their crops on which families relied for income.

Values and Customs

Cultural perspective regarding values and customs of Filipinos can help establish rapport, provide insightful questions to better conceptualize problems and answer the referral question, and understand what treatment recommendations may or may not be followed to completion. Generally, traditional Filipino values can be affected by several factors including collectivism, social acceptance and conformity, and Christianity (particularly Catholicism).

Collectivism, or the value of prioritizing the well-being of the greater community over individual needs, is a common Filipino value. Filipinos often feel uniquely interconnected and desire to do activities with other Filipinos to provide emotional support and promote personal identity. Familism is a type of collectivism emphasizing family obligation including putting ones' family first, caring for ones' elders as they age, and respecting elders including older siblings and parents. Respect for elders, or **paggalang sa nakatatanda**, is commonly shown in Filipino families by calling older siblings or elders by endearing terms or respectful titles, allocating significant weight or deference to parents' opinions, and caring for aging parents by having them move into a family member's home. Often a strong Filipino work ethic will interact with a desire to help family and often lead to sacrifice (e.g., family members in the United States working hard to send money back to the Philippines).

Filipino value for social acceptance and conformity leads to interconnectedness within families and communities. **Pakikisama**, often means maintaining relationships within and outside of the family dynamic to avoid confrontation, going along with group opinions, or behaving in socially acceptable ways to not show opposition or anger in order to maintain harmony. In a healthcare setting, this may produce a deference to authority figures (e.g., medical providers) and avoidance of asking questions. For example, Filipino patients may say yes and indicate understanding during the feedback session even if they do not fully grasp a diagnosis or other information discussed. This may also lead a patient to not ask particular questions to clarify uncertainty. Further, if a patient does not feel connected to the clinician (e.g., culturally) there may be less trust, and the patient may not share important information. In addition, negative comments made by the evaluator during testing may have undesirable consequences since many Filipinos are generally sensitive to criticism because of a high pride or **amor propio** and the notion of "saving face." Therefore, it can be helpful for providers to attempt to gauge the patient's understanding during the feedback session.

Spirituality and Religion

About 82%–85% of Filipinos are Christian and mostly Roman Catholic, followed by followers of Islam and tribal religions. My (MFD) grandmother in the Philippines had a large Mother Mary statue in her front yard that also served as her physician's clinic in the countryside. This symbolized the interaction and importance of Catholicism in her home and work life. Since many Filipinos are spiritual, their approach to managing medical issues may often be faith-based. A Christian values-based system would include goodwill toward others (helping people), indebtedness (e.g., a child feeling obligated to their parents for their upbringing), specific types of help-seeking behavior (e.g., seeking pastoral counseling), and faith-based healing (e.g., attending a healing mass, prayer). One faith-based coping mechanism is the expression "**bahala na**" or "Leave it in God's or fate's hands." While this can help reduce anxiety and rumination, it may also lead to not seeking medical help for serious problems.

Health Status

Cardiovascular disease (e.g., heart disease and stroke) and vascular risk factors, including diabetes mellitus, hypertension, and hyperlipidemia, are among the most common medical conditions impacting Filipinos. Other common conditions include cancers and chronic pulmonary conditions.[14,15] A common thread among these conditions is that they are noncommunicable diseases with a number of preventable causes, including poor/unhealthy diet, limited exercise, and tobacco and other substance use.[14] Dietary habit may be one area of focus, as Filipino gatherings typically consist of sharing meals that can contribute to overeating foods high in sodium and fat. Additionally, Filipinos have higher rates of smoking compared to other Asian groups.[14] Increasing health literacy, education, and prevention or reversal opportunities (e.g., prediabetes) is important starting at an early age. Discussing these important issues and providing practical information and recommendations about relevant lifestyle changes becomes an integral part of the neuropsychological feedback session.

Mental Health Views

Compared to other Asian groups, Filipinos are least likely to utilize mental health services.[16] There are a number of possible reasons for this including limited access to mental health resources in the Philippines; stigma related to mental health issues; and lack of identification with and perceived inaccessibility of mental health providers. In the Philippines, a majority of mental health providers and treatment facilities are in Manila or other major urban areas. Along with high costs for services, accessibility to individuals living in more rural areas and from lower socio-economic backgrounds is limited.[17] Beliefs about the root causes of mental illness also significantly impact from whom Filipinos seek care. For example, spiritual causes, like the belief that hardship or illness is a punishment from God for something they had done in the past, may lead to seeking care from traditional healers or clergy.[18,19] In one study, highly religious Filipino Americans sought help from religious clergy more often than mental health professionals due to perceived accessibility, concerns about loss of face, and difficulty understanding English.[19] Help-seeking behaviors are also impacted by stigma related to mental health issues, which may stem from the aforementioned concern about loss of saving face and *hiya*, or embarrassment.[18,20] Additionally, the concept of **ibang tao**, or outsider, may be another barrier to seeking help from or being completely forthcoming with mental health professionals. The perception of a mental health provider as an outsider or not "one of us," has been shown to impact rapport, trust, and feelings of acceptance.[18,21] For example, my (KAA) patient's wife stated that they first sought help from a Filipino deacon in their church for the patient's behavioral changes due to frontotemporal dementia. They expressed feeling most comfortable and trusting in this deacon because they got to know him at weekly masses over the course of many years; he was of a similar age to the patient and his wife was originally from the same region in the Philippines, and he spoke the same language.

Assessment Needs

Careful assessment of the multifaceted nature of a patient's medical and psychosocial history discussed in the previous sections is vital to establishing rapport, test interpretation, norms selection, and provision of feedback and recommendations. One model for ensuring a thorough and valid clinical interview and neuropsychological assessment proposed by Dr. Daryl Fujii involves attempting to collect information regarding education, culture and acculturation, languages spoken and English proficiency, economic issues, communication style, testing situation involving level of patient comfort and motivation, intelligence value, and context of immigration (ECLECTIC framework).[20] It is important during the clinical interview and with questionnaires to ascertain the patient's level of acculturation including how long the person has lived in the United States, age when immigrated, community integration level, and level of assimilation to mainstream US culture. There are a number of predominantly Filipino communities in various US cities where many Filipino patients interact in their native language in stores, restaurants, and churches and watch Filipino channels on television. This allows maintaining customs and culture and leads to less familiarity and acculturation to mainstream American customs and culture.

Few neuropsychological tests have been normed for Filipino and Filipino Americans. There are some exceptions of tests and questionnaires created and normed in the Philippines [21-24] and several Western-based instruments that have been translated into Tagalog.[25-30] A full listing of these instruments can be found in Appendix.

Section II: Case Study — "This Might Be God's Punishment"

Presenting Problems

I (Dr. Romero) evaluated "Cecil," a 6-year-old second-generation Filipino American boy who was referred by his principal due to having significant receptive and expressive language deficits. Instructions needed to be repeated several times, but Cecil often still did not understand the instructions or expectations. Expressively, while he was able to speak in simple sentences, he mostly used instrumental/conventional gestures and one- to two-word utterances. Additionally, he had notable articulation difficulties impacting intelligibility. Given his communication deficits, his teacher reported difficulty in gauging Cecil's learning acquisition due to his limited speech and comprehension.

Cultural and Language History

Cecil currently lives with his paternal grandparents, his aunt, and his older sibling. His parents are both second-generation Filipino Americans. Both Cecil and his sibling had been living with his grandparents shortly after his parents separated but only received legal guardianship recently. Delays were due to limited resources and not knowing how to navigate the system. Cecil's grandparents moved to the United States in the 70s. Both his grandparents graduated college in the

Philippines but are currently unemployed and receive social security and veteran supports. Their family struggles to make ends meet. His aunt contributes financially but supports her own college education. Neither parents provide child support. Cecil had not seen his mother since she left three years ago and intermittently sees his father, who lives with his new family in a neighboring city.

The family lives in the city, within a big Filipino community. They attend Catholic services weekly. Cecil listens to English music and watches both American and Filipino television shows. However, his grandparents predominantly watch Filipino shows. His biological parents, sibling, and aunt speak predominantly English but understand Tagalog. At home, his grandparents mostly speak Tagalog (dialect from their province). His grandparents have conversational skills in English but admitted to not being proficient. While they communicate better in Tagalog, they try to speak in both languages to Cecil inside and outside of the home. He reportedly responds in English. Aside from his grandparents, no one else speaks with him in Tagalog.

Cecil reportedly has many friends in school. Given the composition of his school's population, his friends are from different races/ethnicities.

Health and Developmental History

Cecil was born full-term via normal delivery and weighed eight pounds. I was also informed of possible exposure to substances prenatally. His grandfather reported that Cecil's parents used drugs in the past, so exposure to drugs in utero was very likely. At three months old, he was brought to the hospital due to seizures and was in and out of the hospital for four months. Initial seizure episode was thought to be due to an accidental hit on the head by his older sibling. Details of the accident were unknown as Cecil's grandfather was vacationing in the Philippines at that time. Cecil has not had any seizure episodes since then. Early developmental milestones for gross motor and speech/language were reportedly delayed. His grandfather believed that Cecil started walking at age 2 and started talking at age 4. His family thought he was deaf and mute because he was very quiet and did not speak. Cecil's first language is English since both of his parents only spoke English. His grandfather stated Cecil understands both English and Tagalog but has very limited expressive communication in both. Other developmental issues were denied. He was otherwise physically healthy with occasional viral colds and fevers. Hearing and vision were normal based on school physical exam at the beginning of the school year. He does not take any prescribed medication.

Educational History

At the time of the evaluation, Cecil started first grade at a private school, where he and his older sibling receive educational funding. According to his teacher, Cecil previously received some 1:1 intervention and peer tutoring for language arts and pre-academic math classes. His grandfather reported that Cecil benefited from the tutoring but was unsure why it was discontinued as they are unable to pay for a private tutor. While he was unable to read and had poor phonological awareness, he could recite his letters and numbers and write numerals up to 100. His grandfather reported that it had been very difficult to teach Cecil at home because he could be "stubborn" and often claimed to be "tired."

Social, Emotional, and Behavioral Functioning

Cecil is quite shy, which was attributed to his communication difficulties. Cecil was described by his grandfather as friendly, loving, cheerful, and obedient. Cecil's teacher described him as a sweet and playful boy who was well liked by his peers. Behaviorally, he could be inattentive during school, but there were no other concerns at home and in school.

Daily Functioning

Cecil enjoys spending time with his family. Due to his young age, they do not expect him to do chores; therefore, they do everything for him. At home, he can perform daily living activities independently; however, his grandmother checks on him to ensure he does things correctly. He can feed and dress himself.

Previous Test Findings

Last year, Cecil underwent a pre-academic screening, which resulted in below-age performance across the board. Specifically, his expressive language skills were very low, while his receptive skills were slightly better but still well below average. Letter knowledge was well below average, while his number sense was below average. Poor vocabulary and mild articulation difficulty were noted. His fine motor skills were significantly low. A comprehensive developmental evaluation was recommended, including medical (i.e., immediate dental care), speech, and occupational therapy evaluation. Tutoring was also recommended for basic phonics and word decoding.

Classroom Observation

Cecil was observed on three separate occasions at his school in order: during recess, independent class work, and small group. Cecil was noted to reference his seatmate's work almost always to ensure he was correct and also copied his seatmate's answers. Cecil used gestures when communicating and needed prompting to use his words. Throughout my observations, he was very quiet and rarely talked to his peers. He watched and listened but hardly interacted with them. He gazed at me a few times but never engaged.

Testing Behavioral Observations

I evaluated Cecil on two different occasions at his school. Cecil was polite, enthusiastic, and cheerful; he easily developed and maintained rapport. While he was quiet and never initiated any conversations with me, he responded to my questions, which was expected in the Filipino culture (i.e., respond when spoken to). His eye contact was good. The evaluation was completed in English as his spontaneous speech/expressive language was only in English. Even when questions were asked in Tagalog, his responses were in English. He needed prompts and directions repeated. When items were easy, he was confident and responded quickly. In contrast, when items were difficult, he looked up, pretended to think but did not respond. On a few verbal tasks, he responded with "Don't know" without really thinking about the questions. During these times, I tested limits by translating words in Tagalog or allowed him to respond in Tagalog to see if it would make a difference, which it did not. He seemed to know fewer words in Tagalog based on informal assessments and observation. When provided with multiple-choice answers in both English and Tagalog, he provided correct answers based on recognition and process of elimination. To note, he did relatively better in English than in Tagalog. Overall, he put forth sufficient effort; thus, the results of this evaluation were thought to be accurate.

Test and Norm Selection

There are no translated or validated tests for Filipino children. I selected a test battery based on his history of developmental delays, his utilization of English than Tagalog, and what would best capture his strengths and weaknesses: Wechsler Intelligence Scale for Children—Fifth Edition, Wechsler Individual Achievement Test—Third Edition, NEPSY—Second Edition,

Expressive/Receptive One-Word Picture Vocabulary Test, Bender-Gestalt Test, Beery Buktenica Visual-Motor Integration, Behavior Assessment System for Children—Third Edition. While none of the following tests have been culturally validated with Filipino or Filipino American children, results were interpreted with these considerations in mind and thought to still adequately represent his current functioning based on his use of English more than Tagalog and familiarity with US-based testing systems.

Test Results and Impressions

Neuropsychological evaluation revealed significant variability in his performance/skills. Cecil's cognitive functioning was variable; he had better developed nonverbal reasoning abilities (low average) than his verbal/language skills (very low). Relative strengths were noted in recreation of block designs, identification of missing details of a picture, and transcription of symbols. Significant weaknesses were noted in nonverbal abstract reasoning, as well as in expressive (picture naming and oral-motor sequencing) and receptive (picture naming and comprehension of instructions) language. While Cecil made progress in the past year, his language skills remained deficient, falling significantly below his peers.

Language-based academic skills were generally below expectations. This includes rapid automatic naming, word reading, reading comprehension, and spelling. Regarding memory, sentence repetition and list-learning were borderline, while memory for faces was above expected levels. These were consistent with his performance on the cognitive test. Results of the rating scales indicated average adaptive and emotional/behavioral functioning.

Overall, this neuropsychological profile revealed a pattern of weakness with verbal/language skills. Considering the above, Cecil met diagnostic criteria for Language Disorder (mixed receptive and expressive). While testing was done in English, his Tagalog proficiency was also poor. In fact, he knew less words in Tagalog based on informal assessments/observation. As such, I recommended Speech and Language therapy to address his deficits in this area. I gave him an additional diagnosis of Academic Problems, given his language-based academic weaknesses. While he currently did not meet full criteria for a Specific Learning Disability, he is experiencing significant difficulties and would need to be followed. I encouraged his grandfather to request classroom accommodations, instruction modifications, and resume one-to-one tutoring at his school. He also demonstrated vulnerabilities in graphomotor skills. He was not given an additional diagnosis at this time based on variability in fine-motor and visual-spatial tasks; however, it is important that this is monitored. Occupational therapy evaluation was also suggested. Additionally, I recommended a neurological evaluation given his history of seizures and prenatal exposures to drugs.

Feedback and Follow-Up

I discussed the results of this evaluation and Cecil's strengths and weaknesses and explained the pattern of deficits in verbal/language skills with his grandfather, who was confused about the diagnosis of Language Disorder as Cecil can be quite talkative at home. After explaining the concepts and differences between basic interpersonal communication skills and cognitive academic language proficiency, he appeared to understand Cecil's vulnerabilities and how these affected his functioning. I further explained how Cecil's language disorder was impacting his learning at school. I provided examples of his academic difficulties and how he is at-risk for further lagging behind his peers if not addressed.

Cecil's grandfather inquired about possible causes of Cecil's problems, specifically asking about his mother's drug use or his seizures during infancy. He also stated that this might be God's punishment due to the patient's parents' drug use. While being affirming, I provided psycho-education on brain development and neuropsychology. His grandfather also expressed feeling ashamed for not being aware of these deficits. They did not think something was "wrong" with Cecil as he understands both English and Tagalog. I described the different measures and testing of limits that I used to determine whether his performance would improve with Tagalog. However, I found the opposite. He also asked why he had never heard of this diagnosis before. I normalized his concerns and further explained that neurodevelopmental disorders affect individuals from different backgrounds. I explained that it may be less diagnosed in Filipinos as we tend to focus on physical illness rather than developmental delays or may view language difficulties as benign when learning two languages and believing that children will eventually catch up.

Cecil's grandfather brought up many valid concerns such as financial issues and "cures" for Cecil's challenges. This exemplified how Filipinos tend to search for the "cure" and have a mindset that developmental delays will be overcome/resolve on their own. This thinking sometimes prevents families from seeking services in the hopes and belief that the child will somehow "grow" out of the delays. He and his wife supported their grandchildren using minimal income, and he was very concerned about the costs of these interventions. We discussed different options such as transferring to a public school and utilizing the free services through the public-school system and insurance. I also provided them with specific interventions they could do at home to help improve his language and reading skills, as well as activities to improve fine-motor/visuospatial skills.

The feedback session was conducted in both English and Tagalog as some concepts do not have direct Tagalog translations. For example, the direct translation for Language Disorder is **karamdaman ng wika**, which can be back translated to "illness of language." This translation does not fully capture the concept of a child having speech and communication problems. Similarly, sensorimotor and visual-spatial skills have no direct translations. Hence, English terms were used with a Tagalog explanation of the concepts. His grandfather expressed his gratitude to me for speaking in Tagalog.

Neurodevelopmental disorders are not likely to be discussed or familiar to Filipinos. While they may know of or may have heard of intellectual disability, attention deficit hyperactivity disorder, or autism, language disorders and learning disability are less "popular" constructs, and deficits in these areas may be thought to be related to intellectual or general cognitive slowness. Having a Tagalog-speaking neuropsychologist explain these less "popular" constructs, which may not necessarily have a direct Tagalog translation, contributed to a meaningful feedback session with Cecil's grandfather. It may have also facilitated the grandfather's willingness to pose clarifying statements and questions to the neuropsychologist in light of the above discussion about values of *ibang tao* or outsider, and *pakikisama* or smooth interpersonal relationships to maintain group harmony.

Section III: Lessons Learned

- The Philippines is a diverse country with influences from Asian, Spanish, and American cultures as a result of trade routes and colonization. Filipino history and culture may be more similar to those of Latin countries that were also under Spanish rule compared to other Asian countries.
- There are distinct regions with specific languages and dialects spoken. Tagalog and English are the two national languages. Therefore, assessment of language proficiency in the clinical interview is an essential component of the clinical interview to determine appropriate test and norms selection, interpretability of data, and overall assessment of cognitive ability.
- There is likely to be significant variability in education level influenced by socio-economic status, region, and education reforms. Questions surrounding number of years of formal

education, quality of education, and education/school resources, and accessibility are also essential.

- The ECLECTIC model established by Dr. Daryl Fujii provides an excellent framework for assessing important cultural components when working with diverse patients.
- Translating psychological terms and concepts into Tagalog, or other Filipino languages or dialects, can be difficult as some terms do not have direct translations. Alternatively, one may explain the concept rather than translate word for word. Providing a report summary in the patient's native language can be helpful for patients and family.
- Few neuropsychological tests have been normed for Filipino and Filipino Americans, and these tests are usually adapted from US-based tests, with a few exceptions. There are no appropriate measures available for Filipino children.
- Negative comments made by the examiner during testing may have undesirable consequences since many Filipinos are generally sensitive to criticism because of high self-esteem.
- Filipinos are known to be religious/spiritual. Thus, when it comes to locus of control, patients and family members may believe that a patient's vulnerabilities are punishment by God because of some past wrongdoing rather than biological or medical reasons and may therefore seek religious means to resolve problems. Others may adopt a *bahala na* attitude in which they leave it to fate or the hands of God.
- The concept of *ibang tao*, or outsider, may be a barrier to seeking help from or being completely forthcoming with mental health professionals. The perception of a mental health provider as an outsider, or not "one of us," can impact rapport, trust, and feelings of acceptance. Filipinos may be more comfortable or forthcoming with providers that are Filipino or Filipino American or with the use of an interpreter that speaks Filipino.
- Filipinos tend to show a deference to authority figures or shy away from disrupting group harmony and may therefore say yes or indicate understanding toward medical professionals despite not fully understanding the information presented.

Glossary

Amor propio.   Self-pride leading to sensitivity to criticism.

Bahala na.   Leaving one's future to fate or to God.

Economic turmoil.   Post WWII national development struggles included peasant unrest, communist rebellions, and Moro liberationists amidst land reforms and trade restructure.[30]

Ferdinand Magellan.   A Portuguese explorer who organized the Spanish expedition from 1519 to 1522.

Ferdinand Marcos.   Philippines head of state from 1965 to 1986, initially as president but then established martial law.

Filipino (language).   One of the national languages of the Philippines, declared in the Philippine Constitution of 1987, that is generally based on and evolved from Tagalog.[31]

Ibang tao.   Outsider.

Karamdaman ng wika.   The direct translation for Language Disorder, which can be back translated to "illness of language."

Paggalang sa nakatatanda.   Respect for elders.

Pakikisama.   Going along with group opinions and behaving in a way to maintain harmony within the group or family.

Pensionados.   Children of prominent Filipino families.

Sakadas.   Filipino laborers.

Tago ng tago.   Always hiding; a term used for undocumented Filipino immigrants.

References

1. The World Bank. Population, total—Philippines [Internet]. World Bank Group: 2020. Available from: https://data.worldbank.org/indicator/SP.POP.TOTL?locations=PH
2. Nadal KL, Monzones J. Neuropsychological assessments and Filipino Americans: cultural implications for practice. In Fujii DEM, editor. The neuropsychology of Asian Americans. New York (NY): Psychology Press; 2011. p. 47–70.
3. Agbayani-Siewert P. Assumptions of Asian American similarity: the case of Filipino and Chinese American students. Social Work. 2004;49:39–51.
4. Gov.ph. About the Government [Internet]. Available from: https://www.gov.ph/about-the-government.html
5. Gallardo LK, Batalova J. Filipino immigrants in the United States [Internet]. Migration Policy Institute: 2020. Available from: https://www.migrationpolicy.org/article/filipino-immigrants-united-states
6. Kitano HH, Daniels R. Asian Americans: emerging minorities. 2nd ed. Englewood Cliffs, New Jersey: Prentice Hall; 1995.
7. Posadas BM. The Filipino Americans. Westport, Connecticut: Greenwood Press; 1999.
8. U.S. Congress. U.S. Congressional serial set (Volume 6200) [Internet]. Government Printing Office: 1912. Available from: https://hdl.handle.net/2027/ucl.b3992101
9. Espiritu YL. Filipino American lives. Philadelphia: Temple University Press; 1995.
10. Montoya, CA. Living in the shadows: the undocumented immigrant experience of Filipinos. In Root MPP, editor. Filipino Americans; transformation and identity. Thousand Oaks (CA): Sage Publications; 1997. p. 112–120. doi:10.4135/9781452243177
11. Lopa-Ramos MR, Ledesma L. Neuropsychology in the Philippines. In Fujii DEM, editor. The neuropsychology of Asian Americans. New York (NY): Psychology Press; 2011. p. 285–291.
12. UNESCO Institute of Statistics. Philippines [Internet]. UNESCO Institute of Statistics: 2020. Available from: http://uis.unesco.org/en/country/ph
13. Macha W, Mackie C, Magaziner J. Education in the Philippines [Internet]. World Education News + Reviews: 2018. Available from: https://wenr.wes.org/2018/03/education-in-the-philippines
14. Abesamis CJ, Fruh S, Hall H, Lemley T, Zlomke KR. Cardiovascular health of Filipinos in the United States: a review of the literature. J Transcult Nurs. 2016;27(5):518–28.
15. Almagren O, Duque F, Weiler GA. Time for action to stop the deadliest diseases in the Philippines [Internet]. World Health Organization: 8 May 2018. Available from: https://www.who.int/philippines/news/commentaries/detail/time-for-action-to-stop-the-deadliest-diseases-in-the-philippines
16. Abe-Kim J, Takeuchi DT, Hong S, Zane N, Sue S, Spencer MS, et al. Use of mental health–related services among immigrant and US-born Asian Americans: results from the National Latino and Asian American study. Am J Public Health. 2007;97(1):91–8.
17. Tuliao AP. Mental help seeking among Filipinos: a review of the literature [Internet]. Faculty Publications, Department of Psychology: 2014. Available from: http://digitalcommons.unl.edu/psychfacpub/792
18. Abe-Kim J, Gong F, Takeuchi D. Religiosity, spirituality, and help-seeking among Filipino Americans: religious clergy or mental health professionals? J Community Psychol. 2004;32(6): 675–89.
19. Fujii, DEM. Developing a cultural context for conducting a neuropsychological evaluation with a culturally diverse client: the ECLECTIC framework. Clin Neuropsychol. 2018;32(8):1356–92.
20. Pasco ACY, Morse JM, Olson JK. Cross-cultural relationships between nurses and Filipino Canadian patients. J Nurs Scholarsh. 2004;36(3):239–46.
21. Julom, AM. The development and validation of a neuropsychological assessment for mild cognitive impairment of Filipino older adults. Ageing Int. 2013;38:271–327.
22. Ledesma LK, Diputado BY, Ortega GO, Santillan CE. Development of the De-Westernized Dementia Screening Scale. Philipp J Psychol. 1993;26(2):30–8.
23. Javier SB, Luna-Reyes OB, Walter RT, Ledesma LK, Reyes TM. The Manila motor-perceptual screening test: its development and field investigation. St Tomas J Med. 1988;37:126–69.
24. Dominguez JC, Phung TKT, de Guzman MFP, Fowler KC, Reandelar M, Natividad B, et al. Determining Filipino normative data for a battery of neuropsychological tests: the Filipino Norming Project (FNP). Dement Geriatr Cogn Disord Extra. 2019;9:260–70.

25. Ligsay A. Validation of the Mini Mental State Examination in the Philippines. Manila: University of the Philippines Manila; 2003.

26. Dominguez, JC, Soriano JR, Magpantay CD, Orquiza MGS, Solis WM, Reandelar MF, et al. Early detection of mild Alzheimer's disease in Filipino elderly: validation of the Montreal Cognitive Assessment-Philippines (MoCA-P). Adv Alzheimer's Dis. 2014;3:160–7.

27. Coffey DM, Javier JR, Schrager SM. Preliminary validity of the Eyberg Child Behavior Inventory with Filipino immigrant parents. Child Fam Behav Ther. 2015;37(3):208–23.

28. Rohlman DS, Villanueva-Uy E, Ramos EAM, Mateo PC, Bielawski DM, Chiodo LM, et al. Adaptation of the Behavioral Assessment and Research System (BARS) for evaluation neurobehavioral performance in Filipino children. Neurotoxicology. 2008;29(1):143–51.

29. Ty WEG, Davis RD, Melgar MIE, Ramos MA. A validation study on the Filipino Geriatric Depression Scale (GDS) using Rasch Analysis. Int J Psychiatr Res. 2019;2(7):1–6.

30. Weekley K. The national or the social? Problems of nation-building in post-World War II Philippines. Third World Q. 2006; 27(1):85–100.

31. Rubrico JGU. The metamorphosis of Filipino as National Language [Internet]. Language Links Foundation, Incorporated. Available from: https://citeseerx.ist.psu.edu/viewdoc/download?doi=10.1.1.693.5187&rep=rep1&type=pdf

Japanese

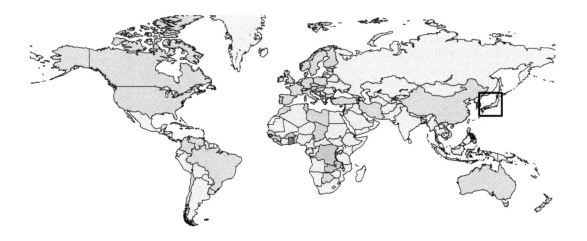

15 Neuropsychological Considerations with Japanese Patients

Nicholas Thaler and Maiko Sakamoto Pomeroy

Section I: Background Information

Terminology and Perspective

Individuals born in Japan are referred to as Japanese or Japanese Nationals in the United States. Japanese Americans are individuals of Japanese descent who live in the United States. First-generation Japanese Americans are referred as Issei. Subsequent generations are chronologically referred as Nisei, Sansei, Yonsei, and Gosei. Individuals who are of mixed-race ancestry are often referred to as Haafu.

I (NT) am a Nisei Haafu, that is, a second-generation born half-Japanese American. I am also a clinical neuropsychologist who was trained in the west coast of the United States. I grew up in a bilingual and bicultural household; importantly, my Japanese grandmother, who spoke no English, helped raise me as a child. This has provided a foundation of my familiarity with the Japanese language, culture, and customs.

I (MSP) am a native Japanese and moved to the United States with a vision to study at the fore of clinical psychology. I attended graduate school in the east coast and trained in the west coast of the United States to become a neuropsychologist. I am bilingual, with Japanese as my native tongue and English as my second. I regularly conduct neuropsychological tests in both languages. I currently reside in Japan and work in both university and hospital settings serving as an educator, researcher, and clinician.

Geography

Japan is an archipelago comprised of over 6,800 islands located in the Pacific Ocean. Four major islands comprise Japan, including Honshu (the largest), Hokkaido, Shikoku, and Kyushu. As of 2020, Japan has a population of 125,960,000 individuals, of which an estimated 97.8% are of Japanese ethnicity. This highlights the homogenous nature of Japanese society, although differences within regions and even cities persist.

The west coast of the United States is an attractive tourist spot for Japanese travelers given that it is directly across the Pacific Ocean. Perhaps not surprisingly then, many Japanese Americans, including my grandparents, made their homes in California. Hawaii is another popular tourist and immigration destination for Japanese nationals and is the site of this chapter's clinical case. In some ways, Hawaii was a chance to revisit my roots, as my maternal grandfather was a second-generation Hawaiian-born Nisei who grew up on the island of Kauai (NT: Note that I adopt my own Nisei status as my mother was born in Japan).

DOI: 10.4324/9781003051862-31

History

There are various theories regarding the original inhabitants of Japan. These include the Ainu, who are associated geographically with regions of Northern Honshu, Hokkaido and even some Russian territories. Other various immigration waves include descendants from the Ryukyu region and the Korean peninsula. Others suggest that the Japanese are descended from Mongolians or that the Japanese have indigenous roots similar to the Ainu. Japanese mythology posits that Emperor Jimmu, a descendent of the sun goddess Amaterasu, ascended the throne as the first emperor around 660 BC.

Whatever the origins, Japan had established itself as a feudal nation comprised of domain lords, known as daimyo, who fought and retained territory over numerous centuries. Japan was ostensibly ruled by a Japanese emperor, although his actual power fluctuated from generation to generation. Japan was largely an isolationist country allowing only minimal trade with Europe up until the year 1853 when the United States Commodore Matthew C Perry sailed his ships to the coast of Japan. Japan subsequently opened up commerce with the rest of the global economy and quickly transformed into a modern industrialized nation in a period known as the *Meiji Restoration*. In the following decades, Japan was involved in multiple conflicts with other nations. The first half of the twentieth century saw an aggressive expansion of Japanese imperialism, which culminated in their defeat in 1945, marking the end of World War II.

Japan has since been rebuilt as a world power, with significant economic prosperity through the 1980s. However, a severe recession in 1991 has slowed the country's growth, which is yet to fully recover from its losses from this period.

People

Japanese culture is internationally known to focus on aspects of honor, respect, and courtesy that has garnered the interest of many foreigners abroad. However, like all people, individual Japanese vary in their beliefs and backgrounds and have their unique perspectives in life. Furthermore, putting a "halo" over the ideas of Japanese honor, respect, and so forth silences the possible psychological challenges that come with living in a collectivist society. With that caveat, there are general cultural facets of Japanese culture that do influence people in their day-to-day interactions.

As stated, the Japanese are a collectivist society that emphasizes harmony within the group over individual achievement.[1] A special loyalty is often expected from children to their elders. Such loyalty historically extends toward a worker's relationship with their boss, as some Japanese companies still guarantee lifetime financial security in exchange for one's devotion.[2] However, this old culture has been changing, especially after the economic bubble burst in the 90s, and younger generations are seeking out better job opportunities while enjoying hobbies and personal interests outside of work to maintain a sense of happiness and well-being.

Due to the emphasis on collectivism typically taught from school-age onwards, Japanese society prioritizes maintaining interpersonal harmony over direct confrontation. This undoubtedly can lead to challenges in conflict resolution among individuals in a social circle and within a family unit.[3] The saying "The nail that sticks up is hammered down" reflects the predominant mentality encouraged by Japanese society, such that dissenters from the group are expected to internalize their disapproval for the betterment of the group.

Immigration and Relocation

Many Japanese nationals immigrated to the United States in the early 1900s, following an agreement between the Japanese and United States governments. Many early immigrants settled in Hawaii to work in agriculture, including my own grandfather's family (NT). However, Japanese immigration temporarily ended after the Immigration Act of 1924, which has had downstream effects on generational cohorts up until the Immigration and Nationality Act of 1965. Because of the Immigration Act of 1924, most Japanese Americans living in the United States during World War II were of Nisei status.

Issei and Nisei Japanese Americans were subjugated to internment in relocation camps across the west coast during World War II. My (NT) own grandfather was subject to the camps and also then imprisoned by the United States government after refusing to serve for the country that stole his legacy. He was among the no-no boys, a subgroup of Japanese American men who refused to denounce the Japanese emperor to the United States government. My grandfather's bitterness toward the United States led him to immigrate to Japan, a country he had never lived in before after World War II ended. It was there that he married my grandmother, eventually returning to the United States with two daughters in tow to resume life in California.

I never did learn much about the undoubtedly mixed feelings my grandfather held toward the United States, his country of birth and natural citizenship. But if he was like many Japanese Americans at the time, he likely felt a sense of betrayal with aspects of shame sprinkled into his cultural identity. He may never have felt like he fit in in Japan—after all, one must adhere to the Japanese way of life to be accepted there and in the end, he was American-born. Yet, this duality of straddling two cultures and experiencing rejection by both must have brought about its own form of trauma, one that would be felt generationally. Similar tales of intergenerational trauma permeate through many immigrant families across cultures.

More recent immigrants to the United States come as students or for vocational purposes. Unlike some other Asian cultures, fewer immigrants come now for the purposes of reuniting with family or to escape from harsher circumstances. These immigrants, of course, are quite distinct from the generations of Japanese Americans who grew up in the United States, of who many now identify primarily as Americans.

Language

Growing up in a bilingual household, I was exposed to the Japanese language from early on (NT). I spoke it daily with my grandmother and other relatives and was fully immersed in the language throughout my childhood up until my early 20s. In addition, I minored in the Japanese language in college and formally studied *kanji*, which is a written language originated in Chinese, in my early thirties. I say all this not to boast but to point out that despite all this experience, my Japanese proficiency was adequate at best and middling by most standards (as it is presently).

The Japanese language is complex. While certain phrases and even casual conversational ability can be relatively simple to learn, it is extremely challenging to master for all but the most savant polyglots. Some of this lies in the complexity of context; that is, the way you speak varies tremendously among and across groups. You may speak a certain way at work to your boss than to your coworkers and subordinates, yet a distinct way to your friends, your confidants, your spouse, and your children. Individuals who are interested in pursuing Japanese studies can seek out the Japanese Language Proficiency Test (JLPT), which has five levels of difficulty.

Further confounding matter is the often bidirectional nature of this language barrier. Many Japanese nationals find English challenging and intimidating to learn and speak. Despite the fact that all Japanese students spend years learning English in school, many do not have the confidence to speak it in Japan. This is perhaps related to the fact that Japanese nationals tend to have stronger "academic" English skills, including reading and writing, than their conversational abilities.[4] Of course, this varies from individual to individual and fluency improves for Japanese who are living abroad. However, the neuropsychologist who expects to assess Japanese nationals must be prepared to find an interpreter, which can be challenging in itself. As of 2021, there remains a paucity of neuropsychologists who can test fluently in Japanese.

Education

Education is prioritized in Japanese society, with well over 95% of the population graduating from high school. Much of the educational system is built around standardized national exams, which determine a student's eligibility for advanced education. Only the top-scoring students are eligible to attend the most prestigious universities, and thus by extension, secure the more competitive jobs in the labor market. Graduate education prioritizes the STEM fields, with comparatively fewer students enrolling in the humanities and arts.

Due to the value that Japanese society places on education and, in particular, prestigious academic credentials, the competition for university placement can be fierce. Students will spend inordinate amounts of time "cramming" for entrance exams while trying to juggle other responsibilities in their life. There is often little free time granted to Japanese adolescents, which is a likely risk factor for mental health struggles. Such struggles are all the more compounded when a child is born with learning differences.

The educational system in Japan overall has paid marginal attention to children with special educational needs. However, like other countries, the number of children with developmental disorders is increasing, possibly due to the broadening of diagnostic criteria to include a spectrum of behavioral and functional limitations, improving developmental screening and access to diagnostic and treatment services, and improving knowledge and awareness of developmental disorders in society. While the Japanese government has recognized the right for students with disabilities to receive a fair education under the Basic Act on Education, the actual implementation of practice remains mixed (to be fair, this is similar to the challenges faced in the United States and many other countries).

The Act on Support for Persons with Development Disabilities (発達障害者支援法), which became effective in 2005, aimed for early detection and intervention and providing financial and educational support for individuals with developmental disorders. To date, children with special needs (physical, mental and/or developmental disabilities) have options on whether they attend either classes catering to those needs at a regular school or a school for disabilities with medical/educational professionals' careful evaluations. Children attending these classes at regular schools receive close attention from teachers in small classrooms that range from one to three students. Children generally belong to their "parent" or "communication" classes where they take some regular lessons and interact with children without disabilities. Additionally, children with disabilities can attend after-school programs (20–23 days/month, including holidays and weekends). This costs an estimated 4,600 yen (approximately 44 dollars) per month as this service is insured by the government. With great and long effort by families of children with special needs and schoolteachers, the Japanese educational system has been improving gradually but surely.

I (NT) recall the case of a girl in her twenties who likely had a severe language delay growing up, as well as a possible mild pervasive developmental disorder. She described years of teasing and abuse by her peers. She stated that her teachers stuck her in a classroom where she had to copy sentences over and over again with little instruction, adding that the teachers would "scream" at her if she ever stopped. Her parents, who were quite invested, ultimately moved to the United States, where they hoped she would have an easier time fitting in. Sadly, the girl continued to exhibit signs of trauma while recounting her childhood in Japan, at times pausing to bite her tongue and cry during the interview.

This case is an example of the challenges that children with special needs must navigate in Japan. Such challenges are inherently linked to the pressures of Japanese society toward academic excellence. Such excellence is expected of the dutiful child in honoring their family and their society, with failure often interpreted as a characterological flaw. Thus, the high standards of academic prowess and output that characterize the Japanese educational system must be viewed within the context of the individual cost that comes for those who fall by the wayside.

Literacy

The Japanese reading and writing system relies on three systems; hiragana, katakana, and kanji. Kanji can be read from their original Chinese or indigenous Japanese pronunciations. There are currently 2,136 regular-use kanji which are considered necessary for high school literacy. Along with kanji are two phonetic alphabets: *hiragana* which breaks up all Japanese words into their phonemic components, and *katakana* which breaks up imported words into their phonemic components. *Katakana* is often used for loan words which have no direct Japanese translation, such as foreign names and titles. Most elementary-school children can read hiragana and katakana by the end of their first year of school.

One can posit that kanji is difficult to learn for students with learning differences. Referring back to the girl with the language delay we discussed in the prior section, I recall that she could not read even the simplest of kanji on a mental status examination (e.g., "father"). This was unlikely related to volitional factors, as she passed the effort measures, but highlights the near illiterate status she had despite spending her childhood years in the Japanese school system. Research on the impact that learning disabilities and other delays in educational advancement has on Japanese literacy remains lacking.

Socio-Economic Status

Most Japanese nationals can secure basic needs such as housing, education, and medicine, and an estimated 90% of the population are considered to be in the middle class. However, despite some degree of evident security provided, cracks exist. It has become increasingly difficult for adults to strike out on their own, with increasing numbers of Japanese men and women in their 30s and 40s still living with their parents. Women used to be expected to sacrifice their education and career when starting a family; however, the culture is changing. More and more women attend college and remain working after marriage to contribute to essential family needs, such as their child's education and college funding, housing loans, and so forth. The Act on the Promotion of Women's Participation and Advancement in the Workplace (女性活躍推進法), the law which aims to create a better working environment for women, became effective in 2016. Given declining birth rates and a super-aging society, the Japanese government is trying to use the women's labor force by providing opportunities to both work and have children.

Values and Customs

Traditional Japanese values follow many other Asian values, which highlight collectivism, respect, honor, humility, and hospitality. Doctors often are viewed as absolute authorities in their field, with expected deference toward their expertise (it is perhaps no coincidence that doctors are referred to as sensei, or teacher, in Japan). However, this deference does not necessarily reflect a positive experience for the patient, and practitioners must be mindful that their words and advice can be taken poorly if delivered in a harsh or insensitive manner. Furthermore, patients may not always self-advocate their needs if they feel that the doctor will judge them. Even Japanese patients who feel comfortable with their provider may still withhold information due to an internalized pressure to remain stoic about one's ailments.

Many psychological symptoms in Japanese patients might emerge as somatic physical and cognitive complaints, which are typically viewed as more acceptable to share due to their "medical" basis.[5] The astute clinician must be aware when their patients present with a host of ailments that essentially serve a sign of psychological distress, or as it manifested in my patient, grief.

Gender and Sexuality

Japan remains a patriarchal society, with such values taught in early childhood. Following Confucian values, the eldest son is often the favored child as he is expected to carry on the family legacy. With such attention comes the pressure to academically and financially thrive and eventually care for his family. Although this culture is swiftly fading, daughters and younger sons typically receive less of this undivided attention, with daughters in particular encouraged to primarily prepare for a domestic lifestyle. As discussed earlier, more women keep jobs after having a family; however, the expectation of raising the children and keeping the house still remains. As a result, this unbalanced expectation has led to a reluctance toward marriage for some women. Men, in turn, face the burden of providing for a family with little time to actually bond with them, and so also may find marriage undesirable. There is also a unique situation with Japanese couples, where they experience long-distance marriages (単身赴任), in which the husbands relocate to different prefectures for business purposes, and wives and children remain in their current location due to educational and financial reasons.

Unfortunately, Japanese society is at times still quite inimical toward women's rights. Sexual assault is often silenced and women who speak out may find their career opportunities dry up. Systemic issues still persist, with a pervasive gender wage gap and disparate job prospects. Outright scandals, including a test scandal that weighted scores in favor of boys, highlight the institutionalized sexism sometimes tolerated in Japan. Such lingering intolerance in a first-world country is perhaps explained by the pressure that Japanese people have against speaking out for their needs and rights. On the positive side, sexism in Japan has been getting more attention and acknowledgment by the media and government.

The patriarchal foundation in Japan has allowed for disparities in sexual activities as well. Married men have been allowed and at times encouraged to engage in prostitution, while pornography is widely tolerated, even finding itself in comic books and video games. Homosexuality has been largely met with disapproval, though perhaps less hostile than that seen in Judeo-Christian societies. However, Confucianism does frown upon homosexual activity and many gay and lesbian Japanese still elect to hide their sexuality, with some entering traditional marriages to maintain a façade of "normalcy." However, homosexual activity has never been outright outlawed in Japan and in modern times, laws recognizing transgender rights have passed.

One area that has received media attention is the decreasing sexual activity observed in Japan. The reasons for this are likely multifaceted. Adults struggle maintaining a work-life balance and may simply have few opportunities to meet partners. The diminishing prospects of marriage, as viewed by modern-day men and women, have already been discussed. In addition, there is some indication that pornography has served as a substitute for actual sexual activity in younger people.[6] The longstanding implications of decreasing sexual activity, with a corresponding declining birth rate, raise some concerns for the future.

Spirituality and Religion

In general, the Japanese follow a more spiritual rather than explicitly religious path. The two primary faiths that Japanese follow are Shinto and Buddhism, which have overlapping yet distinct features. Per the Agency for Cultural Affairs, approximately 65%–70% of Japanese nationals report that they follow one or both of these faiths, in contrast to 1.5% who identify as Christian and 6.2% who identify with other religions. Somewhat curiously, other surveys have suggested that up to 70% of the country self-reported that they do not follow any particular religion. This highlights the contrast between the cultural and customary practices of Shinto and Buddhism and the more traditional organized religions often seen in other cultures.

Shinto is the original indigenous religion in Japan that focuses on kami, or "spirits" that rest in virtually all physical forms. Buddhism is a global religion that the Japanese likely adopted from China. The dual beliefs of Shinto and Buddhism align with several aspects of Japanese culture. There is a sense of "letting go" tied to these religions, such that material objects and indeed life itself are deemed transitory, while spirits and gods beyond our understanding dwell in the very rocks we step on. In this sense, some Japanese may turn to religion to help cope with the stresses of modern life or otherwise find solace and meaning in a world that may be filled with, at times, arbitrary and restrictive rules and customs.

Acculturation and Systemic Barriers

When considering neuropsychological practice with a Japanese national, I (NT) think back to my early visits to Japan as an adult. In my opinion, there are few places in the world that are simultaneously so familiar and yet so different from the United States as Japan. As a Westerner might feel a familiar yet alienating feeling when exploring Japan, so might a Japanese national feel the same while exploring the United States. Consider the unacculturated patient who works with a Western doctor. There is already an inculcated deference toward physicians that likely would apply to the neuropsychologist. Testing is both familiar and yet unfamiliar, as testing in Japan is typically academic in nature and designed to separate groups by ability. This may not transfer as readily to neuropsychological tests, which are designed to assess for and diagnose pathology.

Health Status

Life expectancy in Japan is about 84 years, longer than in many developed countries. By contrast, the United States currently has a life expectancy of 78 years. Diet and low obesity rates likely contribute to the longer lifespan of Japanese citizens. Furthermore, Japan has one of the lowest levels of dementia in the world.[7] Of concern in Japan is the high incidence of suicide rates throughout the country, with an estimated 30,000 suicides a year. Excessive alcohol and tobacco use are also public health concerns in the country.

Mental Health Views

Mental health awareness in Japan has improved over time, although some gaps still persist. Japanese medicine is a highly respected field of study and physicians often are the initial providers who detect mental illness in the general population. However, more acute psychiatric illnesses, such as schizophrenia and bipolar disorder tend to receive more medical attention, in part because of the usual need for psychopharmaceutic intervention. This "medicalization" of mental illness carries over the stigma that individuals with a psychological disorder must have a particularly severe one. Thus, milder cases of depression and anxiety may be overlooked (or even met with disapproval as a "characterological weakness") and untreated. Mental awareness has increased of late, perhaps in response to the spread of culturally bound syndromes such as *hikikomori*, (i.e., severe social withdrawal and self-isolation) observed in some Japanese youth.

History of and Approach to Neuropsychological Evaluations

Neuropsychology arrived in Japan along with the rest of Western medicine in the late 1800s.[8] However, the process of credentialing neuropsychologists is still absent. Doctoral-level psychologists in Japan primarily do research and the only neuropsychologists who received doctoral training likely trained outside of Japan. Their role there is often based in research with little opportunity for clinical practice. Indeed, most "neurocognitive" examinations completed in Japan are carried out by physicians and their technicians. Their exposure to neuropsychology training, including psychometrics, is not yet at the level of Western standards.[8]

The careful clinician is encouraged to monitor the comfort level of the patient in the testing environment. It may be worth spending additional time ensuring that patients fully understand the nature and purpose of the tests so that they do not feel pressured to attempt a "perfect" score. Anxiety may manifest through a reluctance to guess or a proclivity to give up early, as disengagement may be "safer" than a wrong answer. I (NT) recall working with at least one older patient who would silently shake their head when they felt their capacity had met. Only quiet encouragement and patience elicited further responding, though it remains unknown if the patient's full capacity on some tests was accurately ascertained.

Section II: Case Study—"… and he Talks Like a Cartoon Character Now"

Note: Identifying information and other details have been altered to protect the family's identity. As with the rest of this chapter, the following case study is an admixture of narrative and fact.

Background and Behavioral Observations

I (NT) received word from a colleague that there was a need for a medical-legal pediatric neuropsychologist who speaks Japanese. A young boy, "Ken," was visiting Hawaii with his family from Japan when he was struck by a motor vehicle, resulting in a traumatic brain injury (TBI) with lesions to the left hemisphere about three years prior, when he was three years of age. At that time, my Japanese was about as proficient as it ever would be, and I recently had the privilege of assessing several Japanese patients at the University of California, Los Angeles medical center, as well as in my private practice. I had memorized approximately 1,500 kanji and had administered batteries developed in Japan for Japanese populations. Thus, I felt equipped to approach this evaluation with the caveat that we would still rely on an interpreter for the parent interview.

I considered whether or not to rely on an interpreter for this case. I had used them before with my clinical cases, but there were times that no interpreter was readily available, in which case I worked with my own Japanese skills. I was at that time fluent enough to carry on conversations with friends and colleagues and was reading books at about an eighth-grade level. At the same time, I was not born in Japan and had not lived in the country for years. My familiarity with the language was primarily academic (e.g., stiff, not up to date on colloquialisms), and I felt some reservation about conversing with parents about something as intensely emotional as their son's tragedy and making a verbal error.

So, with interpreter in tow, the assessment commenced. The parents were highly educated and worldly; the father owned several businesses that often took him overseas and Ken had an older sister who was in graduate school. Of interest, the boy also attended an international school in Japan that exposed him to the English language. Right away, it was clear that this was a family of a higher SES status, which granted them some of the privileges associated with wealth including education and travel.

It is worth taking a minute to consider the medical-legal nature of this assessment. Japanese nationals, in general, are not particularly litigious in the personal injury arena. This ties with the cultural beliefs discussed in this chapter about accepting one's personal loss for the good of the community. One can imagine that the parents may have felt pressure to accept the insurance company's initial offer as not to stir waves. Instead, as many parents would, they sought outside counsel. I would further posit that some things, such as parental outrage, transcend all cultures.

The parents were polite and deferential. The interview went well, with them taking their time to consider before answering each question. "He's different now," said the mother at one point. "He used to be so sweet. Now he's angry all the time, yelling and hitting me, saying the worst things. He doesn't listen and can't sit still. And," she added with some confusion in her voice, "he talks like a cartoon character now." When pressed for more information, she was specifically speaking of Doraemon, a Japanese cartoon robot cat from the future who assists a feeble, bullied boy by using futuristic gadgets. Doraemon's voice is famously idiosyncratic, often speaking bluntly and with a nasally and raspy tone. In those words, she captured the essence of how she viewed her son since his TBI. The father was no less descriptive. "I can't help it," he said at one point. "I spoil him so much now. I feel so guilty for what happened. What could I have done? Now," he added, "now, I give him everything."

Ken was a delight. At six, he carried the exuberance and joy many of his same-age peers possess. He had a cherubic quality, with a hint of mischief in his actions. He was also completely unable to focus on anything for more than a minute. Japanese children are taught to respect their elders, to defer to teachers and doctors and never question them. This boy, within seconds, started to treat me as a favored uncle, cackling and running around the table, at times trying to climb into my lap or smack my stomach. Despite his attentional issues, he was enthused enough with the tests that he completed many of them rapidly, if in a somewhat disorganized and haphazard fashion. He espoused a real joy with the testing process and clearly worked very hard, with little concern for motivational factors. Of course, attentional issues undoubtedly impacted his test scores.

Test and Norm Selection

The battery included the Japanese Wechsler Intelligence Scale for Children, Fourth Edition (JWISC-IV[9]), which was designed and normed for students living in Japan (of note, some subtests such as Comprehension and Picture Completion are fascinating cultural glimpses into the differences between Western and Japan beliefs). The rest of the battery relied on a somewhat cobbled together battery of measures normed in the United States and translated into Japanese. The Test of Memory Malingering (TOMM[10]) was used as a measure of effort. The California Verbal Learning Test for Children (CVLT-C[11]) was translated into Japanese yet scored with English norms.

This boy's academic exposure in an international setting allowed for some testing in English as a comparison; thus, the Wide Range Assessment of Memory and Learning, Second Edition (WRAML-2[12]) was administered in its entirety in English. Academic testing was limited, although some of the reading and mathematical subtests in the Woodcock-Johnson Tests of Achievement, Fourth Edition (WJ-IV[13]) were administered. Other measures included the Connor's Continuous Performance Test, Third Edition (CPT-3[14]), the Developmental Neuropsychology Assessment, Second Edition (NEPSY-II[15]) subtests, the Rey Complex Figure Test (RCFT[16]) and the Beery Visual-Motor Integration (BVMI[17]) test were administered. In this manner, a mix of Japanese-normed, Japanese-translated, and visual measures were administered. Parent reports included a translated adaptation of the Behavior Assessment System for Children, Third Edition (BASC-3[18]), while a BASC-3 in English was sent to Ken's teacher.

Test Results and Impressions

Ken performed in the average range on the JWISC-IV Verbal Comprehension Index and Working Memory Index. In contrast, his Processing Speed Index was in the low average range, with the

Coding subtest falling below expectations. His Working Memory Index was in the low average range, with average performance on the two subtests. Furthermore, the Picture Completion subtest fell well below expectations.

Scores on the neuropsychological measures confirmed struggles on measures of sustained attention and visuospatial functioning. Ken's struggles on visuospatial testing generally supported that he had difficulty processing the details of images rather than the overall gestalt; for example, he flipped Block Design images, had distorted details within the RCFT, and could not complete the Picture Completion subtest. His processing speed was highly variable, fluctuating from the 5th to 75th percentile across subtests with more trouble on highly visual subtests (e.g., Coding). Japanese verbal and English reading skills were within expectations. Memory testing in Japanese and English generally reviewed struggles in free recall with better recognition scores. Motor testing was bilaterally within expectations. Parent and teacher-rating scores converged to support significant externalizing problems; furthermore, Ken's mother rated severe anxiety and atypical behaviors in her son.

Overall, there was considerable evidence that Ken had developed cognitive struggles in visuospatial and the frontal/executive systems. Of particular note, Ken was reportedly using his right hand prior to the accident yet switched to his left hand upon recovery. This type of "pathological left-handedness" often emerges in youth who sustain left-hemisphere lesions at a very young age. Research supports that the language systems switch over to the right hemisphere, "crowding out" visuospatial skills.[19] This laterality was seen with Ken (although not on fine motor testing). Social skills can also be impacted, which may explain some of Ken's overfamiliarity with me during testing.

Diagnostically, I determined that Ken met the criteria for a Mild Neurocognitive Disorder secondary to his TBI with neurobehavioral features including impulsivity, emotional lability, and a personality change.

Treatment Considerations

If Ken lived in the United States, there would be some straightforward recommendations to provide. Assuming he attended a public school, an Individualized Educational Program (IEP) would be recommended so that he could have access to a specialized learning environment with smaller class sizes. If he attended a private school, as he did in Japan, then the school would work with the family to determine if Ken could stay or if he would require a different setting. Ultimately, I learned that Ken's family was asked to leave the international school he was attending as the principal felt that his needs would be better suited elsewhere. Japan does have specialized schools for children with neurodevelopmental disorders, and it is possible that Ken enrolled in one of those. Alternatively, as the parents were of a higher SES, they may have had access to additional resources.

His visuospatial struggles are of some concern for his academics. Two kanji may differ only by a single stroke yet have completely different meanings. Ken had yet to learn much kanji given his age, but with his visuospatial struggles, one could imagine that he might have an acquired reading disability that is specifically linked to his written language. His frontal/executive struggles, of course, have profound implications in a society that emphasizes blending in. Children, in particular, are expected to obey without question, and so Ken's prognosis in the strict setting of his home country could be poor without adequate interventions and accommodations.

In some ways, Ken has a number of advantages including invested parents of a higher SES who are well-traveled (indeed, their cosmopolitan lifestyle likely led them to me in the first place). He likely will receive adequate medical care, educational support, and, if necessary, assistance when he is an adult. At the same time, his TBI clearly has both immediate and long-term implications for his cognitive and emotional functioning. The degree to which he and his family will be able to navigate the complexities of Japanese society remains to be seen.

Section III: Lessons Learned

- Japan is a relatively homogenous and collectivist society that emphasizes group harmony over the individual.
- This has the advantage of providing a safe and organized society, yet the disadvantage of overlooking or dismissing the needs of those who do not fall easily within its boundaries.
- Effects of this collectivist attitude are felt in the family, which remains patriarchal and deferential to elders, the school system (which emphasizes conformity and obedience) and the workplace (which expects lifelong loyalty to the company).
- The Japanese language is highly contextual, where the way you phrase something carries enormous weight in how it is communicated. In addition, language must consider the audience, whether you are speaking to a superior, colleague, inferior, intimate, etc.
- Japanese patients are likely to be deferential to doctors, to the point where their ailments may easily be missed or dismissed if the clinician is not carefully attuned to their own cultural biases.
- Like many East Asian cultures, psychological language is often absent or inadequate in capturing the subtleties of a person's distress. Somatic ailments may be a common expression of psychological distress.
- On the other hand, psychological distress may be minimized in an effort to maintain a stoic attitude and avoid disrupting the harmony of their community. Further confounding this is the misconception that mental illness is by definition severe and debilitating (e.g., uncontrolled schizophrenia).
- Neuropsychological testing may prove a familiar avenue for Japanese patients, as they are likely to accept the medical basis for such tests and have been regularly exposed to examinations throughout their schooling.
- However, clinicians must take care to ensure that the patient does not confuse the scholastic aptitude nature of the tests they took in school with the diagnostic testing used in our assessments.
- Patients may find testing to be anxiety-provoking or elect to give up or profess ignorance rather than risk a wrong guess.
- At this time, there remain relatively few neuropsychological measures normed for Japanese patients. However, some IQ and additional batteries are available through testing companies.
- Pertaining to the above point, a mixed model of using both Japanese and English-normed tests is required to obtain a comprehensive neuropsychological evaluation. However, this comes with numerous limitations, highlighting the need for developing additional neuropsychological tests for Japanese populations.
- While the cognitive aspect of testing may be accepted by the medical community, the psychological aspect may not be. Confounding this issue are the roles that psychologists play in Japan, as they are typically Master's level clinicians who defer to the medical doctors.
- Pediatric testing comes with its own challenges. Ken's case was striking for some of the universal medical findings that emerged from his case (e.g., pathological left-handedness) along with the cultural issues that he and his family will have to navigate with his long-term cognitive and neurobehavioral deficits.
- Japanese-normed adaptations of common neuropsychological assessments are available at https://www.nichibun.co.jp/english/products/

References

1. Kagawa-Singer M, Chung R. Toward a new paradigm: a cultural systems approach. In Kurasaki KS, Okazaki S, Sue S, editors. Asian American mental health: assessment theories and methods. New York (NY): Kluwer Academic/Plenum Publishers; 2002. p. 47–66.
2. Roland A. In search of self in India and Japan: toward a cross-cultural psychology. Princeton (NJ): Princeton University Press; 1988.
3. Doi T. The anatomy of the self. Tokyo: Kodansha; 1985.
4. Tsushima WT, Tsushima VG Fujii D. Neuropsychology of Japanese Americans. In Fujii DM, editor. The neuropsychology of Asian Americans New York (NY): Psychology Press; 2011. p. 107–29.
5. Hwang WC. The psychotherapy adaptation and modification framework: application to Asian Americans. Am Psychol. 2006;61:702–15.
6. Padgett VR, Brislin-Slütz JA, Neal JA. Pornography, erotica, and attitudes toward women: the effects of repeated exposure. J Sex Res. 1989;26(4):479–91.
7. Britnell M. In search of the perfect health system. London: Palgrave; 2015. p. 18.
8. Sakamoto M. Neuropsychology in Japan: history, current challenges, and future prospects. Clin Neuropsychol. 2016;30(8):1278–95. doi:10.1080/13854046.2016.1204012.
9. Wechsler D. (2010). Technical and Interpretive Manual for the Wechsler Intelligence Scale for Children [K. Ueno, K. Fujita, H. Maekawa, T. Ishikuma, H. Dairoku, H., O. Matsuda, trans.] Original Work Published 2003. 4th ed. Bloomington (IN): NCS Pearson, Inc.
10. Tombaugh TN. Test of Memory Malingering (TOMM). New York (NY): Multi-Health Systems, Inc.; 1996.
11. Delis DC, Kramer JH, Kaplan E, Ober BA. CVLT-C: California Verbal Learning Test. 1994.
12. Sheslow D, Adams W. Wide range assessment of memory and learning. 2nd ed. Psychological Assessment Resources, Inc.; 2003.
13. Schrank FA, Mather N, McGrew KS. Woodcock-Johnson IV Tests of Achievement. Rolling Meadows (IL): Riverside; 2014a.
14. Conners CK. Conners Continuous Performance Test. 3rd ed. Toronto (ON): Multi Health Systems, Inc.; 2014.
15. Korkman M, Kirk U, Kemp S. NEPSY-II: a developmental neuropsychological assessment. San Antonio (TX): The Psychological Corporation; 2007a.
16. Meyers J, Meyers K. Meyers scoring system for the Rey Complex Figure Test and the Recognition Trial. Odessa: Psychological Assessment Resources; 1994.
17. Beery K. Developmental test of visual-motor integration. Cleveland (OH): Modern Curriculum Press; 1989.
18. Reynolds CR, Kamphaus RW. Behavior assessment system for children. 3rd ed. San Antonio (TX): Pearson; 2015.
19. Satz P, Strauss E, Hunter M, Wada J. Re-examination of the crowding hypothesis: effects of age of onset. Neuropsychol. 1994;8(2):255.

Nepali-Bhutanese

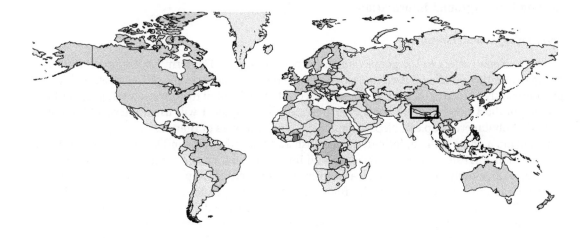

16 Neuropsychological Considerations with Bhutanese Refugees of Nepali Ethnicities Residing in the United States

Katrina E. Belen and David Lerner

Section I: Background Information

Terminology and Perspective

The term Nepali refers to the people/language/food of Nepal.[1] The term Lhotsampa translates as "people from the south" and is often used to refer to the Bhutanese people of Nepali ethnicities who predominantly resided in the southern-most part of Bhutan. Most of them are now refugees of Bhutan residing in the United States.[2] For the purposes of this chapter, I will use the terms "Bhutanese-Nepali", "Bhutanese people of Nepali ethnicities," and "refugees of Bhutan."

I (KB) am a white woman, bilingual in English and Spanish, living in Dallas, Texas, and I often evaluate non-English speakers and people with limited to no formal education. When I was asked to evaluate an elderly man for a medical waiver for his US citizenship application in 2015, I had no prior interactions or awareness of the Bhutanese-Nepali languages or culture. I quickly learned that the Bhutanese-Nepali community was very new to the United States, the literature concerning them was sparse, and the only interpreters were Nepali and not from Bhutan. Fortunately, I was able to work closely with a Nepali law intern, originally from Kathmandu, and together we learned about the community and evaluated about 100 adult Bhutanese refugees of Nepali ethnicities.

This chapter is based on the training I have received in multicultural assessment, reading of the literature, advice from mentors, and personal interactions with Bhutanese refugees and their families in Texas. It is my hope that this chapter will lead to a discussion that fosters the inclusion of the Bhutanese perspective. I additionally aim to provide an example of one way to approach novel populations with regard to neuropsychological assessment.

Geography

Bhutan is a landlocked country, about one-half the size of Indiana, that lies at the base of the Eastern Himalayas between China and India.[3,4] At its north lies the highest unclimbed mountain in the world, the Gangkhar Puensum (7,570 m), and only 150 km south are subtropical broadleaf forests.[3,4] The weather in the north is like the arctic, and the weather in the south is tropical. Most of the population of Bhutan resides in the north, east, and west. The low-lying foothills of the southern border are home to the Bhutanese people of Nepali ethnicities.[2,5]

People

There are about 156,000 Bhutanese people of Nepali ethnicities. They are a linguistically and ethnically diverse group with ancestral roots in Nepal and the Nepali-speaking part of Darjeeling in

DOI: 10.4324/9781003051862-33

West Bengal. They have close ethnic and cultural ties to parts of India and predominantly follow the Hindu religion, with some belonging to the highest castes.[2,5,6] Most are descendants of peasant farmers.

History

The Bhutanese nation has a diverse past of multi-ethnic, multicultural, and multi-religious identity, and the issue of "who arrived in Bhutan when" is important to refugees of Bhutan. Some claim Nepali presence in Bhutan as far back as the seventeenth century. Most of the migration occurred after the Anglo-Bhutanese wars of 1864–1865 and lasted through the 1930s.[4] Nepali workers settled in southern Bhutan, cleared the land, established agrarian communities, and became valuable contributors to agriculture and commerce.[2,5]

The modern concept of citizenship was introduced for the first time in Bhutan with the Citizenship Act of 1958, which granted Nepali inhabitants' equal rights as citizens. Some citizens of Nepali ethnicity rose to influential positions in society, and the king and ruling elite feared the group could overrun the majority. In the late 1970s and beginning of the 1980s, the Bhutanese government initiated a movement toward a homogenous Bhutanese cultural identity: the *One Nation One People* policy.

Laws were enacted that systematically disenfranchised Bhutanese people of Nepali ethnicities. The Marriage Act placed penalties on Bhutanese citizens who married ethnically non-Bhutanese individuals including disqualification from receiving state benefits such as land, medical care, and education. A new Citizenship Act in 1985 nullified the Citizenship Act of 1958. Households were required to provide proof of legal Bhutanese residence by way of a 1958 Land Tax Receipt. The Bhutanese of Nepali ethnicities were mostly farmers with limited education and did not keep documents. When they did, Bhutanese authorities usually refuted them.

On January 6, 1989, the king issued a royal decree requiring all inhabitants of Bhutan to follow the elite **Drukpa** religion and language. The policy enforced national standards for dress, etiquette, and cultural practice. Schools and seminaries in southern Bhutan were closed, and the Nepali language was removed from the curriculum. People were fined, imprisoned, forced into labor, and refused state services if they did not wear the traditional Drukpa dress, which was expensive and incompatible with the tropical climate of southern Bhutan.

In 1990, there were widespread demonstrations against the government, which responded with brutal retaliatory measures including mass arrests and violence. There are over 2,000 documented instances of physical torture, consistent with the World Medical Association's definition.[7] Homes, lands, and belongings were destroyed or redistributed to people of other communities and many cities were re-named.

The exiled Bhutanese of Nepali ethnicities first sought refugee status in West Bengal, India, but they were turned away. Bengali authorities deported them to Nepal, where the local government constructed refugee camps with the help of the United Nations High Commissioner for Refugees (UNHCR). By 1992 up to 500 individuals arrived in the refugee camps daily. In all, over 100,000 refugees were expelled from Bhutan, an estimated sixth of the total population.[2,5,6]

Between 2008 and 2016, the United States accepted the largest number of refugees of Bhutan among all nations that received them—a total of about 90,000.[6] The first large group accepted was sent to Dallas, Texas, in 2009, followed by waves in Pennsylvania and Ohio. New York and Georgia also received smaller groups of refugees. Due to internal secondary and tertiary migration, Central Ohio now has the highest population, estimated at around 30,000. Australia, Canada, New Zealand, the Netherlands, and Denmark received about 15,000 refugees all together. As of December 1999, only around 7,000 people remained in the refugee camps located in Nepal.[8]

244 Katrina E. Belen and David Lerner

The UNHCR drastically cut funding to the camps in 2021, and the refugees who remain there are being referred to Nepali public services.[9]

Knowledge of the history and context just described can contribute considerably to a clinician's ability to establish rapport and provide accurate diagnoses and treatment recommendations. For example, an individual who emigrated from Bhutan earlier may have experienced years without permanent residence or social services. Alternatively, an individual who emigrated later may have been exposed to more severe trauma. In particular, children born between 1988 and 1993 are likely to have been exposed to high levels of maternal stress and disease and to have received poor pre- and post-natal care. An evaluator must also consider the condition of the camp to which the examinee was assigned, as there is considerable variability in this experience as related to education, medical care, nutrition, and trauma history.

Immigration and Relocation

Understanding the circumstances surrounding Bhutanese refugees' relocation is important, as those who moved to the United States earlier may have had little support upon arrival, and those who left camps later may have had uncontrolled medical conditions or may have spent time in camps alone without the support of extended family. Intergenerational disagreements likely complicated the decision for many families to leave Nepal as well. Although younger generations who had spent most of their lives in the camps were generally excited at the prospect of new opportunities, older generations were intimidated by the relocation process and hoped for a return to the home they once knew.[2,5,6]

Language

Most refugees of Bhutan speak Nepali and many speak multiple other languages including Hindi, Tamang, and **Dzongkha**.[2,5] Younger generations who grew up in refugee camps in Nepal were regularly exposed to English as well.[10] However, although the UNHCR estimates that about 35% of Bhutanese refugees have some functional English abilities, 90% require interpreters for medical screening examinations,[11] which has important implications for clinicians. Additionally, a clinician should consider that some refugees are deaf or hard-of-hearing; although special support was available in some camps to teach lip reading and sign language, the quality of this training varied substantially among camps. After arrival to the United States many have begun to learn American and Nepali Sign Language.

Communication

Younger refugees of Bhutan were born in refugee camps and educated in English. As such, they are typically much more comfortable communicating with it than older individuals, who require an interpreter. A clinician should be aware that older individuals generally prefer to rely on family members in this role. Familiarity with the traditional greeting, *Namaste* (I greet the god within you), may help with rapport building. This salutation may be used for both hello and goodbye. Typically, Bhutanese refugees press their palms together in the prayer position when offering a greeting. Refugees of Bhutan make eye contact during all types of communication, including greetings. As it is in many cultures, pointing directly at people is considered impolite. The right hand is used when handing things to people and eating since the use of the left hand is considered impolite.[9]

From my experience, I have observed that adult children typically speak on their parent's behalf. Older individuals are often hesitant to speak with me directly during evaluations and usually require encouragement from family. This may also be partially attributable to distrust of authority figures and, more broadly, White, English-speaking individuals.[12] Elderly parents expect that their adult children will communicate on their behalf and may become angry if they do not; as such, a clinician should be flexible about allowing family members to participate in the evaluation process more extensively than is typical.

Education

Bhutanese citizens of Nepali ethnicities who grew up in Bhutan generally had little to no formal education. Ironically, despite limited access to academic resources, Bhutanese people of Nepali ethnicities had higher levels of literacy compared to their nativist Drukpa counterparts due to their close proximity to India, where their children sometimes attended school.[2,5,10]

After their expulsion from Bhutan and subsequent resettlement in refugee camps, Bhutanese refugee school-aged children received formal education through the Bhutanese Refugee Education Program (BREP) administered by the international Catholic charity organization CARITAS, who also sponsored the Child Play Centre for younger refugee children and the Youth Friendly Center for 18- to 21-year-learners. The teachers themselves were also refugees living in the camps.[10] Although the quality may have varied in the camps, in general, the standard of English education was higher than that in the rest of Nepal. All subjects were conducted in English except the Nepali and Dzongkha language classes. After completion of the 10th year of study, students could sit for a Nepali national exam required to earn the *School Leaving Certificate* (SLC), the Nepali equivalent of a high school diploma. There were very few educational opportunities beyond this for residents of the refugee camps.

Literacy

The literacy rate among Bhutanese refugees of Nepali ethnicities was estimated between 65% and 85% in 2000.[10,11] However, these statistics apply to younger individuals who received education in the refugee camps. Most of the older refugees that I have evaluated grew up in Bhutan, did not participate in any sort of formal education, and had no ability to read or write.

Socio-Economic Status

After resettling in the United States, the Bhutanese refugee community primarily obtained employment in the service industry or by working in factories.[6] Young members of the community appear to have quickly acclimated to the United States and are rapidly advancing to higher socio-economic levels; many are completing university degrees and are obtaining professional careers.[13] When living in Bhutan, people of Nepali ethnicities lived an agrarian lifestyle. As refugees, they had limited food rations and experienced nutritional deficiencies. Housing generally consisted of bamboo huts with thatched roofs and lacked electricity, indoor plumbing, and running water.

Values and Customs

When evaluating and treating Bhutanese refugees of Nepali ethnicities, there are many cultural factors and customs of which a well-informed clinician should be aware in regards to religion, social organization and hierarchy, disability and illness, marriage customs, and privacy. Bhutanese people of Nepali ethnicities have traditionally followed a formal caste system, with status often denoted by family name. Today, however, although some older individuals still maintain an awareness of such a system, younger individuals are far less observant of caste status. In general, the clinician should also be aware that those who still adhere to the social and behavioral mores of a caste system are unlikely to discuss them with outsiders.[14]

The average household is multigenerational and includes elderly individuals as well as the spouses and children of younger members. In general, household members remain close throughout life events. As discussed earlier, the social structure of Bhutanese refugee families and communities may be considered interdependent with a patriarchal social hierarchy. Younger generations assume the responsibility of caring for aging relatives, who are, in turn, considered to bring good fortune to the home. Sons are expected to care for their parents, and daughters-in-law are obligated to care for their mothers-in-law.[9]

I have observed this dynamic during my evaluations of Bhutanese refugees of Nepali ethnicities. Adult children often report providing 24-hour care to a parent and sharing supervisory responsibilities with other adult peers in the community. Adult children nearly always attend their parents' doctor's appointments, manage their medications, and assist with their parents' personal needs. There appeared to be no family pressure for these designated care partners to maintain employment in the community.

Another important cultural factor for clinicians to keep in mind is that Bhutanese refugees consider deafness and disability to be a karmic form of punishment for the family. As such, caring for a family member with a disability is a spiritual endeavor that serves to purge the household of karmic burden, and Bhutanese refugees are hesitant to delegate this responsibility to individuals outside their immediate household. Because of this, teasing apart the details of an individual's true functional capacity within the context of cultural expectations is difficult. Additionally, older Bhutanese people of Nepali ethnicities often consider sickness to be related to an imbalance of mind, body, and spirit (perhaps caused by engaging in behavior discordant with their traditional values) or the result of evil spirits. Traditional healers called **dhami-jhakri** focus on re-establishing balance through methods such as reading rice, recommending special diets, and performing blessing rituals.[14] The use of home remedies is also common.

Refugees of Bhutan have several other cultural factors bearing mention including household customs, marriage practices, attitudes toward authority and privacy, and the conceptualization of time. Like many Eastern and Northern European cultures, Bhutanese refugees typically remove their shoes when entering or visiting homes. I have observed in my practice that many elderly refugees of Bhutan experiencing cognitive decline have removed their shoes upon entering my office while their families did not, suggesting reduced awareness or confusion. In general, refugees of Bhutan are vegetarian, and staple foods include rice and **dal**. Also, prayer rooms and kitchens are considered sacred spaces and should not be entered without permission. Traditionally, marriages were arranged when a boy reached the age of 7 or 8, and polygamy was an occasional practice.[14] Another practice within this context was the custom of encouraging a young man to marry his wife's close relatives of similar age if one of them experienced a chronic illness or disability.[4,14] This is relevant to clinical practice, as Bhutanese refugees often use late marriage as a proxy for intellectual impairment or disability. For example, I have observed that collateral interviewees use the age of marriage as a gauge of premorbid capacity, with higher age signifying lower levels of functioning.

Bhutanese refugees are hesitant to trust people in positions of authority. Many are leery of the police and are afraid to call them for assistance due to their traumatic experience with authority figures in Bhutan (the police, the military, and government officials).[14] In my experience, patients who are refugees of Bhutan have often shown distrust for evaluative and immigration processes, and some have verbalized distrust of non-Bhutanese Nepali interpreters. Taking the time to explain the evaluation process and answer all questions is an important part of building rapport, not just with the identified client but also with their family. Efforts should always be made to obtain a Bhutanese-Nepali interpreter. When not available, communicating your understanding of the challenges and being open to alternatives, including family participation, is helpful.

Additionally, I provide a comfortable and safe place for larger groups to collect if necessary, as patients are often accompanied by large groups of extended family and community members several hours prior to their scheduled appointment time. I also stream a live Nepali language radio station in the waiting room, which helps with comfort and rapport building.

A final, very important consideration when working with refugees of Bhutan is that one should prepare office mates, staff, and security personnel ahead of time to receive these individuals, as cultural differences regarding hygiene, time, and family involvement may be disruptive.

Gender and Sexuality

Gender roles are clearly defined within the culture of refugees from Bhutan—women are expected to take responsibility for household chores and parenting, and both genders are equally expected to participate in work outside the home. Men traditionally hold decision-making authority in the family and community.

Traditionally, sexuality is a taboo subject among Bhutanese people of Nepali ethnicities, and most older individuals are hesitant to discuss sex-related topics. A clinician should be aware that women will consciously avoid discussing the experience of sexual violence due to fear that they will be ostracized by their family and peers. In Bhutanese-Nepali cultural practice, the experience of rape is attributed to sins committed in a past life and considered karmic retribution. Although many Bhutanese refugee women experienced sexual violence during their expulsion, they are frightened of reporting incidence of trauma, torture, and rape in fear that they will be further punished by family and peers. A clinician should be sensitive to these factors when probing for a history of trauma; I have noticed that sometimes older women euphemistically refer to sexual violence as "ill-treatment," "mistreatment," and "misbehavior." As younger Bhutanese Nepali women are more open to discussing sex-related topics among themselves and with providers, collecting collateral information is vital to the assessment process. However, the clinician should also keep in mind that even young Bhutanese refugee women remain hesitant to discuss sex and related topics with elders, men, or family members.[14]

Spirituality and Religion

There is religious diversity within the Bhutanese refugee community; around 60% of refugees are Hindu, 27% are Buddhists, 10% are **Kirat**, and some are Christians.[11,15] *Brahmins*—or Hindu priests—provide prayer leadership and officiate ceremonies **puja**, among other responsibilities. Worship takes place at Hindu temples and prayer is regularly carried out in the home. Formal transition to adulthood occurs at seven for girls and eight or nine for boys. Girls are given their first **sari** before puberty and boys receive a **jennoi** (a holy thread worn throughout life) from the *Brahmin* in their community.[14] Birthdays and festivals are celebrated according to the Hindu calendar, and a clinician may find it useful to have a Hindu calendar on hand for evaluating orientation.

Acculturation and Systemic Barriers

Prior to relocating to the United States, the International Organization for Migration (IOM) provided classes to dispel stereotypes and orient refugees to US culture. Educational topics included how to use a seatbelt, maintain proper personal hygiene, manage a misbehaving child, and use a Western-style toilet.[7,10]

Limited access to medical care was another systemic barrier that Bhutanese refugees of Nepali ethnicities faced after they arrived in the United States; federal resettlement benefits only provided eight months of financial assistance to pay for medical services following relocation. As a result, many older adults often lacked medical insurance and received limited medical care until they obtained citizenship and access to Medicare. With regard to mental health services, MacDowell et al.[12] found that over one-third of refugees reported having problems accessing care. Individuals over the age of 55 had the most difficulty accessing services due to limitations in their ability to read, speak, and write English.

Refugees faced many additional systemic and cultural barriers to acculturation in the United States. For example, many had never been formally employed and were not accustomed to associated responsibilities such as punctuality, time management, and autonomous work. Additionally, prior to relocation, refugees had never rented or owned their own homes and were unaccustomed to maintaining them and paying rent in a timely manner. These factors combined with family separation and limited social and governmental support made the transition to life in the US challenging.[16]

Despite these barriers, refugees of Bhutan display many resilience factors including a strong sense of connection to their families, community, and spirituality. Bhutanese refugees have also initiated annual events to bring the community together and have recently formed formal social organizations including the Bhutanese American Sports Council (BASC), the United Bhutanese Community of Texas, and the Bhutanese Community Association of Akron.

Mental Health Views

As in many Asian cultures, refugees of Bhutan associate mental illness and its treatment with social stigma, particularly older individuals.[12] Because there are high rates of psychiatric illness and suicide among the Bhutanese refugee community both within camps in Nepal and in the United States,[16-8] the clinician should be aware of stigma-related barriers, cultural tendencies to conceal emotions, and idioms of distress including **aatmahatya** and **jhundera maryo**.[19-22] Familiarity with common spiritual and cultural beliefs, in addition to related idioms of distress, may reduce obstacles and facilitate improved treatment. *Idioms of distress* refer to colloquial methods by which individuals of a certain culture communicate the experience of negative emotions. For example, in English speaking cultures expressions such as "feeling down" or "feeling blue" are idioms of distress.

Most Bhutanese refugees follow the Hindu faith system in which the self is understood as the interaction of **man** (heart-mind), **dimaag** (brain-mind), **jiu/saarir** (physical body), **saato** (spirit/soul), and **ijjat** (honor).[22] Knowledge of these concepts allows one to be sensitive to idioms of distress that can guide corresponding treatment options.

For example, a Bhutanese refugee expressing problems related to *ijjat* may be concerned about social shame and stigma; corresponding treatment modalities can include social inclusion activities and relationship counseling.[21,22] Likewise, when patients and families disclose *dimaag*/brain-mind-related problems, this may suggest symptoms of psychosis, anger, and substance abuse. The *man*/heart mind is considered the center of desire, emotion, and memory, and related problems include suffering, sadness, despair, worry, and memory symptoms such as flashbacks.[21,22] In such cases, a clinician can encourage support from friends and family, participation in talk therapy, and participation in traditional healing rituals.[23] Speaking from my personal experience, when I first interviewed a refugee from Bhutan, I asked whether he felt sad. The interpreter laughed, explained that the patient would never admit to that, and appeared uncomfortable himself at the suggestion. I would likely have been able to receive an honest answer by asking about problems with *man*/heart-mind, a Bhutanese-Nepali idiom of distress. Another important source of information is collateral interviews with patients' younger care partners, who generally manage their older relatives' medical appointments. These individuals are much less averse to discussing and seeking mental health services.[12]

Nepali refugees of Bhutan do not hesitate to endorse problems related to physical health (*jiu/saarir*). However, the clinician should be aware that persistent somatoform disorders and medically unexplained pain are common among Bhutanese refugees.[11,24] Notwithstanding, physical health problems should be taken seriously and warrant referral to appropriate medical providers.

Approaches to Testing

Because younger and older generations have had distinctly different cultural, language, and educational experiences, the clinician will need to tailor the testing approach based on individual needs. In general, refugees under 30 years of age were born inside refugee camps and received more consistent education including instruction in English. Conversely, older individuals born prior to the *One Nation, One People* movement are far less acculturated and, as such, require flexibility in regards to the testing approach.

As always, when conducting a neuropsychological examination, the clinician should include a thorough interview with the family, a behavioral exam, functional testing, and corroborating information such as academic and medical records. In particular, collateral interviews with younger individuals, who generally care for their elders, are likely the clinician's best resource in case conceptualization. Young men are most typically the individuals arranging medical appointments and completing medical paperwork for their parents and also other senior members of the community. In general, seniors never complete these tasks unassisted. Even with input from younger care partners, uncovering the onset and course of symptoms in older individuals can be a challenge. Younger persons are often unaware of their parents' developmental, educational, and trauma histories. Although they may be able to recall their elders' level of functioning in the refugee camps, life there involved few of the functional demands that are required for the transition to the United States. For example, they seldom used money in the camps to purchase goods, which were rationed. Additionally, purchases were made with Indian Rupee bills, for which a larger physical size denotes higher value. As a result, older individuals did not need to acquire number sense (the magnitude of numbers and their relation to each other). As such, the clinician should determine whether the examinee grasps this concept, which is necessary to make purchases using the US Dollar. This can also give the clinician an idea about the examinee's ability to learn new and abstract information. Speaking from personal experience, I have observed many older Bhutanese-Nepali display significant limitations in numbers sense and who cannot count above the number 5. Likewise, tasks involving reading or using writing instruments may be unfamiliar for older examinees and even perceived as threatening. The clinician should be familiar with alternative methods of examination such as the match stick test, which requires the examinee to copy a simple figure by using matches as opposed to drawing with a pen or pencil.[25]

Orientation is another important aspect of cognition, as some older Nepali-Bhutanese individuals may use the Hindu calendar but not the Gregorian calendar. The Hindu calendar has a cycle of 60 years and the New Year usually begins at the end of April according to the Gregorian calendar. As such, one should be aware of the Hindu date and related alternate responses to support recognition cuing for orientation. Likewise, the clinician is encouraged to be familiar with recent and upcoming holidays and festivals to guide inquiry into orientation to time and the functional aspects of episodic memory, as measured, for example, by the CDR® Dementia Staging Instrument (CDR[26]).

Motivation and effort is another factor to keep in mind when providing evaluations for refugees of Bhutan. In my experience, I have observed that some Bhutanese Nepali individuals feel pressure to perform poorly so they can secure citizenship, and with it, access to medical services. Suboptimal test performance can be an indication of distrust. To assuage patient and family concerns, the clinician should enlist the support from trusted leaders within the Bhutanese refugee community (who are generally younger, educated, and familiar with the US medical system) to help explain the process to examinees. One more thing to keep in mind is that although Nepali interpreters are available, refugees of Bhutan are culturally distinct from them, and differences in language use and terminology can not only introduce error but also erode trust. As such, one is encouraged to use a Bhutanese-Nepali interpreter.

Section II: Case Study — "She Speaks a Strange Language"

Note: Possible identifying information and several aspects of history and presentation have been changed to protect patient identity and privacy.

Reason for Evaluation

In October 2020, I evaluated Ms. Rai, a 65-year-old refugee of Bhutan, who was seeking US Citizenship. In my experience, all of the Bhutanese individuals of Nepali ethnicities that I have evaluated were seeking accommodations for the US Citizenship Evaluation, and my role was to determine eligibility for such accommodations. Her son arranged the appointment and completed all of the intake paperwork in English. He told me that although Ms. Rai's best language is Nepali, she sometimes "speaks in a strange language that nobody knows." With this knowledge, I wanted to ensure I had access to an interpreter who could potentially identify and understand other languages spoken in Bhutan (e.g., Hindi, Tamang, and Dzongkha), and this was only available telephonically. Prior to the evaluation, I met with the interpreter and discussed the evaluation procedures, including the importance of interpreting with a more concrete approach that might reveal expressive communications deficits including aphasia. I also emailed the interpreter validated Nepali versions of the standard measures (i.e., PHQ-9, RUDAS, etc.) that I typically use for these types of evaluation.

Background and Behavioral Observations

Ms. Rai arrived at her appointment one and a half hours early, accompanied by several members of her family including her younger brother, 27-year-old son, and daughter-in-law. Although her family conversed casually in both Nepali and English in the waiting room, she did not participate in any social interaction and instead stared at the floor. Ms. Rai did not respond when I initially greeted her and invited her into my office; her daughter-in-law prompted her to return my greeting and also guided her by hand during ambulation, which was characterized by a slow and antalgic gait.

After her brother and extended family crowded into my office together, I asked her if she wanted their company. She appeared confused and was unable to confirm her preference until the interpreter and I tried a variety of wordings, and she continued to appear alternately overwhelmed and apathetic throughout the interview process. She frequently looked to her son and daughter-in-law for reassurance; her son generally spoke for her and her daughter-in-law provided emotional support. After a simplified explanation of my role and the purpose of the assessment, she provided consent. The details were reviewed more thoroughly with her family and each member verbalized consent and understanding.

Based on her family's report, Ms. Rai was born in Bhutan and experienced no developmental delays or problems with adaptive functioning during childhood. Her first language was Nepali, and she received no formal education. She married at about age 13, had four children, and occupied her time following marriage with domestic and aggregrarian activities. Her husband was arrested for political reasons during her fourth pregnancy, and she was forced to leave Bhutan as a condition of her husband's release. She subsequently emigrated together with her family to Nepal, where she was eventually reunited with her brother in a refugee camp. Her husband was fatally injured after a fall about five years after they arrived in Nepal.

In terms of psychiatric history, Ms. Rai's son reported that she had experienced "mental problems" on occasion before leaving Bhutan. However, he explained that they did not interfere with culturally relevant instrumental activities of daily living (IADLs) including agrarian and domestic activities. Her brother denied having observed Ms. Rai present with psychiatric problems prior to marriage, though he had little interaction with her following that time.

When asked to explain Ms. Rai's "mental problems," her son reported that she experienced "attacks," characterized by seizure-like symptoms, that occurred about once a month. These episodes included falls followed by full-body spasms lasting several minutes, subsequent confusion, and states of alternating agitation and hypersomnolence that lasted from hours to days afterward. He also reported that she retained no memory of the falls or spasms themselves. These episodes interfered with domestic-related IADLs, for which she received support from her sister-in-law and older children. She also neglected hygienic activities for days following these episodes and seemed unaware of any problem. Her family reported that although she was prescribed medication in Nepal, they were unclear as to the purpose. They were also unaware whether she visited a traditional healer during this time. She did not bring medical paperwork with her when she relocated to the United States in 2015.

Ms. Rai's family reported that she experienced a severe seizure-like episode six months following her arrival to the United States. During this episode she fell, displayed disorganized speech and combative/aggressive behavior. Briefly thereafter, she lost consciousness and could not be roused. Her son took her to the emergency room, and she was hospitalized for three days. After staff could not identify the cause of her episode, she was referred to a physician who prescribed her risperidone and quetiapine; although these appeared to reduce the severity of subsequent attacks as well as associated behavioral symptoms, they did not eliminate the seizure-like episodes themselves.

At the time of assessment, Ms. Rai's family reported that she did not recognize familiar people or remember their names. She displayed considerable regression for IADLs including her ability to make simple purchases, prepare meals, and contribute to maintaining the home. She also displayed considerably reduced initiative. Formerly social with neighbors and friends in the community, she became uncharacteristically withdrawn, spending most of her time sitting in her room and staring out a window. Her reduced level of motivation and initiative also markedly impacted basic ADLs. For example, she no longer requested food and only ate when meals were placed in front of her, and she also did not initiate other self-care skills including dressing and hygienic activities.

Appearance and Behavior

Ms. Rai appeared undernourished and disheveled; she was hastily dressed in a mismatched combination of traditional and Western attire (she wore a sari, **tikka**, and bangles, with a dirty sweatshirt and wool-hat despite temperate weather). Her voice was hoarse and raspy, and she spoke with low volume. Language content was limited in Nepali; she spoke in single words and short phrases. As detailed above, Ms. Rai had difficulty understanding the purpose of her evaluation; notwithstanding she appeared to understand that the evaluator was a medical professional, as she pointed to places on the right side of her body where she experienced pain. She required significant encouragement, demonstration, and prompting throughout her evaluation. Her daughter-in-law was included in the testing session and provided emotional support and encouragement after agreeing not to offer answers or direct help. Ms. Rai displayed a tendency to give up quickly, which may have suggested suboptimal effort. This was considered during case conceptualization. Her family carried all her personal effects including her identification card.

Test and Norm Selection

All measures were reviewed with a Nepali-Bhutanese interpreter prior to the appointment and administered together with the interpreter. The battery included the following tests:

- CDR® Dementia Staging Instrument (CDR[26])
- Informant Questionnaire on Cognitive Decline in the Elderly IQ-CODE—Short[27]
- Common Objects Memory Test (COMT[28])
- Rowland Universal Dementia Assessment Scale, Nepali version (Nepali-RUDAS[29])
- Patient Health Questionnaire, Nepali adaptation (PHQ-9[20])

Test Results

Ms. Rai was completely disoriented to time when administered the CDR, and she remained disoriented to time with the provision of a Hindu calendar. She was also disoriented to place, and she was unable to recall her address or city of residence despite having lived there for the past five years. Notwithstanding, she was able to recognize her state of residence from among three options.

When administered the Nepali-RUDAS, Ms. Rai struggled with a basic praxis examination, she was unable to return a demonstration of basic hand movements, and she could not differentiate between right and left. She required five attempts to repeat a list of four items and could not recall them after a brief distraction. She could repeat simple three-word sentences and follow simple one-step commands. She was only able to follow the final step of two and three-step commands, suggesting a recency effect. On a measure of list generation, she was able to name 3 animals in 60 seconds. She was able to successfully duplicate a simple geometric pattern with match sticks.

Confrontational naming and short-term memory were measured using the COMT. On the confrontational naming portion of the examination, she was only able to name two out of ten everyday objects when presented with them initially. Although she was able to repeat the names of the remaining objects with demonstration, she was unable to name them spontaneously on second and third trials of confrontational naming. When asked to recall these items from memory after a delay, she could remember none of them. Notwithstanding, she accurately identified nine of the ten objects and had only one false positive error when offered recognition cues, which suggested good effort and some level of functional carryover of new information.

Ms. Rai was unable to understand the concepts presented on the PHQ-9 despite the provision of considerable non-standardized assistance from her daughter-in-law and the interpreter. Ms. Rai's son endorsed marked decline from prior levels of functioning in episodic memory, orientation, problem-solving, basic financial skills, decision making, and receptive and expressive communication on a questionnaire addressing cognitive abilities and IADLs (IQ-CODE).

Impressions

Ms. Rai's clinical course and symptoms as reported by her family included seizure-like episodes beginning with falls, evolving into full-body spasms that last a minute or two, and resolving into protracted episodes of confusion, amnesia, disorganized speech, and agitation or hypersomnolence. These clinical symptoms strongly suggested an epileptic syndrome. I requested a release of information so that I could obtain her medical records from the hospital, her primary care physician, and her psychiatrist. The hospital records indicated a diagnosis of seizure disorder and status epilepticus, but there was no documentation of follow up with EEG or brain imaging. Her family and primary care physician appeared completely unaware of her hospital diagnosis. According to records, her primary care physician referred her to psychiatry after her son reported concern regarding "mental problems" as he did with neuropsychology. Psychiatry diagnosed Ms. Rai with Major Depressive Disorder with psychosis. Although Ms. Rai was provided with a Nepali interpreter, her family was barred from participation in the interview process with psychiatry, likely due to a naive attempt to protect her privacy and confidentiality. Like with primary care, psychiatry appeared to have had no knowledge of her seizure diagnosis from the hospital.

Ms. Rai's overall neurobehavioral profile suggested global cognitive decline, highlighted by marked problems in both receptive and expressive communication, memory loss, and general functional impairment. Her progressive deterioration of language and other cognitive skills in the context of her clinical history strongly suggests an epilepsy syndrome, which would clearly interfere with her ability to learn the information and demonstrate the language skills necessary to pass the US citizenship test. Ms. Rai's level of difficulty on direct testing was such that she could complete very few standardized formal measures, and implementation of non-standardized procedures provided better clinical utility by testing limits. Using non-standardized techniques helped garner important information that would assist Ms. Rai to receive an appropriate diagnosis, medical treatment, and her citizenship.

Feedback and Follow-Up

I provided feedback to Ms. Rai and her family with the same telephonic interpreter that assisted with the evaluation. Given her neurobehavioral profile and the information I obtained from medical records, I provided basic education regarding seizures and a referral to a Nepali-speaking seizure specialist in the area. In March, 2021 Ms. Rai's family called to inform me that she had been diagnosed with symptomatic epilepsy due to underlying neurocysticercosis, was granted citizenship, and with it, Medicare. She was receiving treatment with anticonvulsant medication and had not had any seizures for several months. Neurocysticercosis is a parasitic infection caused by the tapeworm Taenia solium and is contracted through the consumption of undercooked pork, water contaminated with the tapeworm egg, or through poor hygienic practices, and is the most common underlying pathology for epilepsy in Nepal.[30,31]

This example illustrates the number of barriers Bhutanese refugees face in receiving treatment for medical and psychiatric problems, including poor understanding of medical terminology, social stigma related to neurobehavioral symptoms, suspicion of authority figures, and problems communicating with providers. As such, sensitivity to cultural beliefs including idioms of distress is important in establishing rapport so that a clinician can obtain an accurate history of symptoms and be enabled to provide effective feedback and education that will help refugees of Bhutan become stronger self-advocates in the US healthcare system.

Section III: Lessons Learned

- Culturally adapted tests (in other words, tests that are not simply translated) are essential for questionnaires regarding health, mood, and beliefs about health. For example, the PHQ-9 has not only been translated into Nepali but also includes idioms of distress. Also, clinicians should stay up to date with new adaptations, translations, and research for diverse populations in order to use the most valid and reliable instruments possible.
- Clinicians must be flexible and adapt their approach to best serve people for whom our traditional measures of neuropsychological functioning are of limited utility. This means liberal use of non-standardized procedures—qualitative data is likely of much greater value than normative data.
- There are many sources of relevant data beyond traditional neuropsychological test scores, especially medical records and behavioral observations. Likely the most valuable assessment

technique is a thorough interview with collateral sources combined with sensitivity to cultural factors. In the present case, good communication with the family, detailed collateral interview, and the obtaining of medical records allowed for the client to obtain the correct diagnosis, and with it, effective treatment.

- In general, the meaning ascribed to physical and psychiatric problems is culturally bound, and it is important to know cultural idioms of distress. For example, for the Bhutanese refugee population, a clinician should understand that stigma and implied guilt may be associated with certain medical and psychiatric conditions. Older Bhutanese refugees may view trauma as the result of bad **karma**, and, as such, they may be less likely to endorse these types of symptoms. Again, building a strong rapport with both the client and family combined with detailed collateral interviews is crucial to arriving at an accurate diagnosis.
- Although cultural beliefs may present barriers to accessing mental health services, these can be protective factors as well. For example, among refugees of Bhutan, participation in purification rituals may help survivors of trauma to let go of negative memories and move past the experience.[21] This may be an excellent adjunct to treatment.
- Among refugees of Bhutan and similar groups, community and peer counselors can be very effective in facilitating the acquisition of mental health support. For example, in the case sample above, the participation of younger individuals who were fluent in English and were viewed as community leaders was crucial in both rapport building and obtaining client history.

Acknowledgment

I would like to thank Sunil Gupta for his dedication to the Bhutanese refugee community, and for being my guide, interpreter, and friend as we navigated through so many evaluations with Bhutanese-Nepali individuals.

Glossary

Aatmahatya. The Hindi word for suicide.

Dal. A soup prepared from lentils, peas, or beans (pulses) considered a staple food in South Asian countries.

Dhami-jhakri. Traditional healer or shaman.

Dimaag. The brain-mind; the seat of thoughts, the pragmatic mind that acts according to social norms and is responsible for controlling behavior and thinking. Includes many symptoms of mental illness including psychosis and alcoholism.[22]

Drukpa. The term collectively refers to the Buddhist peoples of Bhutan with Mahayana Buddhism as the religion and Dzongkha as the language.[5]

Dzongkha. The national language of the Kingdom of Bhutan.

Ijjat. Honor or reputation, is the link between the person and the social world and is indicated by social status and respect. Behaving in a manner consistent with the caste hierarchy and social norms is essential to maintaining ijjat.[22]

Jhundera maryo. The term used to describe suicide and suicidal behavior among Bhutanese refugees. Literally meaning "to hang oneself."[17]

Jennoi. A holy thread given to a young man by the Brahmin in their community that is worn throughout life.

Jiu/saarir. The physical body and site of physical pain. Related to diseases and injuries.[22]

Karma. A term used in Hinduism and Buddhism that refers to the sum of a person's actions in this and previous lives and is viewed as deciding their fate in future lives.

Kirat. A religion practiced by some Bhutanese individuals of Nepali ethnicities. People who practice Kirat worship ancestors and nature, such as trees, rivers, animals, and stones.

Man. The heart-mind; the seat of desires, referring to opinions, intentions, and personal feelings.[22]

Puja. A cleansing ritual performed by a Hindu priest.

Saato. The spirit or soul, presence of mind, and consciousness. The soul helps protect the body from supernatural forces. Symptoms of psychological distress may include frightening easily, lack of energy, and fatigability.[22]

Sari. A brightly colored garment worn by women made of several yards of lightweight cloth draped so that one end forms a skirt and the other a head or shoulder covering.

Tikka. A Hindu traditional blessing made of red powder that is placed on the forehead between the crown of the nose and the hairline.

References

1. National Geographic style manual, National Geographic; 2021. Available from: https://sites.google.com/a/ngs.org/ngs-style-manual/home/N/nepali-nepalese
2. Venkat P. The Lhotsampa people of Bhutan: Resilience and survival. New York (NY): Palgrave Macmillan; 2016.
3. The World Factbook 2020. Washington, DC: Central Intelligence Agency; 2020. https://www.cia.gov/library/publications/resources/the-world-factbook/index.html
4. Savada AM, editor. Bhutan: a country study. Washington: GPO for the Library of Congress; 1991.
5. Hutt M. Unbecoming citizens: culture, nationhood, and the flight of refugees from Bhutan. New Delhi: Oxford University Press; 2003.
6. Pedicord S. (2015). The long journey home: a brief overview of Bhutanese refugee resettlement. *Masters Essays,* 28 [dissertation]. John Carroll University, Carroll Collected. Available from: http://collected.jcu.edu/mastersessays/28
7. SAARC Jurists Mission on Bhutan, International Center for Law in Development, Informal Sector Service Centre. The Bhutan tragedy, when will it end?: human rights and inhuman wrongs; first report of the SAARC Jurists Mission on Bhutan. Kathmandu: Informal Sector Service Centre; 1992.
8. Maharajan U. Status of Bhutanese refugees. [Internet]. 2019, December 19. Available from: https://risingnepaldaily.com/opinion/status-of-bhutanese-refugees
9. United Nations High Commission for Refugees, The UN Refugee Agency, Global Focus UNHCR Operations Worldwide. 2021 Planning summary, Operation: Nepal; n.d. https://reporting.unhcr.org/sites/default/files/pdfsummaries/GA2021-nepal-eng.pdf. Retrieved February 5, 2021.
10. Ringhofer M. Bhutanese refugees history and present situation with emphasize on education. Lifelong Education and Libraries. 2002;2:43–72. Available from: http://hdl.handle.net/2433/43617
11. U.S. Department of Health and Human Services Centers for Disease Control and Prevention, National Center for Emerging and Zoonotic Infection Diseases, Division of Global Migration and Quarantine. Bhutanese refugee health profile; 2014.
12. MacDowell H, Pyakurel S, Acharya J, Morrison-Beedy D, Kue J. Perceptions toward mental illness and seeking psychological help among Bhutanese refugees resettled in the U.S. Issues Ment Health Nurs. 2020;41(3):243–50. https://doi.org/10.1080/01612840.2019.1646362
13. Schultze ML. Bhutanese refugees are finding their place in Ohio. Huffington Post [Internet]. 2018 Apr 6. Available from: https://www.huffpost.com/entry/akron-ohio-bhutanese-refugees_n_59ca88cfe4b0cdc773353640#:~:text=As%20many%20as%205%2C000%20Nepalis,here%20during%20the%20last%20decade
14. Maxym M, Upadhayay P, Dhital M. Nepali-speaking Bhutanese; 2010. Downloaded 2020 Sept 18 from https://ethnomed.org/culture/nepali-speaking-bhutanese/
15. Van Ommermen M, Sharma B, Komproe I, Poudyal BN, Sharma GK, Cardeña E, de Jong JT. Trauma and loss as determinants of medically unexplained epidemic illness in a Bhutanese refugee camp. Psychol Med. 2001;31:1259–67. DOI:10.1017/S0033291701004470

16. Hagaman AK, Sivilli TI, Ao T, Blanton C, Ellis H, Lopes Cardozo B, Shetty S. An investigation into suicides among Bhutanese refugees resettled in the United States between 2008 and 2011. Journal Immigr Minor Health. 2016;18(4):819–27. doi:10.1007/s10903-015-0326-6

17. Meyerhoff J, Rohan KJ, Fondacaro KM. Suicide and suicide-related behavior among Bhutanese refugees resettled in the United States. Asian Am J Psychol. 2018;9(4):270–83. doi:10.1037/aap0000125

18. Ao T, Shetty S, Sivilli T, Blanton C, Ellis H, Geltman PL, Cochran J, Taylor E, Lankau EW, Lopes Cardozo B. Suicidal ideation and mental health of Bhutanese refugees in the United States. J Immigr Minor Health. 2016;18(4):828–35. doi:10.1007/s10903-015-0325-7

19. Ellis BH, Lankau EW, Ao T, Benson MA, Miller AB, Shetty S, Lopes Cardozo B, Geltman PL, Cochran J. Understanding Bhutanese refugee suicide through the interpersonal-psychological theory of suicidal behavior. Am J Orthopsychiatry. 2015;85(1):43–55. doi:10.1037/ort0000028

20. Kohrt BA, Luitel NP, Acharya P et al. Detection of depression in low resource settings: validation of the Patient Health Questionnaire (PHQ-9) and cultural concepts of distress in Nepal. BMC Psychiatry. 2016;16:58. doi:10.1186/s12888-016-0768-y

21. Sharma B, van Ommeren M. Preventing torture and rehabilitating survivors in Nepal. Transcult Psychiatry. 1998;35(1):85–97. doi:10.1177/13634615980350010

22. Kohrt BA, Harper I. Navigating diagnoses: understanding mind-body relations, mental health, and stigma in Nepal. Cult Med Psychiatry. 2008;32(4): 462–91. doi:10.1007/s11013-008-9110-6

23. Vonnahme LA, Lankau EW, Ao T, Shetty S, Cardozo BL. Factors associated with symptoms of depression among Bhutanese refugees in the United States. J Immigr Minor Health. 2015;17(6): 1705–14. doi:10.1007/s10903-014-0120-x

24. Van Ommeren M, de Jong JT, Sharma B, Komproe I, Thapa SB, Cardeña E. Psychiatric disorders among tortured Bhutanese refugees in Nepal. Arch Gen Psychiatry. 2001;58(5):475–82. doi:10.1001/archpsyc.58.5.475

25. Baiyewu O, Unverzagt FW, Lane KA, Gureje O, Ogunniyi A, Musick B, Gao S, Hall KS, Hendrie HC. The Stick Design Test: a new measure of visuoconstructional ability. J Int Neuropsychol Soc. 2005;11(5):598–605. doi:10.1017/S135561770505071X

26. Besser L, Kukull W, Knopman DS, Chui H, Galasko D, Weintraub S, Jicha G, Carlsson C, Burns J, Quinn J, Sweet RA, Rascovsky K, Teylan M, Beekly D, Thomas G, Bollenbeck M, Monsell S, Mock C, Zhou XH, Thomas N, … Neuropsychology Work Group, Directors, and Clinical Core leaders of the National Institute on Aging-Funded US Alzheimer's Disease Centers. Version 3 of the National Alzheimer's Coordinating Center's uniform data set. Alzheimer Dis Assoc Disord. 2018;32(4):351–8. doi:10.1097/WAD.0000000000000279

27. Perroco TR, Damin AE, Frota NA, Silva MM, Rossi V, Nitrini R, Bottino C. Short IQCODE as a screening tool for MCI and dementia: preliminary results. Dement Neuropsychol. 2008;2(4):300–4. doi:10.1590/S1980-57642009DN20400012

28. Kempler D, Teng EL, Taussig M, Dick MB. The common objects memory test (COMT): a simple test with cross-cultural applicability. J Int Neuropsychol Soc. 2010;16(3):537–45. doi:10.1017/S1355617710000160

29. Nepal GM, Shrestha A, Acharya R. Translation and cross-cultural adaptation of the Nepali version of the Rowland Universal Dementia Assessment Scale (RUDAS). J PatientRep Outcomes. 2019;3:38. doi:10.1186/s41687-019-0132-3

30. Rajbhandari KC. Epilepsy in Nepal. Le journal canadien des sciences neurologiques. 2004;31(2): 257–60. doi:10.1017/s0317167100053919

31. (10 facts about neurocysticercosis. World Health Organization [Internet]. 2017 April; Available from: https://www.who.int/features/factfiles/neurocysticercosis/en/

Pakistani

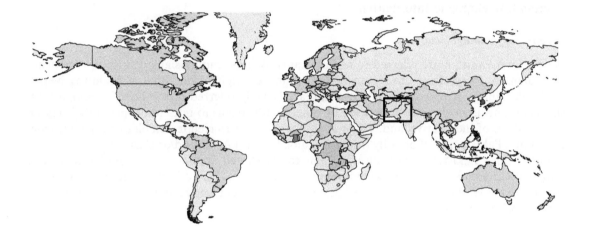

17   Asian Communities of Pakistani Origin

Sanam J. Lalani, Farah Hameed, and Louise F. Wheeler

Section I: Background Information

Terminology and Perspective

People from Pakistan are referred to as Pakistanis, Asians/South Asians, Pakistani American/ Canadian, etc. People from this region in South Asia (i.e., Afghanistan, Bhutan, Maldives, Nepal, Sri Lanka, India, Bangladesh, and Pakistan) are broadly referred to as "Desi," meaning from this land. This is a colloquial term used by other South Asians to refer to people of their region when outside of their native land. The first author's (SJL) preferred terminology for people from Pakistan is Pakistani or, if broadly from the region is South Asian and/or Desi.

I (SJL) am a Pakistani American who came to the United States (US) at age nine years as a bilingual Urdu and English-speaking immigrant. I (SJL) was raised in the American South and trained on the West Coast of the United States, where I am currently a practicing neuropsychologist in a private outpatient setting.

Geography

Pakistan is located in South Asia and borders India to the East, Afghanistan, and Iran to the West, the Arabian Sea to the South, and China to the Northwest. Pakistan is four times the size of the United Kingdom, with a population of over 216.5 million in 2019.[1] It includes the most youth in the world; the majority of the population in Pakistan is under the age of 30.[2] It is the fifth most populated country after China, India, United States, and Indonesia.[1] The capital of Pakistan is Islamabad, with a population of 1 million people.

History

The history of Pakistan begins with the glory of the Muslim kingdom dating back to the 700s. By the 1400s, competition for global dominance and wealth led to colonization and myriad cultures and religions lived peacefully in the Indian subcontinent for centuries. More recently, following the British colonization of India from 1858 to 1947, the minority Muslim population won its independence and separated (known as Partition) itself into a democratic and predominantly Muslim nation of The Islamic Republic of Pakistan on August 14, 1947. Initially, Pakistan consisted of West and East Pakistan, that later became Bangladesh in 1971.[3] The process of Partition displaced 10–12 million people along religious lines, creating a disordered and violent refugee crisis.[4] The history of this traumatic event has led to a complicated and distrusting relationship between

DOI: 10.4324/9781003051862-35

India and Pakistan.[5] Although the result of the shifting borders has led to many commonalities between the cultures, it is important to note that the religious identity of people from India and Pakistan are generally distinct. In addition, the complex geographical history has also resulted in multiple disputed territories. For example, control of the Jammu and Kashmir region remains under dispute with India occupying Jammu and Pakistan occupying the Kashmir region.

People

I (SJL) was born in Karachi, Pakistan, in the 1980s and raised there for the first nine years of my life. The city of Karachi contains more than 15.7 million people and is projected to be the third-largest city in the world by 2050. Karachi consists of 18 towns (i.e., suburbs) surrounding the city and many diverse boroughs within the city.

I grew up in an intergenerational home in a middle-class borough. Some of my earliest memories are of playing with my neighbors. I can recall the drive to visit our family who lived by the sea and can still remember the striking Spanish tiles decorating the roads along the drive. My cousins and I would run around inside the spacious home and play in the singular air-conditioned room. When playing outside, the smell of jasmine floated through the gardens. We also visited family in the lower socio-economic boroughs; I recall playing on the unpaved roads as motorbikes whizzed past and street vendors and animals meandered about.

In the late 1980s, while under Martial law, I snuck out of the gates of our apartment complex to visit a friend down the street. Although I was young, I knew enough to hide behind parked vehicles and avoid detection by the passing military armored trucks. Suffice it to say, the family of my friend was horrified by the risk I took to visit. Luckily, our community took care of one another, and my parents were notified immediately. It is the diversity, the sense of community, and the feeling of belonging in the face of hardship that I admire most about the Pakistani people.

Immigration and Relocation

The first phase of immigration from Pakistan to the West occurred before Pakistan was independent. This wave of immigration included young men from British India (the province of Punjab) who settled predominantly in California.[6] Following the 1965 US Immigration and Naturalization Act, Pakistani immigrants were highly educated and affluent professionals entering on employment-based visas.[7] Immigration in the 1980s included family sponsorship. In the 1990s, immigration included the US Diversity Program (also knowns as the "lottery"), a program created to increase immigration from underrepresented minority groups within the United States.

The Diversity Program is notably different from the prior immigration patterns of other cultures that had a financial selection bias in that it allowed Pakistani immigrants without higher education or financial stability to move to the United States. Therefore, exploring each patient's immigration history may allow for a richer understanding of their current circumstances.

The current make up of Pakistanis in the United States is 2% of the total Asian population (~1 million) and the seventh largest immigrant population. As such, Pakistanis no longer qualify for the Diversity "lottery" Program and it is difficult to achieve residency in the United States.[7] By 2015, 67% of American Pakistanis were foreign born, with varying naturalization and residency statuses, and many (approximately 35%) lived in multigenerational households that predominantly spoke English in the home.[8] While Pakistanis live in all 50 states, areas of concentration exist in the Northeast (New York City; Washington DC), the South including Texas

(Houston, Dallas) and Georgia (Atlanta), the Midwest (Chicagoland area), and California on the West Coast.[8]

There are many reasons for immigration. My family left Pakistan in 1990 in pursuit of sociopolitical safety and financial stability. The presence of a preexisting Pakistani community eased our transition, but it was still a stressful experience. For this reason, assessing a person's immigration history including the presence of immigration-related trauma, changes in socio-economic status, English language fluency, and level of acculturation to the dominant culture, could help contextualize the patient's concerns.

Language and Communication

Urdu is the national language of Pakistan and is the primary medium of communication throughout the country. However, only 8% of the local population speaks Urdu as their first language.[9] Pakistan is culturally divided into four provinces, each with their own provincial language: Punjabi is spoken in Punjab and is the most widely spoken language in the country, Sindhi is spoken in Sindh, Pashto is spoken in Khyber Pakhtunkhwa (formerly Northwest Frontier Province), and Balochi is spoken in Balochistan.[10] Gilgit-Baltistan, located in the Northeast part of the Khyber Pakhtunkhwa province, has semi-provincial status in Pakistan and has been proposed to become the fifth Pakistani province. There are several local languages spoken in this region, and Shina and Urdu are the official languages.

Spoken Urdu is similar to Hindi (a language spoken in India), but Urdu characters are based in Arabic—as such, Urdu is written from right to left. Due to the colonial history of Pakistan, government documentation is in English and Urdu. Moreover, many well-respected and private academic institutions provide English instruction. Therefore, many Pakistanis have some level of English proficiency. In America, 64% of American Pakistanis have been in the United States for over ten years and 72% speak English to some degree in home.[11] Unfortunately, there are few formal measures available to determine English proficiency in Urdu speakers. Therefore, understanding a patient's level of acculturation may be a useful proxy. For example, inquiring about the language of academic instruction, the number of years lived in the English-speaking country, languages spoken at home, work, or in social situations, and how English was acquired (formally or informally) may all be helpful considerations.[12] In the event an Urdu interpreter is necessary but unavailable, a Hindi-speaking interpreter may be helpful.

Outside of speaking English, effective communication requires an understanding of the meaning and context behind the patient's words and is necessary to build rapport, elicit accurate information, deliver effective feedback, and increase the chances that the patient will implement the recommendations made. See the following case example.

> An elder Pakistani woman presented to her cardiologist. Distressed, she relayed to the physician that her chest hurt, she experienced heart palpitations, and felt as if she could not breathe. The physician, taking the patient at her word, ordered a cardiac work up which showed minor abnormalities and prescribed the patient medication to improve her heart function. The patient reported that thereafter, she presumed she had heart problems and her medical record reflected the same. Years later, she presented to the emergency department distressed and reported similar symptoms (e.g., palpitations, shortness of breath). During this visit, a culturally sensitive physician obtained a detailed medical and social history from both the patient and a family member who was present. The patient was subsequently diagnosed with social anxiety and the appropriate treatment recommendations were explained to the patient and her family caregiver. In this example, the physician was able to contextualize all

of the data to fully appreciate that the reported symptoms as somatic complaints, confirmed by ruling out medical comorbidities, and begin appropriate treatments.

Similar to other South Asian communities, Pakistani communication generally tends to be polite and indirect to avoid conflict. Direct eye contact is less common and reserved for personal relationships; therefore, lack of eye contact should be considered in context. Conflict avoidant language is common and includes responses such as "Inshahallah" which means "god willing" when too polite to reject a recommendation, or "what can you do?" when unsure/confused about something. Rather than asking a clarifying question, they opt to "save face" and avoid confrontation. The complementary nonverbal gesture for non-committal responses has been described elsewhere in this text as a "head shake/wobble." A mix between a nod "yes" and a nod "no," the head shake is an ambiguous gesture that reflects acknowledgment but does not always reflect the agreement. Therefore, if there is a question around the patient's understanding, the provider is encouraged to probe comprehension with open-ended questions. Direct communication, on the other hand, is reserved for close relationships and, in particular, for men or younger people who are considered to be more "Westernized."

A few general considerations that may be helpful include showing respect for elders regardless of the situation; therefore, the eldest in the room should be addressed first or the elder may require deference during a family conference/feedback session regardless of their level of involvement. Getting buy-in will likely go a long way in compliance. Also, doctors are highly revered by Pakistani people, and therefore patients and family members may not directly express any concerns, which could lead to non-compliance. When Pakistani patients in England were provided the reasoning for a prescription rather than just being told to take the medication, compliance improved.[13] Lastly, haggling is commonplace in Pakistani culture and may need to be addressed, particularly in outpatient or out-of-pocket settings. Similar discussions around time management may also be necessary. While the perception of time in Western cultures is linear and limited, Desi cultures interpret time as cyclical and endless, and therefore patients may arrive late to scheduled appointments, following "Desi standard time." The neuropsychologist may choose to send appointment reminders to ensure timeliness.

Socio-Economic Status, Education, and Literacy

Vast socio-economic disparities exist across the provinces that are worse in rural areas and have widened over time.[14] These socio-economic disparities contribute to inequity in access to and quality of education in Pakistan, in particular for girls in rural areas who are unlikely to attend school.

The Pakistani education system consists of elementary (grades 1–5), middle (6–8), and secondary education, which is divided into lower secondary (9–10) and higher secondary (11–12). It was common to complete one's education at grade 10 (not 12); thus, clarification may be warranted. Secondary education can be followed by vocational or technical education (1.5–2 years) or with traditional higher education (bachelor's, master's, or doctorate level degrees). Traditional higher education degrees were previously awarded earlier relative to international standards but this has been updated.[2] Given the cultural values of norm adherence, respect for authority, and a sense of community, Pakistani education tends to require rote learning vs. critical thinking ability.

The Pakistan literacy rate is ranked 113 out of 120 countries but can be as high as 75% in some urban cities, similar to neighboring Asian countries. In contrast, rural areas have literacy rates as low as 9%.[15] Education disparities include the language of instruction. Public education may be offered in a local language, while private education may include either English, the local languages, or a combination thereof. The quality of instruction also varies, from the qualifications of the teacher to the classroom itself. Children educated in rural areas may be taught in a room without furniture, textbooks, or writing tools, while children in affluent areas may have well-qualified teachers, air-conditioned classrooms, desks, and access to Western textbooks. Education is commonly pursued for financial security and this privilege is largely reserved for boys who will later provide for their families. For those who were unable to pursue an education, it may be prudent to assess work history as a proxy for literacy. Educational attainment by Pakistani Americans is similar to other Asian Americans in the United States. However, relative to all Americans, Pakistanis are more likely to obtain bachelor's and advanced graduate degrees.[8]

Religion and Views on Mental Health

About 97% of Pakistani's are Muslims (people who practice Islam). The majority of Muslims in Pakistan are Sunni (76%), and the remainder are Shia. Christians, Hindus, Sikhs, Zoroastrians, and Baha'i make up the remaining 3%.[16] Islam is a monotheistic religion that follows Abrahamic traditions. Muslims traditionally pray five times per day, and Friday is considered the holy day. Common religious customs include abstaining from pork and alcohol and giving to charity. Ramadan, a holy month, is celebrated by daily fasting (i.e., abstaining from food and water), beginning at dawn until sunset. In addition to teaching obedience and discipline, fasting develops empathy toward the suffering of others. The end of the month is celebrated with a festival called Eid-ul-Fitr.

Religion plays an important role in psychiatric beliefs in the Muslim community. In Islam, homosexuality and suicide are traditionally considered a sin. However, individual interpretation of the scriptures varies. Rather than make assumptions, the clinician may respectfully ask the patient's preferences. Related influences include the consideration of religious oppression or persecution in treating religious minorities. And discussing the impact of 9/11 on the patient may also be relevant. The semester of the 9/11 attack, I was a student at a public university. The sharp increase in on-campus crimes against all brown-skinned students, Muslims, and non-Muslims alike led me to take that year off for fear of my safety. These instances of violence against Muslims persist and inquiring about potential hate crimes may be important.[17]

Spirituality also plays a role in psychiatric beliefs. When experiencing a hardship, a patient may believe "god willed it" and it is their responsibility to "bear the burden" rather than seek refuge in treatments. Therefore, events such as seizures may be explained away spiritually. A culturally normative explanation includes the involvement of a "djinn" (a supernatural being). Additionally, chronic illnesses may turn family members into primary caregivers, and as a result, a patient may not present to their physician until symptoms have progressed. The increased level of severity and related limitations in treatment could confirm the cultural belief that Western medicine is unhelpful. Thus, exploring family stressors for early detection and psychoeducation could play an important role in de-stigmatization and clinical care.

Common medical treatments may include homeopathy or ayurvedic treatments rather than Western medicine (allopathy) because conventional medicine is not consistently available. This results in limited resources, poor medical sophistication, and poor compliance. It is common for Pakistanis to not dispose of unused medications for fear of losing access and this can lead to off-label use of medications. Similarly, over-the-counter medicines, such as acetaminophen, can be misused (e.g., taken as a portion of the recommended dose) and/or referred to as a panacea, presumably referring to a placebo response. Notably, prescribed medications are typically accessible over-the-counter in Pakistan, making this a more affordable option for persons living abroad.

Regarding mental health, Desis may not directly refer to depression or anxiety; rather, concerns with mood may present physically described as frustration, fatigue, unease, pain in the mind/headache, chest pain, heart palpitations, or shortness of breath, without insight into the broader relationship between these experiences and low mood. Discussing the symptoms, rather than naming the disorder, is a culturally sanctioned method of expressing distress, likely reinforced over time due to the stigma associated with experiencing mental health disorders. Therefore, patients may first present these physical complaints to their primary care physician or to specialties such as cardiology rather than directly to psychiatry/psychology. While mental health may not have been a priority in the Pakistani culture, the authors do believe the tide is turning.

Values and Customs

The collectivistic nature of Pakistani culture is reflected in its values and customs. Pakistanis value their faith and show honor and respect for their family and their community. Thus, decision making involves considerations beyond the self and includes the effect on the family and broader community. On the other hand, awareness of the patient's values can aid the clinician in validating the patient's interdependent sense of self with their family. The clinician should be cautious in sharing individualistic values to prevent any rupture in rapport.

Common customs reflecting Pakistani values begin with the initial greeting. One will always greet the elders in the room first. While men greet one another physically (e.g., hug), a common greeting can include a handshake or a simple right hand placed over the heart. Men and women may not be comfortable making physical contact (including a handshake) with the opposite sex.[16] Opposite-sex providers should ask permission before physical contact. Customs such as arranged marriages and multigenerational households continue to exist; however, love marriages are increasingly valued, and it is becoming less common to live in the same household as the groom's family. That said, these cultural practices can lead to intergenerational conflict, as well as internal conflict, as one attempts to reconcile traditional and progressive values.

Acculturation and Systemic Barriers

Acculturation in the context of neuropsychology is defined as "the similarity of a client's culture and experiences to, and adoption of, mainstream culture."[18] The level of acculturation has previously been shown to have a direct impact on neuropsychological test performance as these tests are developed to measure Western constructs and values.[19] Objective measures to quantify the level of acculturation exist,[20–22] but few are specific to the Desi culture in the United States.[23] The good news is that level of acculturation can be estimated with a clinical interview. Birman and Simon[24] suggest that one aspect of acculturation is language proficiency. It is notable that children may pick up the dominant language faster than an adult immigrant and integrate it more fully than the adult counterpart. Another method may be to determine to what degree one identifies with their American versus Pakistani identity. Considerations of shifts in behavior such as grocery shopping at an American grocery store or watching English-language television could also be helpful.

While there are cultural barriers preventing appropriate recognition and treatment of psychiatric disorders, the respect Pakistanis feel toward physicians who treat "biological" conditions can be leveraged. As neuropsychologists, we are uniquely qualified to be the bridge between psychology and medicine. One way I (SJL) like to implement this into practice is by rephrasing the patient's presenting concerns into language reflecting brain-behavior relationships.

Health Status

Cardiovascular disease is a significant health concern in the Pakistani population. Relative to other ethnicities in the United States, there is a higher prevalence of risk factors for cardiovascular disease such as obesity, type II diabetes, hypertension, and dyslipidemia, which results in higher rates of myocardial infarction and stroke.[25-29] While South Asians make up approximately 25% of the world's population,[30] they make up 60% of the world's cardiovascular cases (masalastudy.org). Exploring the effects of health on cognition will be important in the Pakistani population.

Approaches to Neuropsychological or Psychological Evaluations

A detailed and culturally sensitive interview is necessary to identify the underlying cognitive and/or psychosocial causes. However, some cultures may feel the process is intrusive and taking time at the start to explain the purpose of the assessment and highlighting the differences between neuropsychology and medicine could be helpful. Reiterating a focus on confidentiality could also reassure the patient that we value their privacy and create a safe space. For example, a young adult may be accompanied by a parent. If the young adult engages in recreational drug use, alcohol consumption, or has a significant other outside of marriage, they may not feel comfortable sharing that information in the presence of a family member. The ECLECTIC framework is a helpful tool to keep in mind during *all* interactions with our patients, but it is particularly useful during the clinical interview.[20]

For those patients with low English fluency, the evaluation may require an interpreter. Interpreters themselves can have an impact on testing and should be utilized carefully for cognitive assessments.[31] Family members should not be interpreters. In working with interpreters, I (SJL) have found taking time prior to the start of the evaluation to acquaint the interpreter has been helpful. The interpreter receives a copy of the forms and is encouraged to take notes. Emphasis is placed on standardization so there is no change in meaning or cognitive load of the test items.

Prior to the start of testing, I consider the cultural and linguistic appropriateness of the measures I have selected. Because there are few cognitive measures translated in Urdu and many lack appropriate normative data for Pakistani populations, it is important to accurately gauge the patient's level of acculturation[32] and English proficiency[33] whether administering in English or with an interpreter. In addition, it is also important to consider familiarity with basic test taking, comfort with the testing environment, and familiarity with paper/pencil versus computer-based tests to data collection is valid. Finally, it is important to identify these limitations in the report. In my experience, reporting my thought processes around test selection and data interpretation has been instrumental in assisting other providers with understanding my conclusions and recommendations.

During the feedback session, patients may expect "prescriptions" for the next steps. This desire to follow doctor's orders may be moderated by the patient's cultural/spiritual beliefs. A sensitive touch may be helpful when delivering a new diagnosis. For example, if diagnosing a family member with Alzheimer's disease, it may be important to specifically outline each family member's role and identify concrete treatment goals. Without such psychoeducation, it may be easier for the family to "leave it up to god."

Regarding specific recommendations, warm hand-offs are advised when possible. For example, if the evaluation requires a referral, the clinician may find it helpful to enter the referral or make the initial phone call for the patient to increase the likelihood of a follow-up. A discussion may be necessary with the patient and/or their family to address the stigma associated with treatment for neuropsychological disorders.

Section II: Case Study — "Racing Heart, Racing Mind"

The patient presented in this case study was seen for a presurgical workup. His information was de-identified and shared with the authors for use as a case example. Potential identifying information was changed to protect the patient's identity.

Relevant Demographics

Mr. Khan was a 62-year-old, right-handed, bilingual (Punjabi primary/native; English secondary) Pakistani male. He immigrated to the northeast region of the United States in the 1980s and has resided there for 24 years. His early education was completed in Pakistan in English and Punjabi; he earned an associate's degree in the United States. He has been gainfully employed and is involved in his community. He was diagnosed with Parkinson's disease (PD) for 11 years and presented for a presurgical evaluation for consideration of deep brain stimulation (DBS) surgery.

Presenting Concerns

Mr. Khan's initial symptoms were typical for PD, and he was successful with Sinemet for ten years. Unfortunately, the disease continued to progress, and he lost his job this year (approximately ten years after being diagnosed). He continues to experience PD-related symptoms. He also endorsed recent occasional shortness of breath and fast/irregular heartbeat. He endorsed difficulties falling asleep, stating his mind wanders and he cannot control his thoughts. He denied other physical or sensory concerns. He denied depression, anxiety, or compulsive behaviors but endorsed occasional low mood, particularly when thinking about his recent job loss and how he may be perceived by his community. He understood the risks and benefits involved with DBS surgery. He reported being independent in all activities of basic and instrumental daily living with the exception of driving, which he stopped three years prior to the evaluation.

Health History

Prior medical history was remarkable for fainting twice over many years and rare postural hypotension. Cardiovascular risk factors included diabetes and mildly elevated blood pressure, which were well controlled. Family history was unremarkable for Parkinsonism or neurodegenerative disorder. Psychiatric history was denied.

Social History

Mr. Khan was a married man with two adult children who lived independently. He did not consume alcohol and rarely smoked cigarettes. His primary role in the community was as the fundraiser at the local mosque.

Behavioral Observations

Mr. Khan arrived alone and was appropriately dressed for the appointment. He primarily spoke English and occasionally conversed in Punjabi. Motor movements were consistent with PD. He was alert and oriented to person, place, time, and situation. No sensory concerns were reported or observed. His comprehension was intact based on his responses during the evaluation. His speech was accented and fluent, with no concerns observed. Speech content was topic specific. His mood was neutral, with a mildly anxious affect. He demonstrated a restricted range of facial expressions. He denied any current hallucination, delusions, suicidal, or homicidal ideations. Overall, Mr. Khan was cooperative, engaged, and appeared to put forth a good effort. Therefore, the attained scores were believed to be an accurate reflection of his current neurocognitive functioning.

Test and Norm Selection

Language dominance was assessed using a semantic fluency measure and obtaining a detailed linguistic history. Results reflected English-language dominance (Animal Naming, Punjabi = 9 Raw vs. Animal Naming, English = 17 Raw). As such, given the widespread availability of English measures and his understanding of the English language, English language-based tests were used. Instructions were translated into Punjabi by a Punjabi-speaking neuropsychologist, as needed. Unfortunately, there were no ideal normative comparisons available, and because these tests are normed on native English speakers that are educated in American schools in English, some scores *may* have underestimated his true abilities. However, every effort was made to interpret the results within the patient's linguistic context.

The test battery included a comprehensive neuropsychological battery typically used for pre-DBS evaluations and included emotional functioning.

Test Results and Impressions

Abbreviated test results and impressions are presented below.

Mr. Khan's performance was intact on a task assessing broad cognitive functioning and he performed in the average range for his age on premorbid estimations of intellectual functioning. Most notably, his performance on tasks assessing language reflected an impoverished English lexicon rather than problems with language, per se. In that context, his performance on the remainder of the neuropsychological battery reflected a pattern consistent with PD. Mr. Khan did not meet criteria for dementia. From a neuropsychological perspective, Mr. Khan was a viable candidate for DBS surgery.

Although his responses on measures of emotional functioning did not reach clinical significance, in our conversation, we were able to connect reports of recent chest pain and difficulty breathing to the negative thoughts related to the recent job loss. His wife was invited to the feedback session and psychoeducation was provided to teach them how to monitor changes to his mood or levels of anxiety. They were provided resources both within and outside of their community to help improve his current mood state and prevent further deterioration.

Notably, he appeared more open to the discussion around mood when a biological link with PD was presented as a potential etiology. As his comfort increased, so did his wife's and she became more involved in the discussion. She noted he was quieter and less physically active but had thought it was best not to comment in order to not upset him further. She had no idea how concerned he had been about the community's reaction to his job loss. She was able to provide examples in the moment that provided an alternative perspective and challenge his negative thoughts. As a result, he had a more balanced perspective. A plan was made to include more pleasant activities in his day and use positive reinforcement when engaged in the community. Had his wife not been present, neither party would have developed insight into the observed changes in mood. Instead, both parties left feeling hopeful and empowered.

In summary, Mr. Khan received culturally sensitive care. His linguistic and educational background were considered to contextualize his neuropsychological functioning and prevent over-pathologizing. Cultural awareness allowed early detection of depressed mood. Finally, the strategic inclusion of a family member in the feedback session allowed recommendations to be made within the patient's cultural context and improve outcomes and compliance with medical recommendations.

Section III: Lessons Learned

- Pakistan is a country rich in history and diversity that is highlighted by the provinces and their respective languages. We hope the information presented in this chapter serves as a primer on Pakistani culture. We also hope to convey the importance of assessing each Pakistani patient as a unique individual with their own belief systems.
- Pakistani immigration patterns are varied, and each immigrant has a unique story that deserves exploration to receive culturally sensitive care.
- Urdu is the official language of Pakistan, but only a minority of Pakistanis speak it as their first language. However, due to a colonial past and potential immigration patterns, English is an important part of Pakistani culture.
- Assessing the level of acculturation and English language proficiency is important. Helpful questions to understand the level of acculturation and language proficiency include asking the number of years they have lived in the English-speaking country, which languages are used frequently, and how English was acquired?
- Effective communication requires an understanding of the meaning behind the patient's words and can aid in building rapport, eliciting accurate information, delivering effective feedback, and increasing recommendation compliance.
- Pakistanis respect medical providers and may avoid asking for clarity. Clinicians should gauge understanding of the information provided.
- If an interpreter is necessary and an Urdu-speaking interpreter is unavailable, a Hindi-speaking interpreter may also be helpful.
- Clinicians should clearly communicate expectations regarding clinic policies as the approach to time varies across cultures.
- Based on varying levels of education and experience with test taking, Desi individuals might not be familiar with the testing environment and may need additional guidance to become more comfortable with the process.
- Religion plays an important role in a Pakistani person's perception of mental health. It is important to be mindful of these beliefs so as to not under/over pathologize and make culturally appropriate recommendations.
- Cultural factors often impact symptom presentation (e.g., presenting with somatic concerns related to mental health difficulties that do not fit within the dominant culture's expectations) and adherence to treatment recommendations. Understanding their experience is influenced by their family, the community, and their faith will help clinicians to provide individualized recommendations.
- In the neuropsychological report, a cultural considerations section that outlines the decision making around test selection, data interpretation, and recommendations may be helpful. This information could help current and future providers to fully appreciate the patient's cultural context.

Acknowledgments

The authors would like to thank Dr. Jasdeep S. Hundal for providing the case study and Ambreen Musani and Sajida Jivani for sharing their insights as two Pakistani immigrants from different provinces.

References

1. The World Bank. Pakistan [Internet]. The World Bank; 2020 [cited 2020 Sep 15]. Available from: https://data.worldbank.org/country/pakistan

2. Hunter R. Education in Pakistan [Internet]. World Education News and Reviews; 2020. Available from: https://wenr.wes.org/2020/02/education-in-pakistan

3. Stein B. A history of India. 2nd ed. Arnold D, editor. West Sussex: Wiley-Blackwell; 2010. p. 466.

4. Talbot I, Singh G. The partition of India. Cambridge, UK: Cambridge University Press; 2009. p. 224 (New Approaches to Asian History).

5. Dalrymple W. The great divide: the violent legacy of Indian Partition [Internet]. The New Yorker; 2015 Jun 22; Available from: https://www.newyorker.com/magazine/2015/06/29/the-great-divide-books-dalrymple

6. An introduction to South Asian American history [Internet]. South Asian American Digital Archive; [cited 2020 Sep 15]. Available from: https://www.saada.org/resources/introduction

7. Moore KM. Pakistani Immigrants. In: Bayor RH, editor. Multicultural America: an encyclopedia of the newest Americans [Internet]. Santa Barbara (CA): Greenwood; 2011. Available from: https://www.religion.ucsb.edu/wp-content/uploads/4148-321-1pass-Pakistani.pdf

8. Pakistanis in the U.S. fact sheet [Internet]. Pew Research Center Social & Demographic Trends; 2017 [cited 2020 Sep 15]. Available from: https://www.pewsocialtrends.org/fact-sheet/asian-americans-pakistanis-in-the-u-s/

9. Population by mother tongue [Internet]. Pakistan Bureau of Statistics; 2006 [cited 2020 Sep 15]. Available from: https://www.pbs.gov.pk/content/population-mother-tongue

10. Sawe BE. Provinces of Pakistan [Internet]. WorldAtlas; 2019 [cited 2020 Sep 15]. Available from: https://www.worldatlas.com/articles/provinces-of-pakistan.html

11. About Pakistani Americans [Internet]. American Pakistan Foundation; [cited 2020 Sep 15]. Available from: https://www.americanpakistan.org/pakistani-americans

12. Díaz-Santos M, Hough S. Cultural competence guidelines for neuropsychology trainees and professionals: working with ethnically diverse individuals. In: Richard Ferraro F, editor. Minority and cross-cultural aspects of neuropsychological assessment: Enduring and emerging trends, 2nd ed. Philadelphia (PA): Taylor & Francis; 2016. p. 11–33. (Studies on neuropsychology, neurology, and cognition.).

13. Ali N, Atkin K, Neal R. The role of culture in the general practice consultation process. Ethn Health. 2006 Nov;11(4):389–408.

14. Zulfiqar K, Gillani DQ. Socio-economic disparities and an imperative for inclusive economic growth in Pakistan. J Res Soc Pak. 2019;56(1):73.

15. Rehman A, Jingdong L, Hussain I. The province-wise literacy rate in Pakistan and its impact on the economy. Pac Sci Rev B Humanit Soc Sci. 2015 Nov 1;1(3):140–4.

16. Evason N, Memon I. Pakistani culture [Internet]; 2016. Available from: https://culturalatlas.sbs.com.au/pakistani-culture/pakistani-culture-core-concepts

17. Disha I, Cavendish JC, King RD. Historical events and spaces of hate: hate crimes against Arabs and Muslims in Post-9/11 America. Soc Prob. 2011 Feb 1;58(1):21–46.

18. Fujii DEM. Conducting a culturally-informed neuropsychological evaluation. Washington (DC): American Psychological Association Press; 2016.

19. Fujii DEM. Developing a cultural context for conducting a neuropsychological evaluation with a culturally diverse client: the ECLECTIC framework. Clin Neuropsychol. 2018;32(8):1356–92.

20. Gim Chung RH, Kim BS, Abreu JM. Asian American multidimensional acculturation scale: development, factor analysis, reliability, and validity. Cultur Divers Ethnic Minor Psychol. 2004;10(1):66.

21. Stephenson M. Development and validation of the Stephenson Multigroup Acculturation Scale (SMAS). Psychol Assess. 2000;12(1):77–88.

22. Anderson J, Moeschberger M, Chen MS, Kunn P, Wewers ME, Guthrie R. An acculturation scale for Southeast Asians. Soc Psychiatry Psychiatr Epidemiol. 1993;28(3):134–41.

23. Ghuman PAS. Acculturation of south Asian adolescents in Australia. Br J Educ Psychol. 2000;70(3):305–16.

24. Birman D, Simon CD. Acculturation research: Challenges, complexities, and possibilities. In: Leong F, editor. APA handbook of multicultural psychology. Washington (DC): American Psychological Association; 2014. p. 207–30.

25. Raza Q, Doak CM, Khan A, Nicolaou M, Seidell JC. Obesity and cardiovascular disease risk factors among indigenous and immigrant Pakistani population: a systematic review. Obes Facts. 2013;6:523–35.

26. Shah AD, Vittinghoff E, Kandula NR, Srivastava S, Kanaya AM. Correlates of pre-diabetes and type 2 diabetes in US South Asians: findings from the Mediators of Atherosclerosis in South Asians Living in America (MASALA) study. Ann Epidemiol. 2015 Feb;25(2):77–83.

27. Gany F, Levy A, Basu P, Misra S, Silberstein J, Bari S et al. Culturally tailored health camps and cardiovascular risk among South Asian immigrants. J Health Care Poor Underserved. 2012 Nov;23(4 Suppl):1–4.

28. Kanaya AM, Kandula N, Herrington D, Budoff MJ, Hulley S, Vittinghoff E et al. Mediators of the Atherosclerosis in South Asian Living in America (MASALA) study: objectives, methods, and cohort description. Clin Cardiol. 2013 Dec;36(12):713–20.

29. Gunarathne A, Patel JV, Gammon B, Gill PS, Hughes EA, Lip GY. Ischemic stroke in South Asians: a review of the epidemiology, pathophysiology, and ethnicity-related clinical features. Stroke. 2009 Jun;40(6):e415–23.

30. Worldometers.info [Internet]. [place unknown]; [cited 2021 Mar 20]. Available from: https://www.worldometers.info/world-population/southern-asia-population/#:~:text=Countries%20in%20Southern%20Asia&text=The%20current%20population%20of%20Southern,among%20subregions%20ranked%20by%20Population

31. Casas R, Guzmán-Vélez E, Cardona-Rodriguez J, Rodriguez N, Quiñones G, Izaguirre B et al. Interpreter-mediated neuropsychological testing of monolingual Spanish speakers. Clin Neuropsychol. 2011 Dec 20 ed. 2012;26(1):88–101.

32. Marin G, Gamba RJ. A new measurement of acculturation for Hispanics: the Bidimensional Acculturation Scale for Hispanics (BAS). Hisp J Behav Sci. 1996;18(3):297–316.

33. Ali S, Elliott L, Biss RK, Abumeeiz M, Brantuo M, Kuzmenka P et al. The BNT-15 provides an accurate measure of English proficiency in cognitively intact bilinguals–a study in cross-cultural assessment. Appl Neuropsychol Adult. 2020;1–13.

South Korean

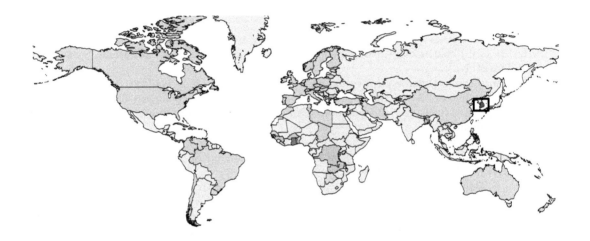

18 Cultural Considerations in the Neuropsychological Assessment of South Koreans

Land of the Morning Calm Meets K-Pop

Dongwook David Lee and Mi-Yeoung Jo

Section I: Background Information

Terminology and Perspective

The Korean language is an East Asian language, spoken by approximately 77 million people. It has been traced to the Altaic language family, which includes the Turkic, Mongolian, and Tungusic language families. The written language (called Hangeul) was created by King Sejong the Great during the **Chosen Dynasty** in the 15th century. Prior to this, the written language in Korea was based on the Chinese language. We (authors) will use the term "Korean(s)" for those who primarily use the Korean language (spoken and/or written) in informal and formal settings. For the purposes of the clinical case presentation, we focus on monolingual Koreans whose English proficiency is limited.

Both authors of this chapter are multilingual, Korean-American neuropsychologists who were born in South Korea. One of the authors (DL) was trained in the southern and midwestern United States and currently practices in an outpatient clinic setting in the southeast. The other author (MJ) was trained in the northeastern United States and currently practices in a private outpatient setting on the West coast.

Geography

The Korean peninsula is located in North-East Asia and divided into North Korea (Democratic People's Republic of Korea) and South Korea (Republic of Korea). The closest neighboring counties are China, Japan, and Russia. South Korea is approximately the size of the US state of Indiana. Korea has four distinct seasons. The biggest city is Seoul (9.73 million in population) and the second largest is the southern port city of Busan (3.43 million). Non-stop travel from the United States to Korea takes approximately 12 hours by plane from the West Coast (Los Angeles) and 14 hours from the East Coast (New York). Many major US cities offer direct flights to Seoul Incheon International Airport, one of the largest and busiest airports in the world.

History

Ancient Korean history began with the establishment of the legendary prehistoric kingdom of Gojoseon in 2333 BCE. Koreans are proud of their long historical heritage ("history of 5,000 years"). Various kingoms appeared and disappeared in the Korean peninsula and surrounding vicinities without much contact with the Western culture until the 19th century. Frequent contacts and

DOI: 10.4324/9781003051862-37

trading with the Western culture can be traced back to the late Chosen Dynasty (1392–1910 CE), whose cultural impact, such as **Confucianism**, still can be felt in many aspects of modern Korean life. After 45 years of Japanese colonial rule (1910–1945), modern Korea was formed when Japan surrendered to the Allies in 1945. Because of the geopolitical interests of the United States and the Soviet Union, Korea was temporarily divided into North and South; this temporary division was consolidated further following the Korean War (1950–1953). The two countries (South which followed the Western model of capitalism and North which followed the model of communism) remained antagonistic after the Korean War. In more recent years, limited trading and cultural exchanges began between the two countries, but the relationship between South and North is still precarious at best. Unless noted separately, "Korea" denotes "South Korea" in this chapter.

People

Koreans are a highly homogeneous ethnic group, which has helped in defining unique cultural values and promoting a strong national identity. On the flip side, this can also contribute to xenophobic attitudes and differential practices toward those that are seen as "other." As Korea becomes a more multicultural society with its recent rise in immigration, there are hints of change, if not outright calls, to challenge the homogeneous mindset in favor of a more contemporary outlook.[1]

There are approximately 52 million South Koreans living on the Korean peninsula as of 2020, and approximately 1.8 million South Koreans living in the United States.[2] Starting in the early 1970s, South Korea began developing into a prosperous capitalistic society and underwent tremendous social and cultural changes. The generational gap between old and young Koreans can be quite significant. The lifestyle and viewpoint of the younger generation can be very similar to that of Western society, while the older generation remains more traditional and conservative in their cultural perspective. Koreans living in the United States can also be quite different in their world views and customs from their counterparts living in Korea.

It is possible for acculturation to the mainstream US culture to be delayed due to the widespread availability of the internet, social media, and mobile devices in the Korean language. Before the age of the internet and smartphones, international phone calls were expensive, and many Koreans living in the United States had no family or relatives locally. Therefore, except for activities in the local Korean communities, there was little exposure to the Korean culture, which forced many Korean immigrants back then to find ways to adapt to their new country faster than they would have otherwise. Nowadays, younger Korean immigrants or visitors are armed with tremendous electronic resources and information in Korean via smartphones that allow them to connect easily with their friends and family. Most information and entertainment in Korea, such as news, music, and movies, are simultaneously accessible in the United States and in Korea. Therefore, if one chooses to, one would not necessarily have to adapt to the American lifestyle or struggle with learning English. This delay in acculturation amid globalization is an ironic phenomenon observed in recent years.

Immigration History

Generally speaking, Korean immigration to the United States can be divided into three major waves that began in 1903 with mostly men who came to the United States as field or farm laborers and settled in Hawaii or the West Coast. The second wave consisted of women who married American soldiers and children adopted into American families. The third wave of Koreans, beginning in the mid-1960s, came under the occupational and family reunification preferences of the Immigration and Naturalization Act of 1965. Many Korean immigrants from the 1970s to 1980s were more educated than previous groups, and there have been a more diverse group of immigrants in recent years, including employees of Korean corporations with US factories. The number of temporary visitors from Korea to the United States has been increasing in recent years due to the VISA Waiver Program implemented in 2008. This program allows South Koreans to travel to the United States for 90 days or less without obtaining a visa. Although most Koreans living in the United States still reside in large Korean immigrant communities in areas such as Los Angeles, New York/New Jersey, Washington, DC/Virginia, Chicago, Seattle, and Atlanta, there are many Koreans who live in small communities throughout the United States.

It is important to note that there are significant variations among Koreans living in the United States. Depending on their initial immigration status (e.g., student vs. business), marriage (e.g., mixed or single ethnicity), and generation (e.g., 1st vs. 2nd generation), worldviews and value systems can be very different. There are also large individual differences among those who were not born in the United States, depending on when they immigrated (e.g., 1970 vs. 2010) and where they were in their stage of life at the time of immigration (e.g., before teenage vs. late adulthood). Additionally, those who were born and grew up in Korean families in the United States have unique qualities and cultural viewpoints compared to other Koreans who were born in Korea and moved to the United States.

Language

The modern Korean educational system includes English as a major subject, and it is expected that most Koreans born after the 1960s achieve a certain level of proficiency in the English language. However, the emphasis is primarily on spelling, reading, and grammar; therefore, many Koreans may not be fluent in speaking and writing. This may lead to a false sense of English proficiency among Korean patients if the clinician just uses performance from a word reading or sentence comprehension measure. It is possible that a patient may not have difficulty following written instructions but may struggle to understand simple oral instructions. It is also important for clinicians to understand that a patient's reliance on an interpreter does not necessarily mean that he/she does not comprehend English at all. In fact, it is possible that the patient follows and understands much of the communication between the clinician and the interpreter. Despite this, the patient may still choose to use an interpreter because he/she is not comfortable speaking English, particularly when having to convey complex medical issues. An interpreter may also be accepted out of respect to the clinician.

There are local variations in the Korean language called "satoori," which can include unique local phrases/words, pronunciations, and accents (similar to the southern accent in the United States). When arranging for an interpreter, it could be useful to request one who understands a particular local satoori for the patient. However, this may not be necessary because most satoori are mild regional variations that most Koreans would be able to understand.

Literacy and Education

Korea's literacy rate in 1945 was one of the lowest in the world (22%), but this changed dramatically with the industrialization and modernization of the country. It reached 98.3% in 2008.[3] The simplicity of the Korean alphabet contributes to the high literacy rate, but at the same time, it also prevents development of a reading test to measure premorbid functioning due to its lack of silent letters. While complete illiteracy among Koreans is rare nowadays, it is possible to encounter older Koreans who may not have complete command of reading and writing in Korean.

As the country became more modernized and economically developed, a stronger emphasis was placed on education. With the increase in household income and improvement in socio-economic status, mere survival ceased to be the main issue for many families. Parents poured enormous resources into educating their children, with the primary aim of obtaining a degree from a prestigious college. For most families in Korea, a college degree from a prestigious institution is the guaranteed path to occupational opportunities and success. Academic excellence supersedes every aspect of a student's life. The over-emphasis on education in recent decades could provide important information in a clinical evaluation. If a patient in her 40s reports that she did not finish high school, this can be clinically meaningful and may deserve further inquiry. Since dropping out of school without a high school diploma is rare in modern Korea, this may mean a significant personal life event. Currently, the school system in Korea consists of 12 years of compulsory education: elementary school (1st to 6th grades), middle school (7th to 9th grades), and high school (10th to 12th grades). English is one of the primary subjects taught beginning in middle school; however, most students receive some type of English education starting in their early years from a for-profit private institution ("hagwon"). Hagwon is very prevalent in Korea, and it is equivalent to the Sylvan Learning Center or Kumon in the United States.

Korea has an international reputation for having a high-quality educational system, and it consistently ranks among the best in the world.[4] Practitioners in the United States can be assured that the educational practices within the Korean educational system are comparable to the United States minimizing threats to test validity when utilizing Western assessment approaches with Korean-speaking patients.

Socio-Economic Status

Korea's socio-economic status has changed rapidly in the past half-century, and South Korea's economy is now the 12th largest in the world. While there are still disparities between rich and poor, the majority of Koreans do not worry about daily food supplies and safe shelter. The older generation went through tremendous socio-economic and political changes in their lifetime, whereas the younger generation mostly lived in a rather stable and economically established society. The typical lifestyle of younger generation Koreans is not much different from those in the United States.

The perception of the general public in the United States toward Korea has evolved significantly over the past decade. Because of products from large Korean companies, such as automobiles, smartphones, and electric gadgets, as well as influence from the Korean entertainment industry (*K-Pop*), past memories from the Korean War have been replaced with vastly different modern images. It is very common to see Korea depicted as a poor, underdeveloped, farming country in US movies from the 1980s, but this is no longer true. Travelers to Korea often comment that they are impressed by both the traditional and modern cultures coexisting side by side in Korean society.

Values and Customs

As with other Asian cultures, Koreans traditionally value honor, loyalty, humility, and a collectivistic attitude. Family is considered more important than the individual in general. Although Koreans value family, community, and peer groups more than those from Western cultures, it is important to recognize that there is a wide range of differences among Koreans in their worldviews. While extended families (e.g., three or more generations living together) still exist, the composition of the modern Korean family typically includes only two generations (parents and children). Aging parents could live in proximity of other family members, and extended families often exchange visits during major holidays, such as Chuseok (Korean Thanksgiving) and Seolnal (New Year's Day).

Elders are respected in the family and community, and Koreans use specific language/terms to relate to their elders or social superiors. The Korean language includes numerous terms and expressions to reflect the hierarchical social structure. Elders, teachers, doctors, and bosses are treated with respect, and juniors/younger people carefully choose their language and demeanor in interactions. To call a superior by their first name is culturally inappropriate. Bowing is the primary way to greet someone, followed by a handshake. Typically, a person with lower social status bows first, and they are expected to use both hands for handshakes. Direct eye contact is considered impolite and rude, particularly when interacting with someone with higher social status. Hugging is not a norm but is allowed among very close friends, spouses, and family members. While Koreans are generally humble and reserved in interactions with superiors or those they are unfamiliar with, they can be very friendly, boisterous, and social with friends and family.

It was not unusual in earlier times in Korea to register a newborn after their actual birthdate, sometimes months or even years after. Reasons for this include the high infant mortality rate in the past and availability of local resources for registering the child's birth on time. Koreans also traditionally consider a newborn child to be one year of age at birth (to account for the nine months spent in the womb), and to further confuse matters, some Koreans follow both solar and lunar calendars when keeping track of their birthdates. Because the difference of even one year can have an impact on the choice of norms and clinical decision-making, it is important to clarify the date of birth as part of the initial evaluation process with an older Korean patient.

Gender and Sexuality

Traditionally, gender roles in Korean society followed the stereotypical expectations of men working in the field and taking care of business ("outside") and women raising children, preparing meals, and maintaining the home ("inside"). Married couples even referred to each other as the "person for outside" and the "person for inside." The traditional roles of women in the family have evolved as Korean society has developed and become more Westernized. While older women tend to be conservative, younger women are more vocal in challenging restrictive and conservative gender stereotypes. In 2001, the Korean government established the Ministry of Gender Equality to promote women's policy and advance women's rights and status, which later changed to the Ministry of Gender Equality and Family in 2010.

Sexuality is a complex subject in Korean culture and is typically not discussed openly in public. Large generational gaps between conservative (traditional) and liberal (modern) views exist on the topic of sexuality. Discussions about sexual activities or sexual health can be difficult even in clinical settings, particularly for older patients. Views on issues such as prostitution and homosexuality/LGBTQ are heavily influenced by Confucian traditions. Same-sex marriage is not recognized in Korea. According to the *Organisation for Economic Cooperation and Development* **(OECD)**, Korea lags behind other countries when it comes to the acceptance of homosexuality.[5] Very recently, Korean television dramas and shows have started to include LGBTQ characters into the storylines, which would have been unheard of even a few years ago, reflecting changes in public views of LGBTQ issues.

Religion

Based on the 2015 national census, 56% of Koreans reported no formal affiliation with organized religion. However, many still observe traditional Buddhist and **shamanic shamanism** based practices. Nowadays, native shamanistic beliefs and ideals of Confucianism coexist with formal religions in the form of cultural practices rather than as organized religions. Buddhism (16%) and Christianity (Catholics—8%, Protestants—20%) are now the dominant formal religions in Korea. A minority of Koreans (less than 1%) practice Islam, Taoism, and other religions. The influence of Christianity in Korea became noticeable starting in the 19th century and grew rapidly from the mid- to late 20th century. In recent years, however, the number of Christians has declined due to growing public criticism against Christians on various social and religious issues.

Many Koreans living in the United States have strong affiliations with Protestantism (71%)[6] and attend church regularly. It has been suggested that the responsiveness of Christian churches to immigrants' needs, their communal nature, as well as social pressure from other Koreans are the main reasons for the high affiliation. Many Korean churches have English ministry for mostly second-generation Koreans who may not be fluent in Korean. The church is influential in daily life for many Koreans living in the United States and meets the various social and ethnic needs of its congregants, including providing Korean language education for children as well as providing a sense of identity and belonging.

Healthcare and Mental Health Views

Westernized medicine is the primary healthcare practice among Koreans; however, Eastern medicine is still popular among older Koreans. Practitioners of Eastern medicine in Korea, referred to as Hanbang, receive post-graduate/doctoral training, equivalent to that of Western medicine. Acupuncture, herbs, and **cupping** are common treatment modalities. Both Western and Eastern medicine approaches are respected, and it is not uncommon for older Korean patients to use both to treat or manage medical conditions.

Family members, such as adult children of older patients, may accompany the patient to an evaluation, particularly if the patient's English is limited. Because of reluctance to discuss culturally sensitive matters (e.g., mental health issues, sexuality, etc.), a separate interview with the children could yield more detailed and valid information. Depending on family dynamics, English proficiency, and the patient's preference, multiple sessions (with/without family members) may be necessary to gather more complete background information.

The health care system in Korea is considered among the best in the world. It is a universal and government-mandated single-payer system that provides coverage for the entire nation. In Korea, hospitals are usually equipped with modern diagnostic technologies (e.g., CT and MRI) and access to care and patient satisfaction is generally high.

There is significant stigma regarding mental health issues in Korea. Much of this comes from influences from Confucianism, where hard work, individual will, and self-discipline are emphasized. Seeking mental health treatment is generally considered dishonorable in the Korean culture. The homogeneous cultural mindset discussed earlier can also contribute to the shame and stigma of mental health concerns. Some reports indicate that less than 10% of those affected by mental illness seek psychiatric help. The universal health coverage affords medication and other treatments for mental illness for the majority of Koreans, but stigma often discourages individuals and families from utilizing this aspect of their healthcare coverage. In the past ten years or so, Korea has seen its suicide rate skyrocket, and it now ranks first among the OECD countries. Koreans are under significant stress from a young age because of academic, social, and cultural pressures. Data from the Health Ministry shows that mental illness, particularly depression, is the most significant cause of suicides in Korea.

Neuropsychology in Korea

The first neuropsychology laboratory in Korea was established in 1994 at the Department of Neurology of Samsung Medical Center. With increased awareness, understanding, and acceptance of the importance of psychological principles in promoting one's well-being in Korean society and with government support for brain research, neuropsychology in Korea has enjoyed much growth since its beginnings in the early 1990s. There are formal, university-based training programs in clinical psychology, through which one has the opportunity to specialize in neuropsychology. While the number of professionals involved in neuropsychology in Korea is steadily growing, those who can be identified as neuropsychologists (50% or greater time in practice, teaching, and/or research) still remain quite low when compared to the United States. Nevertheless, Korean neuropsychologists actively conduct research and regularly publish in well-respected scientific journals. There are multiple neuropsychological measures that have either been translated into Korean from the US version or have been developed and standardized for the Korean population. Considering its relatively short history, neuropsychology in Korea has seen much advancement in the past 20–30 years. With the increasing demand for neuropsychological services in Korea, there is much promise for continued growth and advancement of the field in the country.[7]

Section II: Case Study — "I Have No Plans to Retire"

Note: Identifying information and some aspects of history and presentation have been changed to protect patient identity and privacy.

Reason for Referral

Mr. Park was referred for neuropsychological evaluation by his neurologist after suffering a mild right-sided stroke with residual left hemiparesis four months prior to the evaluation. He had been hospitalized for eight days and then released home to the care of his wife.

Mr. Park's official medical record indicated that he was 79 years old, but he reported during the clinical interview that his real birthday was one year earlier, which made his actual age 80 years instead of 79 years. This information was taken into account when selecting tests with appropriate norms.

Behavioral Observation

Mr. Park arrived early with his wife and son for his appointment. Arriving early is the norm for many Korean patients and conveys respect for the doctor and his/her time. Mr. Park was personable and cooperative. He and his wife expressed appreciation for being able to speak to a clinician who was fluent in their preferred language, and this appeared to facilitate positive rapport quickly. Mr. Park walked slowly with a three-point cane. He had left-sided weakness and was observed not to use his left hand during testing. Mr. Park spoke fluently and was able to express himself in Korean without difficulty, but he tended to be quiet and allowed his family to speak for him during the clinical interview. When he did participate in the interview, he was observed to be forgetful and repetitive at times. For example, he asked the examiner's name a few times, sometimes just minutes after being told. During the mental status exam, Mr. Park was unable to recall the date or place correctly. Mr. Park reported his mood to be "okay," but his affect was observed to be flat. He was slow to initiate tasks at times and required prompts or cues. He tended to give up easily. Other times, he was impulsive and attempted to start tasks before instructions were given. Instructions had to be repeated at times. He complained of fatigue after approximately two hours of testing, consistent with behavioral observation, but was agreeable to continue to complete the evaluation.

Presenting Concerns

Mr. Park initially denied any significant cognitive problems but later acknowledged that he could not remember things as well as he used to. He and his wife owned a dry-cleaning business, and he was still involved in overseeing the finances of the business. Mr. Park's family reported that his memory had worsened since his stroke, and he was also slower overall to speak and respond. Mr. Park had not driven since his stroke but expressed a strong desire to resume driving. Physically, he reported weakness in both legs, especially on the left. He fell at home after his stroke and started using a cane after that. His family had noticed that he was physically slower with "everything" and also seemed to have decreased energy. Mr. Park was receiving physical therapy and weekly acupuncture treatment at the time of the evaluation, with reports of some improvement as a result. He was also taking traditional Korean herbal medicine.

Daily Functioning

Mr. Park and his wife lived by themselves in an apartment building. Mr. Park was able to manage all basic self-care activities without assistance. He had a shower chair installed after his stroke for fall prevention. As is typical in traditional Korean families, Mr. Park's wife did all the cooking and cleaning, as well as management of household finances. Mr. Park was managing his own medications. Socially, Mr. Park was still meeting with friends regularly, mostly from church. He and his wife attended church weekly, and they cited religion as an important part of their daily life.

Health History

Mr. Park reported that he was healthy as a child. He developed diabetes in his 30s, presently managed with diet and medication. He had otherwise been in good health prior to his stroke. Mr. Park did not report a preference for traditional vs. non-traditional medicine approaches and had been utilizing both since his stroke (herbal medicine, acupuncture, physical therapy, neurology follow-ups). Mr. Park had a significant family history of stroke. Both his parents died from stroke-related complications in their mid- to late 80s.

Educational and Occupational History

Mr. Park completed high school and college in Korea. He reported that he was a good student and did well in school. He studied accounting and worked as an accountant in Korea prior to immigrating to the United States in his 40s. In the United States, Mr. Park owned a small fashion shop for a few years before purchasing a dry-cleaning business. He and his wife managed the business together. Mr. Park had started to cut back his work hours prior to his stroke, with one of his children helping out as needed. Mr. Park stated that he still did not have any plans for retirement, and it was his intention to return to work once he recovered from his stroke.

Language Proficiency

Mr. Park completed all of his formal education in Korea. While he had been in the United States since his 40s and had conversational fluency in English, Korean was his preferred language. It was the language that he used almost exclusively at home and when socializing with friends. As such, evaluation procedures were selected that would minimize bias due to cultural and language factors.

Cultural History

Mr. Park was born and raised in Seoul, South Korea, as the oldest of eight children. As the eldest son in a traditional Korean family, Mr. Park would have enjoyed the privileges that came with this position, but he also would have had many expectations and burdens and would have functioned essentially as another parental figure to his siblings. This early role appeared to continue to influence him even into the present as he was recovering from his stroke. As head of household, he saw his primary role as being the provider, and hence, he had no plans to retire and intended on returning to work when he could.

Mr. Park and his wife immigrated to the United States in the early 1980s. His cultural outlook and mindset were still primarily traditionally Korean, but in his almost 40 years of living in the United States, Mr. Park appeared to have found a good balance between keeping to his Korean traditions and assimilating into the larger mainstream culture, as evidenced by his successful work history in the United States and his use of both traditional and non-traditional health care approaches.

Emotional Functioning

Mr. Park denied any mood symptoms. His family also agreed with this initially and stated that they had not noticed any depression or anxiety. However, further questioning revealed more mood symptoms than what Mr. Park or his family had initially been willing to acknowledge. When mood difficulties were normalized in the context of his recent stroke, Mr. Park opened up and admitted that he had been more easily tearful than before. His family also added that he seemed more emotional and sensitive than what was typical for him. They also reported noticing some apathy with certain hobbies he used to enjoy, such as *baduk* (Korean board strategy game). When his family mentioned this, Mr. Park admitted that playing *baduk* was more cognitively difficult now than before his stroke.

Preliminary Formulation

Cognitive/neurological sequelae related to Mr. Park's recent stroke were expected, but the presence of a mood disorder as a sequela not just of the neurological event but of post-stroke adjustment difficulties moderated by cultural variables was also considered. Considerations were made that this may have resulted in minimization of mood problems and denial or unawareness of the contributions of mood to post-stroke adjustment and recovery for Mr. Park and his family.

A neuropsychological test battery that could assess Mr. Park's cognitive and emotional functioning in a culturally fair manner was selected and administered.

Test and Norm Selection

A battery of tests that could be administered in Korean was selected. Test instruments included several neuropsychological instruments from Korea, as well as several US-developed neuropsychological measures.

1 Korean Mini-Mental Status Exam (MMSE-KC, from the CERAD neuropsychological assessment battery).
2 Korean Elderly Memory Disorder Scale (EMS).[8] The EMS is a battery of tests that assesses verbal and visual memory, auditory and visual attention/working memory, naming skills, and visual-spatial ability. It is similar to the Repeatable Battery for the Assessment of Neuropsychological Status (RBANS).[9] For clinicians practicing in the United States without

access to the EMS, translating the US RBANS subtests may be an acceptable substitute based on the authors' experience. However, usual caveats apply in terms of acknowledging the limitations of the normative database and introduction of possible errors when translating tests, particularly language-based tests. As an alternate to translating the verbal list learning test from the RBANS, the Korean Auditory Verbal Learning Test is available.[10]

3 Korean Wechsler Adult Intelligence Scale-IV (K-WAIS-IV).[11] The K-WAIS-IV is modeled after the US version and has all the same subtests. The US WAIS-IV performance-based measures and norms may be appropriate to use for an older Korean patient based on the authors' experience.

4 Korean Stroop Color-Word Test for Senior.[12] The procedures for the Korean version of the Stoop Color-Word Test are the same as the Golden version of the Stroop test.

5 Brief Visuospatial Memory Test-Revised.[13]

6 Color Trails Test 1 and 2.[14] As an alternative to Color Trails, Trail Making A and B with the English alphabet can be used for Korean patients with 13 or more years of education.[15]

7 Line Orientation and Semantic Fluency subtests from the RBANS.

8 Grooved Pegboard Test.[16]

9 Category Fluency: Animal fluency; Tombaugh et al. (1999) norms, which are stratified by age and education, were used with Mr. Park.[17] Older adult Korean norms for category fluency and letter fluency have been published, which were unavailable to the examiner at the time of Mr. Park's assessment.[18,19]

10 Wisconsin Card Sort Test-64.[20]

11 Korean Beck Anxiety Inventory (same cut-off scores as the US version).[21]

12 Geriatric Depression Scale[22]—Korean translation (same cut-off scores used in the United States).

Test Results and Impression

Mr. Park's premorbid level of functioning was estimated to have been in the average range based on his educational and occupational history. His test results revealed mildly impaired mental status, including impaired orientation to date and place. Additional deficits were found in memory, visual-spatial skills, processing speed, aspects of executive functioning (cognitive flexibility, problem solving), and left-sided fine motor control. Despite these deficits, there was no evidence of decline in intellectual functioning from baseline levels based on his K-WAIS-IV scores. Mr. Park obtained very strong scores on measures of auditory attention/working memory. He scored at expected levels on measures of visual attention/working memory, reasoning, and response inhibition.

Mr. Park did not endorse any significant mood symptoms on formal mood measures, but given clinical observations as well as his and his family's reports during the clinical interview, it was determined that Mr. Park had a mild mood disorder secondary to post-stroke adjustment difficulties characterized by increased emotionality, increased sensitivity, mild anxiety, and mild apathy.

Mr. Park was still independent with basic and instrumental daily living activities and was given diagnoses of Mild Vascular Neurocognitive Disorder and Unspecified Adjustment Disorder. Recommendations were made for cognitive rehabilitation, with the acknowledgment that this may be difficult to access for an individual like Mr. Park, given the language barrier. Individual and family counseling with a Korean-speaking therapist were also recommended, as well as considerations for future consultation with a Korean-speaking psychiatrist for medication management if mood symptoms persisted.

Feedback Session and Follow-Up

The feedback session was held with Mr. Park, his wife, and his son. Mr. Park and his family were not surprised to hear about his cognitive deficits but were relieved to hear that he did not have dementia, which is something they had all feared. Education was provided about stroke-related symptoms and the stroke recovery process, which was information they had not received previously from any of the other doctors they had seen. Mr. Park and his family were also not surprised at the mood diagnosis as that was something they had suspected even though they had initially denied any mood difficulties. A discussion ensued of the importance of addressing mood issues and how this could affect the recovery process, which they seemed to understand and appreciate. While open to this discussion, Mr. Park and his family still appeared to receive the recommendation for counseling with some hesitation, indicating that their faith was what they preferred to turn to. It was left as an option for them to consider for the future, which they were agreeable to. They expressed appreciation that Korean-speaking counselors were available in their community. We also discussed the issue of retirement in the context of minimizing stress going forward. Mr. Park was receptive to the idea of retiring and acknowledged that it might be time for him to step back and allow his family to help. Getting reassurance from a medical professional appeared to help Mr. Park give himself "permission" to step back. His son reiterated support for the idea of retiring, adding that he and his siblings would be there to help out as needed. The importance of pursuing healthy lifestyle habits was also emphasized. A follow-up evaluation in approximately one year was also recommended, and Mr. Park and his family were agreeable. In the end, they again expressed their gratitude for being able to work with a clinician who could communicate with them in their preferred language.

Section III: Lessons Learned

- It is important to recognize that there is a wide range of differences among Koreans living in the United States. Worldviews and value systems can be very different depending on one's generation, age, time of immigration, immigration status, profession/career, birthplace, and religion, among others.
- Given the unique values and customs among Koreans, a cultural broker can be helpful for clinical evaluations in understanding various socio-economic, cultural, and linguistic factors. A cultural broker can be a local psychologist/clinician or a community member who can provide advice and guidance regarding Korean social and cultural practices, which can influence clinical outcomes.
- Elders, parents, doctors, and teachers hold positions of respect in Korean society. Patients and families appreciate it when a doctor (neuropsychologist) spends extra time to listen to their stories, review test results, and provide recommendations.
- There has been a lot more acceptance of the importance of mental health in the Korean community, but much stigma still remains, particularly in the older, more traditional generation. Rather than asking direct questions such as "Are you depressed?" asking questions such as "Are you stressed?" or "What worries you?" or normalizing it in the context of a medical condition may yield more information about mood.
- Religion, especially Christianity, plays an important role in many Korean families in the United States. Many Koreans forgo recommendations for formal counseling in favor of seeking out church elders, praying, and/or reading the Bible.
- The language barrier continues to limit access to counseling and rehabilitation programs for many Koreans, especially those of the older generation. More research, funding, and culturally competent clinicians are needed to bridge the gap.

- Norms developed in South Korea may not be the most accurate for a Korean individual who has been living in the United States for most of his/her adult life. Having separate norms for Koreans living in the United States vs. Koreans living in Korea would be ideal. None are available currently, to the authors' knowledge, but this would be an important area for future research.
- While there are Korean tests and norms commercially available, they can be difficult for general US practitioners to gain access to. Further research into more appropriate norms and methodology are necessary to meet the needs of an increasing Korean-speaking population in the United States.

Glossary

Chosen Dynasty (also transcribed as Choson or Joseon). The Chosen Dynasty was a Korean dynastic kingdom in the Korean peninsula that lasted for five centuries (1392–1897). It was founded by the military commander Yi Seong-Gye after the Goryeo Dynasty. He established the capital at Hanyang (now Seoul) and allied himself with a group of reform-minded Confucian scholars. Teachings of Confucius became the guiding principles of the government as well as the general public, rather than the Buddhism of the Goryeo Dynasty. The legacy of the Chosen Dynasty can still be felt in many areas of modern Korean life, including language, cultural norms, social roles/expectations, and family life. The kingdom lasted until it became the Korean Empire in 1897, which was later colonized by Japan in 1910.

Confucianism. Confucianism is a system of philosophical and ethical teachings, founded by Confucius in the 6th century BCE and further developed by Mencius in the 3rd century BCE in China. It is considered a religion by some and a social and ethical code by others. Confucianism believes that human beings are inherently good, and it advocates strict ethical codes and rituals to achieve peace and prosperity in life. While the influence of Confucianism decreased over the past decades, it can still be felt in many aspects of life in Korea, such as close family ties, respect for the elderly and teachers, hierarchical social interactions, and stereotypical gender roles.

Cupping. Cupping is a practice in Eastern medicine that involves placing cups on the skin of the patient. By warming the air within the cup, a vacuum is created, and the skin is drawn up into the cup. The major benefit of cupping is increased blood flow and loosening of connective tissue. Cups are typically placed on the back, neck, and shoulders. It is similar to a deep tissue massage.

K-Pop. K-Pop refers to Korean popular music that originated in South Korea. K-Pop music in its current form started in the 1990s and was popularized in the 2000s. It includes genres of rock, hip hop, rap, and electronic music. K-Pop idols are groups of young artists and musicians, typically formed by entertainment companies. These idols often begin their career in their teens and train for years to become a member of an idol group. K-Pop melodies are simple and catchy, with perfectly in-sync choreographies. K-Pop idols often enjoy megastar status with their physically fit physique, attractive appearance, and unique styles.

OECD. The Organisation for Economic Co-operation and Development (OECD) is an international organization with 37 member countries. It was founded in 1962 to promote world trade and to build better policies. OECD members consist of high-income countries and are considered as developed countries. It publishes influential economic data and evaluations/rankings of member countries, although it does not have the power to enforce its decisions. The headquarters is located in Paris.

Shamanism. Shamanism is not tied to any single culture or religion. The religious practice involves a shaman who is believed to have special powers to interact with souls or spirits and influence them. One of the common beliefs in shamanism is that everything/everyone is inter-connected. Evidence of shamanistic practices has been found in Scandinavia, Siberia, Mongolia, Korea, Japan, China, Inuit, and First Nations tribes of North America.

References

1. Kim-Bossard M. Challenging homogeneity in contemporary Korea. EAA. 2018;23(2):38–41.
2. Pew Research Center. Social & demographic trends: Koreans in the U.S. Fact Sheet [Internet]. 2015. Available from: https://www.pewresearch.org/social-trends/fact-sheet/asian-americans-koreans-in-the-u-s/#korean-population-in-the-u-s-2000-2015
3. National Institute of Korean Language, Republic of Korea. Literacy Rate Report (in Korean). 2008. Available from: https://www.korean.go.kr/front/board/boardStandardView.do?board_id=6&mn_id=19&b_seq=208
4. Pearson. New global education index shows Asian superpowers excel in learning [Internet]. 2014. Available from: https://www.pearson.com/news-and-research/announcements/2014/05/new-global-educationindexshowsasiansuperpowersexcelinlearning.html
5. Organisation for Economic Cooperation and Development (OECD). Society at a glance—OECD social indicators [Internet]. 2019. Available from: https://www.oecd.org/publications/society-at-a-glance-19991290.htm
6. Pew Research Center. Religion & public life: Asian Americans: a mosaic of faiths [Internet]. 2012. Available from: https://www.pewforum.org/2012/07/19/asian-americans-a-mosaic-of-faiths-religious-affiliation/
7. Kim M, Chey J. Clinical neuropsychology in South Korea. Clin Neuropsychol. 2016;30(8):1325–34.
8. Choi JY. Elderly memory disorder scale. Seoul: Hakjisa; 2007.
9. Randolph C. Repeatable battery for the assessment of neuropsychological status. San Antonio, TX: The Psychological Corporation; 1998.
10. Cheong SS, Woo JM, Kim E, Yeon BK, Hong KS. Development of Korean auditory verbal learning test. J Korean Neuropsychiatr Assoc. 1999;38(5):1016–25.
11. Whang ST, Kim JH, Park KB, Chey JY, Hong SW. Korean Wechsler Adult Intelligence Scale-IV. Daegu: Korea Psychology Corporation; 2012.
12. Lee DY, Suh EH. Korean Stroop Color-Word Test for senior. Seoul: Hakjisa; 2016.
13. Benedict RH. Brief Visuospatial Memory Test-revised. Lutz (FL): Psychological Assessment Resources; 1997.
14. D'Elia L, Satz P, Uchiyama CL, White T. Color Trails Test. Odessa (FL): Psychological Assessment Resources; 1996.
15. Jang J, Kim K, Baek M, Kim S, Jang J. A comparison of five types of trail making test in Korean elderly. Dement Neurocogn Disord. 2016;15(4):135–41.
16. Klove H. Clinical neuropsychology. In: Forster FM, editor. The medical clinics of North America. New York (NY): WB Saunders; 1963.
17. Tombaugh TN, Kozak J, Rees L. Normative data stratified by age and education for two measures of verbal fluency: FAS and animal naming. Arch Clin Neuropsychol. 1999;14(2):167–77.
18 Ryu SH, Kim KW, Kim S, Park JH, Kim TH, Jeong HG et al. Normative study of the category fluency test (CFT) from nationwide data on community-dwelling elderly in Korea. Arch Gerontol Geriatr. 2012;54(2):305–9.
19 Kim BJ, Lee CS, Oh BH, Hong CH, Lee KS, Son SJ et al. A normative study of lexical verbal fluency in an educationally-diverse elderly population. Psychiatry Invest. 2013;10(4):346–51.
20. Kongs SK, Thompson LL, Iverson GL, Heaton RK. Wisconsin Card Sorting Test-64 card version. Lutz (FL): Psychological Assessment Resources; 2000.
21. Kim JH, Lee EH, Hwang ST, Hong SH. Korean-beck anxiety inventory. Daegu: Korea Psychology Corporation; 2014.
22. Yesavage JA, Brink TL, Rose TL, Huang V, Adey M, Leirer VO. Development and validation of a geriatric depression screening scale: a preliminary report. J Psychiatr Res. 1982;17(1):37–49.

Taiwanese

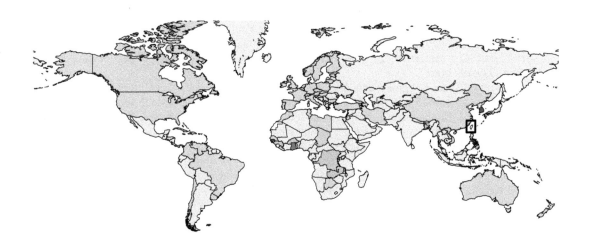

19   Taiwan—The Island That Embraces the Pan Chinese Culture

June Yu Paltzer

Section I: Background Information

This chapter focuses on the most pertinent topics in neuropsychological assessment conducted by a US-trained neuropsychologist with a Taiwanese/Taiwanese-American examinee.

Terminology and Perspective

People from Taiwan, home of the 2023 INS mid-year conference, are referred to as Taiwanese, though a heterogenous group is represented. For the purpose of this chapter, identification as Taiwanese is established through self-assessment. Many residents in Taiwan are originally from mainland China due to the 1949 mass exodus. Depending on whose research you read, a high number of inter-marriages between the native Taiwanese and Chinese is present.[1] Many families have been regularly touring back and forth between Taiwan and China since 1987, when such travel became permissible.

I am a grateful Taiwan-born Chinese daughter of now retired diplomats who are ethnically Chinese. While I grew up in various countries, my parents and grandparents instilled in me strong Chinese cultural values. On a daily basis, I continue to listen, speak, think, read and write in Chinese at the most advanced level. More will be discussed in the Language section below regarding the written language which unites Chinese (including the Taiwanese) people, as well as the importance of reading and writing in the Pan Chinese culture.

Geography

Taiwan is an island country off the southeastern coast of China. In the 1500s, Portuguese sailors discovered this island and named it "Formosa," which means "beautiful" (island). If Taiwan were one of the United States, it would be the third largest by population at 23 million: smaller than California and Texas but larger than New York or Florida. By economic output (GDP), Taiwan would fall behind California, Texas, and New York, but ahead of each of the other states in the United States. By area, Taiwan would be the 42nd largest state, larger than only relatively small states like Maryland, Hawaii, and Massachusetts. Taiwan is about 7,000 miles from California, so flying there from the United States takes just about a full day. The subtropical climate is similar to Hawaii and ideal for growing colorful fruits, vegetables, and tea. If you visit Taiwan's capital city of Taipei, you must see the vibrant Taipei 101 building, currently the world's 11th tallest building (and formerly the world's tallest from 2004 to 2010). Email me if you are disappointed by the food inside Taipei 101.

DOI: 10.4324/9781003051862-39

History

It is a daunting task to write a good summary of Taiwan's history. I will focus on people and topics most likely to be encountered in a neuropsychological assessment in the United States.

As early as 220 AD, Taiwan was explored, occupied, or governed at different time periods by some of the following groups: The Three Kingdoms (between the transition from the Han to the Jin Dynasty), the Dutch, the Portuguese, the Aborigines (aka the indigenous High-Mountain group), the Hoklo from China's Fujian province, the Hakka Hans, the Japanese, soldiers and followers of the Nationalist Party who retreated to the island around 1949, and finally new immigrants from South-Eastern Asia and elsewhere since the 1990s. Taiwanese people have long embraced many adventures, challenges, traditions, and influences. Please forgive me if I did not include a group that is personally significant to you.

The more recent Taiwanese history is as follows. Taiwan became the first colony of Japan after the defeat of the Qing in the Sino-Japanese war of 1895. This led to a 50-year occupation by Japan from approximately 1895 to 1945. As a colony of Japan, Taiwan participated in World War II, with Taiwanese men being conscripted into the Japanese military. When Japan surrendered at the end of World War II, Taiwan was formally placed under the governance of the new leadership there. However, the United States was active in the reconstruction of both Taiwan and Japan and temporarily provided governance ostensibly until China could take control.

In 1949, the then dominating political party in China, known as the Kuomintang (the Chinese Nationalist Party), was defeated by the Communist Party and forced to move to Taiwan. Using my family as an example, my maternal grandparents and their then seven-year-old child, my mother, followed the leaders of the Nationalist Party and moved to a small city near Taipei. My father's family had more involvement in the Chinese civil wars and separated from each other earlier in mainland China. My father survived and entered a foreign language school that later helped him to enter the Taiwan diplomatic corps. Strong work ethic, value on doing (vs. speaking), and family pride pushed my parents to work hard. This is consistent with Chinese philosophy and history of many growing up in Taiwan: "There shall be no impossibility if one works diligently" (一勤天下无难事).

In 1979, the United States opened diplomatic relations with the People's Republic of China (PRC) as there was a heightened sense of concern over the growing threat of the nuclear super-power that was the USSR. It was then that the United States recognized the PRC's claim to Taiwan officially, and United States relations with Taiwan transitioned to informal and unofficial. However, the United States has continued to trade with Taiwan and has routinely sold military defense equipment to Taiwan to enable Taiwan to maintain a sufficient self-defense capability. Today Taiwan is effectively governed as an independent country, known as the Republic of China (ROC), while the PRC still considers Taiwan to be part of its "One China."

Values and Customs

Readers are reminded that the main goal of this chapter is to assist the interested neuropsychologist to gain a better appreciation of the Taiwanese culture in order to provide services to their client. Taiwan is a progressive and democratic country. As evidence of this, Taiwan is one of approximately 23 countries in the world that, as of this writing, has a female President. You might not immediately find such data because China insists on the name "Chinese Taiwan" under the "One China" policy. Despite its political stalemate with the PRC, Taiwan is closely tied to the Pan Chinese culture. "Chinese" is a heterogeneous group, and China is the motherland of other ethnically Chinese-influenced countries, including Taiwan. To reiterate, it is beyond the scope of this chapter to describe the long and complex sub-cultural attributes. Taiwan continues to embrace cultures and influences of many origins including various Chinese groups (e.g., the indigenous Taiwan, Han, Man, Miao, Hakka, etc.), as well as other influences such as the Dutch, Japanese, and American! If I were to name two main distinct characteristics of the Taiwanese (as opposed to the Chinese), they would be (1) their education level being more homogenous i.e., Taiwanese-Americans are generally well educated and (2) that they are adventurous, resourceful, friendly, and open to learning and benefitting from other cultures and ways of living.

Taiwan attracts tourists from all over the world as well as American businesses, more so than China. On an everyday bus or subway train in a larger city, such as Taipei, one finds not only traditional Taiwanese and Chinese restaurants but also McDonald's, Kentucky Fried Chicken (KFC), Starbucks, as well as other international cuisine and cafes. One sees signs as well as writing in both Chinese characters and English. Spoken English along with the two primary dialects spoken in Taiwan, Mandarin and Taiwanese, can be heard routinely. On a high-speed train to the other cities in Taiwan, one hears a combination of languages and dialects: Mandarin, Taiwanese, Hakka, and English. In the Chinese culture, a dialect represents a common way of speaking for a community (usually a province or in geographically larger provinces, a specific region), admitting to only minor variations in structure; language consists of a continuum of dialects and usually refers to the written characteristics.

Chinese people share many cultural characteristics stemming from Confucian teachings emphasizing action (doing), reading and writing (vs. speaking), education, family, specific role of various family members, and physiological/somatic (vs. psychological expressions).[2] A neuropsychologist who is familiar with the nuances of the Chinese and Taiwanese culture and history is equipped to consider many of the pertinent psychosocial factors and is more likely to be able to obtain a relatively more coherent history of an examinee and their family.[3] As illustrated in the case study below, Mr. Yang's uncle was not only a semi-famous entrepreneur in Taiwan but also had a unique surname. The moment Mr. Yang mentioned his uncle's history, I identified who his uncle was. Another example is the actress mentioned in the case vignette who won the "Oscar of China" for Best Actress also has a unique name that tells a learned Chinese person that she is of mixed Chinese and Mongolian heritage. In sum, invaluable history of a Taiwanese (or Chinese) examinee can be inferred by their name alone. If using an interpreter, consider asking him/her if there is any significance or insight to be gained from the examiner's name.

For more information regarding the importance of cultural nuances, such as food in the Taiwanese tradition, refer to the movie Wedding Banquet by the two-time Academy award-winning director, Ang Lee, who was born in Taiwan, educated in Taiwan and United States, and socio-culturally identified as Chinese because his parents were born and raised in China.

As noted in a previous publication,[3] at least five specific cultural values are pertinent to neuropsychological assessment of Taiwanese-American examines. These are described below.

Language

The official spoken language in Taiwan is Mandarin, and residents of Taiwan can understand spoken Mandarin, even though they may speak a combination of Mandarin and Taiwanese or other Chinese dialects. Just like most Chinese individuals, a Taiwanese person usually learns to speak several dialects while growing up with parents and grandparents in the same house. It is common to have grandparents from both sides who speak different dialects. Thus, Chinese and Taiwanese speakers are trained at an early age to "code-switch" from one dialect to another. It is important to note that Chinese dialects generally differ in cadence and are fairly similar, particularly those from neighboring provinces. Typically, one can communicate easily in a dialect from a neighboring province but not as well from a distant one, unless the individual makes a dedicated effort to consistently learn and practice another dialect. Generally, it would be a mistake to ask a Taiwanese person: "Do you speak Mandarin or Cantonese?" Cantonese is only one of the 30+ dialects spoken by the Chinese and is not a particularly common dialect among the Taiwanese.

Chinese characters are largely uniform, with the traditional version of Chinese written language consisting of about 50,000 characters being used in Taiwan, while the simplified version, making up of about 8,000 characters, being used in China. Of more relevance to assessment of cognitive functions and changes is that Taiwanese-Chinese culture tends to value written language over spoken language. Reading and writing skills in English and Chinese in an educated Taiwanese individual are typically more developed than spoken language (English or Chinese) due to cultural differences. Indeed, there is a common saying that is very similar to "Silence is golden" (言多必失) which indicates the cultural value of silence.

An examiner with an understanding of a specific dialect, non-verbal aspect of the language communication,[4–6] a knowledge base of Taiwanese history, and an effective command of writing skills will be able to catch things that would be lost in a verbal/oral interpretation via writing.[3]

In light of the high level of education a Taiwanese-American generally has, a neuropsychological examiner should possess university-level linguistic skills to assess a wide range of examinees in all five areas of language: listening, speaking, thinking, reading, and writing.[7,8] If the examiner can merely speak a language but cannot read or write it, then he/she is unable to independently conduct a portion of the neuropsychological test battery in the examinee's preferred language due to these limitations. The neuropsychologist who asserts she has Chinese language proficiency should share her certificates, just as a clinical neuropsychologist displays his/her board certification (Lidia Artiola i Fortuny, personal communication, 10/16/2019).

For clinicians who are not of Taiwanese heritage or do not possess cultural and linguistic proficiency, effective rapport can be similarly established (see suggestions below). A burden should be on the neuropsychologist to verify that a non-family member and professionally trained translator or medically certified interpreter is being used to promote accuracy of the interpretation (typically related to the spoken/oral language) and translation (related to the written language), as well as protection of the examinee's privacy.[9]

Education

Education is highly valued in Asian culture in general and in Chinese culture specifically. Approximately 51% of Asian-Americans (Asians living in the United States) have at least a bachelor's degree[10,11]; 21% of Asian-Americans over the age of 25 have an advanced degree, including Master's, MD, PhD, or JD degrees.[12] More specifically, data from the 2018 Program for International Student Assessment (PISA) show a high level of education and test scores by Taiwanese students.[13] According to 2018 to and 2019 data, Taiwan was seventh in the number of international students entering US universities, while China was the first.[14] The higher education system in China, South Korea, and Taiwan ranks among the best in the world.[15] However, this is not to say that every Taiwanese individual has an opportunity for higher education. As an example, the educational system in Taiwan during Mr. Yang's parents' developmental years was still being developed as at that time Taiwan was adjusting to the integration of the immigrants from the many provinces of China. The need to develop an educational system in the Mandarin (vs. Taiwanese) dialect was pressing and immediate.

Many Taiwanese immigrated to the United States (and other parts of North America, Asia, Australia, and Europe) typically for educational and potentially better occupational opportunities. The region of origin in Taiwan is also a factor. A person from the capital city, Taipei, such as

Mr. Yang, generally will have more education in Taiwan prior to moving to the United States than his age-related peers from other geographic regions.

Approach to Neuropsychological Evaluations

Just like many Americans do not know exactly what a neuropsychological assessment entails, a Taiwanese-American client initially might not be aware of the purpose and value of neuropsychology. However, Taiwanese individuals can often be easily informed,[3] particularly given the fact that they tend to be highly accomplished educationally and occupationally. Many have had advanced training in science and/or engineering. Using myself as an example, prior to studying neuropsychology, I majored in physics and studied neuroscience.

A number of strategies can be used to assist with establishing rapport with a Taiwanese examinee and the examinee's family. These are discussed in more detail with a case illustration in a previously published chapter.[3] One strategy involves affirming an examinee's decision to attend the neuropsychology consultation with a statement such as "I'm glad you came. As a neuropsychologist, I assess brain functions but am not here to probe your private feelings. I think that neuropsychology can be of help to you and your family." Descriptions of neuropsychology's interdisciplinary relationship with neurology, neuro-ophthalmology, as well as with rehabilitative services, such as physical therapy, occupational therapy, and speech therapy, can help to underscore the unique role and contribution of a neuropsychologist. Neuropsychologists should reassure the examinee of their professional training and experience by displaying their diploma/credentials in neuropsychology and language proficiency. Use of a certified translator or linguist is highly recommended if the neuropsychologist does not have cultural and linguistic proficiency. Neuropsychologists should reassure the client and his/her family of confidentiality as well as limitations to confidentiality. Modification of standard test procedures is sometimes necessary (as the contents of some tests might not readily apply to the Chinese culture), and the neuropsychologist should be flexible in doing so. The neuropsychologist should share his/her current and/or past scientific research program(s), publications, and/or university affiliation(s), highlighting the relationship between neurophysiology and neuropsychology, as well as emphasizing the predictive and heuristic values of neuropsychology. This reassurance of credibility also helps to build rapport.

Until rapport is more strongly established, it is helpful to first ask questions about an examinee's physical health before inquiring about psychological distress. Finally, whenever possible, a culturally and linguistically competent neuropsychologist should make use of Chinese proverbs and/or famous stories to assist with recommendations. This approach is later illustrated in the case vignette below.

Section II: Case Study — "Now That I've Sustained a Concussion, I Need to Work Hard to Get Back on My Feet. I Need More Food and Oolong Tea to Heal!"

Note: Clinical details below have been modified to maintain patient confidentiality. All names are fictitious.

Presenting Problem

Mr. Yang is a 52-year-old Taiwanese-American, right-handed computer engineer, referred for a neuropsychological evaluation following a motor vehicle accident (MVA). When driving to work, his car was hit by a large truck. He was alert and frightened when the ambulance arrived but was unsure if he lost consciousness. He sustained minor injuries to his neck and right shoulder.

Mr. Yang refused to be taken to the hospital, insisting that he drive himself to work, which would take him only another 15 minutes. He was also observed to be apologizing profusely to a new co-worker, Mr. Lin, who was following Mr. Yang to work that day, as Mr. Lin was unfamiliar with the geographic area. Mr. Lin witnessed the accident and has since reported symptoms associated with post-traumatic stress disorder (PTSD).

After driving himself to his office, Mr. Yang worked a full day and went home feeling tired and still frightened. He began to develop headaches and nausea the next day. His neck and shoulder pain also worsened. However, it was his mother's 80th birthday celebration in two days, and he did not want to tell his parents (who live nearby) about his MVA nor seek medical attention. His symptoms persisted after one week. He had nightmares of car crashes and being chased by animals, and he experienced insomnia. His wife decided to take him to the emergency department of a local hospital. There he had a normal neurological exam and was diagnosed with "post-concussive syndrome (PCS), cervical (neck) strain, shoulder pain and PTSD." He had minor avoidance of the intersection where he had the accident, though this was substantially resolved. He was instructed by the ER physician to take Tylenol as needed and to follow up with his primary care physician (PCP).

Six months after Mr. Yang's MVA, he still suffered from "headaches, neck pain, shoulder pain, disrupted sleep, difficulty focusing attention, fatigue, inability to work without taking several short breaks a day, as well as arguments with his wife and sometimes his 20-year-old son." His PCP ordered a brain MRI scan which was normal. His physician again diagnosed him with "PCS, neck strain, and PTSD" and referred him to an occupational therapist (OT) and a mental health counselor. Mr. Yang followed up with the OT for six sessions, and they agreed to reduce the frequency of visits to once a month. Mr. Yang canceled the follow-up appointment after one additional session, citing a conflict in his work schedule. He met with an individual counselor twice and discontinued. His wife and son saw a family counselor three times after his MVA to discuss their psychological distress and found the counseling to be helpful.

Nearly 15 months after Mr. Yang's MVA, concerns about persisting post-concussion symptoms prompted referral to a neurologist at a local university medical center who found nothing untoward on examination and subsequently referred Mr. Yang for neuropsychological assessment with a Mandarin-speaking neuropsychologist.

Behavioral Observations

Mr. Yang was accompanied by his wife to my office. The assessment was conducted using a combination of Mandarin, Taiwanese, English, and written Chinese. Based on his responses, Mr. Yang showed no difficulty understanding either Chinese or English. He was alert and cooperative. He spoke rapidly and sometimes loudly. His conversational speech was characterized by word-finding pauses.

Mr. Yang was fully oriented. No evidence of a thought disorder was observed. His predominant mood was anxious, and from time to time, he showed flashes of irritability particularly when he felt that his wife was being critical of him. He noted that "people did not seem to appreciate the degree of impact my accident had produced."

Mr. Yang's vision and hearing were both intact. He is right dominant. No fine motor difficulties were detected.

Mr. Yang showed a perfectionistic approach and often watched my reactions and asked how he did.

History was given by both Mr. and Mrs. Yang during a collateral interview which was conducted prior to the individual interview and neuropsychological testing.

Mr. Yang's surname and family history reminded me of a semi-famous pioneer entrepreneur from Taiwan who built a company in a metropolitan city on the East Coast, United States, in the 1970s. Upon further inquiry, he shared that the person is his paternal uncle. I shared that my parents were diplomats posted in the same city around the same time period.

Family History/Background

Mr. Yang was born in a suburb of Taipei, Taiwan. His father is a native Taiwanese, while his mother was born in the Hebei province of China. Mr. Yang is the eldest of three children. He learned the Baoding dialect of Hebei and Taiwan dialect before preschool and heard all three dialects (Baoding dialect, Taiwanese, and Mandarin) prior to going to school. Consistent with my professional and personal experiences, he said that most of his neighbors, extended family members, and friends all speak Mandarin. The formal education he received was in traditional Chinese (written language).

As noted previously, Mr. Yang's paternal uncle was working on the east coast. Mr. Yang and his younger brother were sent to live with his uncle and aunt and spent three years, where he attended a local US elementary school from the age of 9–12. Then he returned to Taiwan. Living with relatives for a period of time is common in Chinese culture.

Mr. Yang has been married to his wife for 21 years, and they have two children (son, 20 and daughter, 17). He moved to the United States in the early 1990s for graduate school and met his wife, who is also a native of Taiwan but immigrated to the United States with her parents when she was a first-grader.

Mr. Yang disclosed a normal developmental history. Per available medical records and self-report, Mr. Yang's medical history prior to his MVA was unremarkable. His family medical history was significant for type II diabetes in his father.

Mr. Yang acknowledged social drinking while denying any history of illicit substance use. He and his wife concurred over a prior history of mild anxiety, along with occasionally minor verbal arguments with his wife and sometimes colleagues. However, he said he did not experience significant sleep problems before the accident.

Mr. Yang obtained a BS degree from a highly prestigious university in Taiwan, majoring in computer engineering. He described himself as a "B+" student. He said that his favorite subjects in school were "math, all sciences and sports." He denied having had a concussion while playing sports. He obtained an MBA degree from a university in the San Francisco Bay Area. According to his recollection, Mr. Yang's mother completed high school. His father obtained a degree that resembles a GED in the US educational system from a "professional government-management school."

Upon receiving his MBA degree, Mr. Yang worked as a programmer for a start-up computer company for a year in the Bay Area. Later, one of his colleagues there recruited him to join the leadership team at his current company, where he has worked for 14 years. After his accident, he was allowed to work from 9 to 3, granted he attends essential team meetings and completes projects. He did not always need this accommodation and worked diligently. About eight months later a younger female manager was hired by his company. Mr. Yang stated the belief that she has been scrutinizing his work and attempting to take away his flextime. According to his wife's observation, he had become more stressed and irritable.

Prior to his accident, Mr. Yang's hobbies were "playing a variety of sports and doing things with his family and friends." Now he takes walks either alone or with his wife and watches football and sometimes movies on TV. He and Mrs. Yang concurred that he has been fully independent in his activities of daily living and instrumental activities of daily livings (ADLs and IADLs). For example, he assists her with cooking and takes the lead in managing the household's finances. A concern expressed by his wife was that after his accident, he self-initiated drinking a larger quantity of oolong tea. He responded by saying she had got him hooked on tea after she took note of his fatigue upon his return to work.

When asked, Mr. and Mrs. Yang reported that they converse with each other in a combination of Mandarin, Taiwanese, and English. Mr. Yang rates his spoken and written English as "good." He had not had an opportunity to consistently use written Chinese but is able to read because the diversity in the Bay Area affords him an opportunity to continue to read in Chinese (e.g., at local shopping malls). He occasionally watches Chinese TV in Mandarin or Taiwanese. When specifically queried, he said he thinks in a combination of Chinese and English. His wife agreed that he has a good command of spoken and written English as he participates in weekly meetings with his co-workers without difficulty. She also praised his oral Mandarin and Taiwanese and observed that he has a cordial relationship with his friends of Chinese and Taiwanese descent. On certain occasions, he appears to be more polite and closer to them than to her and their children. When asked to elaborate, Mrs. Yang said that Mr. Yang seems to forget things she and her children have recently said to him and becomes irritable with them.

I asked Mr. Yang about his favorite football team, and he replied the San Francisco 49ers. He also mentioned a few quarterbacks in the NFL history he particularly likes. I shared with him my familiarity with football including knowledge of his favorite players. Later I said to him that although he may feel like a benched quarterback, he is still a pivotal part of his family. As he probably knows, many football players have ups and downs in their careers. He then spoke of a Chinese film that won critical acclaim at the Golden Rooster Awards the weekend before when he saw my laptop photos from the award ceremony. We chatted about a few other Chinese and Taiwanese movies that involve sports, music, and life lessons.

Tests and Procedures Used

A sufficient number of neuropsychological tests have been appropriately translated to Chinese and normed for the Chinese (including Taiwanese). A number of reliable and valid tests have been developed and normed specifically for the Chinese. Those were used in conjunction with my interviews, behavioral observations, and records review.

Assessment Results

Results suggest that most of Mr. Yang's cognitive functions, including simple attention, episodic memory, concept formation, problem-solving, and fine-motor skills, were at or near pre-accident levels. He showed subtly reduced performance on tests assessing complex attention and processing speed.

When he was alone with me, he reported racing thoughts, worries about his critical new manager who is a younger female, irritability, occasional nightmares (of being pushed off tall buildings and chased by animals, and recently hiking accidents), disrupted sleep, and anger at his wife. When I observed that he repeatedly spoke of "scaring" his co-worker with his accident rather than expressing his feelings of guilt over his family, Mr. Yang was close to tears. He later said it was less intense to speak of an "outsider" (that is, his new co-worker is not a family member) than those who are emotionally close to him.

Mr. Yang took an objective psychological measure in Chinese and produced a valid protocol. According to both Chinese and American norms, his profile suggested a high level of anxiety over his physical symptoms (e.g., headaches, shoulder pain, disrupted sleep). Mr. Yang became emotional when responding to items in his native language. He said that the questions "drove the matter home" and brought him both affirmation of his pain and at the same time sadness. He said that even his own family members do not seem to appreciate his unseen pain and stress but tell him to "stay strong like a man should be." One of his extended family members told him: "Head injuries in Taiwan typically result from motorcycle accidents. It's hard for us to relate to someone who has had your type of accident!" Mr. Yang has been worried that he might not be able to hold onto his job full time to provide for his family and fulfill his duties as a son, husband, and father. I reminded him how quickly he returned to work after his accident, attesting to his high level of responsibility and integrity. His everyday functioning appeared to suggest intact neuropsychological status. He beamed and replied in Chinese: "There is always a taller mountain" (一山比一山高). When asked to elaborate, he said he thought his wife was amazing at juggling family and career, especially after his accident. He said he appreciated my compassion and professionalism. He also offered to bring oolong tea to me.

Conceptualization/Impressions

I diagnosed Mr. Yang with "Unspecified Anxiety Disorder." During the feedback meeting with him and his wife, I reassured them that his "PTSD" symptoms were resolving.

I explained to Mr. Yang and his family that the findings were consistent with overall intact cognitive functions, though he could benefit from specific recommendations to ameliorate his psychological distress as outlined below. I emphasized that his distress stems in part from his strong sense of responsibility related to his culture.

Using the aforementioned "story-telling" technique, I shared that another computer engineer with a similar MVA whom I worked with a year ago called recently with the great news that he has recovered and accepted his company's offer to work 50% from home. Then I invited Mr. Yang to consider that the scrutiny he experiences with his new supervisor was possibly related to systemic changes rather than personal factors. Even those who have been working for twice as long as he has can still make mistakes at work. Therefore, he might not need to be concerned with every criticism she makes. At this time, Mr. Yang appeared to be acknowledging that what I said was making sense to him, saying: "You're a professor!"

Recommendations

In line with Mr. Yang's current needs and cultural values, the following recommendations were made:

1 Mr. Yang should consult a nutritionist about having a healthy diet on a regular basis. While current research shows that the Mediterranean diet is rich in anti-oxidants and ideal for promoting brain hygiene, the Taiwanese diet similarly contains a large amount of fish, vegetables, fruits, nuts (especially peanuts), etc. Integrating these two should be of benefit to him.
2 Mr. Yang should consider reducing tea intake as it contains caffeine which can interfere with his sleep.
3 Continued daily non-strenuous physical exercise (e.g., 30-minute walk, once to twice per day) is recommended. Similarly, participation in physical exercises (e.g., tai chi, pilates, or yoga) to build up relaxation skills, increase social support, and regulate his daily schedule should be beneficial to him.
4 Given his impressive intellect, Mr. Yang should consult literature on concussion recovery strategies. The work by Mittenberg and colleagues[15] was recommended to him. The following tips were punctuated during our feedback meeting:

    a   Eight specific tips that are helpful to alleviate symptoms are: rest, graded resumption of activities, cognitive restructuring, thought stopping, relaxation exercises, reducing distractions, writing things down, and development of problem-solving skills.

   b   When having a headache, try the following: "take a break, reduce your work day, engage in relaxation to reduce tension and rest."

   c   When feeling anxious, try the following: "schedule pleasant activities, stop thinking negative thoughts, and ask yourself if the negative thoughts are really true."

5 According to evidence-based research, participation in mindfulness meditation, CBT, and CBT-i can be helpful in promoting emotional regulation, better sleep, and ultimately increased mental health. It should be explained to Mr. Yang and his family (at least his wife) that symptoms of concussion and PTSD improve over time while acknowledging his high level of motivation, diligence, sense of responsibility, and devotion to his family.

Section III: Lessons Learned (Reminded) and Summary of Pertinent Cultural Factors

- Many people in Taiwan are Chinese, and the Taiwan sub-culture is part of the Pan Chinese culture.
- The official language in Taiwan is Mandarin (like in mainland China and Singapore). Importantly, many, if not most, people in Taiwan converse in two or more dialects.
- Because education, science, and professionalism are valued in the Taiwanese culture, an examiner should strengthen rapport and collaboration in the assessment process by emphasizing the scientific and inter-disciplinary aspects of neuropsychology.
- A scientific approach in assessment with the Taiwanese includes a combination of neuropsychological testing, review of available records (e.g., medical, educational, and occupational records), and interviews of multiple collateral sources, especially family members.
- The educational system in Taiwan during Mr. Yang's parents' developmental years was still being developed such that his parents' educational history might not be an accurate reflection of their intellect.
- Interpreting psychological testing data could be problematic to be used with Taiwanese examinees due to differences between Western and Taiwanese/Chinese cultures. For example, I disagree with several diagnoses translated from English to Chinese. PTSD is currently translated literally as "obstacles following injury/unspecified trauma," neglecting a patient's emotional experience. Autism is currently translated as "self-limiting disorder" or "self-closure disorder." Current psychological measures were developed based on Western cultural values (e.g., individualism, expressions of feelings). They should be used to only elicit clinical data. Formal diagnoses, such as PTSD, anxiety, and Autism Spectrum Disorders should only be made with a thorough review of the examinee's records and history, a clinical interview with the examinee, behavioral observations, as well as collateral interviews with family and individuals who know the examinee in the everyday situation.
- A neuropsychologist performing an assessment with a Taiwanese examinee is encouraged to not only display but also explicitly discuss their credentials including any and all certifications in neuropsychology and language proficiency at the outset of a meeting with the examinee and the examinee's family. This helps to build credibility. As an example, I display my certificates in Clinical Neuropsychology, as well as in Chinese (HSK Certificates for Higher Educational and Professional Purposes, highest level in listening, speaking, reading, and writing).
- If it is not possible to find a neuropsychologist who has cultural and linguistic proficiency, then the use of a certified translator is ideal when working with a Taiwanese examinee, though currently this might not be realistic due to scarce availability. A certified medical interpreter, rather than the examinee's family or clinic staff, should be used.

- A client's premorbid history is a highly relevant component of the neuropsychological assessment and important in making recommendations for interventions. Mr. Yang's experience with both the Taiwanese and American educational systems is a good example.
- Taiwanese people tend to focus on somatic or physical complaints rather than psychological complaints. In Mr. Yang's case, it was easier for him to talk about his physical injuries as opposed to his initial post-traumatic stress.
- A Taiwanese examinee's duty to their parents and family takes precedent over their own needs. Instead of seeking treatment for his headaches, nausea, and pain, Mr. Yang chose to focus his attention on his mother's birthday celebration.
- As a group, my Asian examinees (including Taiwanese examinees) tend to start drinking (more) tea in order to re-energize themselves following a concussion. The act of drinking tea signals a physiological type of coping and a plea for attention and help from the family. Taiwanese clients have easy access to premium Oolong tea, which may contain a high amount of caffeine. I have found it helpful to gently remind them of caffeine's interference with sleep.
- Taiwanese as a group are well educated and likely will expect professional explanations of the neuropsychology of neurological and psychological conditions (e.g., concussion, PTSD). A neuropsychologist is encouraged to prepare written information in advance for the Chinese-American examinee and their family.
- Like Mr. Yang, some Taiwanese Americans have lived and obtained formal education in other countries (e.g., European and other Asian countries). Openness to this phenomenon and an appreciation of a client's educational and social background can be helpful in building an effective rapport.
- A Taiwanese client without multiple abnormal neuropsychological findings such as in the case of Mr. Yang should be told so. Many, if not most, Taiwanese clients prefer results with no abnormal findings and prefer to be told that no medications are needed. Instead, they are still able to return to work or school and continue to demonstrate their competence. Additionally, natural interventions (e.g., physical exercise and nutrition from food and water) are welcome.
- In accordance with APA ethical and AACN practice guidelines, a neuropsychologist should explicitly document limitations in level of rapport, uncertainty over communication accuracy including both verbal and non-verbal communication, any modification of test administration, lack of ethnicity corrected norms, etc.
- In addition to a formal assessment of language proficiency, assessment of everyday language and communication can be easily conducted in a few minutes by discussing current news in any Chinese country (e.g., Taiwan or China), artwork displayed at the professional office, and/or mutually liked music. I often hum currently popular Taiwanese and/or Chinese songs during break time and the examinee's "ability" to join me in singing affords an added opportunity to assess his/her cultural and linguistic proficiency.
- Skills training and goal-oriented methods (e.g., CBT) tend to be better received by the Taiwanese than feeling-based psychological interventions.

References

1. Cheng C. A study of inter-cultural marital conflict and satisfaction in Taiwan. Int J Intercult Rel. 2010 Jul;34(4):354–62.
2. Guo T, Uhm SY. Society and acculturation in Asian American communities. In: Davis J, D'Amato RC, editors. Neuropsychology of Asians and Asian-Americans. New York (NY): Springer; 2014. p. 55–76.

3. Paltzer JY. Assessment of age-related cognitive changes and dementia in Chinese and Chinese American older adults. In: Smith GE, Farias ST, editors. APA handbook of dementia. Washington (DC): American Psychological Association; 2018. p. 125–40.

4. Casas F, Sarriera JC, Abs D, Coenders G, Alfaro J, Saforcada E et al. Subjective indicators of personal well-being among adolescents. Performance and results for different scales in Latin-language speaking countries: a contribution to the international debate. Child Indic Res. 2012 Mar 1;5(1):1–28.

5. Llorente AM, Williams J, Satz P, D'Elia L. Children's color trails test 1 & 2 manual. Lutz (FL): Psychological Assessment Resources; 2003.

6. Manly, J. Assessment of cognitive function among culturally diverse adults. Paper presented at: American Academy of Clinical Neuropsychology. 12th Annual Conference of the American Academy of Clinical Neuropsychology; 2014 June; New York, NY.

7. Artiola i Fortuny L, Mullaney HA. Assessing patients whose language you do not know: can the absurd be ethical? [abstract]. Clin Neuropsych. 1998 Feb 1;12(1):113–26.

8. Rivera-Mindt M, Arentoft A, Coulehan K, Byrd D. Considerations for the neuropsychological evaluation of older ethnic minority populations. In: Ravdin LD, Katzen HL, editors. Handbook on the neuropsychology of aging and dementia. New York (NY): Springer; 2013. p. 25–41.

9. American Psychological Association. Ethical principles of psychologists and code of conduct [Internet]. Washington (DC): American Psychological Association; c2002–2017 [updated 2016; cited 2020 Sep 30]. Available from: https://www.apa.org/ethics/code

10. US Census Bureau News. Asian/Pacific American Heritage Month: May 2012 [Internet]. Washington (DC): United States Department of Commerce; 2012 Mar 21 [updated 2012 May; cited 2020 Oct 10]. Available from: https://www.census.gov/newsroom/releases/pdf/cb12ff09_asian.pdf

11. Wong TM. Neuropsychology of Chinese Americans. In: Fujii DEM, editor. Neuropsychology of Asian Americans. New York (NY): Taylor & Francis; 2011. p. 29–46.

12. Le CN. Asian nation: the landscape of Asian America [Internet]. [place unknown: Asian Nation]; c2001–2020. 14 important statistics about Asian Americans; 2020 [cited 2020 Sep 30]; [about 2 screens]. Available from: http://www.asian-nation.org/14-statistics.shtml

13. OECD Programme for International Student Assessment (PISA). PISA 2018 results Chinese Taipei [Internet]. [place unknown]: Organization for Economic Co-operation and Development (OECD); 2019 [cited 2020 Oct 10]. Available from: https://www.oecd.org/pisa/publications/PISA2018_CN_TAP.pdf

14. International Trade Administration. Taiwan—Education [Internet]. [place unknown]: Export.gov; 2019 Nov 8 [cited 2020 Oct 10]. Available from: https://www.export.gov/apex/article2?id=Taiwan-Education

15. QS Higher Education System Strength Rankings 2018. Retrieved from https://www.topuniversities.com/system-strength-rankings/2018

Vietnamese

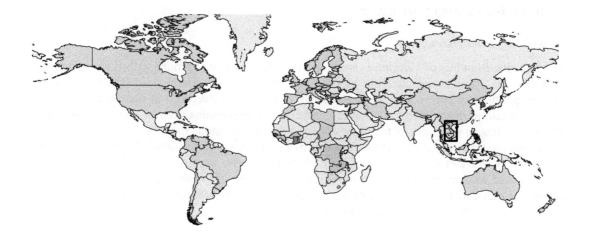

20 Neuropsychological Assessment of Vietnamese Americans

BaoChan Tran, Ann T. Nguyen, Caroline Ba, and Christopher Minh Nguyen

Section I: Background Information

Terminology and Perspective

The Socialist Republic of Vietnam is home to more than 54 ethnic groups with their own unique identities and cultures. People from Vietnam are referred to as Vietnamese. The majority ethnic group, officially known as *Kinh* (**người Kinh**), accounts for over 85% of the population, while Vietnam's ethnic minority population is comprised of indigenous groups—largely the *Khmer*, *Mong*, and *Muong* who have historically settled in the mountainous regions.[1]

Our perspectives are drawn from the clinical experiences of multilingual, first- and second-generation Kinh-Vietnamese refugees and immigrants who assimilated in the Northeastern, Western, and Midwestern regions of the United States. We are early-career neuropsychologists currently practicing in outpatient clinics and inpatient units at academic medical centers and private practices in the aforementioned regions.

Geography

Vietnam is a country in Southeast Asia that borders China to the north, Laos to the northwest, and Cambodia to the southwest. Its maritime border includes the South China Sea along the eastern coastline and the Gulf of Thailand along the southwestern coastline. Vietnam is the 15th most populated country in the world, with over 97.3 million people.[2]

History

Vietnam has a long history of war and conflict, with records dating back to 111 BC when the Han Dynasty from China claimed the territory as part of the Chinese empire. This was the start of a long occupation lasting over 1,000 years.[3] There were numerous revolts against Chinese imperialism, including two notable rebellions led by women: the Trung sisters' rebellion (40–43 AD) and Lady Triệu's revolt (c. 243–248 AD). The revolts were largely unsuccessful until the 10th century when Vietnam gained independence from China in 938 AD, ushering in a succession of dynastic rulers for 900 years, interrupted by periods of Chinese rule and Mongolian invasions. In 1858, Vietnam was colonized by France before regaining sovereignty in 1954 and establishing a demarcation line between North and South Vietnam along the 17th parallel.[3] A civil war began in 1955 between the Communist North and anti-Communist South and ended in 1975 with the defeat of South Vietnam in 1975 and began a mass outmigration of Vietnamese refugees.[3]

DOI: 10.4324/9781003051862-41

Immigration and Relocation

The first wave of Vietnamese refugees immigrated to the United States, Canada, Australia, China, and France at the end of the Vietnam War in 1975.[4] The first wave of immigrants to the United States consisted of 125,000 refugees who were closely affiliated with the US/South Vietnamese government, members of the Vietnamese elite or middle class, and more educated profession-als.[3] From the late 1970s to early 1980s, a second wave of Vietnamese refugees comprised of for-mer military officials and individuals from lower socioeconomic status (SES) backgrounds fled Vietnam due to political instability and economic hardship.[3] These refugees were referred to as "boat people," as many fled on unsafe and overcrowded fishing boats, and experiences such as pirate attacks, sexual assault, starvation, and death were common. Those who survived the jour-ney were rescued and brought to refugee camps in Southeast Asian countries.[5] The third signif-icant wave of Vietnamese immigration to the United States occurred from the 1980s to 1990s and included refugees, political prisoners, and offspring of American servicemen and Vietnamese mothers.[3] Currently, an estimated 2.1 million Vietnamese Americans reside in the United States, which represents the fourth-largest Asian American subgroup behind Chinese, Filipino, and Indian Americans.[6] It has been estimated that Vietnamese immigration has exceeded 3.7 million residing over 100 countries with dense concentrations living in the United States, Eastern Europe, France, Australia, Canada, Germany, United Kingdom, and Northern Europe.[4]

Trauma and Mental Health

Many Vietnamese people have survived traumas associated with the Vietnam War.[7] For example, experiences of pre-migration trauma included the separation and/or loss of family and friends, combat, witnessing and/or surviving massacres, and forced relocation due to the destruction and loss of personal property.[8,9] Refugees who escaped Vietnam on overcrowded and poorly constructed boats in rough waters were often targeted by pirates who killed, robbed, abducted, physically harmed, and/or raped their victims.[10,11] Refugees continued to encounter hardships for years in overcrowded refugee camps under dangerous and unsanitary conditions that led to poor nutrition, starvation, and diseases.[7,12] Resettlement also contributed to post-immigration stressors including acculturation challenges, economic hardship, limited English proficiency, intergenera-tional conflicts, and social stress.[13]

Following the end of the Vietnam War, former military officers and government officials and individuals with ties to the former South Vietnam government were detained and imprisoned in Reeducation Camps (**trại cải tạo**). The reeducation process was both a means of revenge and a sophisticated technique of repression and indoctrination with accompanying hard physical labor, starvation, torture, confinement, and illnesses.[14] In 1989, under the Released Reeducation Detainee Program (also known as Humanitarian Operation), more than 166,000 detainees and their family members arrived and resided in the United States.[15] Due to exposure to war-related trauma and pre- and post-migration stressors, Vietnamese people are at increased risk for developing various psychiatric disorders including depression and posttraumatic stress disorder (PTSD).[3,16] For exam-ple, the rates of clinical depression among Vietnamese Americans in community and primary care settings range from 30% to 50%.[16-18]

Education and Socioeconomic Status

Vietnam's educational system was historically influenced by Chinese and French cultures. The current educational system is similar to those of the American schools' system that includes curriculum from preschool to high school. Trade, technical, and universities are available beyond high school, although the former are likely to be operated by the government.[3] Over the past decades, Vietnam has made significant progress in basic educational systems and has achieved a literacy rate of 92.5%.[19] Regarding educational attainment of the Vietnamese population, a 2005 survey estimated that 52% of Vietnamese born abroad earned the equivalent of a high school degree or less compared to only 21% of US-born Vietnamese.[20] The gap pertaining to English proficiency becomes wider with 34% among Vietnamese born abroad compared to 88% of US-born Vietnamese.[20]

Economically, Vietnam's GDP per capita rank is 152nd out of 228 countries (the United States is ranked 15th).[1] Because of rapid economic growth from increases in economic demand and strong manufacturing exports, Vietnam's real GDP growth rate is ranked 21 in country comparison to the world.[1] Among Vietnamese living in the United States, the poverty rate in 2015 for a US born is at 14.2% in comparison to a rate of 14.3% for a foreign born.[20] Additionally, the median annual household income of a US born is $67,800 in comparison to $58,700 of a foreign born.[20] Lower income levels among Vietnamese born abroad are likely associated with lower English proficiency and a lack of transferable skills upon immigrating to the United States. Specifically, Vietnamese refugees are often employed in manual labor and manufacturing jobs, small industries, or industry jobs with low paying wages (e.g., seamstresses in garment factories, dishwashers, and line cooks in restaurants).[21]

Acculturation

English proficiency among immigrants has been used as a measure of acculturation in the United States.[22] Among Vietnamese refugees, factors such as age, sex, and education in Vietnam significantly impact the level of acculturation in the United States.[17] Vietnamese immigrants from the first wave who belonged to the upper/middle class and attained a higher level of education adopted English more readily and possessed transferable linguistic skills and abilities, which enabled them to assimilate into American society more readily compared to those from subsequent waves of immigration.[23] Limited English proficiency coupled with acculturation challenges present major obstacles for Vietnamese Americans seeking medical and mental health services.[3]

Language

Vietnamese is the official language of Vietnam, while English is increasingly favored as a second language, particularly in educational settings. Other common languages include French, Chinese, Khmer, as well as mountain-area languages such as Mon-Khmer and Malayo-Polynesian.[3] The Vietnamese language has three major dialects classified by geographic regions: **Miền Bắc** (Northern Vietnam), **Miền Trung** (Central Vietnam), and **Miền Nam** (Southern Vietnam). The three dialects differ primarily in phonology, as well as vocabulary and grammar.

Values and Customs

Common religions in Vietnam include Buddhism, Catholicism, Taoism, Cao Dai, and Hoa Hao, although a majority of Vietnamese are non-religious.[3] Awareness surrounding sexuality has increased in Vietnam in recent years, as demonstrated by the lifting of bans on same-sex marriages in 2015, although there is currently no legal recognition of unions.[24]As a patriarchal society, members of the lesbian, gay, bisexual, transgender, intersex, and asexual community can face discrimination and violence, and they do not yet receive protections under the law.

Health Status

The life expectancy at birth is 72.7 years for males and 78.1 years for females in Vietnam.[1] Major infectious diseases include bacterial diarrhea, hepatitis A, typhoid fever, dengue fever, malaria, and Japanese encephalitis.[1] The leading cause of death and disability in Vietnam in 2019 was stroke, followed by ischemic heart disease, diabetes, chronic obstructive pulmonary disease, lung cancer, road injuries, and cirrhosis.[25]

Mental illness in Vietnam is both pervasive and highly stigmatized, afflicting approximately 20% of the population.[26] Common disorders include depression, anxiety, schizophrenia, behavioral issues in youths/teens, as well as alcohol abuse, and drug addiction.[27] However, there is a significant shortage of mental health professionals, particularly the nascent specialization in clinical psychology.[28] As such, neuropsychological services are not yet readily available to Vietnam's aging population.

Approaches to Neuropsychological Assessment

Among Vietnamese-speaking individuals, the neuropsychological assessment is impacted by various factors, as there is a lack of Vietnamese tests, normative data, and culturally/linguistically matched neuropsychologists. While neuropsychological evaluations are ideally completed with culturally/linguistically matched neuropsychologists, this is not always feasible, and thus, interpreters are used as part of the evaluation process. Given the distinct differences across the Vietnamese dialects, it is not only crucial that interpreters are well trained with medical and health-related terminology but also possess a command of the dialect that they are asked to interpret.

The interpretability of neuropsychological test results is limited by the lack of comprehensive normative data; as such, qualitative observations regarding test performance play a significant role in the evaluation process.[29,30] The Cross-Cultural Neuropsychological Test Battery (CCNB)[31] was designed with cultural and linguistic factors taken into consideration to evaluate dementia among five target groups, including Vietnamese Americans. The CCNB is the only comprehensive battery with normative data for Vietnamese Americans (N = 61), with age ranges between 62 and 87 (M = 71.5, SD = 5.8) and education between 0 and 18 years (M = 8.6, SD = 4.1). It was noted that ethnicity and education level were found to be significant contributing factors to performance on several tasks, as education accounted for, on average, 15% of the variance in test scores. This highlights the necessity of comprehensive normative data to include classifications of education level and age for the Vietnamese American population.[32]

Vietnamese Americans are comprised of refugees, immigrants, first-generation (individuals who migrated in their younger years), second-, and third-generation US born individuals with unique experiences. Given the timeline of immigration, older Vietnamese Americans (typically first generation) with war-related traumas are approaching the age in which they are at increased risk of developing dementia. However, due to limited formal education, low language acculturation, reduced health literacy, and disparity in socioeconomic resources, older generations of Vietnamese Americans face greater disadvantages and hardships when obtaining health-related services.[20] Factors such as cultural history, context of immigration, and the individual's unique pre- and post-immigration experiences are important considerations when conducting a culturally informed neuropsychological evaluation.

Section II: Case Study — "Ginseng over Donepezil?"

Mrs. Nguyễn (pseudonym) is a 56-year-old, right-handed, married, Vietnamese woman with 16 years of formal education living in the United States. She was referred for a neuropsychological evaluation by her primary care physician due to concerns of memory decline. In addition to a review of her available medical records, information was gathered from a clinical interview with Mrs. Nguyễn, her husband, and her sister. Of note, Mrs. Nguyễn is bilingual and is proficient in both Vietnamese and English. A bilingual Vietnamese American examiner conducted this evaluation in English per her preference.

Cognitively, Mrs. Nguyễn and her family reported gradually progressive decline in her overall functioning over the past two years. Specifically, she reported increased difficulty recalling details of events, conversations, information discussed during her mother's medical appointments, and names of familiar people. She has also misplaced objects. Her ability to focus has declined and she is easily distracted. She reported decreased multi-tasking skills and difficulty alternating between tasks, which represents a change. She is increasingly dependent upon her children with daily technology-related tasks due to difficulty understanding modern technology. Mrs. Nguyễn reported that she and her husband have recently implemented a morning routine to help organize and orient her after waking, as she has forgotten to complete important tasks during the day. He also purchased a whiteboard to assist her with tracking her family's schedule (e.g., appointments, children's extracurricular activities).

Functionally, Mrs. Nguyễn is independent in her basic activities of daily living (ADLs). In terms of her instrumental ADLs (IADLs), she organizes her medications with reminders from her husband; she denied missing doses. Her husband has historically managed the household finances; however, she manages her mother's finances without difficulty. Mrs. Nguyễn purchases groceries, cleans, and prepares all meals for the family. She currently drives without difficulty and denied any recent accidents, tickets, or missed exits/turns. However, she has gotten lost and increasingly relied on global position systems when deviating from routine routes.

Physically, Mrs. Nguyễn reported a stable appetite and a life-long "sweet tooth," such that she can eat a bucket of ice cream in one sitting. She has dinner with her family every night. She sleeps approximately 5–6 hours and wakes up rested. She wears glasses for distance vision and reading. She reported moderate hearing loss in her right ear at age 10 but denied the use of a hearing aid.

Emotionally, Mrs. Nguyễn reported moderate feelings of anxiety and sadness, particularly regarding her breast cancer history (diagnosed ˜10 years prior). She feels as if she is a burden upon her immediate and extended family due to her cognitive decline. She reported relational strain with her husband and feels similar to a single parent who has had to take on the majority of the parental responsibilities. She takes escitalopram (10mg) for depression and reported always being "naturally sentimental, sensitive to information," and easily moved to tears.

Medical History

Mrs. Nguyen's medical history is significant for left breast cancer status post-chemotherapy in complete remission, hypertension, and hyperlipidemia. She denied any history of head injury or seizures. Genetic testing revealed an APOE genotype of e3/e4. Her family history is significant for Parkinson's disease (father), diabetes mellitus (mother), and cerebrovascular accident (aunt). Recent neuroimaging results are as follows:

- FDG-PET of the brain revealed moderately increased amyloid uptake in the cortical cerebral gray matter involving the frontal, parietal, temporal, and occipital lobes with loss of gray–white matter differentiation in these areas. The scan was positive and reflected moderate to frequent amyloid neuritic plaques.
- PET scan revealed mild cerebral atrophy, most prominently involving the temporal and parietal lobes.
- A brain MRI revealed that temporal lobe volume is at the 22nd percentile and left temporal lobe volume is at the 18th percentile.

Social History

Mrs. Nguyễn was born in a city in the central highlands of south-central Vietnam. Her family relocated to the United States when she was 13 years of age. She is fluent in both English and Northern Vietnamese (**bắc**) dialect. She described herself as a good student. She graduated from a competitive university in California with a Bachelor of Science degree. She was employed as a researcher at a local university for 5–7 years before resigning ~12 years ago to care for her children. She was working part-time (3–4 hours/day) at her sister's dental office. She is married and has two teenage children. Mrs. Nguyễn is highly involved in the parent association at her children's schools.

Behavioral Observations

Mrs. Nguyễn presented to the clinic with her husband and sister, while a younger sister contributed to the clinical interview via telephone. She was appropriately groomed, comfortably dressed, and appeared her stated age. She was alert and oriented to person and situation; however, she was unable to recall the correct date. Gait was unremarkable and no fine motor difficulties were noted. Her speech was normal for volume, rate, tone, and prosody, while articulation was notable for a slight accent. Thought processes were linear and logical. She demonstrated good insight into her cognitive difficulties but was unable to accurately recall important dates (e.g., year of wedding, academic graduations, ages of her siblings). As such, her sister and husband corrected her when necessary. Mrs. Nguyễn appeared visibly distressed and tearful during the first half-hour of the appointment, as she worked to coordinate transportation services for her mother (who had a medical appointment on the same day) and children. Her husband and sister offered to assist with making arrangements after she expressed feeling overwhelmed and emotionally dysregulated. She ultimately regained her composure after reassurance from her family and the examiner and agreed to proceed with the evaluation. For the remainder of the evaluation, Mrs. Nguyễn's mood was euthymic with congruent affect. She denied suicidal and homicidal ideation. No evidence of sensory hallucination or delusional thoughts was observed.

During testing, Mrs. Nguyễn was alert and cooperative on all tasks. She reported feeling fatigued throughout the evaluation process and was provided breaks as needed. She exhibited adequate frustration tolerance during testing; however, she became discouraged on several memory tasks and was concerned with perceived failure/poor performance. The results from the current evaluation appear to provide an accurate assessment of her current cognitive functioning.

Cultural Considerations

Multigenerational Household

Mrs. Nguyễn's living arrangement consists of three generations, with her mother- and father-in-law (both in their early 80s) sharing one bedroom. Within the household, all spaces are shared and doors are typically open with the expectation that members can go in and out freely.

Gender Roles

Mrs. Nguyễn's household is generally patriarchal in structure; her husband is expected to financially provide for the family while she is expected to care for and provide emotional support for her children and in-laws. Specifically, she is her mother's translator and drives her to medical appointments. Mrs. Nguyễn prepares all meals for the entire household with some assistance from her mother. Meals are eaten together at a set time around the dinner table. During the interview, she endorsed feeling overwhelmed by her various familial responsibilities, which has significantly delayed her help-seeking. She often places her needs and health second to those of her family members' and takes on a group-oriented rather than individualist view of self.

Perception of Cognitive Decline

During the interview, Mrs. Nguyễn's husband and sisters reported that the family overlooked initial signs of her cognitive difficulties for several years, as they thought she was "overwhelmed with stress" (**bị áp lực**). Per her husband, Mrs. Nguyễn's mother often attributed her memory lapses to "thinking too much that it makes her go crazy." Mrs. Nguyễn's family members were aware of the 2019 PET scan results indicating a neurodegenerative disease process but had limited understanding that Mrs. Nguyễn's cognitive changes were related. They attributed the observed changes to stress, personality, and cultural factors. She reported that her husband and siblings typically "cover for her" when she has memory lapses or "finish her sentences" when she evidences word-finding difficulty.

Test Selection

The selection of appropriate neuropsychological test battery is essential for valid test interpretations when working with culturally diverse patients. For Mrs. Nguyễn, variables such as years residing in the United States, bilingualism, and acculturation were considered in selection of tests and normative comparison. Based on her social history (e.g., level of acculturation, education, and language proficiency), English language-based tests and Western norms were utilized. The following tests were administered (see Lezak et al.,[33] for further description):

- Boston Naming Test
- Clinical Dementia Rating

- Controlled Oral Word Association Test
- Functional Abilities Questionnaire Geriatric Depression Scale
- Hamilton Anxiety Inventory
- Hopkins Verbal Learning Test-Revised
- Mini-Mental State Exam
- Rey–Osterrieth Complex Figure Drawing Test
- Stroop Color Word Test
- Trail Making Test
- Wechsler Adult Intelligence Scale, 4th Edition (selected subtests)
- Wechsler Memory Scale, 4th Edition, (selected subtests)
- Wechsler Test of Adult Reading
- Wisconsin Card Sorting Task

Summary and Impression

The results from the current neuropsychological evaluation revealed intact auditory attention and visuospatial abilities. Multiple intradomain variations ranging from impaired to average were documented across areas of processing speed, language, and executive functioning. With regard to memory functioning, Mrs. Nguyễn demonstrated largely impaired learning and recall of both visual and verbal information in the context of poor performance across recognition memory trials. She endorsed significantly greater symptoms of depression and anxiety on self-report inventories in contrast to mild symptoms reported during the clinical interview in the presence of family members.

Mrs. Nguyễn is independent in her basic ADLs and most IADLs but requires multiple daily prompts from her husband to stay on schedule. Overall, the results of the evaluation reflected primary deficits in verbal and visual learning and memory, as well as impaired semantic language. Qualitatively, she evidenced difficulty recalling details of her personal history (e.g., year of wedding, academic graduations, ages of her siblings). The nature of her cognitive deficits likely represents a decline based on her high average premorbid estimate, educational attainment, occupational history, and information obtained from the clinical interview.

Altogether, her presentation is most consistent with a diagnosis of Mild Cognitive Impairment (i.e., Amnestic Mild Cognitive Impairment). The etiology is likely secondary to a neurodegenerative process based on the pattern of deficits and neuroimaging findings, which reflected moderate to frequent amyloid neuritic plaques and reduced temporal lobe volume and mild cerebral atrophy with predilection in the parietal and temporal lobes. It should be noted that the presence of mild mood-related symptoms and psychological stressors likely exacerbate Mrs. Nguyễn's cognitive weaknesses but do not wholly account for the magnitude of deficits observed on testing.

Feedback Session and Follow-Up Care

During the feedback session, Mrs. Nguyễn's husband and sisters were informed of her diagnosis, which was supported by the results of the neuropsychological evaluation, details of her genetic analysis, and neuroimaging results. They appeared impassive and matter-of-fact. In a later email, her sister informed the examiner that the family purposefully maintained composure to promote interpersonal harmony and avoid causing alarm or discomfort. Mrs. Nguyễn and her family were provided with the following recommendations:

- *Sharing workload*: Given her cognitive decline, she would benefit from sharing familial responsibilities to reduce her workload. This would alleviate some of the stress and burden of being overworked and overwhelmed.
- *Psychiatry and mood support*: She was encouraged to consult with an ethnically/racially and/or language congruent mental health practitioner with experience in aging to assist her with developing appropriate coping strategies to address difficulties with cognition, mood, and stress. Family sessions may also be appropriate to assist with discussing concepts that are addressed in individual sessions.
- *Family education and support*: Mrs. Nguyễn and her family were provided information for community and national support groups that offer resources related to memory, mood, and aging. These caregiver resources will enable her family to understand the basis of her cognitive complaints and their neurological underpinnings (rather than attribute them to "worrying too much") and to explore how they can assist her in daily functioning that minimizes stigma.

During a one-year follow-up phone call, Mrs. Nguyễn reported that her family continued to attribute her cognitive difficulties to depression rather than cognitive impairment. Her family members also attributed her memory loss to "taking too many Western medicines" that "made her mind hot" and her stress and frustration were interpreted as excess "heat." She was not engaged in psychological services but rather made several dietary changes in an effort to maintain a healthier lifestyle. Her family continued to rely on her with responsibilities and maintained expectations of her to care for her in-laws and children. When she communicated the results of the evaluation with her mother and extended family, they questioned its relevance and did not understand why she sought "outside" help rather than consult with a trusted family physician or herbalist. After much discussion with the provider, Mrs. Nguyễn acknowledged the importance of returning for an 18-month re-evaluation.

Section III: Lessons Learned

Considerations for establishing rapport:

- Vietnamese culture has a strong emphasis on respect based on age and/or status. Therefore, families may be reluctant to share "excessive" details out of respect for the clinician's time and may not correct misconceptions. Ask families to correct interpreters/clinicians at the beginning of the evaluation (e.g., "Please correct us if we misunderstood you or said something incorrectly").
- To prevent unintentional miscommunication that can negatively influence rapport, a common practice in Vietnamese culture is to "ask for forgiveness" at the beginning of the evaluation (e.g., "I apologize in advanced if I misspeak or do something that is insulting as I am not familiar with Vietnamese customs").
- Start the session with a thorough review of privacy policies. Provide examples to establish trust (e.g., "If someone calls and asks for your information, I cannot acknowledge that I work with you without your written permission").

- Non-verbal behaviors that may be welcoming to a Vietnamese patient includes standing up when greeting the patient, inviting the patient to sit first, making eye contact with families and not the interpreter when asking questions, and gesturing to individuals or distal objects with an open hand rather than pointing with the index finger.
- Vietnamese patients who are not familiar with healthcare systems may exhibit mistrust and suspicion about the motives of institutions (e.g., insurance and government programs). Clarifying the clinician's goals and motivations may be necessary in these instances.

Considerations for the clinical interview:

- Clinicians should be aware of the patient's family dynamics and identify key family members who play a role in healthcare decision-making. For example, there may be changes in family dynamics as parents age and the possibility of role reversals, with parents relying on their children to act as healthcare decision-makers.
- Vietnamese patients may be hesitant to disclose medical information due to stigma. In this context, the clinician interview with the patient and family members can occur together and then separately. Interviewing the group as a whole will highlight important family dynamics while interviewing individuals separately will bring to light important information that the patient or family members may be more reluctant to share in a group setting.
- Vietnamese people value the elderly and may be very complimentary toward elders who demonstrate aging ideals, such as aging gracefully in the context of beauty (**đẹp lão**), being insightful and logical (**sáng suốt**), having a keen and shrewd mind (**minh mẫn**), and having an alert/lucid mind (**tỉnh táo**). As such, they may be reluctant to endorsed cognitive deficits or decline to "save face" among their community. Therefore, tailoring the clinical interview to specific symptoms of deficits rather than general concepts of cognitive decline may be helpful in eliciting diagnostic information.
- Cultural beliefs surrounding illnesses may focus on a temperature imbalance, such as ingesting foods or medications that are overly "hot" or "cold." Therefore, illnesses may be perceived as temporary and not worth discussing due to causal links to variables that can be adjusted (e.g., diet).
- Clinicians can reduce the stigma of illnesses by:
  - Acknowledging cultural beliefs, particularly regarding Western medicine, memory, aging, and mental health
  - Validating the family's efforts and reassuring them that one would expect even the "best" of families would require specialist care
  - Encouraging the family to share in efforts to assist the patient
- Vietnamese families may not report the use of Eastern medicines and remedies without direct questioning. Specifically, reliance on alternative medicine (**thuốc bắc**), such as steaming ginkgo biloba, sanshin root, ginseng, ginger, and other herbs to regain the mind-body balance is a common practice.
- Clinicians should query about medication adherence for all prescribed medications. For example, Vietnamese patients may exclusively rely on over-the-counter medications for medical complaints and/or replace prescribed medications with Eastern medicines as discussed above (e.g., reliance on ginseng over donepezil).

Considerations for testing and interpretation:

- While the selection of appropriate neuropsychological test norms is essential for interpretation and case conceptualization, comprehensive norms are not available for Vietnamese patients. Thus, tests with fewer language demands may be more appropriate. While not an exhaustive list, we have included tests in the Appendix section that have translations/norms for the Vietnamese population.
- All assessment data should be integrated and interpreted within the context of the patient's cultural characteristics. For example, results of verbal tests with Western norms likely provide an underestimate of actual abilities if the patient is not proficient in English. In this case, the clinician must rely more heavily on consistencies in the patient's overall presentation rather than focus on "deficits" on select tests.
- If test results are deemed to have poor validity, the clinician may need to emphasize functional abilities described by collateral sources in the interpretation of assessment data.
- Clinicians should clearly document all non-standardized assessment procedures, rationale for the modifications, as well as limitations of test interpretations in the neuropsychological report.
- It is important that clinicians are aware of how patients perceive the testing situation to maximize comfort. For example, a Vietnamese patient may be uncomfortable with the testing situation due to stereotype threat, poor rapport with the examiner, or anxiety related to performance.
- Provide reassurance to patients prior to testing that their results are private and will not be shared without their consent to reduce anxiety about "losing face."
- Flexible test administration and modifications may be necessary. Vietnamese patients may not understand standardized testing procedures and may need examples or modeling to complete tasks. In addition, testing of limits may help ameliorate issues with cultural/language incongruence.

Considerations for feedback and recommendations:

- Families may be agreeable and reluctant to voice their questions, doubts, or confusion. Remind families that they should openly communicate their disagreement and/or concerns.
- Discussion of results and recommendations should use definitive terminology where possible. Using ambiguous terms such as "possibly" or "maybe" can lead to assumptions or dismissing all data.
- Use tangible, short, and personalized action plans. Given language and cultural barriers, families and individuals are easily overwhelmed by paragraphs of detailed recommendations with medical jargon. Present the recommendations as a short list of "to do's" that involves the individual's family.
- Provide culturally congruent recommendations, such as *Tai Chi/qigong* training for physical activity and meditation for stress management.
- Patients may be reluctant to join support groups due to stigmatization and "losing face." Discuss alternative solutions with the family, such as support from individuals in the "inner circle."

- Vietnamese families may perceive placement in retirement communities or nursing homes as a lack of filial piety and loss of love. This can cause significant distress and tension between family members as well as shame and guilt in children.
- It may be worthwhile to discuss the patient's history of reliance on alternative treatments, such as coining, cupping, and use of Eastern medicine. Furthermore, patients should be encouraged to communicate the use of Eastern medications with their prescribing physicians to avoid potential harmful effects.

Glossary

bị áp lực.   Overwhelmed/overburdened with unavoidable stressors.

đẹp lão.   Aging gracefully in the context of beauty.

giọng bắc.   Vietnamese dialect.

Mi`ên Bắc.   Northern Vietnam.

Mi`ên Nam.   Southern Vietnam.

Mi`ên Trung.   Central Vietnam.

minh mẫn.   Having a keen and shrewd mind.

người Kinh.   The majority ethnic group.

sáng suốt.   Being insightful and logical.

thuốc bắc.   Alternative/herbal medicine, such as ginkgo biloba, sanshin root, ginseng.

tỉnh táo.   Having an alert/lucid mind.

trại cải tạo.   Re-education camps.

References

1. Central Intelligence Agency. The World Factbook—Vietnam [Internet]. 2021 [updated 2021 Feb 24; cited 2021 Mar 1]. Available from: https://www.cia.gov/the-world-factbook/countries/vietnam/
2. World Population Review. Vietnam Population 2021 [Internet]. 2021 Feb 27 [cited 27 Feb 2021]. Available from: https://worldpopulationreview.com/countries/vietnam-population
3. Ngo D, Le MT, Le PD. Neuropsychology of Vietnamese Americans. In Fujii DE, editor. The neuropsychology of Asian Americans. New York (NY): Taylor and Francis Group; 2011. p. 181–200.
4. Pham AT. The returning diaspora: Analyzing overseas Vietnamese (Viet Kieu)—contributions toward Vietnam's economic growth. DEPOCEN Working Paper Series No. 2011/20. 2012. p. 1–39.
5 Kelly GP. Coping with America: refugees from Vietnam, Cambodia, and Laos in the 1970s and 1980s. Ann Am Acad Political Soc Sci. 1986 Sept;487(1):138–49.
6. Pew Research Center. Social & demographic trends [Internet]. Washington (DC): Pew Research Center; 2017 Sept 8 [cited 2021 Jan 15]. Available from: https://www.pewsocialtrends.org/fact-sheet/asian-americans-vietnamese-in-the-u-s-fact-sheet/
7. Abueg FR, Chun KM. Traumatization stress among Asians and Asian Americans. In: Marsella AJ, Friedman MJ, Gerrity ET, Scurfield RM, editors. Ethnocultural aspects of posttraumatic stress disorder: issues, research, and clinical applications. Washington (DC): American Psychological Association; 1996. p. 285–99.
8. Matkin RE, Nickles LE, Demos RC, Demos GD. Cultural effects on symptom expression among Southeast Asians diagnosed with posttraumatic stress disorder. J Ment Health Couns. 1996 Jan;18(1):64–79.
9. Hsu E, Davies CA, Hansen DJ. Understanding mental health needs of Southeast Asian refugees: historical, cultural, and contextual challenges. Clin Psychol Rev. 2004 May;24(2):193–213.
10. Cohen R, Hemphill S. No safe port in a storm: the plight of Vietnamese refugees. Harvard Int Rev. 1991 Summer;13(4):32–35.

11. United Nations High Commissioner for Refugees (UNHCR). The state of the world's refugees 2000: Fifty years of humanitarian action—Chapter 4: Flight from Indochina; 2000. p. 27.

12. Sutter RW, Haefliger E. Tuberculosis morbidity and infection in Vietnamese in Southeast Asian refugee camps. Am J Respir Crit Care Med. 1990 Jun;141(6):1483–6.

13. Iwamasa GY. Recommendations for the treatment of Asian American/Pacific Islander Populations [Brochure]. Washington (DC): Council of National Psychological Associations for the Advancement of Ethnic Minority Interests; 2003. Available from: www.apa.org/pi/oema/resources/brochures/treatment-minority.pdf

14. Mollica RF, Wyshak G, Lavelle J. The psychological impact of war trauma and torture on Southeast Asian refugees. Am J Psychiatry. 1987 Dec;144(12):1567–72.

15. Chan S, editor. The Vietnamese American 1.5 generation: Stories of war, revolution, flight, and new beginnings. Philadelphia (PA): Temple University Press; 2006.

16. Lin E, Ihle LJ, Tazuma L. Depression among Vietnamese refugees in a primary care clinic. Am J Med Sci. 1985 Jan;78(1):41–4.

17. Tran TV, Manalo V, Nguyen VT. Nonlinear relationship between length of residence and depression in a community-based sample of Vietnamese Americans. Int J Soc Psychiatry. 2007 Jan;53(1):85–94.

18. Leung P, Cheung M, Cheung A. Vietnamese Americans and depression: a health and mental health concern. Soc Work Ment Health. 2010 Oct;8(6):526–42.

19. The World Bank. UNESCO Institute for Statistics. Literacy rate, adult total (% of people ages 15 and above)—Vietnam [Internet]. 2020. Available from: https://data.worldbank.org/indicator/SE.ADT.LITR.ZS?locations=VN

20. Pew Research Center. Educational attainment of Vietnamese population in the U.S., 2015 [Internet]. Washington (DC): Pew Research Center; 2017 July 6 [cited 2021 Jan 15]. Available from: https://www.pewresearch.org/social-trends/chart/educational-attainment-of-of-vietnamese-population-in-the-u-s/

21. Kula SM, Paik SJ. A historical analysis of Southeast Asian refugee communities: post-war acculturation and education in the US. J Southeast Asian Am Edu Adv [Internet]. 2016 Mar;11(1):1–27. Available from: 10.7771/2153-8999.1127

22. Schumann JH. Research on the acculturation model for second language acquisition. J Multiling Multicult Dev. 1986;7(5):379–392.

23. Yee, BWK. The social and cultural context of adaptive aging among southeast Asian elders. In Sokolovsky J, editor. The cultural context of aging [Internet]. 2nd ed. New York (NY): Greenwood Publishers; 1997 [cited 2021 Mar 1]. Chapter 26.

24. Lewis S. Same-sex marriage ban lifted in Vietnam but a year later discrimination remains. Time [Internet]. 2016 Jan 18 [cited 2021 Mar 1]. Available from: https://time.com/4184240/same-sex-gay-lgbt-marriage-ban-lifted-vietnam/

25. Institute for Health Metrics and Evaluation. Vietnam [Internet]. University of Washington; 2020. What causes the most deaths? Top 10 causes of death and disability (DALYs) in 2019 and percent change 2009–2019, all ages combined. Available from: http://www.healthdata.org/vietnam

26. Nguyen DT, Dedding C, Pham TT, Wright P, Bunders J. Depression, anxiety, and suicidal ideation among Vietnamese secondary school students and proposed solutions: a cross-sectional study. BMC Public Health. 2013 Dec 17;13(1):1–10. doi:10.1186/1471-2458-13-1195

27. Vuong DA, Van Ginneken E, Morris J, Ha ST, Busse R. Mental health in Vietnam: burden of disease and availability of services. Asian J Psychiatr. 2011 Mar;4(1):65–70. Table 1, Prevalence of 10 common mental disorders; doi:10.1016/j.ajp.2011.01.005

28. Weiss B, Dang H-M, Ngo V, Pollack A, Sang D, Lam TT et al. Development of clinical psychology and mental health resources in Vietnam. Psychol Stud. 2011 Jun 1;56(2); 185–91. doi:10.1007/s12646-011-0078-x

29. Tran B, Lawler K. Neuropsychological evaluation of a Vietnamese speaking man with Parkinson's disease and consideration for deep brain stimulation (DBS) surgery: a case report. Poster session presented at: International Congress of Parkinson's Disease and Movement Disorders; 2018 Oct 5–9; Hong Kong.

30. Nguyen CM. A culturally-informed neuropsychological assessment of a Vietnamese patient. In Fujii D. (Chair), Using the ECLECTIC framework for guiding the neuropsychological evaluation process: case studies with Latinx and Asian clients. Symposium presented at: International Neuropsychology Society; 2020 Feb 5–8; Denver, Colorado.

31. Dick MB, Teng EL, Kempler D, Davis DS, Taussig IM. The Cross-Cultural Neuropsychological Test Battery (CCNB): effects of age, education, ethnicity, and cognitive status on performance. In Ferraro FR, editor. Minority and cross-cultural aspects of neuropsychological assessment. Lisse, the Netherlands: Swets & Zeitlinger Publishers; 2002. p. 17–41.

32. Cook WK, Tseng W, Tam C, John I, Lui C. Ethnic-group socioeconomic status as an indicator of community-level disadvantage: a study of overweight/obesity in Asian American adolescents. Soc Sci Med. 2017 Jul;184:15–22.

33. Lezak MD, Howieson DB, Bigler ED, Tranel D. Neuropsychological assessment. 5th ed. New York (NY): Oxford University Press; 2012.

D. Europe

Overview

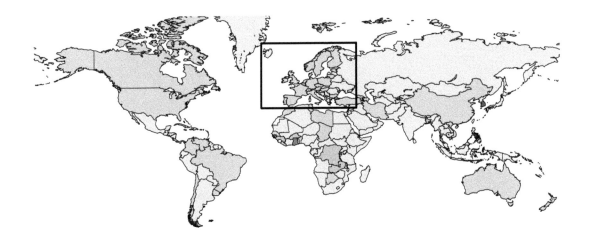

21 Cross-Cultural Neuropsychological Assessment in the European Context

Embracing Maximum Cultural Diversity at Minimal Geographic Distances

T. Rune Nielsen, Sanne Franzen, Miriam Goudsmit, and Özgül Uysal-Bozkir

Clinical Neuropsychology in Europe

Clinical neuropsychology has grown rapidly in Europe over the last 40 years and has expanded into new and wider areas. With the advent of increasingly sensitive multi-modal neurologic biomarker techniques, neuropsychological assessment has shifted from its original role in localizing the lesion to more in-depth characterization of patterns arising from disruptions of brain-behavior relationships.[1] Within healthcare, European neuropsychologists now offer services for patients with cognitive and behavioral symptoms related to neurological, developmental, and psychiatric disorders. The impact of disorders affecting the central nervous system is considerable both in Europe and globally. According to the Global Burden of Disease 2019 study,[2] in the European Union (EU) the burden from neurological diseases is only surpassed by the burden from cardiovascular diseases and neoplasms. The largest burden from neurological diseases in terms of deaths and disability is from stroke, migraine, and Alzheimer's disease, and other dementias, followed by medication-overuse headache, brain and nervous system cancer, and epilepsy. While not responsible for significant portions of deaths, mental disorders represent a large burden in terms of disability.[2] Thus, across Europe there is a great need for healthcare, including neuropsychological services, related to these diseases.

Depending on the definition used, Europe consists of about 50 countries and has a total population of approximately 742 million people, or 11% of the world population. From the later 20th century, "Europe" has come to be widely used as a synonym for the European Union (EU) even though there are millions of people living on the European continent in non-EU countries, mainly in Eastern European countries but also in countries such as Switzerland, Norway and more recently the United Kingdom. Currently, the EU has 27 member countries: Austria, Belgium, Bulgaria, Croatia, Cyprus, the Czech Republic, Denmark, Estonia, Finland, France, Germany, Greece, Hungary, Ireland, Italy, Latvia, Lithuania, Luxembourg, Malta, the Netherlands, Poland, Portugal, Romania, Slovakia, Slovenia, Spain, and Sweden. The EU recognizes 27 official languages, not counting 60 or so regional or EU minority languages and languages spoken by people from other parts of the world.[3] Many European countries have national neuropsychological societies that support specialist education and keep registries of qualified professionals, but their regulatory effect is less well defined. The Federation of the European Societies of Neuropsychology (FESN) was founded in 2008 with the aim of supporting development of scientific and clinical neuropsychology in Europe and currently encompasses 18 national neuropsychological societies.[4] In 2017, a Standing Committee on Clinical Neuropsychology became a permanent body of the

DOI: 10.4324/9781003051862-43

European Federation of Psychologists' Associations (EFPA), aiming to make recommendations for developments in specialization training for neuropsychology.[5]

Legal Status and Role in Healthcare

While most European countries regulate the profession of psychologists, there is large diversity in the regulation of the different fields or specialist areas within psychology.[6] Whereas the general title of psychologist is protected by law in most countries, clinical neuropsychologist is only a protected title in a handful of countries. A license to practice within healthcare from a national authority is the only requirement for clinical neuropsychologists in most countries.[6] There is also wide variability in terms of the healthcare systems and socio-economic situations across the countries. All EU countries, as well as most other European countries, provide universal health insurance or service coverage, or nearly universal coverage, for healthcare through compulsory schemes. While Scandinavian countries (Denmark, Norway, Sweden) have universal public healthcare systems paid largely from taxation, most European countries have systems of competing private health insurance companies, along with government regulation and subsidies for citizens who cannot afford (compulsory) health insurance premiums.[7] However, access to healthcare services, including neuropsychological services, vary greatly by country.[6] Also, there are differences in professional roles so that neuropsychologists in some countries have a subordinate and primarily advisory role concerning diagnosis and treatment planning, while psychologists in other countries have a fully independent role in diagnosis and treatment of patients.[6,8]

Education and Training Models

There is no commonly agreed model for specialization in clinical neuropsychology in Europe and the legal and professional status differs greatly between European countries. Europe mostly follows a common higher educational structure, implemented by the so-called Bologna Process. Programs are offered at three levels, namely bachelor's, master's, and doctoral studies, which are referred to as the three-cycle system.[6] EU programs such as the Erasmus Program have promoted mobility of students within the European community, and many European universities offer psychology and cognitive neuroscience master's and doctoral programs in English. European standards for psychology have been set by the EFPA to serve as the basis for evaluating the academic education and professional training of psychologists across countries.[9] These standards define competencies for psychologists having completed the master's level. Cross-cultural training, awareness, and knowledge are not part of these standards. Psychological specialties are generally less regulated and requirements for study in neuropsychology have not yet been established by EFPA.[6,10]

The specialization models of clinical neuropsychology in Europe and North America are similar in their content and requirements for courses and practice. However, in contrast to the United States and Canada, specialist education in most European countries is related to clinical training and not an academic degree.[10] A survey of 30 European countries[6] found that in one-third of the countries, no commonly agreed-upon model for specialist education in clinical neuropsychology existed and that the duration of specialist education varied from one to five years. Although specialist training can generally only be initiated after completing a master's degree, countries such as Spain only require a bachelor's degree, while the United Kingdom and Ireland require a doctoral degree.[6] As legal regulation is mostly absent and training models differ, those actively practicing clinical neuropsychology have a very heterogeneous educational background and skill level.

Approach to Neuropsychological Assessment

The history and traditions in neuropsychology differ both between and within European countries. Whereas neuropsychology in some countries (or national groups) has historically been dominated by the largely qualitative, flexible, and non-standardized Lurian approach, in other countries the quantitative and highly standardized fixed battery approach introduced by Ward Halstead and Ralph Reitan[1,8] has been more influential. Although remnants of both traditions are still found throughout Europe, as in North America and other parts of the world, European neuropsychologists now generally use a flexible assessment approach,[8,11] meaning that a fairly standardized, fixed set of neuropsychological tests is given to most clients with some flexibility to add or subtract tests given the specific referral question.[12] Often qualitative aspects of performance are considered in the interpretation of test results, and most European neuropsychologists prefer to do the testing themselves rather than relying on test technicians for the collection of neuropsychological data.[13]

In contrast to the United States, in most European countries there is no systematic use of performance validity testing and the issue of formally assessing response bias remains somewhat controversial.[8,13,14] A survey in six European countries[13] found that most neuropsychologists prefer to rely on their clinical judgment, whereas only a minority use performance validity tests in standard clinical neuropsychological assessments (12%). Even in forensic assessments, it is only a minority (45%) who always include a performance validity test.[13] However, there are considerable differences between countries, ranging from 14% in Finland to 70% in the Netherlands, and referral sources are increasingly exerting pressure on neuropsychologists to examine the credibility of symptom reports and the validity of test profiles with formal measures.[13] In cross-cultural assessments, formal performance validity testing has not been validated in many European ethnic minority groups, and the cross-cultural validity of some performance validity tests may be limited in the European context.[15]

Use of Neuropsychological Tests and Normative Data

Although locally developed tests are sometimes used, most of the tests and test batteries used by European neuropsychologists come from the international literature and have Anglo American origin.[8,16] Thus, they have often required translation and cultural adaption to non-English speaking cultures before implementation in clinical practice. Despite the usage of collaborative standardization of batteries such as the Wechsler Adult Intelligence Scale, fourth edition (WAIS-IV)[17] and Repeatable Battery for the Assessment of Neuropsychological Status (RBANS)[18] across Scandinavian countries and the Consortium to Establish a Registry for Alzheimer's Disease (CERAD) neuropsychological assessment battery across German-speaking countries,[19] well-known tests from the international literature have generally required country-specific adaption and standardization.

For instance, it has been necessary to develop Greek and Italian versions of the Trail Making Test as the Greek alphabet differs from the Latin one,[20] and the Italian alphabet does not include the letters "J" and "K."[21] As a result, tests scores are often interpreted using locally developed normative data of variable quantity and quality. Also, across Europe there is a multitude of different education systems that differ considerably in quantity and quality, and general education level and literacy rates also differ between countries.[22,23] This further complicates collaborative test standardization. In most European countries, literacy rates lie between 99% and 100%. However, lower literacy rates are found in some Southern and South-Eastern European countries, including Greece, Malta, and Portugal,[24] mainly driven by low(er) literacy rates in older generations. Although this complicates standardization of neuropsychological tests across European countries, it has also spurred important neuropsychological research. Research groups in Portugal and Greece were thus some of the first to describe associations between illiteracy, cognitive abilities, neuropsychological test performance, and the functional and structural organization of the brain.[25-39] Although rarely considered, key aspects of cross-cultural neuropsychological assessment and test development have thus been central to European neuropsychology since its advent as a modern clinical discipline.

Cross-Cultural Neuropsychological Assessment in Europe

Although a certain degree of diversity has always been present in European countries, ethnic diversity has increased greatly over the last seven decades. This started with the immigration of labor workers from countries outside the EU from 1950 to 1974 and the immigration of people from once-colonized countries, followed by the influx of asylum seekers and refugees in more recent years.[40] Therefore, European countries have had to adjust rapidly to the increasing diversity in their societies. In 2019, non-EU immigrants made up about 5% (21.8 million people) of the total EU population.[41] Several ethnic minority groups in European countries are at an increased risk of medical conditions that are associated with cognitive impairment, such as stroke,[42] diabetes mellitus,[42] and dementia.[43,44] As a result, neuropsychologists in Europe increasingly receive referrals of clients from ethnic minority groups.

Challenges in Cross-Cultural Assessment

Several issues may pose unique challenges to cross-cultural neuropsychological assessment of people from ethnic minority groups in Europe. First, limited proficiency in the host country language is widespread among older people from some ethnic minority groups, including Moroccans and Turks in the Netherlands,[45] South Asians in the United Kingdom,[46] Turks in Germany,[47] and Turks and Vietnamese in Belgium.[47] The language in which neuropsychological tests are administered, as well as the level of formality used, can significantly impact communication, rapport, and subsequent test scores.[48-50] Very few European neuropsychologists speak relevant minority languages, and interpretation through (formal or informal) interpreters is often needed to assess clients in their native language.[15] Several studies indicate that interpreter-assisted neuropsychological assessment may be challenging. The use of relatives as interpreters has been associated with the exclusion of the client from the conversation,[51] problems with adequate translation of medical terminology,[52] obscuring the client's explanatory models, and difficulties in assessing the level of insight.[53] The use of formal interpreters may be challenging as well, especially for tests with high demands on the abilities of the interpreter or when interpreters have received little formal training.[54,55] In many countries, training and licensure of interpreters is not well-regulated. For instance, in Sweden and Denmark, *professional* tends to be used for all interpreters available by interpreter services, irrespective of degree of training.[55] The degree of training of interpreters may therefore range from those who have taken a few courses to authorized interpreters with a medical specialization. Also, access to formal interpreters differs greatly between European countries. For example, in Austria and France, formal interpreters are provided through governmental funding; in Denmark and Belgium there are different rules depending on the specific case and context; and in most other countries there are no government-funded interpreter services.[15] Although general guidelines for psychologists working with interpreters have been published in countries such as the United Kingdom,[56] no specific guidelines are available to European neuropsychologists who generally lack training in working with interpreters.

Second, although the level of education is heterogeneous both across and within ethnic minority groups, low education levels or illiteracy are common among (older) people from various ethnic minority groups in Europe.[45,46] For example, 17%–36% of older Turkish and Moroccan first-generation immigrants in the Netherlands are illiterate, and more than half (50%–90%), especially women, have not completed any form of formal education.[57] Illiteracy, a limited number of years of education, as well as a low quality of education significantly impact neuropsychological tests scores across several cognitive domains.[58–61] Clients who are illiterate may also experience more discomfort in testing situations due to unfamiliarity with the setting, the content of the tests, or differences in what is considered a good response.[62] Also, as the length, quality, and content of the school day and year may vary considerably from country to country and even from school to school in some countries,[58,60] it may be inappropriate or even misleading to apply European norms to immigrants who have their education from a school system that differs greatly from the Western ones.

Third, neuropsychologists in Europe may encounter substantial cultural barriers in their clinical practice. Although ethnic minorities and immigration patterns differ between European countries, the largest ethnic minority groups across Europe originate from South Asian, Middle Eastern, and North African, predominantly collectivist Muslim, cultures.[63] Other significant ethnic minority groups are mainly found in specific European countries, including groups of Sub-Saharan African origin in the United Kingdom and France and of Latin American origin in Spain. Additionally, notable ethnic minorities include the Roma, who are found across most of Europe, indigenous peoples such as the Saami in Sweden, Norway, Finland, and Russia, and Irish Travelers. Acculturation toward the dominant culture differs greatly between and within ethnic minority groups and is closely associated with other factors, such as generation in the country, language proficiency, migration history, and level of education.[64] In particular the "guest workers," who came to Europe as labor migrants in the post-World War II period, may have limited levels of acculturation to the dominant culture as they were initially expected to return to their countries of origin after a number of years—often resulting in a delay of decades in the development of policies promoting social integration and acculturation.[40] The second generation is generally more bilingual and higher educated than the first generation of immigrants, although notable heterogeneity exists within this group. For instance, in the Netherlands second-generation Turks often have poorer Dutch language fluency and are often lower educated than their Moroccan peers.[65] It often poses a significant challenge to European neuropsychologists to determine which tests and normative data are most appropriate for this heterogeneous population.[15] Cultural differences may impact the neuropsychological assessment in several ways. The client may have different expectations of (the purpose of) the assessment, of what is relevant information, and of what information may be shared with a stranger.[66] A neuropsychologist from the majority group may not automatically be trusted. Some clients fear unfair treatment or misunderstanding of their complaints and way of life. For example, if asked about the burden of providing informal care for an older family member, clients from collectivist, family-oriented, cultures may object to this as they do not consider themselves to be informal caregivers. They just do their expected duty as a daughter or son.[67] Additionally, culture influences communication styles, idioms of distress, and the way symptoms may manifest themselves.[62] Also, Al-Jawahiri and Nielsen (2020)[64] showed that lower levels of acculturation are associated with poorer performance on tests of mental speed and executive functioning—even when tests are administered in the person's native language and scores correct for other demographics. Finally, culture and acculturation may influence test scores when tests include "Western items" or when the tests involve culture-specific testing elements and strategies.[68–70]

Cross-cultural neuropsychological assessment could benefit from matching clients from ethnic minority groups with neuropsychologists who are of the same ethnicity and/or are fluent in the client's language. However, in line with the reality in the United States,[71] providing same-ethnicity neuropsychologists to all clients from ethnic minority groups in Europe is currently not feasible considering the number of different ethnic minority groups and the limited ethnic diversity among neuropsychologists in Europe.[15] Instead, there is a general need to improve cross-cultural training, awareness, and knowledge among European neuropsychologists and to increase recruitment of culturally and linguistically diverse neuropsychologists into the field. Cross-cultural training of neuropsychologists has also been identified as a priority in the United States, where "clinicians often lack in-depth training in assessment of ethnic minorities."[72]

In sum, language, (quality of) education, literacy, and culture substantially influence neuropsychological assessment. Cultural and language adaptations, or newly developed, neuropsychological tests for ethnic minority groups in Europe are needed, but such tests are often lacking.[73] Although neuropsychologists in several of the countries of origin of ethnic minority clients are working on the validation of cognitive tests, these initiatives have mostly focused on tests originally designed for (educated) populations in North America and Europe, such as the Trail Making Test[74] or the Montreal Cognitive Assessment[75] in Morocco, and tests from the BİLNOT battery in Turkey.[76] Furthermore, people who are low educated or illiterate are not included in these validation studies or in the normative data samples.

Taking these barriers into consideration, conducting a cross-cultural neuropsychological assessment requires that European neuropsychologists acquire culture-competen competence skills and knowledge. Although some general directions for training of psychologists are presented in the "Guidelines on Multicultural Education, Training, Research, Practice, and Organizational Change for Psychologists" by the American Psychological Association,[77] these guidelines are not specific to neuropsychologists. Despite European and North American neuropsychologists emphasizing that the ability to handle cultural diversity is a "vital functional competency" for clinical neuropsychologists worldwide[78] and, more specifically, "one of the foundational entry-level competencies for neuropsychologists,"[79] no details have been provided on the specific knowledge or skills that European neuropsychologists should acquire to attain sufficient competence to handle the substantial barriers in culture, language, and education.

All these factors pose challenges to the assessment of clients from ethnic minority groups and have initiated recent developments in cross-cultural neuropsychological assessment in Europe. In contrast to North American initiatives that have generally focused on adapting and standardizing well-established tests or batteries for specific languages or ethnic groups (e.g., Hispanics or African Americans),[80–82] European efforts have generally aimed at developing and validating neuropsychological tests and batteries for use across diverse ethnic groups.[83–85]

Advances in Cross-Cultural Assessment

A recent Delphi expert study[15] found that considerable work has been carried out in the development and validation of cross-cultural neuropsychological tests in Europe, but mainly by neuropsychologists working in memory clinic settings. In particular, the European Cross-Cultural Neuropsychological Test Battery (CNTB)[83] and the Rowland Universal Dementia Assessment Scale (RUDAS),[86] which was originally developed for multicultural populations in Australia, are well-validated across European countries. These instruments have been studied in people from numerous minority groups, with a wide variety of education levels, in studies from across multiple European countries (CNTB[64,87–89]; RUDAS[57,90–93]). Together, these instruments measure a variety of cognitive functions including general cognitive functioning (RUDAS), memory (Recall of Pictures Test, Enhanced Cued Recall and recall of a semi-complex figure), language (Picture naming and semantic verbal fluency), executive functions (Color Trails Test, Five Digit Test and

Serial Threes), and visuospatial functions (Clock Reading Test, Clock Drawing Test and copying of simple and semi-complex figures). For some of the other instruments identified in this study, few (if any) validation studies have been published for the target population.[15] However, better cross-culturally validated instruments used in some countries include the Cross-Cultural Dementia screening[85] and modified Visual Association Test[84] in the Netherlands, the computerized EMBRACED battery (unpublished) in Spain, the Multicultural Cognitive Examination[94] in Denmark, and TNI-93,[95] TMA-93,[96] and TFA-93[97] in France.

In order to make them suitable for use across diverse ethnic groups, languages, education, and literacy levels, these instruments were designed without using culture- or language-specific stimuli,[48,68] black-and-white line drawings,[29,30,84] or test elements that require skills learned in school (e.g., Nielsen & Jørgensen, 2013).[61] Generally, the influence of limited education and illiteracy is reduced by using test procedures with higher ecological relevance for people without formal school experience; that is, test procedures relying on elements and strategies from everyday life rather than the classroom.[37,48,73] Often, smaller modifications of existing test paradigms are sufficient to make tests more ecologically relevant. For instance, in the RUDAS the memory subtest requires memorization and recall of a shopping list rather than a list of unrelated words, and in the Multicultural Cognitive Examination the semantic verbal fluency subtest adopts a supermarket category rather than the commonly used animal category. Whereas knowledge about supermarkets is usually obtained through everyday life experience, knowledge about animals and strategies for memorizing and recalling words is largely obtained through formal school experience.[37,58,61] These instruments all represent important contributions to the field of (cross-cultural) neuropsychological assessment in Europe. However, many European neuropsychologists are not familiar with these newer additions to the neuropsychological toolbox, and there is a need for better publication and implementation of the instruments across Europe.[15]

Aside from looking into neuropsychological tests in themselves, European experts in cross-cultural neuropsychological assessment also recognize the importance of taking the cultural context of neuropsychological assessment into consideration.[15] These contextual factors are neatly summarized by the acronym of the ECLECTIC framework[62]: Education and literacy, Culture and acculturation, Language, Economics (e.g., socio-economic status), Communication, Testing situation, Comfort and motivation, Intelligence conceptualization, and Context of immigration. Although this framework has not been formally assessed or implemented in Europe, several key contextual factors have been included in research and clinical practice. For example, an unpublished literacy screening test is used in the Netherlands to determine the quality of the clients' education (E).[15] Neuropsychologists from several European countries make use of short acculturation scales (C) in their research and clinical practice, including a modified version of the Short Acculturation Scale for Hispanics (SASH[98]). Additionally, the effects of language abilities in both native and host country languages (L) are recognized by European experts in the field, as well as the effects of stereotype threat,[99] of being unfamiliar with cognitive testing, and of examinee–examiner ethnic discordance (T) on the assessment.[15] Experts in the field also recognize that it is important to take lifetime (socio)demographic factors and access to and availability of healthcare services into account (E).[15] Some aspects from the ECLECTIC framework, particularly communication styles and intelligence conceptualization, has received less explicit attention among European neuropsychologists. Other specific examples of relevant issues to take into consideration in working with ethnic minority groups in the European context are traumatic experiences, migration-related distress or grief,[100] exposure to discrimination,[101] differences in explanatory models of illness (e.g. van Wezel et al[102], Fazil et al[103]), and differences in symptom manifestation and idioms of distress, such as mixed affective and somatic presentations of depression in Moroccan and Turkish clients.[104] Consistent with this, a survey among European dementia experts found that 84% perceived cultural differences in the presentation of symptoms to frequently affect clinical assessments of clients from ethnic minority groups.[105]

Summary

To sum up, significant work has been carried out in the development and validation of cross-cultural neuropsychological tests in Europe. However, the field of cross-cultural neuropsychological assessment is largely still a developing field, and formal expertise is localized rather than widespread. Despite recent advances in cross-cultural neuropsychological testing and training in some European countries, there is a continuing need for development of cross-cultural tests and normative data, for culture-sensitive training, awareness, and knowledge among European neuropsychologists, and recruitment of culturally and linguistically diverse neuropsychologists into the field. Also, ethnic minority groups are often excluded from scientific research of diagnostic criteria or treatment efficacy for (neuro)psychological therapies because of language or educational barriers.[106,107] More inclusive research with increased efforts to include "hard to reach" ethnic minority groups is needed. Also, the scope of cross-cultural neuropsychological assessment should be widened to include indigenous and transnational minorities such as the Roma across Europe and the Saami across Sweden, Norway, Finland, and Russia.

References

1. Casaletto KB, Heaton RK. Neuropsychological assessment: past and future. J Int Neuropsychol Soc. 2017;23(9–10):778.
2. Diseases GBD, Injuries C. Global burden of 369 diseases and injuries in 204 countries and territories, 1990–2019: a systematic analysis for the Global Burden of Disease Study 2019. Lancet. 2020;396(10258):1204–22.
3. Pan C. Die Bedeutung von Minderheiten-und Sprachschutz für die kulturelle Vielfalt Europas. Europäisches Journal für Minderheitenfragen. 2008;1(1):11–33.
4. Demonet J-F. A new impulse for neuropsychology in Europe: the Federation of the European Societies of Neuropsychology. Amsterdam: IOS Press; 2008.
5. EFPA. Task Force on Clinical Neuropsychology. Introduction & definition [Internet]. EFPA—TF on Clinical Neuropsychology. 2020. Available from: http://clinneuropsy.efpa.eu/
6. Hokkanen L, Lettner S, Barbosa F, Constantinou M, Harper L, Kasten E, et al. Training models and status of clinical neuropsychologists in Europe: results of a survey on 30 countries. Clin Neuropsychol. 2019;33(1):32–56.
7. Jakubowski E, Busse R. Health care systems in the EU: a comparative study. Luxembourg: European Parliament; 1998.
8. Egeland J, Løvstad M, Norup A, Nybo T, Persson BA, Rivera DF et al. Following international trends while subject to past traditions: neuropsychological test use in the Nordic countries. Clin Neuropsychol. 2016;30(sup1):1479–500.
9. Psychology EtECi. EuroPsy regulations [Internet]. 2019. Available from: www.europsy.eu/quality-and-standards/regulations
10. Grote CL, Novitski JI. International perspectives on education, training, and practice in clinical neuropsychology: comparison across 14 countries around the world. Clin Neuropsychol. 2016;30(8):1380–8.
11. Larrabee GJ. Flexible vs. fixed batteries in forensic neuropsychological assessment: reply to Bigler and Hom. Arch Clin Neuropsychol. 2008;23(7–8):763–76.
12. Bigler ED. A motion to exclude and the "fixed" versus "flexible" battery in "forensic" neuropsychology: challenges to the practice of clinical neuropsychology. Arch Clin Neuropsychol. 2007;22(1):45–51.
13. Dandachi-FitzGerald B, Ponds RW, Merten T. Symptom validity and neuropsychological assessment: a survey of practices and beliefs of neuropsychologists in six European countries. Arch Clin Neuropsychol. 2013;28(8):771–83.

14. McCarter RJ, Walton NH, Brooks DN, Powell GE. Effort testing in contemporary UK neuropsychological practice. Clin Neuropsychol. 2009;23(6):1050–66.
15. Franzen S, Papma JM, van den Berg E, Nielsen TR. Cross-cultural neuropsychological assessment in the European Union: a Delphi expert study. Arch Clin Neuropsychol. 2021;36(5):815–30.
16. Maruta C, Guerreiro M, de Mendonça A, Hort J, Scheltens P. The use of neuropsychological tests across Europe: the need for a consensus in the use of assessment tools for dementia. Eur J Neurol. 2011;18(2):279–85.
17. Wechsler D. WAIS-IV. Vejledning del 1. Dansk version. Stockholm: Pearson; 2011.
18. Randolph C. RBANS. Vejledning. Dansk version. Stockholm: Pearson; 2013.
19. Thalmann B, Monsch AU, Schneitter M, Bernasconi F, Aebi C, Camachova-Davet Z et al. The CERAD neuropsychological assessment battery (CERAD-NAB)—A minimal data set as a common tool for German-speaking Europe. Neurobiol Aging. 2000;21:30.
20. Zalonis I, Kararizou E, Triantafyllou N, Kapaki E, Papageorgiou S, Sgouropoulos P et al. A normative study of the trail making test A and B in Greek adults. Clin Neuropsychol. 2008;22(5):842–50.
21. Giovagnoli AR, Del Pesce M, Mascheroni S, Simoncelli M, Laiacona M, Capitani E. Trail making test: normative values from 287 normal adult controls. Ital J Neurol Sci. 1996;17(4):305–9.
22. OECD. PISA 2018 results (Volume 1): What students know and can do. Paris: PISA, OECD Publishing; 2019.
23. United Nations Development Programme. Human Development Report 2019. Beyond income, beyond averages, beyond today: inequalities in human development in the 21st century. New York (NY): United Nations Development Programme; 2019.
24. World Bank. Literacy rate, adult total (% of people ages 15 and above) [Internet]. Washington:World Bank; 2018. Available from: www.data.worldbank.org
25. Kosmidis MH, Zafiri M, Politimou N. Literacy versus formal schooling: influence on working memory. Arch Clin Neuropsychol. 2011;26(7):575–82.
26. Reis A, Castro-Caldas A. Illiteracy: a cause for biased cognitive development. J Int Neuropsychol Soc. 1997;3(5):444–50.
27. Petersson KM, Reis A, Ingvar M. Cognitive processing in literate and illiterate subjects: a review of some recent behavioral and functional neuroimaging data. Scand J Psychol. 2001;42(3):251–67.
28. da Silva CG, Petersson KM, Faisca L, Ingvar M, Reis A. The effects of literacy and education on the quantitative and qualitative aspects of semantic verbal fluency. J Clin Exp Neuropsychol. 2004;26(2):266–77.
29. Reis A, Faisca L, Ingvar M, Petersson KM. Color makes a difference: two-dimensional object naming in literate and illiterate subjects. Brain Cogn. 2006;60(1):49–54.
30. Reis A, Petersson KM, Castro-Caldas A, Ingvar M. Formal schooling influences two- but not three-dimensional naming skills. Brain Cogn. 2001;47(3):397–411.
31. Castro-Caldas A, Petersson KM, Reis A, Stone-Elander S, Ingvar M. The illiterate brain. Learning to read and write during childhood influences the functional organization of the adult brain. Brain. 1998;121(Pt 6):1053–63.
32. Reis A, Guerreiro M, Castro-Caldas A. Influence of educational level of non brain-damaged subjects on visual naming capacities. J Clin Exp Neuropsychol. 1994;16(6):939–42.
33. Castro-Caldas A, Miranda PC, Carmo I, Reis A, Leote F, Ribeiro C et al. Influence of learning to read and write on the morphology of the corpus callosum. Eur J Neurol. 1999;6(1):23–8.
34. Petersson KM, Silva C, Castro-Caldas A, Ingvar M, Reis A. Literacy: a cultural influence on functional left-right differences in the inferior parietal cortex. Eur J Neurosci. 2007;26(3):791–9.
35. Reis A, Guerreiro M, Petersson KM. A sociodemographic and neuropsychological characterization of an illiterate population. Appl Neuropsychol. 2003;10(4):191–204.
36. Folia V, Kosmidis MH. Assessment of memory skills in illiterates: strategy differences or test artifact? Clin Neuropsychol. 2003;17(2):143–52.
37. Kosmidis MH. Challenges in the neuropsychological assessment of illiterate older adults. Lang Cogn Neurosci. 2018;33(3):373–86.
38. Kosmidis MH, Tsapkini K, Folia V. Lexical processing in illiteracy: effect of literacy or education? Cortex. 2006;42(7):1021–7.

39. Kosmidis MH, Tsapkini K, Folia V, Vlahou CH, Kiosseoglou G. Semantic and phonological processing in illiteracy. J Int Neuropsychol Soc. 2004;10(6):818.

40. Van Mol C, De Valk H. Migration and immigrants in Europe: a historical and demographic perspective. In: Garcés-Mascareñas B, Penninx R, editors. Integration processes and policies in Europe. Cham: Springer; 2016. p. 31–55.

41. Eurostat. Migration and migrant population statistics [Internet]. 2020. Available from: www.ec. europa.eu/eurostat/statistics-explained

42. Kunst AE, Stronks K, Agyemang C. Non-communicable diseases. Migration and Health in the European Union. 2011;1:101–20.

43. Parlevliet JL, Uysal-Bozkir O, Goudsmit M, van Campen JP, Kok RM, Ter RG et al. Prevalence of mild cognitive impairment and dementia in older non-western immigrants in the Netherlands: a cross-sectional study. Int J Geriatr Psychiatry. 2016;31(9):1040–9.

44. Adelman S, Blanchard M, Rait G, Leavey G, Livingston G. Prevalence of dementia in African-Caribbean compared with UK-born White older people: two-stage cross-sectional study. Br J Psychiatry. 2011;199(2):119–25.

45. Schellingerhout R. Gezondheid en welzijn van allochtone ouderen. Den Haag: Sociaal en Cultureel Planbureau (SCP): 2004.

46. Blakemore A, Kenning C, Mirza N, Daker-White G, Panagioti M, Waheed W. Dementia in UK South Asians: a scoping review of the literature. BMJ Open. 2018;8(4):e020290.

47. Van Tubergen F, Kalmijn M. Destination-language proficiency in cross-national perspective: a study of immigrant groups in nine western countries. Am J Sociol. 2005;110(5):1412–57.

48. Ardila A. The impact of culture on neuropsychological test performance. In: Uzzell PB, Marcel P, Ardila A, editors. International handbook of cross-cultural neuropsychology. London: Lawrence Erlbaum Associated; 2007. p. 23–44.

49. Carstairs JR, Myors B, Shores EA, Fogarty G. Influence of language background on tests of cognitive abilities: Australian data. Aust Psychol. 2006;41(1):48–54.

50. Boone KB, Victor TL, Wen J, Razani J, Ponton M. The association between neuropsychological scores and ethnicity, language, and acculturation variables in a large patient population. Arch Clin Neuropsychol. 2007;22(3):355–65.

51. Zendedel R, Schouten BC, van Weert JC, van den Putte B. Informal interpreting in general practice: the migrant patient's voice. Ethn Health. 2018;23(2):158–73.

52. Manly JJ, Espino DV. Cultural influences on dementia recognition and management. Clin Geriatr Med. 2004;20(1):93–119.

53. Kilian S, Swartz L, Dowling T, Dlali M, Chiliza B. The potential consequences of informal interpreting practices for assessment of patients in a South African psychiatric hospital. Soc Sci Med. 2014;106:159–67.

54. Casas R, Guzman-Velez E, Cardona-Rodriguez J, Rodriguez N, Quinones G, Izaguirre B et al. Interpreter-mediated neuropsychological testing of monolingual Spanish speakers. Clin Neuropsychol. 2012;26(1):88–101.

55. Plejert C, Antelius E, Yazdanpanah M, Nielsen TR. "There's a letter called ef" on challenges and repair in interpreter-mediated tests of cognitive functioning in dementia evaluations: a case study. J Cross Cult Gerontol. 2015;30(2):163–87.

56. Tribe R, Thompson K. Working with interpreters: guidelines for psychologists. British Psychological Society; Leicester, UK: 2017.

57. Goudsmit M, van Campen J, Franzen S, van den Berg E, Schilt T, Schmand B. Dementia detection with a combination of informant-based and performance-based measures in low-educated and illiterate elderly migrants. Clin Neuropsychol. 2021;35(3):660–78.

58. Ardila A, Bertolucci PH, Braga LW, Castro-Caldas A, Judd T, Kosmidis MH et al. Illiteracy: the neuropsychology of cognition without reading. Arch Clin Neuropsychol. 2010;25(8):689–712.

59. Manly JJ, Jacobs DM, Touradji P, Small SA, Stern Y. Reading level attenuates differences in neuropsychological test performance between African American and White elders. J Int Neuropsychol Soc. 2002;8(3):341–8.

60. Shuttleworth-Edwards A. Generally representative is representative of none: commentary on the pitfalls of IQ test standardization in multicultural settings. Clin Neuropsychol. 2016;30(7):975–98.

61. Nielsen TR, Jorgensen K. Visuoconstructional abilities in cognitively healthy illiterate Turkish immigrants: a quantitative and qualitative investigation. Clin Neuropsychol. 2013;27(4):681–92.

62. Fujii DEM. Developing a cultural context for conducting a neuropsychological evaluation with a culturally diverse client: the ECLECTIC framework. Clin Neuropsychol. 2018;32(8):1356–92.

63. Nielsen TR, Segers K, Vanderaspoilden V, Bekkhus-Wetterberg P, Minthon L, Pissiota A et al. Performance of middle-aged and elderly European minority and majority populations on a Cross-Cultural Neuropsychological Test Battery (CNTB). Clin Neuropsychol. 2018;32(8):1411–30.

64. Al-Jawahiri F, Nielsen TR. Effects of acculturation on the Cross-Cultural Neuropsychological Test Battery (CNTB) in a culturally and linguistically diverse population in Denmark. Arch Clin Neuropsychol. 2021;36(3):381–93.

65. Crul M, Vermeulen H. The second generation in Europe. Int Migr Rev. 2003;37(4):965–86.

66. Greenfield PM. You can't take it with you: why ability assessments don't cross cultures. Am Psychol. 1997;52(10):1115.

67. Nielsen TR, Nielsen DS, Waldemar G. Barriers in access to dementia care in minority ethnic groups in Denmark: a qualitative study. Aging Ment Health. 2021;25(8):1424–32.

68. Ardila A. Cultural values underlying psychometric cognitive testing. Neuropsychol Rev. 2005; 15(4):185–95.

69. Rosselli M, Ardila A. The impact of culture and education on non-verbal neuropsychological measurements: a critical review. Brain Cogn. 2003;52(3):326–33.

70. Ardila A, Keating K. Cognitive abilities in different cultural contexts. In: Uzzell PB, Marcel P, Ardila A, editors. International handbook of cross-cultural neuropsychology. London: Lawrence Erlbaum Associated; 2007. p. 109–25.

71. Elbulok-Charcape MM, Rabin LA, Spadaccini AT, Barr WB. Trends in the neuropsychological assessment of ethnic/racial minorities: a survey of clinical neuropsychologists in the United States and Canada. Cult Divers Ethn Minor Psychol. 2014;20(3):353.

72. Rivera Mindt M, Byrd D, Saez P, Manly J. Increasing culturally competent neuropsychological services for ethnic minority populations: a call to action. Clin Neuropsychol. 2010;24(3):429–53.

73. Franzen S, van den Berg E, Goudsmit M, Jurgens CK, van de Wiel L, Kalkisim Y et al. A systematic review of neuropsychological tests for the assessment of dementia in non-Western, low-educated or illiterate populations. J Int Neuropsychol Soc. 2020;26(3):331–51.

74. Oumellal A, Faris MEA, Benabdeljlil M. The Trail Making Test in Morocco: normative data stratified by age and level of education. Open J Med Psychol. 2017;7(1):1–12.

75. Benabdeljlil M, Azdad A, Mustapha E. Standardization and validation of Montreal cognitive assessment (MoCA) in the Moroccan population. J Neurol Sci. 2017;381:318.

76. Karakaş S, Erdoğan Bakar E, Doğutepe Dinçer E. BİLNOT Bataryası El Kitabı: Nöropsikolojik Testlerin Yetişkinler için Araştırma ve Geliştirme Çalışmaları: BİLNOT—Yetişkin (Cilt I). Konya: Eğitim Yayinevi; 2013.

77. Association AP. Guidelines on multicultural education, training, research, practice, and organizational change for psychologists. Am Psychol. 2003;58(5):377.

78. Hessen E, Hokkanen L, Ponsford J, van Zandvoort M, Watts A, Evans J et al. Core competencies in clinical neuropsychology training across the world. Clin Neuropsychol. 2018;32(4):642–56.

79. Smith G, CNS. Education and training in clinical neuropsychology: recent developments and documents from the clinical neuropsychology synarchy. Arch Clin Neuropsychol. 2019;34(3):418–31.

80. Lucas JA, Ivnik RJ, Willis FB, Ferman TJ, Smith GE, Parfitt FC et al. Mayo's Older African Americans Normative Studies: normative data for commonly used clinical neuropsychological measures. Clin Neuropsychol. 2005;19(2):162–83.

81. Mungas D, Reed BR, Crane PK, Haan MN, González H. Spanish and English Neuropsychological Assessment Scales (SENAS): further development and psychometric characteristics. Psychol Assess. 2004;16(4):347–59.

82. Ponton MO, Satz P, Herrera L, Ortiz F, Urrutia CP, Young R et al. Normative data stratified by age and education for the Neuropsychological Screening Battery for Hispanics (NeSBHIS): initial report. J Int Neuropsychol Soc. 1996;2(2):96–104.

83. Nielsen TR, Segers K, Vanderaspoilden V, Bekkhus-Wetterberg P, Minthon L, Pissiota A et al. Performance of middle-aged and elderly European minority and majority populations on a Cross-Cultural Neuropsychological Test Battery (CNTB). Clin Neuropsychol. 2018;32(8):1411–30.

84. Franzen S, van den Berg E, Kalkisim Y, Van De Wiel L, Harkes M, van Bruchem-Visser RL et al. Assessment of visual association memory in low-educated, non-Western immigrants with the modified visual association test. Dement Geriatr Cogn Disord. 2019;47(4–6):345–54.

85. Goudsmit M, Uysal-Bozkir O, Parlevliet JL, van Campen JP, de Rooij SE, Schmand B. The Cross-Cultural Dementia Screening (CCD): a new neuropsychological screening instrument for dementia in elderly immigrants. J Clin Exp Neuropsychol. 2017;39(2):163–72.

86. Storey JE, Rowland JT, Basic D, Conforti DA, Dickson HG. The Rowland Universal Dementia Assessment Scale (RUDAS): a multicultural cognitive assessment scale. Int Psychogeriatr. 2004;16(1):13–31.

87. Nielsen TR, Segers K, Vanderaspoilden V, Beinhoff U, Minthon L, Pissiota A et al. Validation of a European Cross-Cultural Neuropsychological Test Battery (CNTB) for evaluation of dementia. Int J Geriatr Psychiatry. 2019;34(1):144–52.

88. Nielsen TR. Effects of Illiteracy on the European Cross-Cultural Neuropsychological Test Battery (CNTB). Arch Clin Neuropsychol. 2019;34(5):713–20.

89. Nielsen TR, Segers K, Vanderaspoilden V, Bekkhus-Wetterberg P, Bjorklof GH, Beinhoff U et al. Validation of the Rowland Universal Dementia Assessment Scale (RUDAS) in a multicultural sample across five Western European countries: diagnostic accuracy and normative data. Int Psychogeriatr. 2019;31(2):287–96.

90. Nielsen TR, Jorgensen K. Cross-cultural dementia screening using the Rowland Universal Dementia Assessment Scale: a systematic review and meta-analysis. Int Psychogeriatr. 2020;32(9):1031–44.

91. Goudsmit M, van Campen J, Schilt T, Hinnen C, Franzen S, Schmand B. One size does not fit all: comparative diagnostic accuracy of the Rowland Universal Dementia Assessment Scale and the Mini Mental State Examination in a memory clinic population with very low education. Dement Geriatr Cogn Disord Extra. 2018;8(2):290–305.

92. Nielsen TR, Andersen BB, Gottrup H, Lutzhoft JH, Hogh P, Waldemar G. Validation of the Rowland Universal Dementia Assessment Scale for multicultural screening in Danish Memory Clinics. Dement Geriatr Cogn Disord. 2013;36(5–6):354–62.

93. Nielsen TR, Segers K, Vanderaspoilden V, Beinhoff U, Minthon L, Pissiota A et al. Validation of a brief Multicultural Cognitive Examination (MCE) for evaluation of dementia. Int J Geriatr Psychiatry. 2019;34(7):982–9.

94. Maillet D, Matharan F, Le Clésiau H, Bailon O, Pérès K, Amieva H et al. TNI-93: a new memory test for dementia detection in illiterate and low-educated patients. Arch Clin Neuropsychol. 2016;31(8):896–903.

95. Maillet D, Narme P, Amieva H, Matharan F, Bailon O, Le Clésiau H et al. The TMA-93: a new memory test for Alzheimer's disease in illiterate and less educated people. Am J Alzheimer's Dis Other Dement. 2017;32(8):461–7.

96. Narme P, Maillet D, Palisson J, Le Clésiau H, Moroni C, Belin C. How to assess executive functions in a low-educated and multicultural population using a switching verbal fluency test (the TFA-93) in neurodegenerative diseases? Am J Alzheimer's Dis Other Dement. 2019;34(7–8):469–77.

97. Marín G, Sabogal F, Marín BV, Otero-Sabogal R, Perez-Stable EJ. Development of a short acculturation scale for Hispanics. Hisp J Behav Sci. 1987;9:183–205.

98. Steele CM. A threat in the air: how stereotypes shape intellectual identity and performance. Am Psychol. 1997;52(6):613.

99. Carta MG, Bernal M, Hardoy MC, Haro-Abad JM. Migration and mental health in Europe (the state of the mental health in Europe working group: Appendix 1). Clin Pract Epidemiology Ment Health. 2005;1(1):13.

100. de Freitas DF, Fernandes-Jesus M, Ferreira PD, Coimbra S, Teixeira PM, de Moura A et al. Psychological correlates of perceived ethnic discrimination in Europe: a meta-analysis. Psychol Violence. 2018;8(6):712.

101. van Wezel N, Francke AL, Kayan-Acun E, Ljm Deville W, van Grondelle NJ, Blom MM. Family care for immigrants with dementia: the perspectives of female family carers living in the Netherlands. Dementia (London). 2016;15(1):69–84.

102. Fazil Q, Wallace L, Hussain A. An exploration of the explanatory models of illness amongst Pushtuun families living in the UK who are high attenders in general practice. Divers Equal Health Care. 2006;3:171–81.

103. Sempértegui GA, Knipscheer JW, Baliatsas C, Bekker MH. Symptom manifestation and treatment effectiveness,-obstacles and-facilitators in Turkish and Moroccan groups with depression in European countries: a systematic review. J Affect Disord. 2019;247:134–55.

104. Nielsen TR, Vogel A, Riepe MW, de MA, Rodriguez G, Nobili F et al. Assessment of dementia in ethnic minority patients in Europe: a European Alzheimer's Disease Consortium survey. Int Psychogeriatr. 2011;23(1):86–95.

105. Waheed W, Mirza N, Waheed MW, Blakemore A, Kenning C, Masood Y et al. Recruitment and methodological issues in conducting dementia research in British ethnic minorities: a qualitative systematic review. Int J Methods Psychiatr Res. 2020;29(1):e1806.

106. Shah A, Doe P, Deverill K. Ethnic minority elders: are they neglected in published geriatric psychiatry literature? Int Psychogeriatr. 2008;20(5):1041–5.

Dutch (Moroccan)

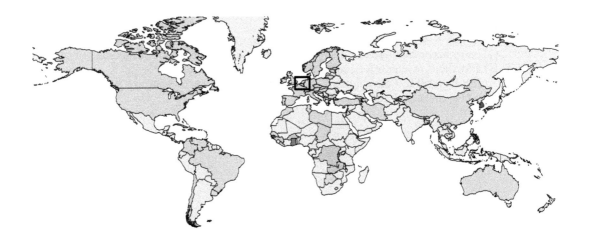

22 Approach to Neuropsychological Assessment of Moroccan Patients in the Netherlands

Özgül Uysal-Bozkir, Sanne Franzen, and Miriam Goudsmit

Section I: Background Information

Terminology and Perspective

People from Morocco in the Netherlands are generally referred to as Moroccans or Moroccan Dutch etc. However, people from Morocco may prefer to be referred to in other ways. For instance, people from the Berber* minority may choose to be referred to as Amazigh or Moroccan Berber. Throughout the chapter, we will use Moroccan to refer to people originating from Morocco's geographical area and only make ethnic distinctions when relevant.

We are clinical neuropsychologists mainly affiliated with public hospitals in two major cities in the Netherlands, where many immigrants live. We have worked with diverse groups in clinical and research studies. Currently, Özgül Uysal-Bozkir (ÖUB) focuses on the work at the university as a researcher and teacher. Sanne Franzen (SF) and Miriam Goudsmit (MG) are both clinicians and researchers. It is essential to notice none of us have a Moroccan background. ÖUB is a Turkish Dutch citizen, and SF and MG belong to the ethnic Dutch majority. We base our knowledge primarily on our experiences working with the Moroccan community.

We will start the chapter by providing some general knowledge of the country of origin to outline a person's possible background present in clinical practice. However, it is essential not to make premature assumptions. Overgeneralization may lead to incorrect assumptions or unfortunate moments, such as in the example below:

> I (ÖUB) was born in the Netherlands, but I spent a lot of time in Turkey, my parents' country of origin. As a 2nd generation Turkish Dutch, I come across prejudice quite often. An example is when the entire team received a bottle of wine as a Christmas gift, and my colleagues subsequently asked me if I wanted to exchange my bottle of wine for something else. They assume that, as a Turkish, and therefore (probably) Muslim, I don't consume alcohol – which is not the case.

Geography

The Kingdom of Morocco is a country located in the Maghreb region of Northern Africa along the Atlantic Ocean and the Mediterranean Sea. Algeria and Western Sahara border it. It also still shares borders with two enclaves considered a part of Spain—Ceuta and Melilla. Morocco's

---

*The word "Berber" may have a negative connotation to some, but in this publication, we use it neutrally and alternated with "Amazigh" for stylistic reasons.

DOI: 10.4324/9781003051862-45

topography varies as its northern coast and interior regions are mountainous, while its coast features fertile plains where much of the country's agriculture takes place. Morocco has a population of approximately 35.5 million people. The capital is Rabat, and the largest city is Casablanca. From the Netherlands you can travel to Morocco by car and ferry, which takes about 2 to 3 days. By plane, the journey takes 3 to 4 hours.

History

Morocco has a long history that has been shaped by its geographic location on both the Atlantic Ocean and the Mediterranean Sea. Its history records a struggle for ascendancy, and from the 18th century, influenced by European powers. Here we briefly outline significant events: From 1667 onward, the Alaouites **dynasty** has been the ruling dynasty of the Moroccan royal family. From the 15th century, there were influences from Europe, such as the Portuguese. At the end of the 19th century, Morocco declared bankruptcy, which was also indirectly the result of repeated attempts to colonize the area. In the Treaty of Fes (1912), Morocco agreed to Spanish and French protection. Morocco gained its independence back from France (1956). From the 1990s, the regime evolved toward more democracy and political reforms. In 1996, Morocco was given a new constitution, and in 1999 Mohammed VI became king. He saw the need to establish closer ties with the West and increase foreign investment in Morocco. The Kingdom of Morocco is a semi-constitutional monarchy with an elected parliament.

Immigration and Relocation

People move from their homeland searching for better personal, social, financial, or political conditions. Common reasons for Moroccan people migrating include economic opportunity and **family reunification**.[1]

After the Second World War, the Dutch industry needed low-skilled labor workers, and many of these first-generation "guest workers" who came to the Netherlands in the 1960s and 1970s were recruited from Morocco. They hoped to earn money in a short time to provide a better future for their family back home. However, most of them did not return because their home countries' economic and political situation remained low, so they stayed in Europe permanently.

From 1975 to 2020, the Moroccan population in the Netherlands grew from 30,481 to 411,000. About two-thirds of the Moroccans in the Netherlands come from the Rif mountain region along the north coast, the south in Agadir (Souss) and Ouarzazate. In the Netherlands, most Moroccans mainly live in the four largest cities: Amsterdam, Rotterdam, The Hague, and Utrecht.

When gathering history, attention should be paid to migration history and acculturation experiences, which can be affected by age at the time of migration, educational backgrounds, worldviews, cultural identity changes, and socio-economic status changes after migration. The decision to relocate to a different country and culture, leaving behind family and friends, is an important and life-changing event. Our experience is that a gracious and sincere interest in this aspect of their lives helps patients feel more comfortable in an unaccustomed situation. Many patients will be pleasantly surprised to find out that the neuropsychologist knows something about their hometown.

Language

In Morocco, a wide variety of languages are spoken. Besides different forms of Arabic (Modern Standard Arabic (MSA) and Moroccan Arabic), French, and Spanish, three Berber languages are spoken. Moroccans learn MSA at school and it is used in administrative offices and schools. Moroccan Arabic is the spoken native *vernacular*, spoken by about 85% of the population. The rest speak one of the **Tamazight** (Berber) languages. Moroccan Arabic, along with Berber, is one of two languages spoken in homes and on Morocco's streets. These languages are not used in writing.

The first generation of Moroccan migrants living in the Netherlands are mostly not educated. About 70–80% of Moroccans originate from the Berber-speaking Rif mountains. Although there may be overlap between dialects, knowledge of one language or dialect does not imply competence in another. This is important to keep in mind when working with interpreters and translators. Accurate gathering of language history in each spoken and written language is critical.

In general Moroccan elderly have limited proficiency in the Dutch language; they rate their command of the Dutch language as bad to mediocre.[2] Second- and third-generation Moroccans master the Dutch language.

MG: When introducing myself, pronouncing my first name (Miriam) rather than the harder-to-pronounce family name (Goudsmit) will often elicit a response of recognition from Moroccan people, since Miriam (or Maryem/Maryam) is a widespread name in Morocco.

Communication

In the Moroccan culture, respect for seniority and age are highly valued. Also, educated persons like medical doctors are authority figures, and it is considered impolite to contradict them. It is essential to acknowledge that a more indirect or "low context" communication style is more common. Older people will not openly disagree with or ask questions about the advice doctors give but may not always follow the advice.

Some communication patterns are tied with religious habits, especially for first-generation Moroccans in the Netherlands. For example, it is not common for women to have contact, or a conversation, with a man who is not part of the family. Shaking hands with somebody from the opposite gender is uncommon.

Education

Until 1963, efforts were concentrated on universalizing education and combating the country's 96% illiteracy rate. The authorities then took concrete measures such as building new schools. Primary education (age 6–12) was made compulsory and free for Moroccan children.

Currently, Morocco's secondary education system is divided into two three-year stages: lower and upper secondary school and a tertiary (higher) education system. Although more than 95% of school-aged children in Morocco are now enrolled in primary school, the education system still faces significant challenges. Drop-out rates are still high, and teacher absenteeism and a multilingual environment at school contribute to Morocco's low literacy rates.[3]

The new law (2019) aims to increase the quality and accessibility of the education system: primary education will be made available from age four. The first stage of secondary education, lower secondary, is currently compulsory.

Not only quantity but also the quality of education should be considered when interpreting neuropsychological test results. Has someone been educated in a small village school or at a private school in the city? There may be large differences between the two. Also, low educational attainment is often based on accessibility or opportunity rather than ability.

Literacy

Illiteracy is relatively widespread among older generations. In rural areas, where most first-generation Moroccan migrants originate, the only educational opportunities were at the primary-school level. Most first-generation Moroccan men do not finish more than primary school or "Quran school", while most Moroccan women have even less schooling or are illiterate.[4] Experience with holding a pen is limited. While neuropsychological testing relies on skills like reading, writing, mental calculation, and drawing,[5] the use of measures with better ecological relevance is necessary.[6-9]

Socio-Economic Status

Over the past decades, substantial development has stimulated the economy and provides opportunities for rural areas. Nonetheless, the difference between rural life and city life remains. Moroccans in the Netherlands generally have a low income and low socio-economic status, with 85% of older Moroccans rating their income as too little to live from.[2] Medical insurance is covered for all citizens in the Netherlands, which significantly facilitates access to care. However, not all care facilities are equally accessible to (older) migrants who might experience language and cultural barriers and have difficulty finding their way in the different care institutions.

Values and Customs

Generally, in traditional Moroccan families, family-centrism, inter-dependence and collectivism, religiosity, respect, and hospitality are essential. The role of the family is important, and medical decisions are generally taken together with family members. Older patients expect their children to care for them, leading to tension between second- and third-generation descendants, who have children, jobs, and parents to take care of.

Spirituality and Religion

Historically, in the period preceding Islam, North Africa came under the influence of both Judaism and Christianity. Morocco has oscillated between periods of religious tolerance and intolerance. Following independence in 1956, Morocco established a constitution that re-established Islam as a state religion. Officially, 99% of the population is Muslim. Paying attention to religion's critical role or spirituality for a Moroccan can help acknowledge worldviews and develop recommendations consistent with those views. Religious and spiritual issues may play a positive role in maintaining health and recovering from illness; for example, when patients experience their disease as a spiritual ordeal, which can generate hope and resilience. On the other hand, diseases might be experienced as a punishment from God, leading to feelings of guilt and despair.[10]

Health Status

In Morocco, the life expectancy at birth rose by seven years between 1990 and 2012 (from 64 to 71 years). Morocco is witnessing a significant shift in its epidemiologic profile with an increasing burden of non-communicable diseases, which currently account for approximately 75% of all deaths in Morocco (cancer, metabolic diseases, including diabetes and cardiovascular disease, account for 40% of the leading causes of death).[11]

Comparable findings are also reported among Moroccans living in the Netherlands. Although literature is scarce, we know that general health problems are higher among (older) migrants and lower wellbeing: experiencing feelings of loneliness and depression.[12] Moroccans are at an increased risk of medical conditions associated with cognitive impairment, such as stroke, diabetes mellitus,[13,14] and dementia.[15]

Mental Health Views

Due to language barriers, limited knowledge on existing (neuro-)psychological services, and cultural differences, many Moroccans in the Netherlands do not seek help for mental health problems. Older Moroccans generally visit their general physician regularly, but they will not be inclined to bring up mental health complaints. Shame or stigma around mental health problems is common. Also, many Moroccan patients fear gossip in their community, which sometimes leads them to refuse an interpreter's help from their community. Clinicians should be aware of differences in idioms of distress, as patients may express stress and other psychological symptoms differently, such as by emphasizing bodily symptoms like headaches.

Approach to Neuropsychological Evaluations

Neuropsychology is a relatively new field of study in Morocco itself. For a long time, professionals wanting to work in neuropsychology could only receive such training abroad (e.g., in France). In 2009 a formal Master's degree program was initiated in Morocco itself, followed by doctorate level training (2012). Neuropsychologists in Morocco often use tests developed in French, but recently, some of these tests have been adapted for Moroccan-Arabic speakers. Administering these tests in French or Arabic allowed for the assessment of higher educated Moroccan patients. Still, patients who are illiterate or are not fluent in these languages remain hard to assess.

In our clinical work in Europe, we mainly see Moroccan patients in a memory clinic setting. Several hospitals in the Netherlands provide dedicated services for patients with a minority background (multicultural memory clinics). In general, the staff are from a majority background, who do not speak the language(s) of their patients. Several multicultural memory clinics therefore provide interpreter services to their patients. Also, since many older patients with a Moroccan migration background have had little education, professionals in these memory clinics are more aware of the importance of ecologically valid data about their daily functioning rather than solely relying on neuropsychological test results. To quantify daily living activities, sometimes an occupational therapist is asked to assess relevant activities of everyday life, such as preparing (Moroccan) tea.

In the SYMBOL study (2010–2013), the Cross-Cultural Dementia (CCD) screening test was validated, with specific norms for Moroccan people.[15,16] The current TULIPA study (2017–2021) aims to adapt and validate international neuropsychological tests and develop several new instruments to provide tools for an in-depth neuropsychological assessment in memory clinic patients with a culturally, educationally, and linguistically diverse background (See Appendix for a list of applicable tests).

To prepare patients for their visit to the memory clinic, we provide an illustrated information booklet developed for first-generation immigrant patients in large, clear, colored images, accompanied by concise and easy-to-understand sentences. Furthermore, patients and their families seem to find it helpful to receive a call a week in advance of their appointment so that they can ask questions about the purpose and practicalities of their visit. These initial phone calls also allow the introduction and planning of an interpreter. Sometimes, children prefer to serve as interpreters for their parents. After explaining that the interpreter is merely present as an additional set of ears and eyes for the neuropsychologist—e.g., helping them look for subtle language changes—most agree with the interpreter's presence.

> I (SF) remember one elderly lady who was unwilling to discuss her previous experiences of physical abuse by her former husband in the presence of their daughter. Once she could speak freely without her daughter present, it turned out she was worried she had acquired brain damage from the physical abuse. We explained that the MRI scan indicated no damage to her brain and conveyed to her how worries, sadness, and anxiety may lead to cognitive symptoms. She agreed to being treated by a psychiatrist to work through some of her past experiences.

The neuropsychological evaluation typically consists of a two- to three-hour session as part of a comprehensive diagnostic work-up. Patients are referred after an initial evaluation by a neurologist or geriatrician in the outpatient clinic. At the neuropsychological assessment, we spend a lot of additional time getting acquainted and building rapport. We know that patients and families might be afraid that a Western-born neuropsychologist will not fully understand their experiences or serve their interests because of negative experiences in society toward foreign-born people or Muslims. We take our time to explain that we will try to understand the patient and their loved ones in their cultural context. In the initial interview, we often rely on questions from the Dutch version of the Cultural Interview[17] to familiarize ourselves with our patients' cultural perspectives, language preferences, and immigration history. Subsequently, we take our time to explain the procedure and possible neuropsychological assessment outcomes to the patient. At first glance, it may be hard for some patients to relate the tests to their complaints about activities in daily life. They may indicate that the tests are childish or decline further testing, stating that they are "not crazy." Therefore, I (SF) explain to my patients that some tests are easier, and others are harder for a reason. I often use the metaphor of getting a car checkup every year. Even though your car may still be running—although with some minor issues—occasionally, you want to check out all of its parts, even if the pieces appear to be in good condition.

Section II: Case Study — "I Know All Prayers by Heart, If Only I Wouldn't Get So Distracted"

Note: Possible identifying information have been changed to protect patient identity and privacy.

Background

In this part of the chapter, we follow one of our typical patients in a multicultural memory clinic.

Behavioral Observations

Mr. Boulahrouz, age 71, was referred to the multicultural memory clinic by his general practitioner. He came with his wife, daughter, and son. Mr. Boulahrouz was neatly dressed and wore a traditional knitted cap called a *kufi*. The present interpreter was a bilingual (Tarifit-Dutch) student of medicine, trained in interpreting during neuropsychological assessments and familiar with the instruments used. Mr. Boulahrouz made an effort to answer in Dutch wherever he could but eased into speaking his mother tongue with the interpreter. Mr. Boulahrouz presented most of his complaints by himself, but his daughter sometimes clarified or corrected his story, often in Dutch, so her father would not understand and she would not unduly embarrass him. It seemed that Mr. Boulahrouz was aware of his cognitive difficulties but sometimes lacked insight.

Although he seemed concerned about his mental problems, he was generally in a good mood. We explained that the neuropsychological assessment consisted of an interview and tests and subsequently asked Mr. Boulahrouz whether he experienced any cognitive complaints.

Presenting Concerns

For a year, Mr. Boulahrouz has been experiencing some memory problems. He sometimes forgets appointments or buying certain items at the grocery store. He needs to write everything down so he will not forget. His daughter is concerned about her father's memory problems, which seem to progress over time. She is afraid Mr. Boulahrouz has dementia, as several of his relatives developed dementia-like symptoms later in life. Mr. Boulahrouz sometimes forgets about major celebrations and seems disoriented in time. He might be surprised at the mosque crowds, not realizing that it is Friday, the most important day of prayer for Muslims. I (SF) then indicated that I know a little about prayer rituals and asked Mr. Boulahrouz whether he has any cognitive difficulties when praying. Although he knows all prayers by heart, he finds that he quickly gets distracted, such as by noises in another room. Sometimes, he loses track of the number of prayer cycles he still has to complete. He does not experience any complaints in other cognitive domains. He can do most of the activities in his daily life by himself. He reports that he can still fix his car when necessary (although his family reports he has not carried out any repairs over the last two years).

Daily Functioning

Mr. Boulahrouz lives with his wife in an apartment in a multicultural neighborhood. Mr. Boulahrouz does not engage in many regular activities. He sleeps in, goes to the mosque to pray and socialize, makes himself a cup of Moroccan tea, and enjoys a good meal at night prepared by his wife. Every once in a while, he goes to the local store to buy groceries. At times, he helps out organizing and cooking at events at his local mosque—he can help come up with a list of dishes to prepare and general planning. Although Mr. Boulahrouz opens the mail and looks at the content, he has always needed help from his children in financial administration and reading difficult letters.

Health History

Although healthy as a young man, the later decades of Mr. Boulahrouz's life have plagued health problems. He experiences pain in his knees from doing heavy labor for years. As a result, he is not very active, has gained weight, and suffers from type II diabetes.

Educational History

As a child, Mr. Boulahrouz went to a "Quranic school" where he learned to recite Quran verses by heart and was first confronted with the Arabic language (although he did not yet learn to read write in it). He spent one year in the local public primary school. However, when his father passed away, Mr. Boulahrouz had to help work so the family could make ends meet. Even though he did not receive any more formal training, he informally learned to read and write in Arabic to a lesser degree.

Language Proficiency

Growing up, Mr. Boulahrouz spoke Tarifit with his family members. While living in the Netherlands, he learned to speak some Dutch. Mr. Boulahrouz can read easy sentences in Dutch and Arabic and read a newspaper (although he does not fully understand it). After retiring from work, he spoke Dutch less and less.

Cultural History and Acculturation

Mr. Boulahrouz grew up in a small rural Berber village in the Rif mountains. He was the second oldest of several brothers and sisters, of which two died at a young age.

Mr. Boulahrouz met his wife through an arrangement that his mother made with his (future) wife's parents. In 1970, one of Mr. Boulahrouz's relatives came to the Netherlands to work. Mr. Boulahrouz became determined to follow in his footsteps and make money to sustain his family by working in Europe. Mr. Boulahrouz and his wife spent only a little time together as a married couple before he was bound for Europe. As his birth had not been formally registered, like many of his peers, he put a fictional date of birth on his official application forms to match the age requirements. In his case, the family estimated that his age as registered was approximately correct.

Mr. Boulahrouz arrived in the Netherlands with two addresses on a paper: his relative's and a location for a guest worker "pension". The inhabitants would work long days. Mr. Boulahrouz mainly did factory work. His peers and relative, who had been in the Netherlands, helped him navigate his way in the Netherlands regarding healthcare and finances. Mr. Boulahrouz saved money to take home with him. He had never expected to stay in the Netherlands. However, when a change in policies made it possible, Mr. Boulahrouz brought his wife over from Morocco.

Now, many years later, Mr. Boulahrouz agrees he sometimes misses his native country. Like many first-generation immigrants, Mr. Boulahrouz spends his long summers in Morocco. Mr. Boulahrouz and his family have noticed a change in recent decades in the level of tolerance toward people born outside the Netherlands. At first, Moroccans were welcomed into the country due to the high demand for labor workers. Currently, many Moroccans feel they are discriminated against based on their ethnic background or Islamic religion.[18] He sometimes struggles because his children have taken on a different lifestyle and hopes his children will honor traditional values and customs. After his death, Mr. Boulahrouz wishes to be buried in Morocco.

Emotional Functioning

During the conversation, Mr. Boulahrouz is in a good mood. He does not experience feelings of depression, anxiety, or loneliness. His daughter agrees that he is generally in a good mood.

Test and Norm Selection

The general practitioner and geriatrician have asked us, neuropsychologists, to determine whether Mr. Boulahrouz may be suffering from a mild cognitive impairment or dementia or whether his memory complaints could be explained by normal aging.

Neuropsychological Assessment 1 (2018)

For his first neuropsychological assessment, we selected the following tests:

- Rowland Universal Dementia Assessment Scale (RUDAS)[19,20]
- CCD[16]

- A literacy screening test (unpublished)
- Modified Visual Association Test, mVAT[21]
- Recall of Pictures Test (RPT)[22]
- Clock Reading Test (CRT)[23]
- Category Fluency Test (animal and supermarket)[24]

Both the RUDAS and CCD have normative data available for the Moroccan population. Besides asking Mr. Boulahrouz about his writing and reading skills and educational history, we estimate these skills through a literacy screening test. We also selected mVAT, a visual-associative memory test in which the original line drawings are replaced with photographs to make them suitable for lower-educated populations. We added a few additional tests for which normative data are available from a sample that includes Moroccans from the European Cross-Cultural Neuropsychological Test Battery (European CNTB), a battery validated in Denmark, namely animal and supermarket fluency, the RPT, and the CRT.[23,24] We examined memory, executive functioning, mental speed and attention, visuospatial functioning, and (to a limited degree) language by selecting these tests.

Test Results and Impressions

As Tarifit is not a written language, we used the (Moroccan-)Arabic version of the literacy screening test. This test showed that Mr. Boulahrouz could point out Arabic letters and read and write letters and short sentences in Arabic. We therefore decided we could administer tests that require a minimal level of literacy. On the RUDAS, Mr. Boulahrouz scored below the cut-off. He especially had difficulties retrieving the items from a grocery list. These memory impairments also showed the delayed recall of the Objects Test (part B) of the CCD, the Recall of Pictures Test, and the mVAT. On tests measuring attention and executive functioning, his performance was variable. It ranged from average on the Sun-Moon Test (attention/mental speed/inhibition) of the CCD to marginally impaired on the Dots Test A (attention/mental speed) and impaired on Dots Test B (executive functioning). In particular, the impaired performance on the Dots Test B was likely influenced by his minimal level of formal education and limited experience with abstract testing material. There were no impairments in verbal fluency, naming, or visuospatial functioning (CRT).

On the MRI scan, white matter lesions without any hippocampal atrophy were seen, pointing in the direction of a vascular origin. The routine lab did not show any abnormalities.

Conclusion: Based on the neuropsychological profile, we concluded that Mr. Boulahrouz had an isolated memory impairment that did not lead to any immediate impairments in daily living activities. As only some executive functioning tests were impaired and memory deficits were most prominent, Mr. Boulahrouz was diagnosed with a Mild Cognitive Impairment, amnestic type (aMCI).

Follow-Up

On finding out about the diagnosis, Mr. Boulahrouz and his family were relieved that he did not have dementia. We then took the time to explain the prognosis for aMCI patients in clear and comprehensible words. In particular, we highlighted the differences between the effects of normal aging and vascular damage to the brain, as some patients and their families may believe that (severe) cognitive impairment is part of "normal" aging instead of a medical condition. After these explanations, Mr. Boulahrouz and his family agreed on scheduling several future visits to follow up on his aMCI every half a year. On the first few visits, Mr. Boulahrouz was doing relatively well, although he did need more and more cues to recall specific information. Two years later, Mr. Boulahrouz explained to the geriatrician that his memory problems increasingly hindered his functioning. After being interrupted in an activity, he had difficulties restarting it. He had concentration difficulties when confronted with background noise. The geriatrician scheduled a follow-up neuropsychological assessment. Aside from repeating the tests that were administered in the first assessment to detect any cognitive decline over time (RUDAS, CCD, mVAT, RPT, CRT, category verbal fluency), several tests were added that had been newly introduced or developed. We now asked Mr. Boulahrouz several questions of the orientation subtest of the Mini-Mental State Exam (MMSE) in his native language—not including the items referring to the season, department, "province," or state, which he probably never learned. Additionally, the following tests were used:

- Naming Assessment in Multicultural Europe (NAME)[25]
- Corsi Block Tapping Test[26]
- Coin-in-the-Hand test[27]
- Stick Design Test (SDT)[28]
- Five Digit Test (FDT)[29]

The SDT and FDT are particularly suitable for low-educated participants, as they rely on skills that most people will have acquired, even without formal education. The SDT is a test of visuoconstruction using matchsticks instead of graphomotor responses, and the FDT, a Stroop-like test, requires patients to count up to five. We added a newly developed naming test, the NAME, a test with culture-sensitive items to determine if there were any severe naming impairments, added the Coin-in-the-Hand test to see if Mr. Boulahrouz was sufficiently able to put in the necessary effort required for testing, and added the Corsi Block Tapping Test to examine his working memory. We supplemented these tests with several questionnaires. We administered the Moroccan-Berber version of the short Geriatric Depression Scale[30] and the short IQ-Code,[31] which we previously examined in a validation study in a multicultural memory clinic sample.[32] We additionally administered the ALD scales[33] and the Caregiver Strain Index+ (CSI+).[34] This last was added to determine whether the caregivers experienced any severe burden. In our experience, informal carers of Moroccan descent emphasize that the care they give is a duty they consider as usual and a fact of life and that they are also proud to return care for their parents. However, in the Dutch society, where second-generation carers often both work, this might lead to a high burden of informal carers.[35]

Test Results and Impressions

Several of Mr. Boulahrouz's test scores had declined, particularly in memory and executive functioning. The short IQ-Code, now indicated that his family members noticed a substantial cognitive decline (average score of 4.3). Given the neuropsychological assessment results, combined with the increasing impairments in his activities of daily living and the findings on an MRI scan of extensive vascular damage, Mr. Boulahrouz was diagnosed with vascular dementia. We explained this to Mr. Boulahrouz and his family, which did not surprise the family or Mr. Boulahrouz. The geriatrician explained that they together needed to monitor his vascular risk factors as much as possible. As the CSI+ indicated that the family did not experience a severe burden of care at this point, telephone follow-ups were planned at low-frequent intervals to check in with the patient and his family.

Section III: Lessons Learned

- Given the influence of Berbers, Arabs, Spaniards, and French on Morocco's history, Moroccan people may come from a very diverse linguistic and cultural background. It is essential to ensure that the neuropsychologist or interpreter and the patient speak the same dialect from the same region.
- It is important for patients with limited experience to be tested to help them prepare for the assessment. This may entail calling ahead to inform patients and caregivers about the practicalities of the visit and an interactive talk at the start of the visit to explain the assessment goals and the use of tests.
- Patients who did not receive any formal education due to a lack of opportunities, access, or financial means may develop literacy skills informally. It is important to ask patients about any informal learning opportunities and take these skills into account when considering which tests are valid and feasible.
- In patients who have long been dependent on others for support in their daily life activities, it is important to take the time to explore which activities are specifically relevant to them (such as performing the prayer rituals). Furthermore, it is crucial to ask the caregiver properly about such impairments through the well-validated short IQ-CODE.
- In our experience, a professional, friendly attitude and genuine interest in the experience of Moroccan elders' complaints helps to establish rapport quickly. Also, it is useful to have knowledge about potentially less direct communication styles. Since many Moroccans in the Netherlands are low educated, health literacy skills are low, so psychoeducation about explanatory models for (mental) health issues is necessary, besides interest in and respect for the patient's explanatory models.

Acknowledgments

We would like to thank Dalila Oulel and Dr. Norah Karrouche for their contribution.

Glossary

Dynasty(ies).   A sequence of rulers from the same family, usually in the context of a monarchical system, but sometimes also appearing in elective republics.

Family reunification.   When children and spouses who were left behind at the time of migration come to join the principal migrant. Family formation is when a migrant comes to the Netherlands to live with their partner for the first time. The latter are often referred to as "marriage migrants."

Tamazight (Berber languages).   Also known as Berber or the Amazigh languages, are spoken by most Moroccans and in some other North Africa countries. In 2011, a constitutional amendment was introduced, giving *Tamazigh*t an official status, recognizing this language and culture as intrinsic components of Moroccan national identity.

Three main groups of Tamazight are distinguished:
- Riffian language, Tarifit or Rif Berber (the Northern Rif mountains);
  - The Tarifit language can be further subdivided into several dialects, such as a Western (Al-Hoceima), Central (Nador), and Eastern (Berkane) dialect. These three regions are less than 200 km apart, yet pronunciation and wording may differ substantially between these regional dialects.
- The Tashelhit (in the South, Region Souss-Massa-Drâa);
- Tamazight (in the Middle-Atlas region).

Vernacular language.   The speech variety used in everyday life by the general population in a geographical or social territory.

References

1. El Bardaï, O. Les Marocains résidant aux Pays-Bas: caractéristiques démographiques et sociales. In: Kabbaj K, editor. Rapport July 2003. Marocains de l'Extérieur, Rabat: Fondation Hassan II pour les Marocains Résidant à l'Etranger. p. 322–73, Rabat.
2. Schellingerhout R. (red.). Gezondheid en welzijn van allochtone ouderen. Tijdschr Gerontol Geriatr. 2005;36(1):250. ISBN 90-377-0191-4.
3. Abdous K. "Privatisation de l'éducation au Maroc—Un système d'éducation à plusieurs vitesses et une société polarisée." Rapport Publié par l'Internationale de l'Education 2020.
4. Crul M, Doomernik J. The Turkish and Moroccan second generation in the Netherlands: divergent trends between and polarization within the two groups. Int Migr Rev. 2003;37(4):1039–64.
5. Nielsen TR, Vogel A, Gade A, Waldemar G. Cognitive testing in non-demented Turkish immigrants—comparison of the RUDAS and the MMSE. Scand J Psychol. 2012 December 01;53(6):455–60.
6. Kosmidis MH. Challenges in the neuropsychological assessment of illiterate older adults. Lang Cogn Neurosci. 2018;33(3):373–86.
7. Nielsen TR. Effects of illiteracy on the European Cross-Cultural Neuropsychological Test Battery (CNTB). Arch Clin Neuropsychol. 2019 July 26;34(5):713–20.
8. Nielsen TR, Waldemar G. Effects of literacy on semantic verbal fluency in an immigrant population. Neuropsychol Dev Cogn B Aging Neuropsychol Cogn. 2016 September 01;23(5):578–90.
9. Franzen S, van den Berg E, Goudsmit M, Jurgens CK, van de Wiel L, Kalkisim Y et al. A systematic review of neuropsychological tests for the assessment of dementia in non-Western, low-educated or illiterate populations. J Int Neuropsychol Soc. 2020 March 01;26(3):331–51.
10. Karbila A. Ziektebeleving bij Niet-westerse migranten "Verklaringsmodellen." Personal presentation 2017, Rotterdam, the Netherlands.
11. World Health Organization. Regional Office for the Eastern Mediterranean. Morocco health profile [Internet]. 2015 World Health Organization. Regional Office for the Eastern Mediterranean; 2016. Available from: https://apps.who.int/iris/handle/10665/253774
12. Conkova N, Lindenberg J. Health and wellbeing of older migrants in the Netherlands: a narrative literature review. Tijdschr Gerontol Geriatr [Internet]. 2018;49:223–31. Available from: https://doi.org/10.1007/s12439-018-0268-2
13. Uitewaal PJM, Manna DR, Bruijnzeels MA, Hoes AW, Thomas S. Prevalence of type 2 diabetes mellitus, other cardiovascular risk factors, and cardiovascular disease in Turkish and Moroccan immigrants in North West Europe: a systematic review. Prev Med [Internet]. 2004;39:1068–76. Available from: https://doi.org/10.1016/j.ypmed.2004.04.009
14. Ujcic-Voortman J, Baan C, Seidell J, Verhoeff A. Obesity and cardiovascular disease among Turkish and Moroccan migrant groups in Europe: a systematic review. Obes Rev. 2012;13:2–16.
15. Parlevliet JL, Uysal-Bozkir O, Goudsmit M, van Campen JP, Kok RM, Ter Riet G et al. Prevalence of mild cognitive impairment and dementia in older non-western immigrants in the Netherlands: a cross-sectional study. Int J Geriatr Psychiatry. 2016 September 01;31(9):1040–9.
16. Goudsmit M, Uysal-Bozkir O, Parlevliet JL, van Campen JP, de Rooij SE, Schmand B. The Cross-Cultural Dementia Screening (CCD): a new neuropsychological screening instrument for dementia in elderly immigrants. J Clin Exp Neuropsychol. 2017 March 01;39(2):163–72.
17. Rohlof H, Ghane S. The cultural interview (Dutch version). In: Rob van Dijk and Nuray Sönmez, editors. Culture-sensitive work with the DSM-IV. Rotterdam, the Netherlands: Mikado; 2003. p. 49–52.
18. Andriessen I, Dijkhof JH, van der Torre A, van den Berg E, Pulles I, en Marian de Voogd-Hamelink JI. (2020). Perceived discrimination in the Netherlands [Report in Dutch]. Institute for Social Research. The Hague, the Netherlands: Sociaal en Cultureel Planbureau.
19. Storey JE, Rowland JT, Basic D, Conforti DA, Dickson HG. The Rowland Universal Dementia Assessment Scale (RUDAS): a multicultural cognitive assessment scale. Int Psychogeriatr. 2004 March 01;16(1):13–31.

20. Goudsmit M, van Campen J, Schilt T, Hinnen C, Franzen S, Schmand B. One size does not fit all. Dement Geriatr Cogn Dis Extra. 2018 August 29;8(2):290–305.

21. Franzen S, van den Berg E, Kalkisim Y, van de Wiel L, Harkes M, van Bruchem-Visser RL, et al. Assessment of visual association memory in low-educated, non-Western immigrants with the modified visual association test. Dement Geriatr Cogn Disord 2019;47(4–6):345–54.

22. Nielsen TR, Vogel A, Waldemar G. Comparison of performance on three neuropsychological tests in healthy Turkish immigrants and Danish elderly. Int Psychogeriatr. 2012 September 01;24(9):1515–21.

23. Schmidtke K, Olbrich S. The Clock Reading Test: validation of an instrument for the diagnosis of dementia and disorders of visuo-spatial cognition. Int Psychogeriatr. 2007;19(2):307–21.

24. Strauss, E, Sherman, EMS, Spreen, O. A compendium of neuropsychological tests. Administration, norms, and commentary. 3rd ed. New York (NY): Oxford University Press; 2006.

25. Franzen, S, van den Berg, E, Ayhan, Y, Satoer, DD, Türkoğlu, Ö, Genç Akpulat, GE et al. The Naming Assessment in Multicultural Europe (NAME): development and validation in a memory clinic. 2021. Manuscript submitted for publication.

26. Corsi PM. Human memory and the medial temporal region of the brain. Dis Abstr Intl. 1972;34:891B.

27. Kapur N. The coin-in-the-hand test: a new "bedside" test for the detection of malingering in patients with suspected memory disorder. J Neurol Psychiatry. 1994;57(3):385–6.

28. Baiyewu O, Unverzagt FW, Lane KA, Gureje O, Ogunniyi A, Musick B et al. The Stick Design test: a new measure of visuoconstructional ability. J Int Neuropsychol Soc. 2005;11(5):598–605.

29. Sedó M. The "Five Digit Test": a color-free, non-reading alternative to the Stroop. Int Neuropsychol Soc Liaison Commit Newsl. 2004;13:6–7.

30. Uysal-Bozkir Ö, Hoopman R, Rooij SE. Translation and validation of the short Geriatric Depression Scale (GDS-15) among Turkish, Moroccan and Surinamese older migrants in the Netherlands. Submitted. Part of thesis, University of Amsterdam; 2016.

31. Jorm AF, Jacomb PA. The Informant Questionnaire on Cognitive Decline in the Elderly (IQCODE): socio-demographic correlates, reliability, validity and some norms. Psychol Med. 1989;19(4):1015–22.

32. Goudsmit M, Van Campen J, Franzen S, Van den Berg E, Schilt T, Schmand B. Dementia detection with a combination of informant-based and performance-based measures in low-educated and illiterate elderly migrants, Clin Neuropsychol. 2021;35(3):660–78.

33. Lawton MP, Brody EM. Assessment of older people: self-maintaining and instrumental activities of daily living. Gerontologist. 1969;9(3):179–86.

34. Franzen, S, Eikelboom, WS, van den Berg, E, Jiskoot, LC, van Hemmen, J, & Papma, JM. Caregiver burden in a culturally diverse memory clinic population: the Caregiver Strain Index-Expanded. Dement Geriatr Cogn Disord. 2021;50:333–340.

35. Ahmad M, van den Broeke J, Saharso S, Tonkens E. Persons with a migration background caring for a family member with dementia: challenges to shared care. Gerontologist [Internet]. 2020;60(2):340–9. Available from: https://doi.org/10.1093/geront/gnz161

Greek

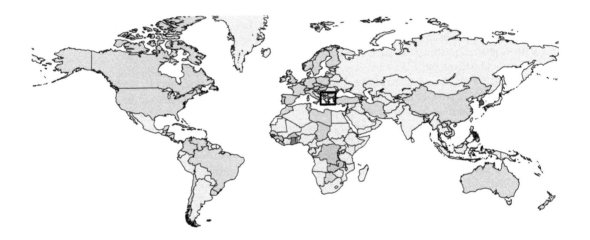

23 Culturally Aware Neuropsychological Assessment with Greek Immigrants

Mathew Staios

Section I: Background Information

Terminology and Perspective

Individuals from Greece are generally referred to as Greeks. First, second, or third generations living in foreign nations often refer to themselves as Greek Australian/American/Canadian. This chapter will use the term Greek to refer to individuals originating from the geographical area of Greece, unless otherwise specified.

I was born in Australia to Greek migrant parents, who arrived and settled in Melbourne during the early 1970s. Melbourne is home to the largest Greek population in Australia. It also has the largest Greek population of any city in the world outside Greece and Cyprus. I attended a bilingual Greek Australian school; I speak Greek fluently and have provided clinical services to the aging Greek Australian community for approximately ten years. Thus, this chapter is based on my clinical experience of working with this group.

Geography

Greece (Ελλάδα), officially the Hellenic Republic, known also as Hellas, is a country located in Southeast Europe. Its population is approximately 10.7 million as of 2018; Athens, the nation's capital, is its largest city, followed by Thessaloniki. The country consists of nine geographic regions, including Macedonia, Central Greece, the Peloponnese, Thessaly, Epirus, Thrace, Crete, the Aegean Islands, and the Ionian Islands.[1]

History

Greece is considered as the cradle of Western civilization, as the birthplace of democracy, Western philosophy and literature, historiography, political science, scientific and mathematical principles, Western drama, and the Olympic Games. The Greek Orthodox Church, which emerged in the 1st century A.D., helped shape modern Greek identity and transmitted Greek traditions to the wider Orthodox World. After falling under Ottoman control in the mid-15th century, Greece emerged as a modern nation-state in 1830 following a war of independence. Throughout the 20th century, Greece was engulfed in political turmoil and economic instability due to World War I (1914–1918), the Greco-Turkish War (1919–1922), World War II (WWII; 1939–1945), the Greek Civil War (1946–1949), and a military junta (1967–1974).

DOI: 10.4324/9781003051862-47

Immigration and Relocation

Throughout the 20th century, millions of Greeks migrated to the United States, Australia, Canada, and Germany, creating a large Greek diaspora. Smaller pockets of Greek migrants also exist in South Africa and South America. While the focus of the chapter will be on Greek Australians, it is worth noting that Greek migrants share similar demographic features and reasons for leaving their country of origin. Therefore, the information provided in this chapter may, to some extent, assist clinical neuropsychologists with broadly understanding and preparing for assessment of this cultural group.

The Greek diaspora is largely concentrated in four nations, namely Australia, the United States, Canada, and Germany. Migration to some of the nations started as early as 1850; however, large waves of immigration started after WWII and the Greek Civil War. The 2016 Australian census recorded 397,431 people of Greek ancestry and 93,740 born in Greece.[2] Between 1945 and 1985, approximately 211,000 Greeks migrated to the United States,[3-5] 100,000 entered Canada,[6] and 274,060 entered Germany.[7,8]

Assessment of Migration Journey

A large majority of Greek migrants fled during or shortly after WWII or the Greek Civil War. These individuals were subjected to a range of traumatic experiences during both of these wars, including famine, malnutrition, physical and psychological torture by foreign and local captors for several years. Following migration to host nations, a number of Greeks were met with xenophobic attitudes, which served to exacerbate underlying trauma and resulted in marginalization.

Gathering information regarding pre- and postmigration history is an important part of clinical assessment and history taking. Factors that warrant consideration can include reasons for relocation, the migration journey, history of trauma, stereotype threat, mistrust in authority figures/government agencies, age at time of migration, visa status, socioeconomic status pre- and poststatus migration, impact of racism, changes in cultural identity.[9] Assessing and understanding these factors can assist with conducting a sensitive and culturally informed interview, leading to accurate interpretation of culturally bound behaviors and attitudes.

Acculturation

Upon migrating to Australia, Greek migrants were faced with the undesirable reality of marginalization and exposure to prejudice. This resulted in Greeks helping other Greeks to find work and accommodation, and in turn, pushed them into ethnic enclaves, residentially, occupationally, and economically.[10] Rosenthal and colleagues[11] noted that Greek Australians retained the collectivistic values while Anglo-Australians demonstrated a more individualistic orientation. Furthermore, Greek Australians displayed only minimal integration of Anglo-Australian cultural values. Research suggests that acculturation to the dominant culture is facilitated by access to knowledge and exposure to mass media.[12] However, given that older Greek Australians had limited English proficiency, they likely did not benefit from such exposures to mainstream Anglo-Australian culture, thus retained Greek values.

Language

Greece is today relatively homogeneous in linguistic terms, with a large majority of the native population using Greek as their first or only language. Among the Greek-speaking population, speakers of the distinctive Pontic dialect came to Greece from Asia Minor after the Greek genocide and constituted a sizable group. Near the northern Greek borders, there are also some Slavic-speaking groups, locally known as Slavomacedonian-speaking, most of whose members identify ethnically as Greeks. It is estimated that after the population exchanges of 1923, Macedonia had 200,000–400,000 Slavic speakers.

Religious Practices

The Greek Constitution recognizes Eastern Orthodoxy as the nation's dominant faith.[13] The Greek government does not keep statistics on religious groups and censuses do not ask for religious affiliation. According to the US State Department, an estimated 97% of Greek citizens identify as Eastern Orthodox.[14] In a 2010 Eurostat–Eurobarometer poll, 79% of Greek citizens responded that they "believe there is a God."[15]

People

While Greeks tend to broadly identify as a homogenous cultural and ethnic group, subtle differences are observed between and within the Nation's nine geographic regions. These differences are due to a combination of factors, including remnants of ancient cultural practices and identity, and the cultural influence of invading forces that have been incorporated into modern Greek identity. Individuals in larger cities tend to share liberal political and worldviews, while those residing in smaller towns or villages tend to be more conservative. In the context of Greek Australian migrants, it has been my experience that attitudes and cultural practices can differ based on educational experience (city or village), spoken language(s), socioeconomic status, values, and customs. For example, individuals from Athens tend to speak only Greek (in addition to a second language, generally English), while some from certain regions in Central Macedonia speak both Greek and Slavic dialects, and thus see themselves as culturally distinct and identify as Macedonian.

Children born to Greek migrants and raised in other nations tend to incorporate customs passed down from their elders, alongside new and sometimes conflicting customs reflected in new cultures, thus resulting in a unique fusion of intergenerational perspectives. These factors often influence a range of psychological processes and warrant careful consideration in the context of a culturally informed clinical evaluation.

Communication

Greeks tend to be indirect communicators. To avoid conflict or confrontation, they often conveying their messages in a tactful manner. In instances where they need to communicate negative information, exchanges are generally conveyed in a noncommittal manner to minimize offence. Verbal communication tends to be quite verbose, expressive, and intense. At times, communication style can be perceived as exaggerated and emotional in tone and expression. They often speak with impassioned, loud voices when talking to each other. This culturally appropriate expression of excitement can often be misinterpreted as a sign of anger by other cultural groups.

Nonverbal communication, greetings, and interpersonal exchanges are equally as important in Greek culture. Greeks tend to be very tactile and openly display signs of affection, such as hugging and kissing. Hand gestures are often used during communication and Greeks tend to be very expressive with overall body language. While Greeks are generally considered to be animated communicators, this varies from person to person. Some may be more reserved upon the first meeting.

Age, seniority, and individuals working as professionals (medical doctor, lawyer) are highly respected in Greek culture. Addressing elders by their appropriate title, for example, "Keerios" (Mr.) and "Keeria" (Mrs.) is expected and seen as a sign of respect. Younger individuals often address elders they are not related to as "Theia" (Aunty) and "Theios" (Uncle). The use of titles, including Dr. or Mr./Mrs, are often used when addressing individuals in professional fields, particularly by older generations. Professionals such as medical doctors are highly respected, leading elderly individuals to not challenge or disagree with opinions, despite having different or conflicting views. This may impact on adherence to an agreed upon medical, therapeutic, or rehabilitation program. Furthermore, details about gender-specific or sexual health history may not be willingly shared with a professional of the opposite sex.

Education and Literacy

Both level and quality of education warrant consideration in neuropsychological assessments, particularly with elderly Greeks. The impact of three consecutive wars had a significant impact on time spent in school and the quality of education attained.[16] Research has also noted gender differences with regard to the level of education, with elderly Greek women not having attended school or only attending for very few years. These differences reflect socioeconomic and gender norms, since they grew up in a poverty-stricken agrarian society during and after World War II when going to school interfered with agrarian responsibilities and household duties, and education was often considered superfluous for girls.[17]

Teaching methods employed in Greece during the aforementioned period were largely didactic in nature, emphasizing rote learning and note-taking methods, thus limiting student participation and capacity for reflection. These methods are in contrast to models and standards of education in English-speaking industrialized nations, which placed an emphasis on problem-solving based learning, mental abstraction, as well as test-taking skills, which are heavily drawn on in traditional IQ tests.[18,19] In the context of clinical assessment, a proportion of elderly Greek migrants are at a significant disadvantage due to the lack of familiarity with testing concepts, limited levels of education, and no prior formal testing experience.

Research exploring the utility of brief cognitive screens, normed in countries of origin, for assessment of migrant peer groups have indicated that they are not appropriate for diagnostic purposes. Plitas and colleagues found that if Greek national cut-off score for the Cambridge Cognitive Examination of the Elderly (CAMCOG) and the Mini-Mental Status Examination (MMSE) were applied to Greek Australians, approximately 66%–72% of the sample would be classified as impaired. Overall, Greek national norms are not applicable to Greek Australians because of high probability of false-positive findings and misdiagnoses.[20] This finding indicates that even when a tool is normed in the country of origin, following the migration process, same language-speaking groups may display disproportionate performances.

Values and Customs

Greeks are a collectivist group who display a strong loyalty to familial and social groups. The cornerstones of Greek values are centered on family, interdependence and collectivism, religiosity, respect, and hospitality. These values also hold true with younger generations, where family loyalty, obligations, and honor are fundamental cultural hallmarks.

Respecting parents and elders are fundamental components of Greek culture, with family often weighing in on significant life decisions, such as choice of career or life partner. Arranged marriages were common practice within Greek culture. In instances where children of migrants married outside of their cultural groups, they often married individuals from other European backgrounds. The custom of arranged marriage is now an outdated cultural practice for younger generations, with younger Greek Australians marrying outside of their ethnic group.

The central societal principles underlying Greek culture, namely interdependence and collectivism, often result in children providing care to an elderly family member. This act is associated with the concept of "philotimo," meaning "sense of honor." With this governing cultural concept in mind, it is not surprising that Greek Australian children take on the role of caregivers to elderly parents. In clinical practice, I have provided support to both patients with dementia and their caregivers, who over time present with symptoms of burnout. While options are available to support their loved one, including Greek nursing homes, this option is seldom considered due to cultural expectations and themes of guilt, failure, and shame. These culturally bound concepts are important factors to consider in the context of providing clinical recommendations and advanced care planning.

It is now well established that speed of processing and a variety of other cognitive constructs are dependent on and vary between cultural groups. The concept of processing speed has been argued to reflect a Western individualist concept, where faster is better. However, for many other cultural groups, this notion is considered contradictory, underlying the assumption that a good outcome is achieved as a result of exercising care and taking as much time as needed.[21] For example, Messinis and colleagues[22] showed that if US normative data were used in Greek nationals (aged 45–59, education level of 9–11 years), a raw score time of 55 seconds for CTT-1 and 122 seconds for CTT-2 would place their performance in the 34th percentile.[23] In contrast, the same raw scores using culturally appropriate normative data would place this performance in the 50th percentile. In other words, the use of US norms would unfairly penalize Greek nationals and possibly other dissimilar groups.

Gender Roles

Traditionally, Greek society has been male dominated. There has been quite a masculine ideal of men cast as the provider. Today, most Greek women receive a high level of education and work to contribute to the household income; however, they are still expected to be responsible for the majority of the household duties.

Mental Health Views and Help-Seeking Behaviors

A number of studies have reported that limited help seeking is related to factors such as previous experiences of racism and prejudice,[24] leading to mistrust in the healthcare system, and a perceived imbalance of power between healthcare professionals and minority groups.[25,26] Thus, it is not surprising that non-English-speaking groups are reluctant to engage with mainstream healthcare services due to a lack of previous experience with cognitive assessment, language barriers, cultural differences, a fear of being misdiagnosed, and culturally stereotyped.[27-29] Poor engagement, high anxiety, and mistrust in examiners are well-known to negatively influence cognitive assessment performances.[30]

LoGiudice and colleagues[31] retrospectively examined the demographic and clinical features of patients from non-English-speaking backgrounds (Greek, Italian, Middle Eastern, and Asian) to those from English-speaking backgrounds who attended a memory clinic in Melbourne, Australia.

Results from this study uncovered that those who were non-English-speaking were more likely to present with a functional psychiatric disorder and showed a greater degree of cognitive impairment compared to their English-speaking counterparts. Differences in health status, lifestyles, and the perception of diseases between ethnic groups can have important implications regarding the use of preventive, curative, and rehabilitative healthcare services.[32-34]

Having worked with a number of aging Greek Australians for several years in both clinical and research settings, I have found that their understanding of mental health and medical conditions is limited. Attitudes toward mental illness and degenerative diseases tend to be met with themes of fear and inferiority, while displaying empathy for those affected. Limited engagement with mental health and medical providers is further impacted by stigmatizing attitudes and fears of personal failure.

Medical Conditions

Data indicates that first-generation Greek-born Australians are the second longest living group in the world, after Japanese-born Hawaiians.[35] Interestingly, elderly Greek migrants were noted to be living longer than their Greek national counterparts.[36] In 2011, they continued to have one of the lowest levels of all-cause mortality, with 35% lower mortality rates arising from cardiovascular disease and cancer, relative to the Australian-born population. However, research indicates a 2–3-fold higher prevalence of obesity, diabetes, hyperlipidemia, hypertension, inactivity, and smoking.[37-39]

Approaches to Neuropsychological Evaluation

In my practice, I see a number of individuals from a wide range of cultural backgrounds. Elderly Greeks make up a large proportion of my referral base, where I provide diagnostic, behavioral support, and rehabilitation services. A large majority of elderly Greeks have not had any previous experience with psychological testing. When they present for neuropsychological assessment, they are often uncertain as to why they have been referred, what to expect, and are unfamiliar with testing procedures. Therefore, I begin by explaining my role and the reason for referral in very simple terms, specifically assessing memory and thinking skills to determine if something is wrong with the brain. I give them examples of what types of tests that I am likely to administer, give them ample opportunity to learn and ask questions, and provide encouragement throughout the session. A large majority of elderly Greeks are not test-wise and therefore guided learning is necessary to ensure that they understand what is required of them during the assessment.

Prior to testing, I often engage in casual conversation as a means of alleviating anxiety and establishing rapport. This seemingly casual conversation allows me to gather information regarding personal history and assess memory at a functional/qualitative level. After rapport has been established, I then delve into subject matter that might be considered more sensitive matters, including medical and psychological history.

Neuropsychological assessment requires the examiner to follow standardized instructions as set out in test manuals, however, this approach has proven to be problematic for some groups. Many Greek Australians tend to be at a disadvantage due to the lack of familiarity with testing concepts, limited levels of education and no prior formal testing experience. In my experience, testing is a foreign concept, and elderly Greeks can be resistant and display anxiety. In instances where they are instructed to complete a timed task without interruption, they tend to start speaking or become easily distracted. For example, I have observed that when completing verbal fluency tasks (supermarket items), a number of elder Greeks tend to engage in conversation about recently named items in reference to what they had for dinner and require redirecting.

Prior to commencing testing, I examine whether commonly used tests and norms are appropriate. At present, domain-specific cognitive tests and normative data do not exist for use in any culturally and linguistically diverse group in Australia. It is now widely acknowledged that the use of Western norms and test content for assessment of cultural minorities is inappropriate. In light of these findings, when assessing elderly Greek Australians, I employ a number of tests that have been standardized in Greece, which are arguably more valid than those from Australia or the United States. For example, I have compared the raw and scaled scores of the US normed WAIS-IV[40] to that of the Greek WAIS-IV[41] adaptation and found a 1 to 1.5 standard deviation difference on a majority of the subtests between the two normative samples, particularly in the elderly groups.

Section II: Case Study — "When You Know the Person Is Your Own, It Is Different, You Feel More Comfortable. I Feel Like I Can Speak to You and You Will Understand What I Am Saying"

NA (pseudonym) was referred for neuropsychological review in August 2017 to provide a second opinion regarding her cognitive status and lifestyle decision-making capacity. This assessment was requested by NA's family following disagreement with medical and neuropsychological services who found that she met criteria for a dementia.

As a result of disagreement among NA's children and medical professionals regarding her diagnosis and required level of care, the case was referred to the Victorian Civil and Administrative Tribunal (VCAT). The main role of VCAT is to provide affordable, timely, and quality access to justice for civil matters. In cases where disagreement is noted among family member with regard to management of medical, financial, or life-style capacity in the context of a cognitively impaired family member, an independent guardian may be appointed to make these decisions.

Family Background and Personal History

NA is an 84-year-old woman of Greek background, born in a village near Thessaloniki, Northern Greece. She has an older sister. She stated that both of her parents worked as farmers and believes that they only attended school for two years.

NA migrated to Melbourne, Australia in 1958 at the age of 25. She reported primarily socializing and living with other Greeks due to her limited English. Approximately one year after her arrival, she met her husband and they were married. Shortly after their union, the couple had three children. Since migrating to Australia, she has not worked and was a stay-at-home mother/homemaker. She has five grandchildren and four great grandchildren. NA and her husband live in their own home, where they have resided for more than 50 years.

Educational and Employment History

NA reported completing five years of primary education in her village in Greece. Time spent in school was inconsistent due to war and economic hardships. She attended school for brief periods during the day/week (between one to three days per week, or none at all). After completing primary school, NA worked as a seamstress in her village until migrating to Australia. Due to caring for her children, she has not engaged in formal employment since migration and stated that her primary role was that of a homemaker. Upon arrival to Australia, she did not attend school or English language classes.

Language Proficiency

NA's dominant language was Greek. Greek was the primary language spoken at home during her childhood and following her migration to Australia.

Emotional Functioning

NA reported a history of anxiety dating back to early childhood, which she believed was related to exposure to war and stresses associated with her migration. She contended with symptoms of anxiety throughout adulthood, however, has not engaged in therapy to address these issues. She stated that services were not available in her language when she arrived to Australia and seeking out the services of a psychologist may have led to individuals within her community perceiving her as "crazy." Overall, NA stated that she managed her anxiety relatively well.

Medical and Health History

NA's medical history consisted of total left and right knee replacement surgery, rheumatoid arthritis, hypertension, and restless leg syndrome. She was admitted to hospital four years prior after a mechanical fall due to cervical myelopathy, and underwent cervical discectomy. During her current admission, she underwent a cognitive screen, using the Rowland Universal Dementia Assessment Scale (RUDAS) and scored a 21/27. Recall was 6/8. Visuoconstructional abilities were not assessed. Following this assessment, she was approved for a bed-based transitional care program. Correspondence provided by her community physician, who has been responsible for her care over the last two years, noted no change in cognition or evidence of impending dementia.

Previous Neuropsychological Assessment

NA was seen for neuropsychological assessment as an inpatient two months prior to my review. It was unclear as to why she was referred for assessment while in hospital. The assessment was conducted with the aid of a Greek interpreter. Results indicated that her neuropsychological profile was notable for impaired executive skills and planning along with significantly impaired insight regarding her cognitive deficits. Furthermore, she responded in a manner to indicate a poor understanding about her ability to manage her household, emergency situations, or adapt her behavior to changing events. The conclusion was that cognitive decline has been longstanding and permanent.

Daily Functioning

During her marriage, NA stated that all financial dealings were generally handled by her husband, including paying bills and managing general financial expenses. NA and her husband have received government assistance for personal care (twice weekly) and domestic care (fortnightly) for a period of five years. These services came into effect following her husband's heart valve replacement surgery. In addition to these services, NA's children support her with personal care, preparing meals, cleaning the house, tending to the washing, and grocery shopping once a week. Prior to their mother's surgery, their parents were managing well with the aforementioned supports in place and did not note any significant barriers or safety concerns.

Corroborative History

NA's youngest son noted that while she presented with moderate/high care needs, and that her mobility had been impacted over the last two years, she is well supported at home. Her home was modified to assist with mobility issues, including ramps and rails. From a functional perspective, she requires support in domestic and personal care due to her noted medical conditions, which has led to progressive muscle weakness. Asides from the mechanical fall that she sustained four years prior, he stated that NA has resided in the community without incident. NA's family stated that her cognitive function is intact. They denied any history of cognitive or behavioral changes.

Preliminary Formulation

Following a review of relevant medical documents, obtaining corroborative history, and interviewing NA, I questioned whether she met criteria for a dementia. It is worth noting that NA's previous assessment was conducted using tests that were not necessarily culturally appropriate, and normative data used for comparisons came from samples in the United States and Australia. These limitations were not noted in the previous report.

Mental State and Presentation

NA was seen for neuropsychological review at her home in Melbourne. She was assessed and interviewed in Greek language by myself. She presented as a polite woman of thin build. Gait was not observed as she was sitting. She was socially appropriate and maintained eye contact throughout the session. She described her mood as "sad" and reported feeling anxious, however, settled as time progressed. Speech output and language content were unremarkable. No word finding difficulties were noted. No cognitive or perceptual disturbance was noted.

Functional memory was intact for personal and autobiographical details. She was able to accurately recall the names of her children, their spouses, her grandchildren, and her great grandchildren. Furthermore, she was able to recall all of her children's home telephone numbers, her own telephone number, and her current address. She was also able to state her date of birth, the year that she migrated to Australia, and the years of her previous knee operations. Functional memory for recent events was also intact. For example, during testing NA recalled the dates of recent surgeries and undergoing cognitive testing.

Test and Norm Selection

A number of standardized neuropsychological tests were administered in Greek to explore NA's cognitive functioning, including:

- Wechsler Adult Intelligence Scale, Greek Adaptation—Fourth Edition (WAIS-IV GR)[41]
    - Similarities
    - Information
    - Matrix Reasoning
    - Visual Puzzles
    - Picture Completion
    - Digit Span

- Kosmidis Story Recall Test[42]
- Kosmidis Verbal Learning Test[42]
- Stroop (Colour Reading)[43]
- Colour Form Sorting[44]
- Greek Naming Test[42]
- Clock Drawing Test[45]
- Semantic Verbal Fluency[46]

Based on NA's educational background, level of acculturation and Greek-speaking dominance, neuropsychological tests were administered using standardized Greek instructions. The scoring of tests was interpreted using normative data derived from age and education matched Greek national peers.

NA's premorbid level of intellectual functioning was conservatively estimated to fall within the Low Average to Average range.

Summary of Results, Feedback, and Follow-Up

NA's neuropsychological profile was consistent with premorbid expectations, falling within the Low Average to Average range. She displayed intact reasoning skills, visuospatial skills, general knowledge, processing speed, attention and working memory, and her ability to encode and recall new verbal/visual information intact. Qualitatively, her ability to shift across mental sets was also intact. Furthermore, no language difficulties or apraxia were noted. Based on the outcome of the assessment, using culturally appropriate neuropsychological measures and normative data, NA did not meet the criteria for a dementia.

NA displayed a good degree of insight into her functional limitations, provided adequate responses to potential emergency situations, demonstrated help-seeking behavior, and practical problem-solving skills.

The outcome of the assessment was presented to VCAT and hospital staff, including the heads of psychology and geriatric medicine. Following a review, it was the opinion of VACT that she did not meet criteria for dementia and was capable of making decisions regarding medical and life-style decisions.

As a result of this incident, NA remained hospitalized for a period of approximately 90 days before her case was heard. During this period, she experienced anxiety and feared that she would be placed into a nursing home against her will. She was subsequently released into the care of her husband and her children.

Section III: Lessons Learned

- Assessment of pre- and postmigration history, psychological trauma, age of immigration, changes in cultural identity, socioeconomic status, acculturation, and prejudice are factors that warrant attention in the Greek community.
- Elderly Greek migrants bring a different set of expectations and knowledge to neuropsychological assessments sessions; thus, may perform more poorly on standardized testing.
- Differences in test-taking are attributed, at least in part, to exposure to Western-style school curricula that foster abstract problem solving and test-taking skills, factors which are heavily imbedded within IQ tests. Given the formal and artificial environments that clients are placed in during assessment, this is a factor that may result in anxiety and underperformance.

- The need to clearly express what is required during the testing processes in essential. Additional guided learning to ensure understanding is recommended.
- The use of norms derived from educated English-speaking groups may not be appropriate for use within a range of Australian ethnic minority groups.
- In an ideal situation, referring clients to a culturally similar neuropsychologist for evaluation of cognitive disorders may assist with errors in communication-related to culturally specific concepts.
- Use of interpreters to assist with conducting neuropsychological assessment does not necessarily result in reducing error. Working with interpreters is a skill that needs to be developed and mastered over time.
- Engaging with neuropsychological or psychological services can be impacted due to limited culture-specific services, stigma, prejudice, shame, and limited information available in target languages regarding healthcare issues.

References

1. Ministry of Foreign Affairs. Government and Politics [Internet]. Retrieved 2020 April 22. Available from: https://www.mfa.gr/usa/en/about-greece/government-and-politics/
2. Commonwealth of Australia; Australian Bureau of Statistics [Internet]. 2020 Retrieved April 23. Available from: https://www.abs.gov.au/websitedbs/censushome.nsf/home/cowsredirect
3. Κατατρεγμένοι Έλληνες από τη Μ. Ασία στις ΗΠΑ [Persecuted Greeks from Asia Minor in the USA] (in Greek) [Internet]. Retrieved 2020 April 23. Available from: https://web.archive.org/web/20040807140929/http://www.mpa.gr/specials/us_hellenes/micra_asia.html
4. Frangos S. "Picture Bride Era in Greek American History." *The National Herald* [Internet]. Retrieved 2020 April 23—via Preservation of American Hellenic History. 2005 March 12. Available from: http://www.pahh.com/frangos/brides.html
5. Diacou S. *Hellenism in Chicago.* Austell, GA, USA: United Hellenic American Congress, The Edwards Brothers; 1982.
6. Statistic Canada. Immigration and Ethnocultural Diversity Highlight Tables [Internet]. Retrieved 2020 April 23. Available from: https://www12.statcan.gc.ca/census-recensement/2016/dp-pd/hlt-fst/imm/Table.cfm?Lang=E&T=31&Geo=01&SO=4D
7. German Federal Office of Statistics [Internet]. Retrieved 2020 April 23. Available from: https://www.destatis.de/EN/FactsFigures/SocietyState/Population/MigrationIntegration/Tables_Persons MigrationBackground/MigrantStatusSelectedCountries.html
8. Fédéral Forgien Office of Germany [Internet]. Retrieved 2020 April 23. Available from: https://www.auswaertiges-amt.de/diplo/en/Laenderinformationen/01-Laender/Griechenland.html#t1
9. Wylie L, Van Meye R, Harder H, Sukhera J, Luc C, Ganjavi H et al. Assessing trauma in a transcultural context: challenges in mental health care with immigrants and refugees. Public Health Rev. 2018;39:22.
10. Dimitreas YE. Social mobility of Greeks in Australia [Unpublished doctoral thesis]. Melbourne, Australia: Victoria University; 1996.
11. Rosenthal DA, Bell R, Demetriou A, Efklides A. From collectivism to individualism? The acculturation of Greek immigrants in Australia. Int J Psychol. 1989;24:57–71.
12. Ardila A. Cultural values underlying psychometric cognitive testing. Neuropsychol Rev. 2005;15:185–95.
13. The Constitution of Greece. Hellenic Resources Network [Internet]. Retrieved 2020 April 24. Available from: http://www.hri.org/docs/syntagma/artcl25.html
14. International Religious Freedom Report 2007. US Department of State, Bureau of Democracy, Human Rights, and Labor [Internet]. Retrieved 2020 April 24. Available from: https://2001-2009.state.gov/g/drl/rls/irf/2007/90178.htm
15. European Commission Special Eurobarometer, Biotechnology; Fieldwork: January–February 2010 (PDF) [Internet]. Retrieved 2020 April 24. Available from: https://ec.europa.eu/commfrontoffice/publicopinion/archives/ebs/ebs_341_en.pdf

16. Noutsos H. The road of camel and the school, the Educational Policy in Greece, 1944–46. Athens: Bibliorama; 2003.

17. Kosmidis MH, Tsapkini K, Folia V, Vlahou CH, Kiosseoglou G. Semantic and phonological processing in illiteracy. J Int Neuropsychol Soc. 2004;10(6):818–27.

18. Nell V. Cross-Cultural Neuropsychological Assessment: theory and practice. Mahwah (NJ): Lawrence Erlbaum Associates, Inc.; 2000.

19. Shuttleworth-Edwards AB, Gaylard EK, Radloff SE. WAIS-III test performance in the South African context: extension of a prior cross-cultural normative database. In: Laher S, Cockcroft K, editors. Psychological assessment in South Africa: research and applications. Johannesburg: Wits University Press; 2013. p. 17–32.

20. Plitas A, Tucker A, Kritikos A, Walters I, Bardenhagen F. Comparative study of the cognitive performance of Greek Australian and Greek national elderly: implications for neuropsychological practice. Aust Psychol. 2009;44(1):27–39.

21. Agranovich AV, Panter AT, Puente, AE, Touradji P. The culture of time in neuropsychological assessment exploring the effects of culture-specific time attitudes on timed test performance in Russian and American samples. J Int Neuropsychol Soc. 2011;17:692–701.

22. Messinis L, Malegiannaki AC, Christodoulou T, Panagiotopoulos V, Papathanasopoulos P. Colour Trails Test: normative data and criterion validity for the Greek adult population. Arch Clin Neuropsychol. 2011;26:322–30.

23. D'Elia LF, Satz P, Uchiyama CL, White T. "Colour Trails Test," in Professional manual. Odessa: Psychological Assessment Resources; 1996.

24. Moodley P. Ethnicity: relationship to stigmatisation of people with mental illness. In: Crisp AH, editor. Every family in the land: understanding prejudice and discrimination against people with mental illness. London: Royal Society of Medicine Press Ltd.; 2005.

25. Ardila A. Cross-cultural neuropsychology. In: Metzger F, editor. Neuropsychology: new research. New York (NY): Nova Science; 2013.p. 59–79.

26. Nell V. Translation and test administration techniques to meet the assessment needs of ethnic minorities, migrants, and refugees. In: Goldstein G, Beers SR, editors. Comprehensive Handbook of Psychological Assessment, Volume 1: Intellectual and Neuropsychological Assessment. New York (NY): Wiley; 2004. p. 333–8.

27. Ahmed A, Wilding MA, HaworthLomax R, McCaughan S. Promoting diversity and inclusiveness in dementia services in Salford [Internet]. Greater Manchester: University of Salford Manchester; 2017. Available from: http://usir.salford.ac.uk/42318/1/C_Salford%20BME_Salford%20BME%20Dementia%20ReportFINAL23032017.pdf

28. Jolley D, Moreland N, Read K, Kaur H, Jutlla K, Clark M. The "Twice a Child" projects: learning about dementia and related disorders within the black and minority ethnic population of an English city and improving relevant services. Ethnicity Inequal Health Social Care. 2009;2(4):4–9.

29. Veliu B, Leathem J. Neuropsychological assessment of refugees: methodological and cross-cultural barriers. Appl Neuropsychol Adult. 2017;24(6):481–92.

30. Kennepohl S, Shore D, Nabors N, Hanks R. African American acculturation and neuropsychological test performance following traumatic brain injury. J Int Neuropsychol Soc. 2004;10:566–77.

31. LoGiudice D, Hassett A, Cook R, Flicker L, Ames D. Equity of access to a memory clinic in Melbourne? Non-English-speaking background attenders are more severely demented and have increased rates of psychiatric disorders. Int J Geriatr Psychiatry. 2001;16:327–34.

32. Jean-Pierre P, Roscoe JA, Morrow GR, Carroll J, Figueroa-Moseley C, Philip Kuebler P et al. Race-based concerns over understanding cancer diagnosis and treatment plan: a URCC CCOP Study. J Natl Med Assoc. 2010;102(3):184–9.

33. Kim Y, Pavlish C, Evangelista LS, Kopple LD, Phillips LR. Racial/ethnic differences in illness perceptions in minority patients undergoing maintenance hemodialysis. Nephrol Nurs J. 2012; 39(1):39–49.

34. Lip GY, Khan H, Bhatnagar A, Brahmabhatt N, Crook P, Davies MK. Ethnic differences in patient perceptions of heart failure and treatment: the West Birmingham heart failure project. Heart 2004;90:1016–9.

35. Young C. Selection and survival: immigrant mortality in Australia. In Studies in adult migrant education. Canberra: Department of Immigration and Ethnic Affairs, Australian Government Publishing Services; 1986. https://searchworks.stanford.edu/view/1644751

36. ABS Death, Australia 2010. ABS category no. 3302.0. Canberra: Australian Government Publishing Service; 2012.

37. Kouris-Blazos A, Wahlqvist ML, Wattanapenpaiboon N. Morbidity mortality paradox of Greek-born Australians: possible dietary contributors. Aust J Nutr Diet. 1999;56:97–107.

38. Itsiopoulos C, Cameron M, Fowler C, Kaimakamis M, Best J, ODea K. Is diabetes less of a coronary heart disease risk factor in Greek migrants. Proc Australian Diabetes Soc. Canberra; 1997.

39. Itsiopoulos C, L Brazionis L, Rowley K, O'Dea K. The Greek migrant morbidity mortality paradox: low levels of hypertriglyceridaemia and insulin resistance despite central obesity. Asia Pac J Clin Nutr. 2005;14(Suppl):S43.

40. Wechsler D. Wechsler Adult Intelligence Scale. 4th ed. San Antonio (TX): NCS Pearson Inc.; 2008.

41. Wechsler D. Wechsler Adult Intelligence Scale. 4th ed. Adaptation for Greece (WAIS-IV GR). Athens: Motibo; 2014.

42. Kosmidis, MH, Bozikas, VP, Vlahou, CH. Neuropsychological Test Battery: Lab of Cognitive Neuroscience, School of Psychology, Aristotle University of Thessaloniki. 2012.

43. Zalonis I, Christidi F, Bonakis A, et al. The Stroop effect in Greek healthy population: normative data for the Stroop neuropsychological screening test. Arch Clin Neuropsychol. 2009;24:81–8.

44. Weigl, E. On the psychology of so-called processes of abstraction. J Abnorm Soc Psychol. 1941;36:3–33.

45. Bozikas VP, Giazkoulidou A, Hatzigeorgiadou M, Karavatos A, Kosmidis MH. Do age and education contribute to performance on the clock drawing test? Normative data for the Greek population. J Clin Exp Neuropsychol. 2008;30:199–203.

46. Kosmidis MH, Vlahou CH, Panagiotaki P, Kiosseoglou G. The verbal fluency task in the Greek population: normative data, and clustering and switching strategies. J Int Neuropsychol Soc. 2004;10:164–72.

Portuguese

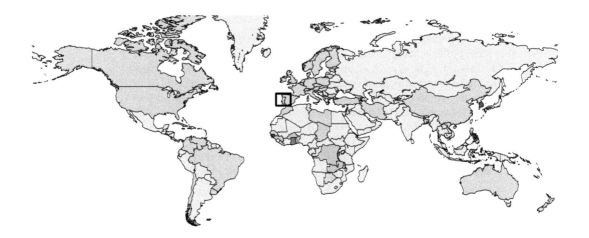

24 Neuropsychology and Rehabilitation in the Portuguese Context

Artemisa R. Dores, Andreia Geraldo, and Sandra Guerreiro

Section I: Background Information

Terminology and Perspective

Persons who live in Portugal are called Portuguese. Our perspective is that of Portuguese neuropsychologists, trained mainly in the North of Portugal and who collaborate with colleagues throughout the country and from various foreign institutions. Additionally, we have links to the Higher Education system in (neuro)psychology, both as Professors with advanced specialization in neuropsychology by the Ordem dos Psicólogos Portugueses (OPP; T.N.: **Portuguese Psychologists Association**) and as PhD students. We share a common interest in research and clinical practice. Thus, our experience of working together reveals our effort to integrate theory (traditionally associated with the academic environment) and practice (traditionally associated with clinical contexts) as crucial to the development and implementation of neuropsychology for high-quality practice in Portugal.

Geography

Portugal is a country in Southern Europe, with a total area of 92,212 km². It is part of the Iberian Peninsula, along with its only neighboring country, Spain.[1] It is located on the extreme southern point of Europe, with a privileged location for import and export. It comprises more than 4 million km² of sea area and is the biggest coastal state of the European Union.[2] Portugal is composed of the continent and two archipelagos, Madeira and Azores. It is organized in 18 districts in the continent and 2 autonomous regions corresponding to the archipelagos.[3]

History and Government

Portugal was founded in 1143 with the celebration of the Zamora Treaty, which recognized the legal status of Portugal as an independent kingdom. Portugal was a monarchy until October 5, 1910, when the first Portuguese Republic was established. Thus, Portugal is one of the oldest nations in Europe, with eight centuries of history. After World War I, a dictatorship settled in the country until April 25, 1974. On this day, a major coup overthrew the dictatorship, and a democracy was established and has been maintained. Portugal was integrated into the European Economic Community (later named European Union) in 1986[4,5] and has since then been integrating and actively contributing to the European Union.

DOI: 10.4324/9781003051862-49

People

Most Portuguese have typical Mediterranean features like brown hair, brown eyes, and a height of less than 6 feet. Characteristics and traces of the Moorish period can be seen in south, in both the physical type and the way of life, and characteristics of Germanic tribes can still be seen in the north of the country, such as some persons being taller, light-haired, and light-eyed.[6] In the course of millennia this mingling between people, combined with the country's isolation from Spain and the rest of Europe, gave rise to a population structure that was homogeneous and distinctively Portuguese, both ethnically and culturally. The Portuguese can be described as easy-going, welcoming, and friendly,[6] who highly value their family and friends with whom they love to celebrate life with around amazing Portuguese food and wine. They are most welcoming to tourists and immigrants, which is one of the main reasons for a mix of cultures and traditions found in Portugal. Traditionally conservative, the younger generations have assumed a much more liberal stance. The attitudes in the northern part of the country are more formal and conservative, while those in the south are generally more casual and relaxed.[6] It is an aging population, due to the decrease in birth rate and to emigration of younger generations. Currently, 10,259,909 persons live in Portugal, of which approximately 14% are younger than 14, approximately 64% are between the ages of 15 and 64, and approximately 21% are older than 65.[7] The period between 2001 and 2019 observed a reduction of the total number of residents in the country under the age of 64, while residents over the age of 65 grew,[7] with a current aging index of 136.2 elderly per 100 young people. This has an impact on late-life brain disorders relevant for neuropsychologists.

Immigration and Relocation

The number of emigrants has been decreasing since 2014 after reaching the maximum value of this century with a peak of more than 130,000 persons exiting Portugal. This is 134,624 in 2014 compared with 77,040 in 2019. In recent years, the Portuguese have emigrated mainly to countries like the United Kingdom, Spain, Switzerland, France, and Germany. Outside Europe, the main destination countries for Portuguese emigration are part of the Community of Portuguese Speaking Countries (CPLP): Angola, Mozambique, and Brazil. There has also been a recent Portuguese emigration tendency to Eastern Europe, with the most common destination being Holland, Luxembourg. France has traditionally been the country in the world with the greatest number of Portuguese emigrants, due to the great wave of emigration in the 1960s/1970s. Countries with strong Portuguese permanence are also Switzerland, the United States, Canada, the United Kingdom, Brazil, and Germany. Several countries have registered a decrease in the last year, such as the United Kingdom, Angola, Brazil, Switzerland, Germany, and France, while an increase was seen in countries like the United States or Belgium.[8]

Language

The official language spoken by residents in Portugal is Portuguese. Portuguese derives from Latin, which was spoken in ancient Rome, and brought to Portugal by Romans. Portuguese is the fifth most spoken language in the world, with around 280 million speakers. Nowadays there are eight countries with Portuguese as their official language (e.g., Angola, Brazil, Cape Verde, Mozambique, São Tomé and Príncipe, East Timor). There are also derivations according to the regions of the country where it is spoken. This is an important aspect for international neuropsychologists to be aware of if they are working with interpreters.

At the beginning of one of the author's professional activity, when taking part in a national team validating children's intelligence tests, the author was confronted with the impact of differences in accents and regionalisms. There was confusion among words such as "abelha and "a velha" ("bee" with "the old woman") or certain objects that have different designations according to the region (e.g., hoe in Portuguese could be enxada, sacho, sachola). This required careful attention with developing, validating, and scoring neuropsychological tests.

Communication

In the past, many health care professionals were trained according to the biomedical model in Portugal. This model prevailed for decades and viewed medical professionals as the main authority responsible for diagnosis and intervention. Today, according to the biopsychosocial model, the importance of a therapeutic relationship, and a patient's active role in their treatment is recognized.[9] Training in verbal and non-verbal communication patterns is carefully attended to when training Portuguese health care professionals to help with therapeutic adherence, patient satisfaction, experience of care, and other biological and functional health outcomes.[10-13] There are communication particularities that should be taken into account when in consult with Portuguese citizens. For example, people in rural areas usually treat health professionals with more reverence, but they tend to be more informal and friendly than in large cities. Men of older generations usually prefer to be treated by their surnames. It is also common to greet with a handshake. Nowadays it is most appropriate to ask by what name they prefer to be treated.

Education and Literacy

The education system in Portugal integrates preschool education (from 3 to 6 years old), basic (from 6 to 14 years old), secondary (from 15 to 18 years old), and university (above 18 years old) education. The state, in particular the Ministry of Education and the Ministry of Science, Technology, and Higher Education, is responsible for regulating the system.[14,15] Currently, compulsory education covers grades 1 to 12. University education is not compulsory or free to Portuguese citizens at the present time. Recently, partly due to the establishment of a higher level of compulsory education, residents in Portugal have obtained higher education levels, with concurrent reduction in school dropout rates and improved mathematical, reading, and sciences competences.[16] Nevertheless, while these improvements have been beneficial for younger generations, adults and older adults who come for neuropsychological assessments may not always have basic or secondary education completed. In 2019, there was a total of 559,800 Portuguese people aged 15 or older without any education, and 1,904,300 had completed up to a fourth-grade education.[17]

In Portugal, the rate of early school dropouts has fallen steadily and is very close to the European target established for 2020 (maximum 10% of young people leaving the education and training system without obtaining a secondary level qualification). This was 10.6% in 2019, compared to 43.6% in 2000. More and more young people are pursuing higher education. In 2019 the figure was 36.2%, which has tripled since 2001.[18] However, the abandonment rate when pursuing a degree is also high at 29%.[19]

In regards to literacy, formal reading and writing in Portuguese language are taught throughout school. The compulsory education is of 12 years. It starts when the student is 6 and ends at age 18. The obligation to learn English in the third year of the first cycle (students who are 8 years old) started officially in the academic year 2015/2016, extending to the fourth year in 2016/2017. The most recent data are from 2011, when 499,936 (340,231 female) Portuguese residents were considered illiterate.[20] This is worth considering when designing a neurocognitive assessment protocol since it can limit the use of some well-established neuropsychological tests (e.g., Trail Making Test, when the education level is under the fourth grade). In the past, we have seen the use of objects available in a clinical office, such as staplers, or graphic representations of objects (e.g., 4 inverted to represent a chair) to test object recognition. In these unstandardized situations, it is important to keep in mind that failed responses could reflect clients' education level and not necessarily cognitive impairment. Also, when there are lower formal schooling levels, it can be difficult to use information and communication technologies and even virtual environments since they might require the use of computers, tablets, or mobile phones that are likely to be out of reach for many.[21,22]

Values and Customs

Portugal is a country that is very rich in traditions and customs. Some of them are exclusive to Portugal. This includes music (e.g., fado), dance (e.g., Pauliteiros de Miranda), gastronomy (e.g., conventual sweets), customs and rituals (e.g., "Caretos de Podence"), and wine (e.g., Port wine). There are several traditions that had fallen out of favor but have been proudly recovered in recent years, even by the younger generations (e.g., certain costumes, fashion props, decorative objects, music, dances). These traditions coexist peacefully with new habits and customs developed from immigration, emigration, and tourism.

Gender

Portugal has a long tradition as a sexist and patriarchal country that has made it difficult for women to access a variety of roles that have typically been considered male responsibilities. Due to the extraordinary impact of the patriarchal and conservative authoritarian regime (from 1933 to 1974), during many years Portugal lagged behind other Western European countries in terms of indicators and policies on gender equality.[23] Despite its young democracy, the country has come a long way and current legislation enshrines values such as equality, freedom, and human dignity, including in relation to gender equality and sexual and reproductive rights. Yet, the process of transposing law into practice has not been always easy or fast. Social change in terms of gender equality and family life started to become evident during the 1980s.[23] Despite machismo being marked in Portugal in the past, this tendency has been attenuated during recent years. Nevertheless, it is worth noting that it is still possible that psychologists have to work with persons who have this norm rooted, especially with older persons.

Spirituality and Religion

Portugal is a secular state. The Catholic religion is the most practiced despite progressive decline since the fall of the fascist regime. The latest major study on religion in Portugal revealed that the number of Portuguese Catholics has decreased in recent years, along with an increase in other religions and non-religious Portuguese.[24] While mainly a Catholic country, it is also pluralistic, with several examples of initiatives that bring together efforts of several religious and non-religious institutions (e.g., **Portuguese Refugee Support Platform**).

Health System

In 1971 a Decree-Law (nr. 413/71 of September 27)[25] declared the lawful right of all citizens to health services and created the Ministério da Saúde e da Assistência [Health and Assistance Ministery] responsible for regulating the role of the state for development and regulation of health politics.[26] In 1979, by the Decree-Law nr. 56/79 of September 15,[27] the National Health Service was established, with main goals of making access to health services universal, general, and free. Currently, this service is a coexistence of public and private entities and is organized in five health regions, namely North, Center, Lisbon, Vale do Tejo, Alentejo, and Algarve, and 18 health sub-regions, corresponding to the districts of Portugal.[25,28] This service is constantly improving, adapted in accordance with the state, institutional, and population's needs. The career of psychologists in the National Health Services has been included in the Superior Health Technicians category since 1994, by the decree-law nr. 241/94.[29] Nonetheless, neuropsychological services are still scarce in the National Public Health System, and mainly under the umbrella of Neurology Services.

Acquired brain injuries (ABIs) are an important public health issue in Portugal since they are one of the main causes of death and disability.[30,31] Cerebrovascular diseases such as strokes caused 11,235 deaths in 2018 and are one of the main causes of disabilities in the country, along with cancer.[32] Higher stroke prevalence rates and high levels of comorbidity have a significant impact on the affected person, their social support network, and the Portuguese society in general.[33] In addition, approximately 275,000 Portuguese suffered a severe traumatic brain injury (TBI) in the past 25 years,[34] mostly related to road traffic accidents, workplace accidents, and falls.[35] Yet, there has been a reduction in TBIs in Portugal over time, with 137 cases per 100,000 residents in 1997 to 65 cases per 100,000 residents in 2014, which is mainly attributed to the preventive measures for workplace and road traffic accidents implemented in Portugal.[35,36] This was also observed in the mortality rates, with higher mortality rates in older adults and higher incidence, hospitalizations, and mortality in males.[35] Finally, brain tumors are also associated with significant consequences to the person itself and their social support networks and represent 2.1% of all cancers in Portugal, with 1,225 new cases every year.[37]

Rehabilitation System

The rehabilitation system in Portugal is strong and aims to provide those with acquired and developmental disabilities with greater participation in social and economic life to maximize autonomy.[38] In the last decades, Portugal has made significant progress in policies and practices for people with disabilities. The road to providing better health and social support care to persons with disabilities started in 1979 with the creation of a rehabilitation and employment service for people with disabilities. This Employment and Vocational Training Institute focused on their professional and social integration. The translation of the International Classification of Impairments, Disabilities and Handicaps for Portuguese, in 1989,[39] provided a conceptual definition of these phenomena and helped both professionals and members of the government to better understand and frame it. From there on, a series of decree-laws[40–44] has focused on improving the quality of life of persons with disabilities, ensuring their rights both at professional, healthcare, and psychosocial levels. The last one was a resolution of the Council of Ministers, in 2010,[45] that defined a National Disability Strategy where the Portuguese State committed to promote, protect, and guarantee decent living conditions for people with disabilities with implications for economic, social, and cultural rights. Despite the progress, it is still possible to identify areas of weakness and optimize the use of resources, including a view to adapting services to citizens, and to increase the number of available interventions and their efficacy, effectiveness, and efficiency.

Neuropsychological Approach

Neuropsychology emerged in Portugal as a clinical discipline toward the end of the seventies/early eighties. Prior to this period, research was focused on diagnosis and treatment of behavioral changes as a result of stroke, with particular focus on language changes. The hiring of professionals from Clinical Psychology to hospitals occurred after 1974 during a period that marked the beginning of democratic life in Portugal. This contributed to the emergence of multi-disciplinary models, which were considered to be technically and scientifically autonomous, among which clinical neuropsychology was born. In the mid-1980s, Neuropsychology Hospital Units emerged and had varying degrees of administrative autonomy, depending on statutes of the Health Units and Hospital Centers; however, neuropsychology's coverage at the national level was reduced. At universities, there was a great investment in neuropsychology in the nineties, with the inclusion of several curricular units in neuroscience and research that contributed to increases in masters and PhDs being awarded.

Currently, *OPP*, a professional public association representing professionals in psychology, created by Law No. 57/2008, recognizes neuropsychology as an advanced specialty in clinical and health psychology.[46] Among the different contexts, Portuguese neuropsychologists focus on health, education, and justice, with roles that extend to different clinical contexts, schools, educational centers, early intervention centers, private institutions for social solidarity, nongovernmental organizations, projects or programs for continuous care, National Institute of Legal Medicine and Forensic Sciences, insurance companies, rehabilitation centers, or courts.

From a training perspective, psychologists who specialize in neuropsychology must, among others, present competencies in assessment and neuropsychological rehabilitation, namely psychometry through the use of clinical interview techniques and standardized instruments, knowledge of psychopathology, and the neurobiological correlates of cognitive and affective phenomena, among others. The advanced specialty in neuropsychology is attributed by the OPP, through a process where the curriculum of each psychologist is evaluated by the specialty board through the following criteria: hours of professional practice, training (congresses, workshops, conferences, and seminars, among others), and other elements (supervision and **intervision** sessions, research projects, internship supervision, among others). Additionally, candidates should present a written report, or a paper published presenting a case study, the assessment of an intervention, or the report of a project that is also assessed by the specialty board.[47] The Portuguese Society of Neuropsychology *[Sociedade Portuguesa de Neuropsicologia (SPNPsy)]* was founded in 2017 and aimed to promote Portuguese neuropsychology and its members' professional and scientific training, and within its legal scope, promote the conditions of good practices in the exercise of the profession.[48] Most of the instruments used in neuropsychological assessment in Portugal were translated and culturally adapted from English language tests, but Portuguese normative data, mainly organized by age and sex groups, are available. Nevertheless, some tests are developed in Portugal.

Section II: Case Study — "I Exist beyond My Diagnosis; Diagnosis Does Not Define Me"

Note: Possible identifying information and several aspects of history and presentation have been changed to protect the patient identity and privacy.

Presenting Concerns

Miguel (fictitious name), male, aged 26 years old, was admitted to CRPG—Centro de Reabilitação Profissional de Gaia [T.N. CRPG—Gaia Vocational Rehabilitation Centre], on October 11, 2019. He came accompanied by his parents, who were both in their 50s and employed full-time. Miguel's father led the interview and explained that his son had been at home since being discharged from the hospital after brain tumor (low-grade glioma in the fronto-temporo-insular region) removal surgery on February 27, 2019.

Miguel initially had two epileptic seizures, and although he did not show focal neurological signs, he showed marked changes in behavior prior to tumor identification. He had disinhibition and high anxiety and was having difficulty performing tasks in the professional context with frequent forgetfulness of requests. After the tumor was identified, he was immediately taken for surgery, but the entire tumor could not be resected. He underwent right pterional craniotomy for partial removal of an astrocytoma. He subsequently showed behavioral frontal lobe dysfunction (impulsivity, irritability, high levels of anxiety, vivid dreams, greater appetite for sweets) and had slightly affected cognitive dysfunction in attention, short-term memory, and executive functions.

Miguel and his family came to CRPG after being referred by a neuropsychologist in a Portuguese Hospital, for support in the rehabilitation process, with a request to emphasize emotional and behavioral cognitive rehabilitation. Specifically, both Miguel and his family reported good physical-functional recovery, without motor sequelae, but had other concerns about his functioning. Post-traumatic epilepsy was still in the medication adjustment phase, so they were concerned about possible crises and Miguel's need to be accompanied. They were also concerned about Miguel's professional work. He was on medical leave without clinical authorization to resume his duties as a cook's assistant, since his work was very demanding, with long schedules and high pressure and stress. As a result, the family was eager to receive professional rehabilitation support and guidance.

Daily Functioning

Miguel's parents noticed that post-surgically, their son had become more irritable, aggressive, and impulsive. They mentioned some unusual behaviors such as gnawing on the cuticles of his hands, shaking his leg, walking from side to side inside the house, greater exaltation, active dreaming, and the emergence of an eating disorder with a greater appetite for sweets. At the cognitive level, they reported difficulties in naming, language comprehension, and attention. Since the surgery, Miguel also did not want to be alone due to fear of epileptic seizures. He went with his father to the studio/**atelier** where he works (family business) or stayed at home with his maternal grandmother. He did not have any structured daily activities, had stopped driving, and was less autonomous even in personal activities of daily living.

Educational and Vocational History

Miguel was a high-achieving student during basic education up to ninth grade. In high school, he chose a science and technology course of study. After completing high school, Miguel entered a public University in Civil Engineering. He tried for two years to be successful with his academics, but since it was a very rigorous program (especially in mathematics and physics), he gave up. In 2016 he decided to join a professional cooking course. After graduating, he worked in several restaurants as a cook. He had an opportunity to work in England but returned home a few months later due to behavioral changes, high anxiety, and difficulties remembering instructions. At the time, these signs were interpreted as difficulties adapting to the new cultural context in England. After returning to Portugal, he started to work in a restaurant where he had previously worked until his diagnosis.

Language Proficiency

Miguel had good language skills, both oral and written, in Portuguese. He spoke English fluently, mainly as a result of his stay in England. As his native language is Portuguese, he was evaluated in this language.

Cultural History

Miguel is original and resident in the North of Portugal. Originally from a working family, his mother works as a secretary and his father is a goldsmith, belonging to average socio-economic status. As an only child he regrets the absence of a sibling in his life.

He presented with strong family ties to his grandparents, uncles, and cousins. His family has been his main social support network through his rehabilitation since social integration at school had been difficult for him, and he had limited social relationships outside his family.

Emotional Functioning

Miguel's adolescence was marked by depression, deep feelings of worthlessness, difficulty in accepting his image, and suicidal ideation. He had panic attacks at school which led to avoidant behaviors, isolation, and rejection by his peers.

At the time of his evaluation, and at the beginning of his rehabilitation program, his most visible traits were high anxiety and impulsivity. He also had fast and repetitive speech, impatience, intolerance to noise, restlessness, and emotional deregulation (intensity and adequacy), for which he had little awareness. These aspects of his personality changes were difficult for him and his family to manage.

Test, Norm Selection, and Results

Miguel arrived at CRPG in October 2019 with a neuropsychological assessment carried out in September of the same year in an inpatient hospitalization context.

The assessment was conducted in European Portuguese, with the European Portuguese version for all tests and Portuguese validation norms. From this previous assessment, we came to knew that Miguel was comfortable with the assessment procedures, was cooperative, and exhibited a satisfactory engagement in all the assessment tasks with no signs of malingering. According to this previous assessment, deficits were found in attention (mainly for visual information), in naming by auditory description, in visuoconstruction abilities with significant difficulties in planning and precision in the copy of Rey's Complex Figure, in visual memory, and in some of the assessed executive functions (reasoning, cognitive flexibility, and perseverative errors in graphomotor sequences). Additionally, a preserved performance was found in tasks that involved visuospatial performance, language (including in verbal fluency tests), learning, verbal memory, and decision-making.

On a self-report scale, high anxiety symptoms were reported, and on a neuropsychiatric inventory, completed by Miguel's parents, mild to moderate symptoms of psychomotor agitation, aggressive behavior, anxiety, disinhibition, aberrant motor behavior (biting nails and cuticles until they bleed), and eating disorder were identified. Cognitive, emotional, and behavioral difficulties were considered significant enough for his integration into a holistic neuropsychological rehabilitation program.

Considering these results, we performed an additional assessment prior to the integration of Miguel on the holistic neuropsychological rehabilitation program provided by CRPG. All the applied tests were in European Portuguese, and the norms used to interpret the scores resulted from Portuguese validations of those tests (for sex, age, and educational level), except for the Wisconsin Card Sorting Test in which the American norms were used. As in Miguel's assessment in the hospital context, in the complementary assessment Miguel exhibited a cooperative and engaged posture in all the assessment tasks, revealing a good comprehension level of the instructions given and no signs of malingering. The results are presented in Table 24.1.

Table 24.1 Neuropsychological assessment results

Domain assessed	Test	Results (M; SD)
Brief Assessment of Mental Status	Montreal Cognitive Assessment (MoCA)[49]	27/30 (M = 27.39; SD = 1.86)
Premorbid intelligence	TeLPI: Teste de Leitura de Palavras Irregulares[50]	Full-scale IQ: 115 (M = 100; SD = 10) Verbal IQ: 116 Performance IQ: 111
Attention and concentration	D2 Test of Attention[51]	Information processing speed: 484 Accuracy: 188 (M = 421.86; SD = 77.61) Overall Performance: 471 (M = 154.09; SD = 37.45) Concentration: 187 (M = 394.09; SD = 74.74) Performance stability: 7 (M = 15.46; SD = 5.53) Precision: 2.7 (M = 6.68; SD = 6.77)
Executive functions	INECO Frontal Screening[52]	20.5/30 (M = 24.6; SD = 2.8)
	The Stroop Color and Word Test[53]	Word reading: 82 (M = 91.1; SD = 28.1) Color reading: 74 (M = 68.3; SD = 21.6) Color-word reading: 49 (M = 42.3; SD = 15.4) Interference: 10 (M = 2.3; SD = 12.6)
	Wisconsin Card Sorting Test[54]	Number of categories completed: 0 (%ile ≤ 1) Perseverative errors: 30 (%ile = 3)
	Trail Making Test (TMT)[55]	TMT—A: 22 s (M = 52; SD = 37) TMT—B: 45 s (M = 113; SD = 71) B – A: 23 s (M = 66; SD = 51) B/A: 2 (M = 2.5; SD = 1.0) B – A/A: 1 (M = 1.5; SD = 1.0) A + B: 67 (M = 160; SD = 96) A × B/100: 9.9 (M = 69; SD = 95)
Memory	Weschler Memory Scale—III; task Faces[56]	Faces I: 4 (M = 10; SD = 1.5) Faces II: 4 (M = 10; SD = 1.5) Retention: 100%
	Weschler Memory Scale—III; task Verbal Paired Associates[56]	Memory Acquisition: 13 (M = 10; SD = 1.5) Delayed recall: 7 (M = 10; SD = 1.5) Recognition: 100%
Working memory	Weschler Memory Scale—III[56]	WM index: 90 (M = 100; SD = 15)
Perception and visual memory	Rey's Complex Figure[57]	Copy: 19.5 (M = 31.17; SD = 3.62) Reproduction: 13 (M = 18.9; SD = 5.41) Type of drawing: III
Verbal comprehension	Token Test[58]	22/22 (M = 21.7; SD = 0.3)
Mood stability	Hospital Anxiety and Depression Scale[59]	Anxiety: 10 (mild symptomatology) Depression: 1 (no symptomatology)
Quality of life	Quality of Life after Brain Injury (QOLIBRI)[60]	Cognitive: 54 (M = 60.6; SD = 20.7) Self: 83 (M = 58.5; SD = 17.4) ADL: 68 (M = 56.3; SD = 20.0) Social: 83 (M = 59.6; SD = 17.9) Emotional: 40 (M = 61.6; SD = 26.1) Physical: 70 (M = 58.7; SD = 14.6) Total: 68 (M = 59.1; SD = 14.6)
Functionality	Glasgow Outcome Scale—Extended (GOS-E)[60]	6—Upper Moderate Disability

Preliminary Formulation

No signs of malingering were identified both on the hospital assessment and on the additional assessment performed in CRPG. Although no stand-alone performance validity test was applied due to the inexistence of signs, the recognition score of the WMS-III Verbal Paired Associates (100%) suggests that Miguel applied is full-effort during the assessment procedures.

Overall, formal testing showed frontal lobe and executive dysfunction. The assessment showed significant evidence of attention and memory difficulties in the work context, especially in situations of stress and pressure.

Ecological assessment was carried out through a guided interview with the client and his parents, which aimed to explore the difficulties in the activities of daily living and in the professional context. From this interview, it became clear that in the professional context Miguel was, at the time of the assessment, unable to respond to the demands of his job function: his work pace was slower, he forgot what he was asked for, and in the face of failures and difficulties he reacted in an impulsive and inappropriate way (catastrophic response). This inappropriate behavior, characterized by mood fluctuations, was reported by the parents at home and confirmed by Miguel. Miguel recognized his difficulties, but he still had difficulty managing his behavior. Associated with these cognitive difficulties were emotional and behavioral changes. The influence of these difficulties was so marked that Miguel was considered unfit to exercise his cook's functions. Cognitive, emotional, and behavioral changes are potentially disabling in a professional context and represented difficulties for Miguel's autonomy in daily living activities. His clinical condition had also not fully stabilized (ongoing adjustment of anti-epileptic medication), and the need for chemotherapy, radiotherapy, or new surgery was being evaluated in case his tumor grew. Our plan was to monitor Miguel's progress and provide psychological support to deal with the uncertainty inherent to his clinical and work status. We agreed that Miguel was a good candidate for our intensive day rehabilitation program.

Rehabilitation Program

Miguel participated in a holistic neuropsychological rehabilitation program from November 2019 until May 2020. Usually, the CRPG program is 23 week-long, but the lockdown due to the COVID-19 pandemic in March 2020 imposed the suspension of services.

The holistic neuropsychological rehabilitation program is an intensive day-care program of 23 weeks with 30 hours per week. The program is focused on neuropsychological and physical rehabilitation with individual and group activities. It includes several structured interventions on neuropsychological rehabilitation, psychotherapy, mindfulness meditation, communication and interpersonal skills training, information and communication technologies skills training, employability, personal and social autonomy, physical therapy, speech therapy, and occupational therapy. The program is based on a therapeutic community with groups of ten patients and a multidisciplinary team.

Miguel's therapeutic goals were to increase emotional regulation, regulate impulsivity, and help him to develop social filter. The program also aimed to manage his attention and memory difficulties, help him develop tolerance, improve autonomy, and redefine his professional work.

Outcomes

Miguel joined the program with a very positive attitude. The context of the therapeutic community among other Portuguese brain-injured residents allowed him to establish a safe space to understand difficulties associated with his brain injury. Adherence to compensation strategies was also achieved as he became a systematic user of external aids for memory and executive functions (for example, electronic calendar, reminders, checklists). Mindfulness techniques allowed him to better regulate his emotions and impulsive behavior. Adjusting his medication for epilepsy also facilitated stability.

Due to confinement at the end of the program, it was not possible to repeat the initial neuropsychological assessment. Notwithstanding, we had the opportunity just before this interruption to reassess his executive functioning skills through the Wisconsin Card Sorting Test (WCST). He completed all categories after 85 trials without any perseverative errors.

Most importantly, Miguel gained autonomy in daily life, which was important for his identity as the only son in a Portuguese family. For instance, he was able to use public transportation on his own and cook family meals. This *post-traumatic growth* reflects the positive mental shift experienced as a result of adversity. Specifically, for relationships, he learned to value friends and family more than he did in the past. For self-esteem, his challenges had given him a deeper inner wisdom, personal strength, and gratitude. The survival experience also helped him accept his vulnerabilities and limitations and change his life perspective in the direction of appreciation, new possibilities, and more flexibility. Both Miguel and his parents reported positive gains after the rehabilitation, primarily regarding his personality since he was more sociable and developed a more positive attitude about his clinical condition. This growth is mirrored in the following excerpt retrieved from a text he wrote for his final celebration during the rehabilitation program: "I exist beyond my diagnosis; the diagnosis does not define me. I learned that my best is not my maximum; I feel like I am a different person after the surgery."

Miguel's progress has been monitored with follow-up sessions. Miguel is currently attending a secretarial course with the goal of working in a back-office context doing professional tasks more appropriate to his current needs.

In addition to the course, Miguel joined an adapted rowing club, where he conducts daily training. He has been feeling well integrated into this group, recognizing both the physical well-being that results from his new sports activity and the emotional well-being that is related to camaraderie and team spirit.

As had happened previously with the rehabilitation program due to the pandemic, it was necessary to switch the training course to an e-learning format. His digital skills have enabled him to fully participate and engage in the course activities in this format.

Currently, the course is being conducted within a b-learning format with success. In addition to academic and professional gains, both Miguel and his parents report stable gains on an emotional level. Disinhibition behavior and changes related to high anxiety are significantly reduced (e.g., Miguel has stopped biting his nails). His participation in the adapted rowing training has also positively contributed to this result. The practice of sport, especially a team sport, has been very beneficial for his physical and mental health. It is expected that Miguel finishes his course next November and engages in a future professional activity.

Section III: Lessons Learned

- As Portugal is a democracy, every citizen should be treated as equal, and their personal values, customs, and beliefs should be respected within the process of neuropsychological assessment and rehabilitation.
- Being a small country, Portugal does not have significant cultural differences between regions, although some of them have different traditions. Nevertheless, some differences in communication styles and in the language (e.g., accents and regionalisms) should be considered when communicating with persons from different regions and when developing, validating, and scoring neuropsychological tests that involve language abilities.
- Most Portuguese citizens have formal education. The educational level of Portuguese people has been growing in the direct way of the establishment of higher levels of compulsory

education. Nevertheless, there are still Portuguese persons who have not completed any formal education (i.e., 12.6% (9.7% female)) nor have completed at least four years of formal education.[20,61] This should be taken into account when designing both neurocognitive assessment and rehabilitation protocols.

- The model that currently prevails in healthcare services in Portugal is the biopsychosocial model, in which the importance of the therapeutic relationship and the patient's active role in their rehabilitation process is recognized.

- It is important to note that the European Portuguese language differs significantly from other versions of the Portuguese language, spoken in Brazil or in other Portuguese-speaking countries such as Angola, Mozambique, Guinea-Bissau, Timor-Leste, Equatorial Guinea, Macau, Cape Verde, and São Tomé and Príncipe. Thus, the instruments are only valid for the country in which they were adapted and validated.

- Changes in emotional and behavioral aspects can be highly disabling due to their repercussions in terms of cognitive functions. In a situation of great anxiety, the person is less able to recruit cognitive functions and often goes into survival mode with a fight-flight or freezing response. It is essential that neuropsychological rehabilitation programs take this issue into account and that they are effective in creating a safe and trusting environment. This includes the development of a therapeutic alliance focused on understanding, acceptance, and support. Understanding these mechanisms of automatic responses facilitates the development of emotional regulation strategies. Throughout the development of our program, we have included mindfulness and self-compassion strategies with good results both in attentional capacity, in emotional regulation, and in acceptance.

- We always learn from our clients, but this time we learn something beyond what we could have imagined: two weeks from completion of the rehabilitation process when we were surprised by the COVID-19 pandemic. We had to restructure our whole life from one day to the next and adapt to this new situation: accepting constraints to keep ourselves safe, managing resources, and taking care of ourselves and of those who need our support. Since then, the clinical team has grown even closer to their clients. Closer by the joint experience of this abrupt and unexpected change to which we are still adapting. Probably some clients have already overcome greater challenges than these and have already been in far more complex and threatening arenas! We learned with their resilience in the face of adversity, we lived with them the limitations of confinement. The expression never seemed so right before: we were all in the same boat.

"If you want to go fast, go alone. If you want to go far, go together" – African Saying

Unpredictability

I had surgery for the removal of a brain tumor on February 27, 2019. After two weeks, I was discharged. A few months later, I underwent a neuropsychological assessment and my neuropsychologist referred me to the CRPG because I needed cognitive rehabilitation.

My rehabilitation process began on November 5, 2019. I learned to deal much better with one of my main problems, which is dealing with the unforeseen.

Some examples of this obstacle are:

- Deal with traffic
- Deal with the unforeseen or something that gets out of my control
- Travel in a cluttered subway
- Understand that the subway might break down
- High-pitched noises

- Children crying
- Places with lots of people
- Very noisy places

All of this causes my brain to suffer too much stimulation and to have an immediate response or to be unable to control my emotions and my behavior.

So, at CRPG I learned some compensation strategies to face the unforeseen more positively, which are mainly:

- Listen to music
- Meditation (act and react)
- Breathing
- Distance:
  - To regulate my internal reaction
  - To provide a more weighted response
  - To be a fuller and kinder human

Some safety signs make me feel calmer and trust what will happen next. These are:

- Feelings of:
  - Group
  - Confidentiality
  - Belonging
  - Tranquility
  - Equality
- To think that I am a normal person, just like the others, despite my difficulties.

Finally, I consider myself to be a different person than the one who started rehabilitation in 2019. I learned that I am not the only one to feel or think in a certain way and that others are going through the same and with whom I can count for support and attention.

I also realized that not everything deserves my attention or dedication. But above all, I accept much better who I was, who I am, and who I will be.

Acknowledgments

The authors wish to thank Miguel for sharing his story, which we expect might contribute to a cross-cultural perspective of neuropsychology in this exciting project. Your resilience is inspiring.

This research was supported by Fundação para a Ciência e Tecnologia (FCT) through R&D Units funding (UIDB/05210/2020), and through a doctoral grant (SFRH/BD/138723/2018) awarded to Andreia Geraldo.

Glossary

Atelier.   Local work of an artist or craftsman that works independently (e.g., architecture atelier or sewing atelier). In some cases, it may also be designated as workshop or studio.

Intervision.   Group sessions where smaller groups of participants (e.g., professionals, trainees, or volunteers) with similar backgrounds exchange experiences without the guidance of a facilitator. The main aims are to learn from the experience of colleagues and peers and address work issues that need clarification or are perceived as problematic by team staff.

Portuguese Psychologists Association (T.N.: Ordem dos Psicólogos Portugueses, OPP). Professional association in which psychologists must be enrolled in order to exercise their professional activity.

Portuguese Refugee Support Platform. Portuguese platform of civil society organizations involved in refugee work in Portugal whose aim is to support the hosting of refugees in the current humanitarian crisis.

Further Readings

Bowden SC. Neuropsychological assessment in the age of evidence-based practice: Diagnostic and treatment evaluations. Oxford: Oxford University Press; 2017.

Gage N, Baars B. Fundamentals of cognitive neuroscience: A begginer's guide. London: Academic Press, Elsevier; 2018.

Guerreiro S, Dores AR, Almeida I, Castro-Caldas A, Barbosa, F. Neuropsychological rehabilitation. In: Cruz-Cunha MM, Miranda IM, Martinho R, Rijo R, editors. Encyclopedia of E-health and telemedicine. Hershey, PA: Medical Information Science Reference; 2016. https://doi.org/10.4018/978-1-4666-9978-6.ch023

Haskings E, Cicerone K, Dams-O'Connor K, Eberle R, Langenbahn D, Shapiro-Rosenbaun A, Trexler L. Cognitive rehabilitation manual: Translating evidence-based recommendations into practice. Virginia, USA: American Congress of Rehabilitation Medicine; 2012.

Kane R, Parsons T. The role of technology in clinical neuropsychology. Oxford: Oxford University Press; 2017.

Koivisto J, Hamari J. The rise of motivational information systems: A review of gamification research. Int J Inf Manage. 2019;45:191–210.

Richards D, Caldwell P. Gamification to improve adherence to clinical treatment advice: Improving adherence to clinical treatment. In: Novak D, Tulu B, Brendryen H, editors. Handbook of research on holistic perspectives in gamification for clinical practice. Hershey, PA: IGI Global; 2016. https://doi.org/10.4018/978-1-4666-9522-1.ch004

Winson R, Wilson BA, Bateman A, editors. The brain injury rehabilitation workbook. London: The Guilford Press; 2017.

References

1. Ministério dos Negócios Estrangeiros (MNE). Sobre Portugal: Dados gerais. [About Portugal: General data] [Internet]. Lisbon: Ministério dos Negócios Estrangeiros; 2020 Oct 19. Available from: https://www.portaldiplomatico.mne.gov.pt/sobre-portugal

2. Plano de Situação do Ordenamento do Espaço Marítimo Nacional (PSOEM). Ordenamento do mar português: Âmbito especial. [Portuguese sea planning: Special scope] [Internet]. 2020 [cited 2020 Oct 20]. Available from: https://www.psoem.pt/ambito/

3. Instituto Nacional de Estatística (INE). Divisão administrativa. [Administrative organization] [Internet]. INE, I.P.: Lisbon; 2020 Oct 19. Available from: https://www.ine.pt/xportal/ine/portal/portlets/html/conteudos/listaContentPage.jsp?BOUI=6251013&xlang=PT

4. European Union (EU). The history of the European Union [Internet]. 2020 [cited 2020 Oct 19]. Available from: https://europa.eu/european-union/about-eu/history_en

5. Ministério dos Negócios Estrangeiros (MNE). História. [History] [Internet]. Lisbon: Ministério dos Negócios Estrangeiros; 2020 Oct 19. Available from: https://ue.missaoportugal.mne.gov.pt/pt/portugal/sobre-portugal/historia

6. GoLisbon. Portuguese people: population characteristics and famous names [Internet]. 2021 May 7. Available from: https://www.golisbon.com/culture/people.html

7. Pordata. População residente: total e por grandes grupos etários. [Resident population: total and by age groups] [Internet]. 2020 Jun 15. Available from: https://www.pordata.pt/Municipios/Popula%C3%A7%C3%A3o+residente+total+e+por+grandes+grupos+et%C3%A1rios-390

8. Pordata. Emigrantes: total e por tipo. [Emigrants: total and by type] [Internet]. 2020 Jun 16. Available from: https://www.pordata.pt/Portugal/Emigrantes+total+e+por+tipo-21

9. Ogden J. Health psychology. 6th ed. London: McGraw Hill Education; 2019.

10. Parker J., Coiera E. Improving clinical communication: a view from psychology. J Am Med Inform Assoc: JAMIA [Internet]. 2000;7:453–61. Available from: https://doi.org/10.1136/jamia.2000.0070453

11. Institute for Healthcare Communication. Impact of communication in healthcare [Internet]. 2011 Jul. Available from: https://healthcarecomm.org/about-us/impact-of-communication-in-healthcare/

12. Rimal RN, Lapinski MK (2009). Why health communication is important in public health. Bull World Health Organ. 2009;87:247–247a.

13. World Health Organization (WHO). Adherence to long-term therapies: Evidence for action [Internet]. Switzerland: WHO Library Cataloguing; 2003. Available from: https://www.who.int/chp/knowledge/publicat

14. Direção-Geral da Educação (DGS). Currículo Nacional—DL 55/2018 [Internet]. Lisbon: Direção-Geral da Educação; 2020 Oct 20. Available from: https://www.dge.mec.pt/curriculo-nacional-dl-552018

15. Ministério da Educação. Educação e formação em Portugal. [Education and training in Portugal] [Internet]. Lisbon: Ministério da Educação; 2007 Sep. Available from: https://www.dgeec.mec.pt/np4/%7B$clientServletPath%7D/?newsId=147&fileName=educacao_formacao_portugal.pdf

16. Conselho Nacional de Educação (CNE). Estado da educação 2018: Edição 2019. [State of education 2018: 2019 edition] [Internet]. Lisbon: Conselho Nacional da Educação; 2019. Available from: https://www.cnedu.pt/content/edicoes/estado_da_educacao/Estado_da_Educacao2018_web_26nov2019.pdf

17. Pordata. População residente com 15 e mais anos: total e por nível de escolaridade completo mais elevado. [Resident population aged 15 and older: total and by highest completed level of education] [Internet]. 2020 Jun 2. Available from: https://www.pordata.pt/Portugal/Popula%c3%a7%c3%a3o+residente+com+15+e+mais+anos+total+e+por+n%c3%advel+de+escolaridade+completo+mais+elevado-2101

18. Pordata. Taxa de abandono precoce de educação e formação: total e por sexo. [Rate of early dropout from education and training: total and by sex] [Internet]. 2020 Feb 6. Available from: https://www.pordata.pt/Portugal/Taxa+de+abandono+precoce+de+educa%C3%A7%C3%A3o+e+forma%C3%A7%C3%A3o+total+e+por+sexo-433

19. Direção Geral de Estatísticas da Educação e Ciência. Percursos no ensino superior: situação após 4 anos dos alunos inscritos em licenciaturas de três anos. [Higher education pathways: situation after 4 years of students enrolled in three-year degrees] [Internet]. 2018 Mar. Available from: https://www.dgeec.mec.pt/np4/%7B$clientServletPath%7D/?newsId=902&fileName=DGEEC_SituacaoApos4AnosLicenciaturas.pdf

20. Pordata. População residente analfabeta com 10 e mais anos segundo os Censos: total e por sexo. [Illiterate resident population aged 10 and over according to the censuses: total and by sex] [Internet]. 2015 Jun 26. Available from: https://www.pordata.pt/Portugal/Popula%c3%a7%c3%a3o+residente+analfabeta+com+10+e+mais+anos+segundo+os+Censos+total+e+por+sexo-2516

21. Dores AR, Geraldo A, Carvalho IP, Barbosa F. The use of new digital information and communication technologies in psychological counseling during the COVID-19 pandemic. Int J Environ Res Public Health [Internet]. 2020;17:7663. Available from: https://doi.org/10.3390/ijerph17207663

22. Geraldo A, Dores AR, Coelho B, Ramião E, Castro-Caldas A, Barbosa A. Efficacy of ICT-Based neurocognitive rehabilitation programs for Acquired Brain Injury: a systematic review on its assessment methods. Eur Psychol [Internet]. 2018;23:250–64. Available from: https://doi.org/10.1027/1016-9040/a000319

23. European Parliament. The policy on gender equality in Portugal [Internet]. 2021 May 7. Available from: http://cite.gov.pt/asstscite/downloads/publics/BA3113937ENC.pdf

24. Centro de Estudos e Sondagens de Opinião, Centro de Estudos de Religião e Culturas. Identidades religiosas em Portugal: Representações, valores e práticas. [Religious identities in Portugal: Representations, values and practices]. Lisbon: Catholic University of Portugal; 2012.

25. Diário da República Eletrónico (DRE). Decreto-Lei n. 413/72 de 27 de setembro. [Decree-Law no. 413/72 of September 17] [Internet]. 1971 [cited 2020 Oct 26]. Available from: https://dre.pt/pesquisa/-/search/632738/details/maximized

26. Sousa, P. O sistema de saúde em Portugal: realizações e desafios. [The health system in Portugal: accomplishments and challenges]. Acta Paul Enferm. 2009;22:884–94.

27. Diário da República Eletrónico (DRE). Lei n. 56/79 de 15 de setembro: Serviço Nacional de Saúde. [Law no. 56/79 of September 15: National Health Service] [Internet]. 1979 [cited 2020 Oct 26]. Available from: https://dre.pt/pesquisa/-/search/369864/details/normal?p_p_auth=JqNc3epD

28. Serviço Nacional de Saúde (SNS). Serviço Nacional de Saúde [Internet]. 2020 [cited 2020 Oct 19]. Available from: https://www.sns.gov.pt/sns/servico-nacional-de-saude/

29. Diário da República Eletrónico (DRE). Decreto-lei n. 241/94 de 22 de setembro. [Decree-law nr. 241/94 of September 22] [Internet]. 1994 [cited May 7]. Available from: https://dre.pt/pesquisa/-/search/604441/details/maximized

30. Kamalakannan SK, Gudlavalleti AS, Gudlavalleti VS, Goenka S, Kuper H. Challenges in understanding the epidemiology of acquired brain injury in India. Ann Indian Acad Neurol [Internet]. 2015;18:66–70. Available from: https://doi.org/10.4103/0972-2327.151047

31. Peeters W, van den Brande R, Polinder S, Brazinova A, Steyerberg E, Lingsma H, et al. Epidemiology of traumatic brain injury in Europe. Acta Neurochir [Internet]. 2015;157:1683–96. Available from: https://doi.org/10.1007/s00701-015-2512-7

32. Instituto Nacional de Estatística (INE). Estatísticas da saúde 2018: edição 2020. [Health statistics 2018: 2020 edition] [Internet]. INE, I.P.: Lisbon; 2020 Oct. Available from: https://www.ine.pt/xportal/xmain?xpid=INE&xpgid=ine_publicacoes&PUBLICACOESpub_boui=257793024&PUBLICACOESmodo=2

33. Ministério da Saúde. Retrato da saúde, Portugal. [Health portrait, Portugal] [Internet]. Lisbon: Ministério da Saúde; 2018 [cited 2020 Oct 19]. Available from: https://www.sns.gov.pt/wp-content/uploads/2018/04/RETRATO-DA-SAUDE_2018_compressed.pdf

34. Cunha B, Costa D, Mota J. Estudo epidemiológico de incidência e mortalidade por traumatismo crânio-encefálico na população portuguesa. [Epidemiological study of the incidence and mortality by traumatic brain injury in Portuguese population] [Internet]. Universidade Católica Portuguesa: Faculdade de Engenharia, Epidemiologia e Saúde Pública. Available from: http://www.novamente.pt/wp-content/uploads/2013/04/Relat%C3%B3rio-ESP.pdf

35. Oliveira E, Lavrador JP, Santos MM, Lobo Antunes J. Traumatic Brain Injury: integrated Approach. Acta Med Port. 2012;25:179–92.

36. Santos ME, Agrela N. Traumatic brain injury in Portugal: progress in incidence and mortality. Brain Inj [Internet]. 2019;33:1552–55. Available from: https://doi.org/10.1080/02699052.2019.1658227

37. CUF. Cancro no cérebro em números. [Brain cancer in numbers] [Internet]. 2020 [cited 2020 Oct 26]. Available from: https://www.cuf.pt/saude-a-z/cancro-do-cerebro

38. CRPG—Centro de Reabilitação Profissional de Gaia & ISCTE—Instituto Superior de Ciências do Trabalho e da Empresa. Mais qualidade de vida para as pessoas com deficiências e incapacidades: Uma estratégia para Portugal. [More quality of life to people with disabilities] [Internet]. Vila Nova de Gaia: CRPG—Centro de Reabilitação Profissional de Gaia; 2007. Available from: https://www.researchgate.net/publication/299393938_Mais_Qualidade_de_Vida_para_as_Pessoas_com_Deficiencias_e_Incapacidades_-_Uma_Estrategia_para_Portugal

39. World Health Organization (WHO). International classification of impairments, disabilities, and handicaps: a manual of classification relating to the consequences of disease, published in accordance with resolution WHA29.35 of the Twenty-ninth World Health Assembly [Internet]. 1976 May. Available from: https://apps.who.int/iris/handle/10665/41003

40. European Union (EU). 86/379/EEC: Council recommendation of 24 July 1986 on the employment of disabled people in the Community [Internet]. [cited 2020 Oct 27]. Available from: https://eur-lex.europa.eu/legal-content/EN/TXT/?uri=CELEX%3A31986H0379

41. Diário da República Eletrónico (DRE). Lei n.° 9/89 de 2 de maio: Lei de bases da prevenção e da reabilitação e integração das pessoas com deficiência. [Law no. 9/89 of May 2—First Basic Law for the Prevention, Rehabilitation, and Integration of People with Disabilities] [Internet]. 1989 [cited 2020 Oct 27]. Available from: https://dre.pt/web/guest/pesquisa/-/search/611899/details/normal?print_preview=print-preview&perPage=50&q=desporto

42. Diário da República Eletrónico (DRE). Lei n.° 38/2004 de 18 de agosto. [Law no. 38/2004 of August 18] [Internet]. 2004 [cited 2020 Oct 27]. Available from: https://dre.pt/pesquisa/-/search/480708/details/maximized

43. Diário da República Eletrónico (DRE). Resolução do Conselho de Ministros n.° 120/2006 de 21 de setembro: I Plano de ação para a integração das pessoas com deficiências ou incapacidade. [Resolution of the Council of Ministers no. 120/2006 of September 21: I Action Plan for the Integration of People with Disabilities or Incapacity (PAIPD)] [Internet]. 2006 [cited 2020 Oct 27]. Available from: https://dre.pt/web/guest/pesquisa/-/search/541782/details/maximized?print_preview=print-preview

44. Diário da República Eletrónico (DRE). Lei n.° 108/2015 de 17 de junho. [Law no. 108/2015 of Jun 17] [Internet]. 2015 [cited 2020 Oct 27]. Available from: https://dre.pt/home/-/dre/67507927/details/maximized?p_auth=h0XwCKYv

45. Diário da República Eletrónico (DRE). Resolução do Conselho de Ministros n.° 97/2010 de 14 de dezembro: Estratégia nacional para a deficiência 2011–2013 (ENDEF). [Resolution of the Council of Ministers no. 97/2010, of December 14: National disability strategy 2011–2013 (ENDEF)] [Internet]. 2010 [cited 2020 Oct 27]. Available from: https://dre.pt/pesquisa/-/search/307186/details/maximized

46. Diário da República Eletrónico (DRE). Lei n.° 57/2008 de 04 de setembro: Ordem dos Psicólogos Portugueses. [Law no. 57/2008 of September 04: Portuguese Psychologists Association] [Internet]. 2008 [cited 2020 Oct 27]. Available from: https://dre.pt/pesquisa/-/search/453992/details/maximized

47. Ordem dos Psicólogos Portugueses (OPP). Orientações para as especialidades: Processo de equiparação. [Guidelines for specialties: matching process] [Internet]. Lisbon: Ordem dos Psicólogos Portugueses; 2018 Jan. Available from: https://www.ordemdospsicologos.pt/ficheiros/documentos/orientaa_aoes_especialidades_neuropsicologia_equiparaa_aao.pdf

48. Sociedade Portuguesa de Neuropsicologia (SPNPsy). Sobre. [About] [Internet]. 2020 [cited 2020 Oct 26]. Available from: http://spnpsy.rf.gd/

49. Simões MR, Freitas S, Santana I, Firmino H, Martins C, Nasreddine Z, et al. Montreal Cognitive Assessment (MoCA, Portuguese adaptation). Coimbra: Faculty of Psychology and Education Sciences of University of Coimbra; 2008.

50. Alves L, Simões MR, Martins C. TeLPI: Teste de leitura de palavras irregulares. [TeLPI: Irregular words reading test]. Lisbon: Editora Hogrefe; 2017.

51. Brickenkamp R. D2: Attention test (Portuguese version). Lisbon: CEGOC Lda; 2007.

52. Moreira H, Lima C, Vicente S. Examining executive dysfunction with the Institute of Cognitive Neurology (INECO) Frontal Screening (IFS): normative values from a healthy sample and clinical utility in Alzheimer's Disease. J Alzheimers Dis [Internet]. 2014;42:261–73. Available from: https://doi.org/10.3233/JAD-132348

53. Fernandes S. Stroop: Teste de cores e palavras (adaptação portuguesa). [Stroop: Colour and words test (Portuguese adaptation)]. Lisbon: CEGOC Lda; 2013.

54. Heaton R, Chelune G, Talley J, Kay G, Curtiss G. Wisconsin Card Sorting Test manual (revised and expanded). Odessa: Psychological Assessment Resources; 1993.

55. Cavaco S, Goncalves A, Pinto C, Almeida E, Gomes F, Moreira I, et al. Trail Making Test: regression-based norms for the Portuguese population. Arch Clin Neuropsychol [Internet]. 2013;28:189–98. Available from: https://doi.org/10.1093/arclin/acs115

56. Wechsler D. Wechsler Memory Scale (WMS-II; Portuguese version). Lisbon: CEGOC Lda; 2008.

57. Rey A. Rey's Complex Figure (Portuguese version). Lisbon: CEGOC Lda; 1998.

58. Coutada, SLB, Albuquerque, CP. Análise dos erros numa versão portuguesa do Token Test. Psychologica [Internet]. 2018;61(1):87–105. Available from: https://doi.org/10.14195/1647-8606_61-1_5

59. Pais-Ribeiro J, Silva I, Ferreira T, Martins A, Meneses R, Baltar M. Validation study of a Portuguese version of the Hospital Anxiety and Depression Scale. Psychol Health Med [Internet]. 2007;12:225–35. Available from: https://doi.org/10.1080/13548500500524088

60. Guerreiro S. Avaliação dos impactos de um programa holístico de reabilitação neuropsicológica: medidas de ativação cerebral, funcionamento cognitivo, estabilidade emocional, funcionalidade e qualidade de vida. [Assessment of the impact of a holistic neuropsychological rehabilitation program: Measures of brain activation, cognitive functioning, emotional stability, functionality and quality of life]. PhD [dissertation] [Internet]. Portugal: University of Porto, Faculty of Psychology and Education Sciences; 2014.

61. INE and Pordata (2021). Taxa de abandono precoce de educação e formação: total e por sexo. [Rate of early dropout from education and training: total and by sex] [Internet]. 2021 Apr 30. Available from: https://www.pordata.pt/Portugal/Taxa+de+abandono+precoce+de+educa%C3%A7%C3%A3o+e+forma%C3%A7%C3%A3o+total+e+por+sexo-433

Spain

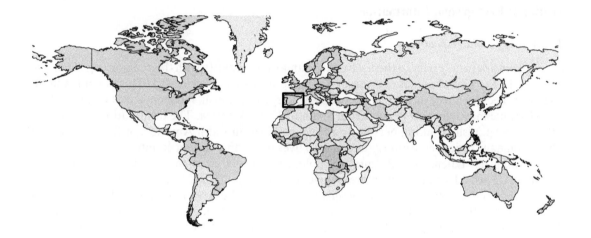

25 Spain, the Land of Diversity

*Laiene Olabarrieta Landa, María Jesús Gómez López,
Isabel González Wongvalle, Diego Rivera, and
Juan Carlos Arango Lasprilla*

Section I: Background Information

Terminology and Perspective

People from Spain may refer to themselves as Spaniards or identify with their region (e.g., Galician, Basque). In the United States, Latinx or Hispanic terms have been used. This is confusing for Spaniards because those terms refer to people who speak Spanish, independent of country of origin. Hispanic may refer to a person from Spain or Latin America. The term Latinx may be used either for a Spanish-speaking person, someone who lives in Latin America, or for an individual whose language is derived from Latin and who lives in Mediterranean countries.

Regarding us, Laiene is a Basque psychologist who works at the Universidad Pública de Navarra (UPNA). Her areas of interest include neuropsychology, brain injury, and bilingualism. Maria Jesus is a Murcian psychologist with a doctoral degree in Clinical Medicine, who is the Director at the Clínica Uner. Diego is a Colombian psychologist who obtained his doctoral degree in psychology in Spain. He is currently working at the UPNA, and his interest lies in methodology and its application to neuropsychology. Isabel, who has lived in the United States for more than 20 years, is a Colombian psychologist who specializes in pediatric neuropsychology. Juan Carlos is a Colombian neuropsychologist who has been living and working as a researcher in Spain since 2002.

Geography

Spain is located on the Iberian Peninsula in southwestern Europe, surrounded by the Cantabrian and Mediterranean seas and the Atlantic Ocean. Peninsular Spain shares borders with France and Andorra to the north and with Portugal to the west. Its territory consists of a large part of the Iberian Peninsula, the Canary and Balearic Islands, and the autonomous cities of Ceuta and Melilla. The country, with Madrid as its capital city, is divided into 17 autonomous communities and 2 autonomous cities, each with unique cultural characteristics.

History

Spain is a compendium of cultures: Iberians, Celts, Tartessians, Carthaginians, Visigoths, Romans, and Arabs have inhabited it, among others. Year 1492 was a key year when Columbus invaded America and the Catholic Monarchs expelled the Arabs from the peninsula. In 1512, Catholic Monarchs conquered the Kingdom of Navarre, unifying all the kingdoms in the peninsula and founding the basis of modern Spain. Therefore, its unitary state identity is fairly recent.

DOI: 10.4324/9781003051862-51

After that, Spain established its empire in regions of America, Asia, Africa, and Europe until the 16th century, which marked the beginning of the progressive decline of Spain's political and economic power.

In 1936, General Franco launched an uprising aimed at overthrowing the country's democratically elected Spanish Republic; this marked the beginning of the Spanish Civil War. In 1937, Nazi planes bombed Guernica as a rehearsal for World War II. It is considered the first air-force attack against civilians, which was repeated again during World War II (e.g., Hiroshima). This inspired Picasso's famous painting, "Guernica." In 1939, Franco won the war and began his dictatorship with political control, banning of political parties, repealing autonomies, and imposing Catholicism. Franco died in 1975, and the transition to democracy began when Adolfo Suárez became president, the Amnesty Law was approved, political parties were legalized, and the first free democratic election took place. The constitution declares Spain as a constitutional monarchy, and from then, several right- and left-wing governments have followed throughout the years. A remarkable milestone was the entry of Spain in the European Union (EU) in 1986.

People

In this culturally complex country, its inhabitants differ per region. For instance, Maria Jesus is from the south, where the people are considered joyful, generous, etc., the prototype of a Spaniard. Laiene, however, is from the north, where the people are considered more reserved and serious. Despite generalizations, both Diego and Juan, who came from Colombia, could notice differences between these regions when they moved to Spain. There are also common features for most Spaniards who tend to be joyful, love sharing with family and friends, and enjoy activities outside the home. Our physical contact often draws foreigners' attention. For example, during her pre-doctoral stay in Toronto, Canada, Laiene shared a house with residents of different countries. Her closest person was her friend from Venezuela. When they got home, they would hug, chat and spend the day together while roommates were silently curious and suspected there was something more than just friendship between them. We needed to clarify that for Spaniards and Latin Americans, physical contact and social relationships are very important and may not necessarily imply love interest. During clinical work, Spaniard neuropsychologists may attend to that need of physical and social contact, especially with children and the elderly. Hugs and kisses, sharing stories, etc., can be a powerful, positive reinforcer that we have found works more effectively than material reinforcements in a testing setting.

Immigration and Relocation

Spain has traditionally been an emigrant country. At the end of the 19th century, there was a migratory flow toward America due to conflict and economic changes. During the Spanish civil war, a forced migration occurred for political and ideological reasons, with most Spaniards relocating to France, Mexico, Argentina or the United States. A third migratory flow occurred during the dictatorship, mainly to Latin America and Europe. The last big migration took place during the 2008–2014 economic crisis. Similar data was never recorded (see Figure 25.1) and was worrisome for many who saw how highly qualified young citizens migrated (and still do) for professional development opportunities. This phenomenon has been called "brain drain" with many psychology colleagues emigrating as they witnessed their research career stall in Spain.

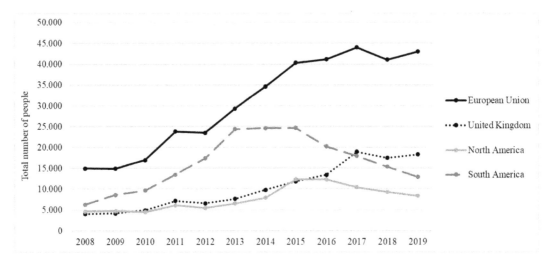

Figure 25.1 Spaniards migration flow abroad (2008–2019 period)

Source: Own compilation with data taken from the INE website: www.ine.es[1]

Acculturation

Culture determines how we express symptomatology, attitudes, and adherence to treatment.[2] Spaniards abroad may miss social relationships and food and time customs (in Spain, lunch and dinner are both very late). Likewise, when they return to Spain, they may suffer "cultural shock" if they find it difficult to readapt to local customs. Maria Jesus met a woman who, after suffering a stroke, decided to return to Spain for rehabilitation. She had gotten married at 23 and emigrated to Holland for work, where she built a family, learned Dutch, and adapted to the country. Upon return to Spain, she no longer liked to be hugged or touched as Spaniards do after becoming acculturated to Dutch values. Emigration circumstances (e.g., age, motives, alone/accompanied, with or without a work/study offer, mastering the language or not) and cultural experience (e.g., discrimination, identity crisis) can all impact outcomes.[3,4]

Language

Spanish is the official language, but co-official languages have recently begun to exist in some autonomous communities (Euskara or Basque, Catalan-Valencian-Balear, Galician, and Aranese). Laiene evaluated a man about 50–60 years old who shared that as a child, he attended a religious school where they recited daily prayers before class. He used to pray in his maternal language, Euskara, but one day the teacher scolded him, saying "Speak Spanish to God; he doesn't understand you in Euskara." In fact, even today, you hear the expression "talk to me in Christian language" if somebody tries to speak in Euskara. At school, it was forbidden to speak in Euskara, and the child who did would receive a finger ring to, in turn, pass on to another child who also spoke in Euskara, thus avoiding punishment.

Therefore, it is important to evaluate the linguistic background and ask in which language the patient prefers to be evaluated. Laiene has encountered three unique situations related to language. First, there are individuals who master Spanish better than their regional language. They have usually been schooled in their regional language but do not use it daily, so they prefer to be evaluated in Spanish. Second, individuals that master their regional language better than Spanish.

For instance, Laiene's grandfather, whose mother tongue was Euskara, communicated worse in Spanish. When dementia was suspected, an evaluation conducted in Spanish did not provide reliable data on his cognitive profile due to his unique linguistic needs. Third, there are individuals who despite having a better command of the regional language, prefer to be evaluated in Spanish. Laiene observed this with Basque speakers older than 45–50 years old who will occasionally indicate their preference for an evaluation in Euskara but, as they start the evaluation, request changing to Spanish (see education section for further discussion). Luckily, today people can be schooled in their regional languages and are encouraged to learn foreign languages such as English. Therefore, Spaniards can easily be trilingual if they speak Spanish, a regional and a foreign language.

Finally, variations of Spanish exist that can make a difference when it comes to expressing emotions/feelings. For instance, "pena" is a Spanish word that in Spain means "sadness" but in Colombia means "shame." Discrepancies exist also within Spain. The Spanish word "fatiga" means "tiredness" in the north, but in the south, it also means "shame." The word "coraje" means "courage," but in the Andalusia region, it also means annoyance/anger. There are also regional words that only residents understand (e.g., **alampar, coscoletas**). We have published guidelines for the administration and scoring of verbal fluency tests by taking into consideration the specific characteristics of the Spanish language.[5]

Communication

Spain is a touristic country where social relationships are essential. Its inhabitants have developed a hospitable character and an open communication style, even with strangers. It is often customary to strike a conversation with strangers as you walk into a place. Silence may feel uncomfortable and avoiding exchanging words may be interpreted as having a lack of education. A direct, fast, loud, and imperative tone of talking, with the use of profanity may be misinterpreted by foreigners as a discussion or anger. However, those profane words may not always a negative connotation. For instance, the word "*hostia*," depending on the context, changes its meaning: "he/she has a bad *hostia*" (he/she is angry), "hostia! How come you're here?" (surprise). Additionally, Spaniards use irony, sarcasm, and jokes that foreigners may find difficult to understand or even misinterpret when paying attention to the content but not the intonation. This can be a problem for patients who have trouble with pragmatics. Maria Jesus remembers a patient who, during rehabilitation, would insist on performing a task in a certain way despite being corrected. The patient lost his patience and addressed the issue using an idiomatic expression: "**pero caes del burro o no?**" (do you fall off the donkey or not?; see Glossary for explanation) and the response was: "soy ingeniero y no tengo burros, vivo en una urbanización" (I'm an engineer and have no donkeys; I live in a community).

On occasion, we use a respectful/formal style of communication ("*usted/ustedes*," formal "you" instead of "*tú/vosotros*," informal "you") with the elderly or certain professionals (e.g., doctors), though this is becoming less common. Visual contact is extremely important; not looking straight in the eye is considered bad education since it is interpreted as a lack of interest in the other person. This is relevant in a healthcare context, where sometimes professionals take notes without engaging in enough visual contact. Therefore, attention must be paid to both verbal and nonverbal communication to fully understand the real meaning.

Education and Literacy

Education is compulsory up to the age of 16 years old. In 2019, most of the population had completed high school level (50.3%) education, with 29.9% completing college. 13% of its population had completed primary education, while 5.3% did not complete it. Lastly, 1.5% were illiterate.[6] Many young people tend to be overqualified and turned down when applying for jobs. This, together with the economic crisis, has contributed to the "brain drain." The rate of young people who neither study nor work (known as *ni-ni*) was higher than in the EU in 2017, and the school dropout rate before completing high school in 2018 was 17.9%, with regional discrepancies (see Figure 25.2). Premature dropout causes are multiple and complex. Here we list some factors to consider during the neuropsychological assessment: low academic motivation/ interest, orientation toward a working life, unstructured families, profession, educational level and employment status of parents, belonging to an ethnic minority or being an immigrant, difficulties with Spanish, educational system unable to attend to the educational needs of students, etc.[7,8]

During Franco's dictatorship, regional languages were prohibited and the vehicular language at school was Spanish. Today, there are different linguistic models in education that differ in the percentage of language exposure. This includes regional and foreign languages, following the EU educational policies.

We previously discussed the cases of those older than 45–50 years old who initially wanted to be evaluated in Euskara but then requested changing to Spanish. This is because despite speaking mostly Euskara on a daily basis and living in a Basque region, many of these individuals

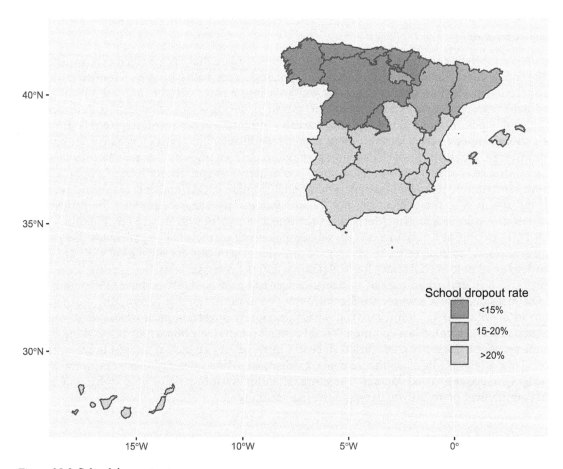

Figure 25.2 School dropout rate

Source: Own compilation with data taken from the INE website: www.ine.es[9]

were taught in Spanish during school, so reading, writing, and arithmetic skills in Euskara tend to be low. In verbal fluency tests, we have noticed some avoid using Basque words that sound like Spanish (e.g., *kartoia-cartón*/cardboard). Since this test is a measure of executive functions, with this intentional behavior, participants spontaneously increase the task's difficulty for themselves and take longer to complete them.[5] Likewise, on verb fluency tasks, some people show trouble identifying and producing verbs in Euskara, despite not showing difficulties in Spanish. Therefore, it is essential to evaluate the influence of education, linguistic competence in various regional languages and Spanish, as well as the interaction between both to adequately interpret results and draw conclusions.

Socio-Economic Status

Socio-economic status affects other areas that, directly or indirectly, influence brain and cognitive development (e.g., healthy nutrition, risk of social exclusion). In 2019, 25.3% of the population was at risk of poverty, and 4.7% suffered severe material deprivation.[10] The Spanish economy is based mainly on the service sector (67.7% in 2018),[11] and the current COVID-19 pandemic has heavily influenced its economy. During the COVID-19 lockdown, between March 14 and June 21, 2020, the non-essential economy came to a standstill. This increased the percentage of homes at risk of poverty/exclusion, and, unfortunately, the Clínica Uner witnessed this impact its patients. A 16-year-old patient who suffers 4 to 6 daily epileptic crises and needs caring for daily functioning lived alone with his mother, who was his main caregiver. The mother, who previously would take advantage of her son's schooling time to work, was laid off, so she had to choose between her child's rehabilitation or eating. They were unable to continue with the treatment and asked for guidelines/exercises they could do at home instead. Finally, it is worth noting that Spaniards tend to become independent later in life, often between the ages of 30 to 40. This is often because the ability to buy a home is prohibitive due to high costs and Spaniards have limited savings capacity due to low salaries and job instability.

Values and Customs

Knowing values and customs enables understanding patients' behaviors and reasons to prioritize some objectives over others. In general, social relationships are extremely important to Spaniards, especially with family and friends. Mealtime is not just to enjoy food but also to share. A traditional custom throughout Spain is to go out to have drinks and bites. The usual expression is "*potear o tapear*." Outdoor group activities are also important: sports, parties, nightlife, etc., and it's customary to value leisure and comfort time more than, say, the job. This could be important in a clinical context because some patients' main objective to recover might be their social life or leisure time rather than aspects that could be more relevant in other cultures (e.g., return to work).

Finally, the notion of time may vary when compared to other cultures. Spaniards are more relaxed and flexible with time and like to take rests (e.g., *siesta*). We may be late for gatherings with family or friends, which can be considered a lack of respect in other cultures. Often, however, we tend to be punctual when it comes to the professional environment or important appointments.

Gender and Sexuality

We conducted a study to evaluate the perception of health workers, including Spanish neuropsychologists, on the sexual activity of their patients with traumatic brain injuries. We discovered that, although most of them (96%) recognized sexuality was fundamental, only 36% approached the subject and 29% would only discuss it if the patient did first.[12,13] Reasons for not approaching the subject included patients not asking about it or not reporting problems and lack of professional training.[13]

Sexuality is an important component of health that must be evaluated. Patients and their partners can be concerned about how their sex life will be affected by a brain injury and how to recover their sexual life. Sexual life has changed, from repression and the perception of sexuality for procreation to its opening and liberation, particularly for women. However, for patients to talk about it, there needs to be a good rapport; otherwise, they will say nothing or, in case they are asked, they may indicate not having any problems due to social desirability.

In the EU, Spain tends to be one of the most accepting of gender diversity and sexual orientation with progressive legislation.[14] Nevertheless, the LGBT collective demands a state law because their rights vary by each community. For instance, the right to change one's name or gender can either require a report from a doctor or clinical psychologist depending on the community. "Conversion therapies" are only expressly prohibited in 4 of the 17 communities in Spain. Therefore, it is essential to know the autonomous community's current legislation to correctly advise the patient and their family about their rights, juridical and rehabilitation services, as well as LGBT associations and institutions. Despite the progress, hate crimes are still being committed based on sexual orientation/identity.

Even though Spain is advancing toward an egalitarian relationship, traditional expressions of femininity/masculinity persist. For instance, many caregivers are women. Expressing emotions/feelings is more difficult for males. Sadly, violence against women exists, and despite increases in complaints, including those for aggression and sexual abuse, only a very small percentage of victims report it. It is already difficult for a healthy woman to complain, but it becomes even more difficult if she has a brain injury. Maria Jesus met a lady that lived with her partner who, after consuming alcohol, physically and psychologically assaulted her. As the suspicion of assault arise, the family was made aware, but they could not do anything because she was not incapacitated and there were no evidence of assault; her decisions had to be respected. In Spain, anyone can call to 016 (attention to victims of abuse due to gender violence) to file a complaint for gender assault; however, despite suspicion of assault, the Justice system will not value the complaint if the victim does not recognize the aggression. Only when someone witnesses the aggression, or conclusive evidence of assault exist (i.e., a bruise), the complaint will be valued by the Justice system, whether or not the victim recognizes the aggression. Therefore, to protect her, work was done toward awareness and decision-making to increase her autonomy and decision-making so that she could report the assault by herself.

Spirituality and Religion

Although no religious belief has state affiliation, the Catholic Church holds economic and educational benefits in Spain. For instance, it is compulsory to offer catholic religion as a school subject, and even taxes can subsidize the Church. Though each family voluntarily decides if they choose religion as a subject for their children. Therefore, it is not surprising that most of the citizens declare themselves Catholics.

In our experience, spirituality may have a great impact on patients and caregivers. Laiene remembers a 50-year-old woman, her husband's caregiver, a gentleman who had recently suffered a severe traumatic brain injury (TBI) and that, additionally, had been suffering from a psychiatric disorder for years. She once shared with Laiene that being a believer helped her overcome adversity. Maria Jesus treated an older woman who suffered a stroke who was a Jehovah's witness follower and loyal to her religion. She believed she was not supposed to follow any medical treatment, so showed no motivation for getting better. Her family tried to convince her to follow the treatment, but she refused until she finally passed away. Therefore, our recommendation, especially for religious individuals, is to value this dimension since spirituality can be an effective coping strategy to help patients and their families make sense of/give a meaning to the event.

Health Status

The public health system in Spain advocates citizens' constitutional right to health protection. It is known for social solidarity and is characterized by universally accessible and deconcentrated (distribution of health services throughout the territory to ensure easy access to the health care system in remote and main cities alike, reducing the concentration of health services in one location), decentralized, and primary care centered. Currently, there is only one health training program based on hospital rotation recognized by the ministry: Psychology Residency Program. This training is focused on clinical psychology, with variable training (depending on the hospital) in neuropsychology. Therefore, there is no public training program for other health fields of psychology, such as neuropsychology. In general, the public health system does not cover neuropsychological evaluations or rehabilitation services. Although, there are autonomous communities where patients may be referred to external centers to receive these services in a subsidized manner (for an established time), as long as the service has been recommended by a doctor specializing in psychiatry, neurology, neurosurgery, or rehabilitation.

The Spanish population is aging due to low birth rates and high life expectancy. For those born in 2015, life expectancy was 80 years for men and 85 for women, while healthy life years were 67 for men and 66 for women, highlighting that Spaniards live around 16 years with some degree of functional limitation.[15] Cardiovascular disease (including stroke) is the most prevalent health condition, followed by cancer.[15] Lung disease, diabetes mellitus, and Alzheimer's disease are also prevalent.[15] Finally, the SARS-CoV-2 pandemic hit Spain very hard, particularly for people over 60 years old, with neurological symptoms that could impact cognitive impairment.[16]

Mental Health Views

Mental health diagnoses often carry stigma, shame, and isolation. Going to a psychologist/psychiatrist can be stigmatized or poorly understood (e.g., if you want to change, you should do it without needing help). Quite often, people go to their primary doctor describing physical symptomatology. When the doctor explains that the cause is psychological, many may resist accepting it and ask for a second opinion. Getting psychological treatment through the public health system can be frustrating since appointments are delayed and treatment time is limited.

Approaches to Neuropsychological Assessment

Neuropsychology was developed in Spain since the 1980s. Most professionals work in hospital environments and their patients (mostly with stroke, TBI, and dementia) are referred by neurologists.[17] Neuropsychology training within undergraduate and postgraduate programs varies considerably. The Official College of Psychologists has a proprietary accreditation in Neuropsychology, which is not recognized by the Ministries of Education and Health. According to Spaniard neuropsychologists, significant problems that impact access to appropriate test instruments are their high cost and lack of normative data.[17] Thus, test selection is often guided by adequate normative data availability (see Appendix for a list of available measures). Due to lack of institutional recognition, the people, and even other professionals, may not fully understand the role of neuropsychologists.

During a neuropsychological assessment, it is advisable to explain the aim of the evaluation. Some people may be comfortable with being questioned about their cognition but be reticent to talk about their emotions. Therefore, it may help to also explain how brain injury can cause direct or indirect sequelae. For instance, family members may understand that apathy may be a brain injury symptom and not a sign of "laziness." It is also recommended to find out how the patient is feeling, how their life has changed, and his/her level of awareness related to their condition. Assessing social support, problems with social relationships, and integration into the community are also important. Additionally, objectives must be established. It is common for Spaniards to pay more attention to physical rehabilitation at the beginning because it enables mobility or because they see physical progress as being faster than cognitive-behavioral-emotional. It is also important to prepare patients (e.g., reminding them to bring glasses), ask them in what language they want to be evaluated, and let them know in advance that there will be tests that require reading and writing.

We also recommend reviewing the report verbally and in written format in front of a trusted person to ensure a proper understanding of the results and the treatment plan. It is recommended to talk to the rehabilitation team members and state who the reference person will be, so they feel confident knowing whom to contact throughout the rehabilitation process.

Section II: Case Study — "The Importance of Family Dynamics in Rehabilitation"

Reason for Referral

RJ was a 57-year-old patient referred to Clinica Uner by his neurologist for a neuropsychological assessment and rehabilitation due to a stroke (ictus) that occurred two months prior to his visit. A neuropsychological evaluation would first need to be conducted and then a rehabilitation program could be developed.

Behavioral Observations

RJ arrived with his wife and eldest son on time for his appointment. He was well-oriented, well-behaved, respectful, excited, and hopeful. Visual problems, such as diplopia, hemianopia, and difficulties calculating distances were observed. Poor balance and hemiplegia were noted. He used a wheelchair for mobility. A good rapport was established since he felt that he had finally found somebody who understood him and was going to help him. During the evaluation, he worked hard and appeared collaborative. RJ presented instances of verbiage and disorganized speech, which complicated the assessment, forcing the evaluator to be more directive. RJ exclaimed that he had never taken so many "exams."

Presenting Concerns

RJ indicated that after his stroke since he could speak, he was expected to recover quickly and without any sequelae. However, after hospital discharge, he began to feel that things were moving too fast and he would easily become overwhelmed by the situation. He realized he needed to have things repeated. He observed that his friends yelled at him, and he couldn't understand why because he could hear them well. Once, while watching a movie, he realized he was crying, and he didn't understand why he couldn't control it. He was surprised because that had never happened before; he grew up with the idea that "men don't cry." A certain degree of anosognosia was detected. Even though he was dependent for all basic and instrumental daily life activities, due to physical and cognitive sequelae, he mentioned he did not know why his family worried about him. There was also concern about his visuospatial functioning, hemianopia, and lack of initiative, egocentrism, and emotional lability.

Daily Functioning

Before the stroke, RJ was a very active man. He used to get up early to go for work until nighttime. His wife would take care of the housework, the kids, and the business paperwork. On Saturdays and Sundays, he would also get up early and go to work but would be back for the family meal. For him, feeling tired was normal because his job demanded great physical effort. After the stroke, his daily functioning changed. This was characterized by an overall lack of initiative and motivation. His wife helped him with his activities of daily living (i.e., bathing, dressing, meal preparation). Similarly, while his family prepared to leave the house, he would wait quietly until he was told it was time to go to rehab. Once in the center, he participated in rehabilitation sessions for three hours each day. At the end, he sat quietly, waiting for his family to pick him up. Upon his arrival home, he would sit and watch TV while his wife did all of the house chores and errands (i.e., cleaning, shopping).

Health History

RJ presented an ischemic stroke of the right middle and posterior cerebral artery, with right cerebral artery dissection (Figure 25.3). He did not report any history of prenatal or congenital health

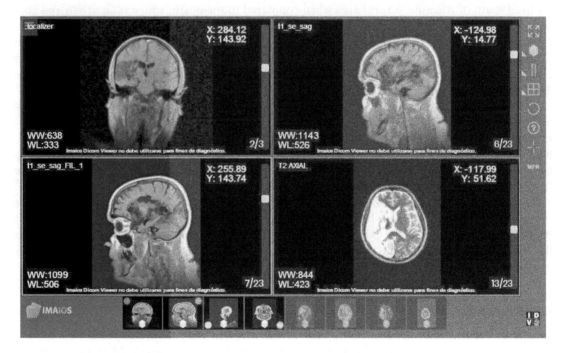

Figure 25.3 Ischemic stroke of the right middle and posterior cerebral artery

problems. He was healthy and did not take any medications. He slept well, had healthy food, and consumed alcohol as a "social drinker." He did not smoke and had never consumed drugs. His father died of a sudden heart attack and no other family pathologies were known. At the time, he was taking Keppra for epileptic seizures and acetylsalicylic acid for coagulation.

Educational History

RJ grew up in the town of Alicante and attended school because his mother forced him to do so. While studying, he helped his father with the family business during vacation time and on weekends. At the age of 14, he finished school and started to work in the family business. He did not continue studying. Following the tradition, he introduced his children to the family business.

Language Proficiency

While young, RJ spoke Spanish at home, but both at school and outside the home he spoke Valencian until the age of 20. In those days, Valencian was the language spoken in inland Alicante, but, as time went by in Alicante, Valencian has been gradually disappearing, while the use of Spanish has been growing. Testing was done in Spanish as he identified Spanish as his preferred language, as well as his primary language for reading and writing.

Cultural History

RJ lived south of Alicante, a rural area when compared to the north, which is an urban and cosmopolitan area. RJ is the eldest of three brothers, born into a humble family in an agricultural region. His birth was received with great joy since his father wanted to keep his last name (in Spain, it is customary for the son/daughter to use their father's last name first) and have his son continue with the family business. Being the eldest son, as a male, he was in charge of the family. The family had no financial issues.

He considered himself to have been a good kid until adolescence, when he started being very naughty with girls, flirting with anyone. At the age of 18, he fell in love with his wife. They got married and she started collaborating with the family business. Shortly after having their first child, his father passed away. He was relieved that he had a son to ensure the continuation of his father's last name. They followed the traditional family pattern, whereby RJ then became the head of the family and his wife supported the family goals.

RJ had a basic level of studies, he was not a regular reader and he did not have cultural hobbies (i.e., cinema, theater). However, he had great knowledge related to agriculture. This is important because this knowledge can be extended to other aspects of his life. In agriculture, you need to be flexible and patient since results are only appreciated at harvest time and do not always come out as expected; therefore, he learned to tolerate frustration.

Emotional Functioning

Emotional functioning was assessed through interviews with the patient and family. RJ did not report a history of any emotional disturbance or required any medication. After the stroke, he recognized he felt out of place and cried for no apparent reason. He worried about his family and felt like he was a burden to his family.

Test and Norm Selection

A flexible battery of tests was prepared to evaluate all cognitive functions, with particular attention to right hemisphere functions. All tests were administered in Spanish. Tools adapted with a
Spanish context and appropriate norms are marked with an asterisk (*).

1 Diller-Weinberg Visual Cancellation Test[18]
2 Benton Right-Left Orientation, Judgment of Line Orientation, Facial Recognition Test, and
   Visual Form Discrimination[19]
3 Corsi Block Tapping[20,*]
4 Brown–Peterson Task of Letters and Numbers[21]
5 Rey–Osterrieth complex figure test[22,*]
6 The Five-Point Test[23,*]
7 Wechsler memory scale-III: logic memory, verbal paired associates, faces, and Family
   Pictures subtest[24,*]
8 Poppelreuter-Ghent's overlapping figures test[25]
9 Hooper Visual Organization Test[26]
10 Clock Drawing Test[27,*]
11 Picture Absurdities subtest of the Terman-Merrill Stanford-Revision of the Binet-Simon
   Intelligence Test[28]
12 The Mental State Examination[29,*]
13 Trail Making Test[30,*]
14 Phonological (M/R/P) and Semantic Verbal Fluency Test (Animals)[31,*]
15 Stroop Color and Word Test[32,*]
16 Wisconsin Card Sorting Test[33,*]
17 Behavioral Assessment of the Dysexecutive Syndrome[34]

Test Results and Impressions

The results of the evaluation indicated that the following functions were impaired: information
processing speed, temporal orientation, visual immediate and delayed memory, visuoperceptual,
visuospatial, and visuoconstructive functions due to the hemianopia, as well as vigilance, selective and divided attention. Abstract reasoning and social judgment were slightly impaired, while
executive functions (verbal fluency, planning, seriation, organization) were moderately impaired.
These deficits accounted for his dependence on others for his daily activities. Verbal immediate
and delayed memory, as well as verbal recognition, were normal-borderline. His understanding
and verbal expression were adequate and helped understand why his family tended to minimize
his cognitive sequelae (e.g., disorganization, lack of attention); RJ typically could express an
excuse for his poor daily issues. Person and place orientation, calculation, ideational and ideo-
motor praxis were preserved. Finally, during the evaluation, anosognosia, disinhibition, mental
rigidity/perseverance, disorganized speech, aprosodia, lack of initiative, egocentrism, confabulation, and emotional lability were observed. RJ's neuropsychological profile indicated the right
temporo-parietal junction was affected.

Feedback Session and Follow-Up

A family session was conducted to explain the results and establish the therapeutic objectives for RJ and his family. Also, RJ was derived to an optometrist in order to evaluate his

visual problems. As RJ was a hard-working family man, his rehabilitation goal focused on acquiring autonomy to continue his daily life independently. He began outpatient rehabilitation sessions with a speech therapist, physiotherapist, occupational therapist, and neuropsychologist. He received rehabilitation services for three hours daily, for a total of 18 months. As part of his rehabilitation, professionals gave his family and friends recommendations in order to help him achieve rehabilitation goals. For example:

- Speak slowly and one by one
- During the time he was wheelchair bound, family or friends were encouraged to explain to him where they were going and give him spatial directions (i.e., now we are going to cross the street). This helped reduce his anxiety and sometimes anger due to his feeling of lack of control over the situation.
- Support his hemianopia: e.g., when RJ began to walk, the family was requested to stand on his left of him during walks to force him to turn his head.
- Work on attention: when he was able to walk, family was encouraged to talk to him while walking because otherwise, he would remain silent.
- Given his tendency to perseverate, the family was told to respond as if it was the first time. If not, RJ responded defensively (e.g., do you see how angry you are with me?)
- Encourage autonomy: involve him in decision-making (e.g., shopping, children, business).
- Activities of daily living: follow the instructions given by the physiotherapists, such as when undressing, first start with the healthy side and continue with the affected side. Another example, give him the time he requires to shower, offering the steps but letting him do it himself. Before rehabilitation, the family used to shower him to do it faster.
- Socialization: avoid leaving him alone at home; invite him to return to socializing to prevent isolation and apathy.
- At the end of the day, help him remember how the day was, what events happened and in what order. This helped to temporarily guide events and organize his speech.
- Finally, the family was contacted with the association of relatives of people with acquired brain damage.

During one of the rehabilitation sessions, Maria Jesus was impacted by a comment of RJ, but, given its content, she did not initially believe it. He repeated the same comment the following day but, this time, through the way he was talking about it, the details provided, and the emotions he expressed, Maria Jesus began to wonder if were true. The reported fact was so intimate that Maria Jesus did not know how to verify the information with his wife. In a subsequent rehabilitation session, his wife, despite the fear of being judged and feeling embarrassed, acknowledged that, after receiving bad news, she could not follow the guidelines to help with her husband's rehabilitation. Maria Jesus suspected it may have been related to RJ's "confabulation" comment earlier. The wife said that another woman appeared in one of her visits to her husband in the hospital, and he acknowledged that he had been leading a double life with that woman. Due to his cognitive state, he was not able to maintain his double life in secret. His lack of inhibitory control pushed him to say what he thought without being aware of the emotional damage that could cause to his wife.

This had a significant impact on the family structure. Rehabilitation became more complicated after a deterioration in the wife's emotional state. She struggled with her husband's brain injury, her sense of responsibility for his care (in Spain, the responsibility of care tends to fall on women, even more in rural areas), and her concern about what their neighbors would say about her husband's affair and a possible separation. Moreover, she was now the head and breadwinner for her family. Treatment then needed to shift focus on helping her. Despite her hardships, RJ's wife managed to comply with her responsibilities, including helping her husband in his recovery. Moreover, she was also concerned about what her neighbors would think if she separated her husband, just when he had suffered a brain injury. Members of the family also completed eight additional family intervention sessions, which presented a mixture of strategies from a cognitive-behavioral family therapy, including structural, narrative, and solution-focused family therapy.[35] It is noteworthy that RJ's wife was only able to begin to rebuild her trust and take on the role of a caregiver after she viewed herself as a "widowed" lady who was taking care of a dependent person. That is, to avoid the gossip of the neighbors, in public, she behaved as RJ's wife and caretaker; however, in private, she assumed solely her caregiver role. This overall intervention helped maintain the family's coexistence.

By the end of his rehabilitation, RJ was autonomous for basic activities of daily living. Although sometimes he required supervision, he could stay alone at home while his wife was running errands. He was able to walk and improved his attention, memory, reasoning, temporal orientation, speech organization, as well as distance calculation. In addition, he got into the habit of looking sideways before crossing the street. It was also possible to reduce his egocentricity: he asked about other's emotions, did not centralize conversations toward him, respected turn taking, etc.

Section III: Lessons Learned

- Although Spaniards share many cultural characteristics, neuropsychologists should understand that Spain is a compendium of cultures and although Spanish is the official language, many people speak other languages.
- Spanish is the official language in Spain, but co-official languages exist in their autonomous communities (Euskara, Catalan-Valencian-Balear, Galician, and Aranese). When possible, neuropsychological evaluation should occur in the primary language of the individual, which may not be Spanish. When assessing bilingual people, it is advisable for the neuropsychologist to know both languages.
- Education is compulsory up to the age of 16 years old. In 2019, most of the population had completed high school-level education.
- Even though Spaniards share many similarities (language, religious traditions, etc.) with individuals from Latin-American countries, there are also huge sociocultural differences relevant for neuropsychological evaluation, for instance, linguistic preferences, quality of education, formalities with respect to the health care professional–patient interaction, folkloric beliefs regarding medicine and treatments.
- Spaniards are very family oriented, for this reason, it is very important to include family as part of the rehabilitation process.
- Social life is very important in Spain, and individuals spend much of their time outside of their homes interacting with others in public places. This aspect should be leveraged and highly considered as a key factor for the success of neuropsychological rehabilitation programs in this population.

Acknowledgments

We are grateful for the confidence shown by RJ, his wife, and his children during recovery time. They learned to live with a brain injury and cope with any disagreements along the way with respect, humility, and generosity. We continue to be in contact with this family and share the fight for Brain Damage.

Glossary

Alampar.   That burns, craves something, that goes very fast.

Coscoletas.   Carrying someone on the back.

"Pero caes del burro o no?".   Literally "do you fall off the donkey or not?" It means acknowledge that you have made a mistake that you have stubbornly persevered on.

Ni-ni.   A person who does not work neither study. From the expression "neither studies nor works."

Siesta.   Midday or afternoon nap.

References

1. Flujo de emigración con destino al extranjero por año, país de destino y nacionalidad (española/extranjera) (24303) [Internet]. INE. 2020. [cited 2020 Nov 29]. Available from: https://www.ine.es/jaxiT3/Tabla.htm?t=24303&L=0
2. Niemeier JP, Kaholokula JK, Arango-Lasprilla JC, Utsey SO. The effects of acculturation on neuropsychological rehabilitation of ethnically diverse persons. In: Uomoto JM, editor. Multicultural neurorehabilitation: clinical principles for rehabilitation professionals. New York: Springer Publishing Company; 2015. p. 139.
3. Gasquoine PG. Variables moderating cultural and ethnic differences in neuropsychological assessment: The case of Hispanic Americans. Clin Neuropsychol. 1999;13(3):376–83.
4. Manly JJ, Byrd DA, Touradji P, Stern Y. Acculturation, reading level, and neuropsychological test performance among African American elders. App Neuropsychol. 2004;11(1):37–46.
5. Olabarrieta-Landa L, Landa Torre E, López-Mugartza JC, Bialystok E, Arango-Lasprilla JC. Verbal fluency tests: Developing a new model of administration and scoring for Spanish language. Neurorehabilitation. 2017 Apr 15;41(2):539–65.
6. Población de 16 y más años por nivel de formación alcanzado, sexo y comunidad autónoma. Porcentajes respecto del total de cada comunidad (6369) [Internet]. INE. 2020. [cited 2020 Nov 29]. Available from: https://www.ine.es/jaxiT3/Tabla.htm?t=6369
7. Romero Sánchez E, Hernández Pedreño M. Análisis de las causas endógenas y exógenas del abandono escolar temprano: una investigación cualitativa. Educacion XX1. 2019;22(1): 263–93.
8. Fernández M, Mena L, Riviere J. Fracaso y abandono escolar en España. Barcelona: Obra Social, Fundación la Caixa; 2010.
9. España en cifras [Internet]. 2019 [cited 2020 Nov 29]. Available from: https://www.ine.es/prodyser/espa_cifras/2019/14/
10. Malgesini G. Poverty Watch 2020. Madrid: European Anti-Poverty Network; 2020.
11. España en cifras [Internet]. INE. 2020. Available from https://www.ine.es/ss/Satellite?L=es_ES&c=INEPublicacion_C&cid=1259924856416&p=1254735110672&pagename=ProductosYServicios%2FPYSLayout&param1=PYSDetalleGratuitas
12. Arango-Lasprilla JC, Olabarrieta-Landa L, Ertl MM, Stevens LF, Morlett-Paredes A, Andelic N, et al. Provider perceptions of the assessment and rehabilitation of sexual functioning after traumatic brain injury. Brain Injury. 2017 Jan 1;31(12):1605–11.
13. Arango-Lasprilla J, Olabarrieta-Landa L, Ertl M, Stevens L, Morlett-Paredes A, Andelic N, et al. Survey on international health professional training and attitudes on sexuality after traumatic brain injury. Sex Disabil. 2017 Dec 1;35(4):473–84.
14. Calvo K, Trujillo G. Fighting for love rights: demands and strategies of the LGBT movement in Spain. Sexualities. 2011;14(5):562–80.
15. Ministerio de Sanidad, Consumo y Bienestar Social—Portal Estadístico del SNS—Estadisticas y Estudios—Informes y Recopilaciones [Internet]. 2020. [cited 2020 Nov 29]. Available from: https://www.mscbs.gob.es/estadEstudios/estadisticas/inforRecopilaciones/indicadoresSalud.htm

16. Fotuhi M, Mian A, Meysami S, & Raji CA (2020). Neurobiology of COVID-19. Journal of Alzheimer's disease, 76(1), 3–19.

17. Olabarrieta-Landa L, Caracuel A, Pérez-García M, Panyavin I, Morlett-Paredes A, Arango-Lasprilla JC. The profession of neuropsychology in Spain: results of a national survey. Clin Neuropsychol. 2016;30(8):1335–55.

18. Diller L, Ben-Yishaym Y, Gerstamn LJ, Goodkin R, Gordon W, Weinberg J. Studies of cognition and rehabilitation in hemiplegia. Rehabilitation monograph N° 50. New York (NY): New York University Medical Center; 1974.

19. Benton AL, Abigail B, Sivan AB, Hamsher KD, Varney NR, Spreen O. Contributions to neuropsychological assessment: a clinical manual. New York: Oxford University Press; 1994.

20. Corsi PM. Human memory and the medial temporal region of the brain. Diss Abs Int. 1972:34(02);891B. (University Microfilms No. AAI05-77717).

21. Peterson L, Peterson M. Short-term retention of individual verbal items. J Exp Psychol. 1959;58(3):193–8.

22. Rey A. Test de Copia de una Figura Compleja—Edición Revisada (De la Cruz M. adaptadores). Madrid: TEA Ediciones; 2012.

23. Sedó M. Test de Los Cinco Dígitos. Madrid: TEA Ediciones; 2007.

24. Wechsler D. WMS-III, Escala de Memoria de Weschsler-III.: Manual técnico y de interpretación—Edición Revisada (Pereña J, Seisdedos N, Corral S, Arribas D, Santamaría P, Sueiro M, ediors). Madrid: TEA Ediciones; 2004.

25. Poppelreuter W. Disturbances of lower and higher visual capacities caused by occipital damage(trans. Zhil J, Weiskranz L, de Die psychischen Schädingungeng durch Kopfschuss im Kriege 1914–1916. Leipzig: Voss; 1917). Oxford (UK): Clarendon; 1990.

26. Hooper HE. Hooper visual organization test manual. Los Angeles (CA): Western Psychological Services; 1983.

27. Cacho J, García-García R, Arcaya J, Gay J, Guerrero-Peral AL, Gómez-Sánchez JC, et al. El test del reloj en ancianos sanos. Revista de neurologia. 1996;24:1525–8.

28. Roid GH. Stanford-Binet Intelligence Scales (5th ed.). Itasca (IL): Riverside Publishing Co; 2003.

29. Lobo A, Saz P, Marcos G, GT Z. MMSE: Examen cognoscitivo mini-mental. Madrid: Tea Ediciones; 2002.

30. Reitan RM. Trail Making Test: manual for administration and scoring. Tucson (AZ): Reitan Neuropsychology Laboratory; 1992.

31. Benton A, Hamsher KS. Multilingual aphasia examination. Iowa City (IA): University of Iowa; 1989.

32. Golden CJ. STROOP. Test de Colores y Palabras—Edición Revisada (Ruiz-Fernández B, Luque T & Sánchez-Sánchez F. adaptadores). Madrid: TEA Ediciones; 2020.

33. Heaton RK, Chelune GJ, Talley JL, Kay GG, Curtiss G. Test de clasificación de tarjetas de Wisconsin–Edición Revisada (De la Cruz M., adaptadores). Madrid: TEA Ediciones; 2001.

34. Wilson B, Alderman N, Burgess P, et al. Behavioural assessment of the dysexecutive syndrome (BADS). Manual. London: Harcourt Assessment; 1996.

35. Flores Stevens L, Lehan T, Segura Durán MA, Olivera Plaza SL, Arango-Lasprilla JC. Pilot study of a newly developed intervention for families facing serious injury. Topics Spinal Cord Injury Rehabil. 2016 Jan 1;22(1):49–59.

Turkish

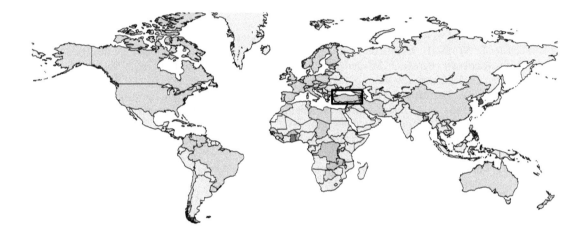

26 Cross-Cultural Neuropsychological Assessment with Turkish Immigrants

T. Rune Nielsen

Section I: Background Information

Terminology and Perspective

People from Turkey are generally referred to as Turkish, Turks or Turkish American/Canadian, etc. However, people from Turkish ethnic minorities may prefer to be referred to in other ways. For instance, people from the Kurdish minority may prefer to be referred to as **Kurdish**, Turkish Kurdish or Turkish Kurd. Throughout the chapter, I will use the term Turkish to refer to people originating from the geographical area of Turkey and will only make ethnic distinctions when relevant.

I am a clinical neuropsychologist who mainly practices in a memory clinic in a public hospital in Denmark. I have worked extensively with the Turkish community in clinical and research studies. However, it is important to notice that I do not have a Turkish background myself but belong to the ethnic Danish majority. Thus, this chapter is based on my experiences working with the Turkish community for several years but will inevitably be from the perspective of an outsider.

Geography

The Republic of Turkey has a population of approximately 82 million people. It is a transcontinental country located mainly on the Anatolian peninsula in Western Asia, with a smaller portion on the Balkan peninsula in Southeastern Europe. It is bound by the Black Sea, the Mediterranean Sea, and the Aegean Sea. Turkey shares borders with Greece, Bulgaria, Georgia, Armenia, the Azerbaijani exclave of Nakhchivan, Iran, Iraq, and Syria.

History

The Anatolian peninsula, comprising most of modern Turkey, is one of the oldest permanently settled regions in the world. At various points in its history, the region has been inhabited by diverse civilizations including the Assyrians, Greeks, and Armenians. The foundation of Turkey began in the 11th century when the **Sunni** Muslim Seljuk Turks began migrating to the area. The region was part of the Ottoman Empire from the late 13th century onward. Following World War I and the Turkish War of Independence against occupying powers, the monarchy was abolished and on October 29, 1923, the Republic of Turkey was established with Mustafa Kemal Atatürk as its first president.

Since 1984, there has been active **Kurdish–Turkish conflict** between the Turkish state and Kurdish separatists, primarily in the southeast of the country. Various Kurdish groups, with the

DOI: 10.4324/9781003051862-53

most known being the **Kurdistan Workers' Party (PKK)**, demand separation from Turkey to create an independent Kurdistan or to have autonomy and greater political and cultural rights for Kurds in Turkey.

People

People from Turkey may have very different cultural experiences and worldviews depending on their ethnicity, spoken language(s), geographic location, educational experiences, religion, economic background, values, and customs. One should never make premature assumptions about cultural experiences or worldviews based on the country of origin. For instance, the experiences of a patient from a Turkish ethnic or religious minority may differ greatly from those of a patient from the Turkish majority. Similarly, a Turkish academic in Istanbul may share more worldviews with an academic in a large city in Western countries than with an unskilled worker from a small Turkish village. For descendants of Turkish immigrants who have grown up in a Western country, the picture is even more diverse as they have their unique mixture of intergenerational worldviews. It is important to not make assumptions based on ethnic or cultural background as there are as many different cultural experiences or worldviews as there are people. It is important to remember that all patients, irrespective of cultural background, bring their unique history and experiences that should be considered during clinical history taking.

Immigration and Relocation

Common reasons for Turkish people to leave Turkey include economic opportunity and family reunification. Significant Turkish populations are found in several countries throughout the world. These populations are constituted of both descendent of Turkish people who settled during the reign of the Ottoman Empire and more recent immigrants. In the United States, modern immigration from Turkey began with smaller numbers of Turkish professionals with Western social values arriving during the 1950s and 1960s. But it was not until after the 1970s that significant numbers of Turkish immigrants (approximately 200,000 people), representing the complex social mosaic of Turkish society, relocated to the United States. However, most Turkish migrants have relocated to Western Europe. Turkish people constitute the largest foreign-born population in Western Europe (approximately 5.5 million people, not counting descendants of Turkish immigrants). Due to significant waves of Turkish migration to Western Europe, Turkish people form the largest ethnic minority community in Denmark, Germany, and the Netherlands and the second-largest minority group in Austria. Other Western European countries also have sizeable Turkish communities.

Modern immigration of Turkish people to Western Europe began with **Turkish Cypriots** migrating to the United Kingdom in the early 1920s after the British Empire annexed Cyprus. Migration significantly increased during the 1940s and 1950s due to ethnic disputes between Turkish and Greek Cypriots. During the 1960s, migration from Turkey to Western Europe increased significantly, primarily due to large-scale Turkish labor migration. Large numbers of so-called guest workers arrived under bilateral Labour Recruitment Agreements between Turkey and several Western European countries. These agreements allowed the recruitment of migrant workers to work in the industrial sector in jobs that required few qualifications. The migrant workers were primarily young unskilled men from semiliterate agricultural backgrounds who left Turkey with a dream to save up enough money to be able to return home and start a small business. By the early 1970s, most of the Turkish migration to Western Europe happened through family reunification programs as many of the migrant workers had settled permanently and were now joined by their families. Starting in the 1980s, politically active and often better educated, socialist Turks and Kurds began seeking asylum in Western Europe and particularly during the 1990s with many Turkish Kurdish asylum seekers coming to Western Europe due to displacement and the violence in the southeast of Turkey. Although there are no official estimates, the number of illegal immigrants in Denmark is generally considered to be very small.

In my experience, paying close attention to the migration history early in the history taking is not only important for gaining information about any pre-migration trauma, changes in socio-economic status after migration and other acculturation experiences, but also for establishing rapport. For most people, the decision to relocate to a different country and culture is an important and life-changing event that many, but not all, feel comfortable talking about. In my experience, a polite and genuine interest in this aspect of their lives as well as being able to ask the "right questions" based on the little knowledge I have about Turkish geography and Turkish immigration to Western Europe has helped me make patients feel more at ease in an unfamiliar situation. However, it may be important to be sensitive to the immigration status of the patient. For instance, asylum seekers may be reluctant to disclose their migration history due to uncertainty or fear that this may affect their asylum claim. Descendants of immigrants from Turkey may not have immigration experiences themselves but may still be affected by their parents' or grandparents' migration and acculturation experiences. This may affect both emotional well-being and test-taking approaches in an assessment. This is especially true for first-degree descendants who may have been raised by parents with little or no formal schooling or knowledge of the majority language.

Languages

Establishing language proficiency and bilingual/multilingual status is important to ensure good communication and valid evaluation of cognitive abilities. The official language in Turkey is **Turkish**, which is the first language of approximately 85% of the population. Approximately 12% of the Turkish population has the Kurdish dialect **Kurmanji** as their mother tongue, while several other languages and dialects are the mother tongues of smaller parts of the population. Turkish and Kurmanji languages have different writing systems that are both based on the Latin alphabet. However, irrespective of their mother tongue, most educated Turkish people read and write in Turkish as this is the official language that is taught in Turkish schools. Consequently, many Kurdish people will have Kurmanji or another Kurdish dialect as their mother tongue but will use Turkish for reading and writing and for common communication. Unlike many other alphabetic writing systems, Turkish orthography is characterized by completely predictable mappings between orthography, and phonology which has implications for the presentation of language disorders, their diagnosis, and rehabilitation.[1] Although there may be some overlap between Turkish and Kurdish languages and between Kurdish dialects, knowledge of one language or dialect does not imply competence in another.

Today, schools in Turkey teach Turkish as well as a foreign language. The foreign language taught differs between schools, but English is most common. In some private schools, a second foreign language such as German or French is also an option.

Communication

Understanding of both verbal and non-verbal communication patterns may help establish rapport, accurate history taking, and effective feedback. For Turkish immigrants in Western Europe, lacking abilities in the majority language can pose a challenge for nuances in communication. Age, seniority, and educational achievements tend to be respected. More formal tones, such as Dr. or Mr./Mrs. are often used with authority figures rather than first names, especially by older generations. Professionals such as medical doctors (and neuropsychologists working alongside those medical doctors) tend to be highly respected, which may be important to recognize as clinical diagnoses or recommendations may appear to be accepted without questioning or criticism, despite doubting or disagreeing with them. This may affect adherence to apparently agreed upon medical, therapeutic, or rehabilitation programs. Also, details about gender-specific medical issues or sexual life may not be readily shared with a professional of the opposite gender.

Some non-verbal communication patterns should also be mentioned. For more devout Turkish Muslims, there may be clearly delineated gender boundaries. Physical contact between genders may be avoided with people outside the family. Turkish people may prefer to simply say hello to someone of the opposite gender instead of shaking hands. The best advice is to take your cue from the other person. If their hand is offered, respond with a simple handshake. It is generally considered rude to refuse an offer, especially if you are a guest. However, traditional communications styles and customs may change due to acculturative influences as well as the general globalization of the world, especially among younger and more urban populations.

I remember an episode with an older Turkish woman who I visited for a normative test research study. She was the third person I visited for the study that day and was the third person to offer traditional Turkish tea and sweets. After politely finishing two cups of tea, I declined a third by smiling and saying, "no thanks, if I keep drinking tea, I'll need to run to the toilet all the time." The male bilingual research assistant who interpreted during the visit looked at me somewhat taken aback and said, "I am not going to say that!" Instead, he politely explained to her in Turkish that "the doctor" did not need any more tea. Afterward, the research assistant explained that remarks about needing to go to the toilet were inappropriate for us to share with an older woman. Also, he taught me that if I did not want any more tea, I should simply leave the cup half full or untouched. Otherwise, a good host would keep bringing more tea.

Education

Quality and quantity of education are important factors to consider when doing neuropsychological assessments of Turkish people. There may be large differences between the quality of education from a small village school and an elite private school in a large city. Also, in the case of older people from rural areas, their educational level (years of education) is not necessarily based on ability but rather accessibility or opportunity. In many rural areas, schools stop after the 5th grade with no options for continued schooling in the area. Many families may not be able to afford to send all their children to school and would only send their boys. The teaching methods were typically based on rote learning rather than the applied emphasis in Western educational systems. This may affect the approach to testing and test-taking style. However, with the modernization of the Turkish educational system, there have been Western influences. In 1997, education reforms in Turkey extended compulsory schooling from 5 to 8 years and there has been a steady increase in the number of people attaining secondary and tertiary or post-secondary education. By 2018, about one-third of Turkey's young adults had attained tertiary education.

Some Turkish migrants have academic degrees or other professional training that is not recognized after immigration. Often these people have had to give up the idea of pursuing a career based on these qualifications in their new country and have instead taken jobs within the service or transport industry or started up small businesses. This may have important implications for their identity and self-esteem, and ultimately their emotional well-being.

Literacy

Whereas illiteracy is uncommon among younger Turkish people, illiteracy is relatively widespread among older generations, especially in rural populations and among women. Thus, the literacy rate among men and women younger than 25 years is higher than 99%, whereas the literacy rate for men and women older than 65 years is approximately 93% and 70%, respectively. Importantly, the reason for illiteracy is generally lack of opportunity rather than lacking intellectual abilities. I clearly remember an older Turkish woman who told me that her parents had not allowed her to go to school as she had to stay at home and take care of her younger siblings, tend to farm animals, and help her parents in the fields. But she was eager to learn and with help from her brothers who attended school, and by reading pieces of old newspapers she picked up in the ditches on her way to the fields, she taught herself to read. Despite having no formal education, in my perspective, she clearly had good intellectual abilities. Although most immigrants who are illiterate function well in their pre-migration context, after migration to a highly literate Western society, lacking literacy can pose a significant barrier for acquiring skills in the new language, obtaining a job, accessing services, and supporting children through their schooling.

Experience from formal schooling and literacy is fundamental for performance on most commonly used neuropsychological tests and cognitive screening instruments. For instance, cognitively intact Turkish immigrants with little or no formal schooling or literacy will often score in the impaired range on the Mini-Mental State Examination (mean performance of approximately 21 points) as they have never obtained the skills required to solve items involving reading, writing, mental calculation and drawing.[2] Generally, educational test bias in unschooled or illiterate people is reduced if assessments are performed with measures with greater ecological relevance.[3-5] See Appendix for a list of tests with greater ecological relevance for people who are illiterate.

Values and Customs

Although the best way of obtaining insights into the norms and values held by individual patients is to ask the patients, some knowledge about commonly held values and norms in Turkish communities may help establish rapport and contribute to culturally sensitive history taking and feedback. Generally, traditional Turkish outlooks build on values of family-centrism, inter-dependence and collectivism, religiosity, respect, and hospitality. Even among modernized urban Turkish people, family loyalty, family obligations, and family honor remain strong considerations. Guests are typically treated with great hospitality, and offerings of traditional drinks, sweets, and food items are common ways to show gratitude and respect.

Respecting your parents or elders is central to Turkish culture, and the family may have a deciding voice in important life decisions, such as the choice of education or marriage partner. Although traditional arranged marriages are becoming less common among urban and younger generations, many Turkish people continue to have marriages planned by parents, with family decisions made cooperatively. The respect for older family members and the weight on cooperative family decisions can also affect decisions about caregiving. I have met several family caregivers of patients with advanced dementia who were unable to make the decision to move the person with dementia to a nursing home, although they hardly coped anymore. This was both out of love and respect for the older family member and due to personal and cultural expectations about caring for older family members. In addition, members of the extended family, sometimes including those living in another country, have opposed the idea of nursing homes. This may be important to have in mind when providing feedback or clinical recommendations.

A focus on inter-dependency and collectivism can translate into taking care of the family and greater good before oneself. Children are generally brought up with a value that individual decisions need to be in harmony with the family and cultural structures. I have observed caregivers and patients who, although acknowledging psychological stress and burden, chose not to follow recommendations for self-help if this meant putting their own needs before those other family members. Descendants of Turkish immigrants or those who immigrated at a very young age may have a different cultural mindset than their parents or grandparents, which may lead to inter-generational conflict. The adoption of more Western individualistic worldviews among younger people can make it hard for the older generations to understand or relate to the lives of their children or grandchildren, which may lead to feelings of cultural isolation and loneliness. This may be important to consider in assessment and recommended treatments of older people as this may affect their emotional well-being.

The great cultural value given to time and speeded performance in individualistic Western societies is less pronounced in traditional Turkish culture. This may affect test-taking approaches and results on timed measures as patients may pay closer attention to precision and detail than performance speed. Although patients with experience from formal schooling and numerous academic tests and exams will typically instantly know what is expected in the test situation and understand the inherent value of speeded performance in many neuropsychological tests, this may not be the case for older and less test-wise patients. I remember an older female Turkish patient who I instructed to connect the numbered circles in the Color Trails Test as fast as she could, but without making any mistakes. She immaculately completed the task in a little more than three minutes, making sure the lines were neat and straight and hit the center of the intended targets. Afterward, I asked her if she was satisfied with her performance. She took a glance at the paper and said: "Yes. I didn't make any mistakes, did I?"

Gender Roles

Understanding values concerning gender roles in Turkish culture may help avoid assumptions during communication and support treatment plans that align with these values. In traditional Turkish culture, men and women generally constitute largely separate sub-societies, each with its own values, attitudes, and perceptions of the other. In traditional families, gender roles are clearly defined, and each gender more or less reigns within its appropriate realm. The husband/father is considered the head of the household and is generally in charge of matters involving household interactions with the public, whereas the wife/mother is in charge of the house and family.

Even among more modern urban people, family honor often remains a strong consideration and gender roles may constrain social relations. For instance, friendships between men and women who are unrelated are generally not considered acceptable. Although it may be accepted that men and women meet socially or date, parents will often try to monitor such relationships and discourage their daughters from becoming involved with a man unless the marriage is expected. Among more traditional families, dating could ruin the reputation of a young woman and dishonor her family.

Although women have been discouraged to wear *hijab*, or headscarves, in public venues by the authorities in Turkey, the use of headscarves has been common in rural areas and among women holding more traditional or religious views. While many younger Turkish women follow the latest Western fashions in clothes and cosmetics, some have readopted headscarves and modest dresses to demonstrate their commitment to Islam. Yet again, others seem to have found a middle way. I often meet young Turkish women who wear headscarves but dress and wear makeup according to Western fashion. Values concerning gender roles are highly individual and seem to be constantly changing and negotiated due to the influences of mass media, education, and acculturation.

Religion and Religiosity

Attention to religious views and religiosity in Turkish patients may help to understand worldviews and develop recommendations in line with those views. Turkey is officially a secular country with no official religion. However, most of the population is Muslim and public schools currently teach mandatory religion classes focusing mainly on the *Sunni* branch of Islam. Most Muslims in Turkey are Sunni, followed by a considerable minority of **Shia-Alevi** Muslims. Among non-Muslim religions, Christianity and Judaism are the largest but constitute only a small minority of the population.

Religiosity differs greatly among Turkish people, with recent polls[6,7] indicating that about half of the population considers themselves religious, whereas about one-third do not consider themselves religious. Although some Turkish Muslims say the **five daily prayers**, others may only say some of the daily prayers or pray even less. To many Turkish immigrants, going to worship at the Mosque on Fridays is an important aspect of both their religion and social life within the Turkish community.

Most Turkish Muslims celebrate the **Ramadan**, a month of fasting, prayer, reflection, and community, during the ninth month of the Islamic calendar. Fasting from sunrise to sunset is obligatory for all adult Muslims who are not acutely or chronically ill, traveling, elderly, pregnant, breastfeeding, diabetic, or menstruating. As the spiritual rewards of fasting are believed to be multiplied during Ramadan, Muslims often refrain not only from food and drinks but also tobacco, sexual relations, and sinful behavior, devoting themselves instead to prayer, recitation of the Quran, and the performance of charitable deeds. The end of Ramadan is marked by the **Eid al-Fitr** celebration, also called the "Festival of Breaking the Fast."

Being aware of the celebration of Ramadan may be important for the planning of assessments and interventions. If assessments are made during Ramadan, these are best scheduled in the morning as studies have shown cognitive functioning to be affected later in the day after several hours of fasting.[8] Also, as oral medications are not allowed during the hours of fasting, this may affect the management of medications. Conditions that require medications taken several times a day or that are affected by food and drink intake (e.g., diabetes) may require adjustment of the treatment.

Mental Health Views

For many Turkish immigrants, there are barriers to accessing specialist health services in the country of migration, including psychological and neuropsychological services. Language barriers and little acculturation may result in lacking awareness about available services or challenges taking contact to such services. Although it may be common to go to their general physician for physical conditions, seeking help from "outsiders" for mental health issues, including cognitive dysfunction, may be considered shameful both to the affected person and the family. There is still a lot of stigma around mental health issues and cognitive dysfunction in the Turkish community.

While most Turkish people primarily adhere to the dominant Western biomedical model of mental illness that posits that mental disorders are brain diseases caused by chemical imbalances, emotional distress may be expressed in more somatic terms, and there may be alternative coping systems involving support from extended family or friends or seeking advice from a religious leader or Imam. This may be more acceptable than consulting a psychologist or participating in support groups. Mental health issues and cognitive decline is still very much considered a family matter that should not be shared with outsiders. Some may believe that cognitive or emotional issues are being due to the will of God, as a test or as a punishment, or as an opportunity to remedy disconnection from God. However, religious explanations of mental illness are generally not seen to conflict with biological or environmental causes. For Muslims, health is considered a gift from God, which should be cherished. Accordingly, they have an obligation to look after their health by seeking advice and receiving treatment.

Among Turkish immigrants in Western Europe, it may not be uncommon for patients to consult or get a second opinion from a medical specialist in Turkey when on holidays in the country. It may be important to be aware of this, particularly if the diagnostic conclusions and clinical recommendations of these specialists differ from those made in the Western healthcare system or if medical treatments have been initiated.

Acculturation

There is large variation among Turkish people in their psychological and social experiences from immigrating to a Western country. Whereas some have coped well with migratory stress and changes in cultural identity and have quickly acquired culture-specific skills, including skills in the majority language, others have been less successful. Especially among the older generations of working migrants, many have struggled with *separation* and *marginalization* in the new country. I have seen several older Turkish patients with five years of schooling or less from a village school in central Anatolia, who had lived in Denmark for more than 40 years but spoke little Danish, only used Turkish media, and had no social relationships outside the Turkish community. Several of these patients had children with post-graduate educations and careers within the Danish public or private sector.

Acculturation is known to affect performance on several neuropsychological measures.[9–11] Among middle-aged and older Turkish immigrants in Denmark, the most robust effects of acculturation have been identified on measures of processing speed and executive function.[12] Any effects on other measures tend to disappear when controlling for the effects of education.[2,12] However, acculturative stress or unsuccessful acculturation patterns may also affect emotional and social well-being, which may in turn influence cognitive functioning. I have seen several patients referred for evaluation of possible dementia who presented with cognitive complaints that, after thorough history taking and assessments, clearly reflected psychosocial stressors related to acculturation. In my work with older Turkish immigrants, I have often encountered issues of social isolation, loneliness, and feelings of "not belonging." They never truly felt at home in Denmark, but at the same no longer felt at home in Turkey since it had greatly changed since they left the country. At the same time, intra-familial differences in acculturation often lead to changes in traditional family roles and dynamics. I remember a young adult Turkish woman told me that she had found it a little hard to wrap her head around the fact that after she had completed a Bachelor of Science in Public Health, she had become the "family expert" on medical issues. Now members of her extended family would consult her, rather than her father or uncles, on all kinds of medical matters.

Attention to acculturation stressors along the life spectrum may be important for understanding the clinical presentation, influence on diagnostic conclusions, and be directive for clinical recommendations.

Approaches to Neuropsychological Evaluation

In my clinical work, I mainly see Turkish patients in a memory clinic setting in a public hospital. The neuropsychological evaluation consists of a 2- to 3-hour session as part of a comprehensive diagnostic workup. Patients are referred after an initial evaluation by a neurologist and specialist nurse in the clinic. After the neuropsychological evaluation, patients have another appointment with the neurologist, who provides diagnostic feedback based on the results from all available clinical and biomarker investigations, including the neuropsychological evaluation. Access to memory clinic services, including clinical and biomarker assessments, follow-up, and support, are free for all legal Danish residents but require a referral from a medical doctor. This generally applies to all specialist medical services, including neuropsychological evaluations, rehabilitation, and treatments.

When Turkish patients present for neuropsychological evaluation, they are often unsure about the purpose of the assessment and what to expect. Thus, I usually begin the evaluation by explaining the purpose and nature of the assessment process. As many patients are also unfamiliar with or insecure about issues of confidentiality, I will normally also explain this, including the limits of confidentiality. As patients may be particularly concerned about confidentiality among interpreters from the Turkish community, I often stress that confidentiality applies not only to me but also the interpreter.

As I speak neither Turkish nor Kurmanji, I will often need to do evaluations with an interpreter. I always insist on using professional interpreters, even when patients ask for a family member to do the interpretation. This is both out of ethical and professional considerations. First, I am concerned about the quality of interpretations done by family members, who are emotionally involved with the patient, usually not trained as interpreters, may not be familiar with or adhere to interpreting ethics, and may not have a sufficient psychological or medical vocabulary in either language. This may be particularly concerning for the validity of the neuropsychological testing but also for the accuracy of the information obtained through history taking. Second, I would like any accompanying family members to be exactly that—accompanying family members. Rather than focusing on communication and language matters, they should be able to provide emotional support to the patient and contribute with their own perspectives.

When using professional interpreters, I always take time to inquire about their experience with (neuro)psychological testing prior to testing and instruct them to interpret what is being said as precisely as possible, unless I say otherwise. Importantly, most interpreters have little knowledge about cognition or neuropsychological testing, and the way we communicate during formal assessments differs greatly from everyday conversation. I remember an episode with an older male Turkish patient who did a naming test as part of his assessments. When shown a picture of a turtle, he responded "kurbağa," which the interpreter translated as "turtle." As I was familiar with the Turkish words for the pictures after using the test for several years, I knew that this was an atypical response. When I asked the interpreter about this and told him that I believed the correct Turkish word for the turtle was "kaplumbağa," he said: "Ah, he did say frog, but he meant turtle." The interpreter obviously did not know that this discrepancy was important in a neuropsychological assessment and was focused more on conveying the *meaning* than *detail*.

Prior to neuropsychological testing, I always evaluate whether commonly used tests and norms are culturally, linguistically, and educationally appropriate to the patient. As this will often not be the case, I typically do assessments with a battery of cross-cultural tests that may be supplemented with commonly used tests that I evaluate to be relevant to the clinical question and appropriate for the patient.

Section II: Case Study — "I've Heard a Stressful Life Can Give Alzheimer's"

Mr. Kaplan was a 57-year-old Turkish patient referred to neuropsychological evaluation due to concerns about progressing memory impairment. At the initial consultation with a neurologist in the memory clinic, he had abnormal performances on the Mini-Mental State Examination (21/30 points) and Addenbrookes Cognitive Examination (63/100 points) that were administered in Danish as part of the routine diagnostic workup.

Behavioral Observations

Mr. Kaplan came to his neuropsychology appointment alone after taking public transportation from his home. He was conversational in Danish but spoke with a slight accent. Mr. Kaplan was evaluated in Danish and initially appeared somewhat quiet, lethargic, afflicted by pain and with low mood. He expressed that he had not slept well the night before the evaluation due to pain and nervousness about the evaluation. His spontaneous speech was slow and due to sudden bursts of back pain, he would often stop in the middle of a sentence without completing it. On a scale from 0 to 10, he rated his level of pain as 5 to 6, indicating moderate pain. As the conversation progressed and I explained the purpose of the evaluation and the process involved in neuropsychological assessment, he visibly relaxed and became more focused. After explaining that I was not trying to be inquisitive but was trying to understand his experiences to be helpful, he described his life situation and current difficulties in detail. He was generally composed but visibly struggled to hold back tears when talking about certain points in his history. He built good rapport but sometimes struggled to discern personal and professional boundaries. For example, he was interested in knowing my political views and inquired about the quality of my family relations. During neuropsychological testing, he stated he was nervous but visibly relaxed after the first couple of tests. He remained focused throughout the testing session, gave a good effort, and showed no signs of fatigue.

Presenting Concerns

Mr. Kaplan stated that he was afraid he was developing "Alzheimer's." One of his uncles was diagnosed with Alzheimer's disease in Turkey about a year ago and based on the family's descriptions and what he could read on the internet, he found that he had many of the same symptoms. He explained that he forgot everything. He mainly had problems with "short-term memory" and could forget his tasks or appointments, to pay the bills, or to remove pots from the stove. Also, he could forget that he had already taken his pain medication resulting in him taking a double dosage and making him "completely messed up." As he had also heard that a stressful life or stressful life events could cause dementia, he contacted his GP, who referred him to the memory clinic. Mr. Kaplan explained that his present difficulties all began after a car accident about two years ago where he suffered multiple injuries. He was unconscious when rescued from the car but did not recall having any cognitive symptoms immediately after the accident while admitted to the hospital. However, after being released from the hospital, he believed he had problems with memory and concentration influenced by "constant pain." Both pain and cognitive difficulties had been progressing during the last year.

Daily Functioning

In his adult life, Mr. Kaplan had managed several smaller Turkish import/export and grocery businesses with various successes. After the car accident, he had been unable to work, and several job-training programs had been unsuccessful. Consequently, he was now receiving cash benefits (government assistance for people who are out of work, not studying, and unable to support themselves financially) and feared being evicted from his apartment as he struggled to pay the rent. Most days, he would go for short walks around the neighborhood, and when he could afford it, he would go to a **Hamam** (Turkish bath) as the heat from the steam bath and the heated marble stones lessened his pains. Most days, however, he would stay at home in front of the TV, but without registering what was on. He was unable to concentrate on reading, which extended to mailed correspondence from his GP. He had some contact to one of his sisters, but during the last years, he had gradually lost contact to his family and friends as he generally avoided socialization.

Health History

Mr. Kaplan was unaware of any problems with his birth or early development. He had been medically healthy until he was involved in a car accident. An MRI scan had verified a herniated disc in his upper back. He stated that he took prescribed pain medication due to chronic pain in his back, shoulders, and arms. Otherwise, his most recent blood work was unremarkable, and a brain MRI ordered at the neurological consultation in the memory clinic was described as normal. He was a current smoker (approximately 20 cigarettes a day) but had no history of drinking or abusing drugs. Most nights he hardly got any sleep as the pain increased during the night, making it hard for him to lie down. Consequently, he always felt tired and often involuntarily took short naps during the day. An uncle had been diagnosed with Alzheimer's disease, but otherwise, there was no known family history of neurological disorders. A sister had a history of mild depression. As far as he knew, his children were healthy.

Educational History

In Turkey, Mr. Kaplan passed middle school (eighth grade) exams. Afterward, he worked with his father as a street vendor. He described himself as an average student who was eager to learn. He did not struggle with any particular subject and did not find it hard to stay focused in school. Upon arrival to Denmark in 1980, he attended weekly Danish language classes and was quick to pick up the new language, passing both oral and written Danish language exams after two years.

Language Proficiency

Mr. Kaplan was multilingual. His dominant language was Turkish, followed by Kurmanji and Danish. Turkish was the main language spoken at home by his family during his childhood. However, his mother and maternal family would also speak to him and his sisters in Kurmanji. He could read and write in Turkish, which was formally taught throughout his schooling. He described himself as being "almost fluent" in Kurmanji but to be unable to read or write in Kumanji. Mr. Kaplan indicated that his Danish language proficiency was "good" for speaking but "suboptimal" for reading and writing.

Mr. Kaplan's dominant language was judged to be Turkish, but he expressed a preference for testing in Danish without involving an interpreter. Although he was conversantly fluent in Danish, this was not sufficient to match age and education-based expectations of available Danish-based neuropsychological tests. However, I found it acceptable to test him in Danish using appropriate cross-cultural neuropsychological measures and normative data that are well validated and matched to his cultural and linguistic background.

Social/Cultural History

Mr. Kaplan grew up in Ankara, the capital of Turkey. He was the youngest child of a mother from the Kurdish minority and a father from the Turkish majority. His parents lived with Mr. Kaplan and his two older sisters in a one-bedroom apartment in a poor area of the city. His parents had both lost one of their parents at a young age and had to "become adults" at an early age. Although they were both Sunni Muslim, their families never accepted their inter-ethnic relationship or marriage. It was never directly articulated by Mr. Kaplan, but these experiences clearly affected his own upbringing and relation to his parents.

Mr. Kaplan's father worked as a street vendor while his mother did not work outside the home. Although his parents were poor, they were always able to provide for their children's needs through his early childhood. None of his parents had any formal schooling and both were illiterate, but they valued education and sent both him and his sisters to school.

Mr. Kaplan revealed that his father had been involved with the socialist political movement. During his youth, there was increasing political unrest and violence in Ankara, and he revealed that he had witnessed several people being killed and himself had been beaten up quite severely. He also revealed that he and his family had experienced periods of starvation as they were afraid to leave home due to his father's political activity and the dangerous situation in the city.

Eventually, Mr. Kaplan's parents left Turkey and sought asylum for themselves and their children in Denmark. When he came to Denmark at the age of 17, he initially struggled with the language barrier and the many things that were done or viewed differently in the new culture. However, his family lived in an urban area with easy access to public transportation and options for participating in sports and social activities. Some of their neighbors were of Turkish background and reached out to them socially to help the family get established in the new country. Over the years, he became increasingly immersed in the dominant Danish culture, paid less attention to Islamic principles and started dating Danish girls. His parents highly disapproved of this and slowly he distanced himself from his family. He indicated that he never became an integrated part of the Turkish or Kurdish community due to his "mixed ethnicity." He had never felt welcome among neither Turkish nor Kurdish people, felt looked down upon from both sides, and had occasionally been met with hostility.

In his mid-20s, Mr. Kaplan fell in love with a Danish woman, got married and had two children. Due to increasing tension and conflict in their relationship, which he partly related to cultural differences, they decided to get divorced after four years of marriage. A couple of years later, he married another Danish woman. This marriage was characterized by "chaos and turmoil" from the beginning and to his great despair their three children were placed in foster care. As he used all his energy on staying in touch with these children, he slowly lost contact with his two children from his first marriage. After the car accident, he lost an insurance claim regarding monetary compensation for loss of earning capacity, lost his girlfriend at the time, and lost contact to his three children in foster care as he was "unable to live up to the requirements" and "did not have anything to offer."

Emotional Functioning

Mr. Kaplan expressed that chronic pain had a significant impact on his mood. He never felt in a good mood, and if the pain increased, he could become angry or even aggressive. He had previously been on anti-depressive medication but had stopped taking the medication due to unwanted side effects. Although he felt guilty and ashamed about his social situation and about abandoning his children, he believed that his low mood was related to the chronic pain. As this had repeatedly been rejected by health and social care workers who had told him that his present difficulties were unrelated to the car accident, he stated that he had probably become somewhat paranoid and lacked trust in people. In some ways, he felt that he had "given up." He expressed that he did not understand why so many bad things had happened in his life and that he often found himself concluding that it must be "a punishment from God." He had never contemplated suicide as this is strictly forbidden in Islam.

Preliminary Formulation

At the end of the interview, I mainly suspected Mr. Kaplan's cognitive difficulties were secondary to emotional disorder and pain. Although some of his symptoms may also be seen in post-concussion syndromes (concentration and memory complaints, irritability and other personality changes, sleep disturbances, psychological adjustment problems, and depression), this was ruled out as the car accident happened two years prior to the evaluation and his present cognitive complaints concerned symptoms that had only developed during the last year. Even though Mr. Kaplan did not recognize or want to acknowledge it, he seemed to suffer from depression. In addition to medically confirmed issues with pain, Mr. Kaplan's personal and family history, including pre-migration trauma and immigration and acculturation-related stressors, clearly contributed to the clinical picture. Mr. Kaplan had struggled to establish a new cultural identity in Denmark. He had been unable to develop or maintain satisfying social relationships, and his current physical and emotional difficulties had further contributed to social isolation.

Despite these considerations, Mr. Kaplan was referred for evaluation of progressing memory impairment. So, to rule out possible organic brain dysfunction, I proceeded to administer a neuropsychological battery that could assess his cognitive functioning in a culturally sensitive manner.

Test and Norm Selection

Based on Mr. Kaplan's educational background, level of acculturation, and language proficiency in Danish, I chose to administer the European Cross-Cultural Neuropsychological Test Battery (CNTB), supplemented with two commonly used Danish-based tests. The CNTB covers several cognitive domains, can validly be applied across several ethnic groups, languages, and educational groups, including illiterate groups, without the need to change the content.[13,14] Also, the CNTB was developed to be applied with an interpreter and is minimally affected by acculturation.[12] None of the tests in the CNTB require reading skills in any language. Published age and education adjusted multi-cultural norms based on 330 healthy middle-aged and older people, including Turkish and Kurmanji speakers residing in Western Europe, are available. I administered the following tests in Danish:

1 Rowland Universal Dementia Assessment Scale.[15]
2 Recall of Pictures Test.[16]
3 Enhanced Cued Recall using a slightly modified version of the original test, using colored pictures.[13]
4 Semi-Complex Figure.[13]
5 Serial Threes.[17]
6 Serial Sevens.[18]
7 Color Trails Test 1 and 2.[19]
8 Five Digit Test parts 1, 2, and 3.[20]
9 Symbol digit Modalities Test.[21]
10 Simple copying tasks.[22]
11 Clock Drawing Test.[23]
12 Clock Reading Test.[24]
13 Category Fluency Test (Animals, Supermarket Items).[25]

Also, I administered a brief mood questionnaire, the 15-item version of the Geriatric Depression Scale (GDS-15,[26]). As there was no obvious secondary gain and Mr. Kaplan presented focused and gave good effort throughout the testing session, I saw no need to conduct formal performance validity testing.

Test Results and Impressions

In contrast to the abnormal performances on commonly used cognitive screening tests at the initial consultation with a neurologist, Mr. Kaplan generally performed in the average range across all administered neuropsychological tests after adjusting for age and education. He had slightly more errors than expected across executive function measures, but performances were formally within the normal range. His performance on one processing speed measure was slightly slower than expected (SDMT, 23rd percentile), but this was based on age and education-based norms for the Danish majority population and was not consistent with performance on other cross-cultural processing speed measures. On learning and memory tests, he had a somewhat unstructured approach during the initial encoding of new verbal and visual material, but his total learning and recall of previously learned material was within the normal range. Delayed recall and recognition were unremarkable. Overall, his cognitive profile was judged to be intact.

Evaluation of mood indicated moderate depression (GDS-15 score of 12). He reported symptoms of persisting feelings of sadness, emptiness, and hopelessness, loss of interest and pleasure in most of his normal activities, and feelings of worthlessness and guilt. He also reported problems sleeping, tiredness and fatigue, and trouble concentrating and remembering things. These symptoms could make even smaller tasks in the home seem unsurmountable, and often he just wanted to stay at home rather than go out to socialize or do new things. He reported that increasing physical pain could result in angry outbursts, irritability, or frustration, even over small matters.

Overall, I diagnosed Mr. Kaplan with moderate to severe depression with the recognition that chronic pain complicated the picture and most likely contributed to and was affected by the depressive symptoms. I also acknowledged the influence of frightening experiences in his childhood, problems related to his social environment, including acculturation difficulties, social exclusion, and discrimination, problems related to his family circumstances, including disruption of his family by separation and divorce, and problems related to employment, housing and economic circumstances.

Feedback and Follow-Up

Mr. Kaplan received feedback immediately after neuropsychological testing. He was anxious to know if he had "Alzheimer's." I shared my impression that he did not have a dementia disorder based on his neuropsychological test profile and the normal brain MRI scan. I provided education about signs and symptoms of dementia disorder and we discussed his worries about developing Alzheimer's disease. I explained that although chronic stress has been found to increase the risk of Alzheimer's disease, Alzheimer's disease is caused by disease in the brain and only rarely affects people younger than 65 years. I also explained how his cognitive difficulties could be understood from an attentional and motivational perspective rather than one involving a degenerative brain disorder. He seemed relieved but at the same time was anxious to know what was then wrong with him.

I then carefully proceeded to explain the effects of pain, sleep deprivation, and emotional distress on cognitive functioning and mood. When I shared my impressions regarding depression, he acknowledged it and stated that the car accident was the "straw that broke the camel's back." He stressed that if it had not been due to chronic pain, he would have been able to manage his psychosocial stressors and shared that he feared a mental health diagnosis would be stigmatizing and label him as "crazy" or as a "weak man." I expressed understating of his beliefs and struggle with the diagnosis. I then continued to explain the neurobiological basis of depression and the mechanism of action of medical treatments for him to understand depression as a medical condition. I also explained that proper treatment of his emotional problems was likely to have a positive effect on the pain and sleep problems.

We briefly discussed options of seeing a psychiatrist or being referred for psychotherapy, which he blankly rejected. He preferred the option of having medical treatment initiated by a neurologist in the memory clinic. Although he expressed that it had been nice to talk to me about his life situation as he was rarely able to do so without it being stressful and uncomfortable, this preference came as no surprise to me given his understanding of his condition.

He also needed support with pain management. I presented the option of getting a referral to an interdisciplinary pain management clinic and explained that in addition to medical treatment, this clinic could help him manage pain through different physical, behavioral, and psychological techniques. He was happy that I acknowledged the significance of chronic pain and promised to consider this option.

When Mr. Kaplan returned to the memory clinic for follow-up three months later, I could read from his medical file that he had taken the prescribed anti-depressive medication and that the treatment had lifted his mood and improved his sleep which had also alleviated some of his cognitive symptoms. Also, I could read that he had actively inquired about help with pain management and left the consultation with a referral to a nearby pain management clinic.

Section III: Lessons Learned

- Most Turkish people are Muslim, and traditional Turkish outlooks build on values of family-centrism, inter-dependence and collectivism, religiosity, respect, and hospitality. However, people of Turkish ancestry may have very different cultural experiences and worldviews depending on their ethnicity, spoken language(s), geographic location, educational experiences, religion, economic background, values, and customs. You should never make premature assumptions about cultural experiences or worldviews based on country of origin. If in doubt, the best solution is always to ask the patient.
- Most Turkish people speak Turkish as their first language, but a large minority have the Kurdish dialect Kurmanji as their mother tongue, while a smaller minority have another language or dialect as their mother tongue. Irrespective of their mother tongue, most Turkish people read and write in Turkish.
- Some Turkish migrants have academic degrees or other professional training, while others have limited or no formal school experience. Illiteracy is uncommon among younger Turkish people, whereas illiteracy is relatively widespread among older generations, especially in rural populations and among women.
- If language barriers necessitate the use of an interpreter, generally insist on using a professional interpreter—even in situations where the patient asks for a family member to do the interpretation. This is both out of ethical and professional considerations. First, accompanying family members should be exactly that—accompanying family members. They should be able to provide emotional support to the patient and contribute with their own perspectives, rather than focusing on communication and language. Second, the quality and validity of interpretations performed by family members are uncertain as they are emotionally involved with the patient, usually not trained as interpreters, may not be familiar with or adhere to interpreting ethics, and may not have a sufficient psychological or medical vocabulary in either language.
- A polite and genuine interest in the migration history and other cultural aspects of the patient's life as well as being able to ask the "right questions" based even on a little knowledge

about the patient's country of origin and cultural background, may help the patient feel more at ease in an unfamiliar situation and establish rapport.

- When selecting the test battery and normative data, educational background, level of acculturation and language proficiency in the test language should always be considered. If you do not have access to validated tests in the patient's dominant language or representative normative neuropsychological test data for the specific minority group, consider using a battery of cross-cultural tests such as the European CNTB.
- Although the matching of patient and neuropsychologist on language and ethnicity is often preferable when this is possible, in the case of Mr. Kaplan, my position as an "outsider," representing the medical system and ethnic majority in Denmark, probably made it safe for him to share intimate details about his cultural experiences, and cognitive, social and emotional difficulties. He may have been less likely to reveal the same information to a neuropsychologist with Turkish or Turkish Kurdish background or if the evaluation was done with an interpreter as he may not have felt reassured about confidentiality with someone from the Turkish community.

Acknowledgments

I wish to thank Dr. Farzin Irani for her excellent editorial work and invaluable assistance in the various stages of the preparation of this chapter. Also, I wish to thank Dr. Özgül Uisal-Bozkir and Mahsum Ilhan for their insightful comments regarding Turkish and Kurdish culture and language.

Glossary

Eid al-Fitr.   *Eid al-Fitr* is the holiday that marks the end of Ramadan and the beginning of the next lunar month. It is declared after a crescent new moon has been sighted or after completion of 30 days of fasting if no sighting of the moon is possible. Eid celebrates the return to a more natural disposition of eating, drinking, and marital intimacy.

Five daily prayers.   *Salat*, ritual Islamic prayer prescribed five times daily (at dawn, early afternoon, late afternoon, at sunset, and at night), constitute one of the Five Pillars of Islam. The other pillars of Islam are *shahada* (confession of faith), *zakat* (almsgiving), *sawm* (fasting, especially during the month of Ramadan), and *hajj* (the pilgrimage to Mecca).

Hamam.   A Hamam or Turkish bath is the Turkish variant of a steam bath. Traditional hammams contain three chambers: a hot room to steam, a warm room to scrub, and a cooler room to relax. Not all hammams have this exact layout, but they all involve a hot marble steam room with a raised circular platform on which bathers can lie to soak in the sweltering heat. A traditional Turkish bath includes traditional body scrubbing with a handwoven wash cloth known as a kese, a foam wash, and a massage. The Hamam is thought to have beneficial properties for people suffering from localized aches and pains since better blood circulation carries more oxygen to damaged areas and results in reduction in pain and more rapid healing.

Kurdish or Kurds.   Kurds are an ethnic group native to a mountainous region of Western Asia known as Kurdistan, which spans southeastern Turkey, northwestern Iran, northern Iraq, and northern Syria. Also, exclaves of Kurds are found in other parts of Iran and Turkey, and a Kurdish diaspora has developed in Western Europe. The worldwide Kurdish population is estimated to be between 30 and 45 million people.

Kurdish–Turkish conflict.   This conflict is an armed conflict between the Republic of Turkey and various Kurdish insurgent groups, which have demanded separation from Turkey to create an independent Kurdistan or to have autonomy and greater political and cultural rights for Kurds inside the Republic of Turkey. The main rebel group is the Kurdistan Workers' Party

(PKK). Although the Kurdish-Turkish conflict has spread to many regions, most of the conflict has taken place in southeastern Turkey, which corresponds with Northern Kurdistan.

Kurdistan Workers' Party (PKK). A revolutionary group, the PKK (Kurdish: Partiya Karkerên Kurdistan) was founded in 1978 by a group of Kurdish students led by Abdullah Öcalan. The initial reason given by the PKK for this was the oppression of Kurds in Turkey. At this time, the use of the Kurdish language, dress, folklore, and names was banned in Kurdish-inhabited areas. Following a military coup in 1980, the Kurdish language was officially prohibited in public and private life. Many who spoke, published, or sang in Kurdish were arrested and imprisoned. The PKK was formed as part of a growing discontent over the suppression of Turkey's ethnic Kurds in an effort to establish linguistic, cultural, and political rights for Turkey's ethnic Kurdish minority.

Kurmanji. Kurmanji is the most spoken form of the Kurdish language. Kurmanji is also termed Northern Kurdish and is the northern dialect of the Kurdish languages, spoken predominantly in southeast Turkey, northwest and northeast Iran, northern Iraq, northern Syria and neighboring regions. Phonological features in Kurmanji include the distinction between aspirated and unaspirated voiceless stops and the presence of facultative phonemes. Kurmanji is written using the Latin alphabet and consists of 31 letters (the 26 letters of the ISO basic Latin alphabet with ç, ê, î, ş, û added).

Ramadan. Ramadan falls during the ninth month of the Islamic calendar and is observed by Muslims worldwide as a month of fasting (sawm), prayer, reflection, and community. The annual observance of Ramadan is regarded as one of the Five Pillars of Islam and lasts 29–30 days, from one sighting of the crescent moon to the next. Fasting from sunrise to sunset is obligatory for all adult Muslims who are not acutely or chronically ill, traveling, elderly, pregnant, breastfeeding, diabetic, or menstruating. During Ramadan, Muslims refrain not only from food and drinks but also tobacco products, sexual relations, and sinful behavior.

Sunni and Shia-Alevi. After the death of the Islamic prophet Muhammad, a dispute arose about his legitimate successor. The Islamic community was divided into those who adhered to Abu Bakr, named Sunnis, and those who sided with Ali, called Shia. Concurrently, people who sided with Ali were called Alevis, defined as "those who adore Ali and his family." Political tensions between Sunnis and Shias continued with varying intensity throughout Islamic history and have been exacerbated in recent times by ethnic conflicts. Today, Sunni Islam is the largest denomination of Islam, followed by 87%–90% of the world's Muslims. Shia-Alevis are primarily found among ethnic Turks and Kurds in Turkey and constitute the second-largest branch of Islam in Turkey (between 10% and 20% of Turkey's population), with Sunni Islam being the largest.

Turkish. Turkish is the most widely spoken of the Turkic languages. Distinctive characteristics of the Turkish language are vowel harmony and extensive agglutination. The basic word order of Turkish is subject–object–verb. Turkish has no noun classes or grammatical gender. The language makes usage of honorifics and has a strong T–V distinction, which distinguishes varying levels of politeness, social distance, age, courtesy, or familiarity toward the addressee. The plural second-person pronoun and verb forms are used referring to a single person out of respect. Turkish is written using the Latin alphabet and consists of 29 letters (q, x, w omitted and ç, ş, ğ, ı, ö, ü added).

Turkish Cypriot. Turkish Cypriots or Cypriot Turks are ethnic Turks originating from Cyprus. Following the Ottoman conquest of Cyprus in 1571, about 30,000 Turkish settlers were given land once they arrived to the island. The influx of ethnic Turkish settlers to Cyprus continued intermittently until the end of the Ottoman period. Today, Northern Cyprus is home to a significant part of the Turkish Cypriot population, but the majority of Turkish Cypriots live abroad, mainly in Turkey and the United Kingdom.

References

1. Raman I, Weekes BS. Acquired dyslexia in a Turkish-English speaker. Ann Dyslexia. 2005;55(1):79–104.
2. Nielsen TR, Vogel A, Gade A, Waldemar G. Cognitive testing in non-demented Turkish immigrants—comparison of the RUDAS and the MMSE. Scandinavian J Psychol. 2012;53(6):455–60.
3. Kosmidis MH. Challenges in the neuropsychological assessment of illiterate older adults. Lang Cogn Neurosci. 2018;33(3):373–86.
4. Nielsen TR. Effects of illiteracy on the European Cross-Cultural Neuropsychological Test Battery (CNTB). Arch Clin Neuropsychol. 2019;34(5):713–20.
5. Nielsen TR, Waldemar G. Effects of literacy on semantic verbal fluency in an immigrant population. Neuropsychol Dev Cogn B Aging Neuropsychol Cogn. 2016;23(5):578–90.
6. KONDA Research Consultancy. Religion, secularism and the veil in daily life. Istanbul, KONDA Research Consultancy, 2007.
7. Pew Research Center. Religion is very important. Global Attitudes Project; 2015.
8. Tian HH, Aziz AR, Png W, Wahid MF, Yeo D, Constance Png AL. Effects of fasting during Ramadan month on cognitive function in Muslim athletes. Asian J Sports Med. 2011;2(3):145–53.
9. Razani J, Burciaga J, Madore M, Wong J. Effects of acculturation on tests of attention and information processing in an ethnically diverse group. Arch Clin Neuropsychol. 2007;22(3):333–41.
10. Tan YW, Burgess GH. Multidimensional effects of acculturation at the construct or index level of seven broad neuropsychological skills. Cult Brain. 2020;8:27–45.
11. Razani J, Murcia G, Tabares J, Wong J. The effects of culture on WASI test performance in ethnically diverse individuals. Clin Neuropsychol. 2007;21(5):776–88.
12. Al-Jawahiri F, Nielsen TR. Effects of acculturation on the Cross-Cultural Neuropsychological Test Battery (CNTB) in a culturally and linguistically diverse population in Denmark. Arch Clin Neuropsychol. 2021;36(3):381–93.
13. Nielsen TR, Segers K, Vanderaspoilden V, Bekkhus-Wetterberg P, Minthon L, Pissiota A et al. Performance of middle-aged and elderly European minority and majority populations on a Cross-Cultural Neuropsychological Test Battery (CNTB). Clin Neuropsychol. 2018;32(8):1411–30.
14. Nielsen TR, Segers K, Vanderaspoilden V, Beinhoff U, Minthon L, Pissiota A et al. Validation of a European Cross-Cultural Neuropsychological Test Battery (CNTB) for evaluation of dementia. Int J Geriatr Psychiatry. 2019;34(1):144–52.
15. Storey JE, Rowland JT, Basic D, Conforti DA, Dickson HG. The Rowland Universal Dementia Assessment Scale (RUDAS): a multicultural cognitive assessment scale. Int Psychogeriatr. 2004;16(1):13–31.
16. Nielsen TR, Vogel A, Waldemar G. Comparison of performance on three neuropsychological tests in healthy Turkish immigrants and Danish elderly. Int Psychogeriatr. 2012;24(9):1515–21.
17. Ostrosky-Solis F, Ardila A, Rosselli M. NEUROPSI: a brief neuropsychological test battery in Spanish with norms by age and educational level. J Int Neuropsychol Soc. 1999;5(5):413–33.
18. Folstein MF, Folstein SE, McHugh PR. "Mini-mental state." A practical method for grading the cognitive state of patients for the clinician. J Psychiatr Res. 1975;12(3):189–98.
19. D'Elia LF, Satz P, Uchiyama CL, White T. Color Trails Test. Odessa (FL): PAR; 1996.
20. Sedó MA. Five Digits Test: Manual. Madrid (Spain): TEA Ediciones; 2007.
21. Smith A. Symbol Digit Modalities Test. Los Angeles (CA): Western Psychological Services; 1991.
22. Strub RL, Black FW. The mental status in neurology. 2nd ed. Philadelphia (PA): F.A. Davis Company; 1988.
23. Schmidtke K, Olbrich S. The Clock Reading Test: validation of an instrument for the diagnosis of dementia and disorders of visuo-spatial cognition. Int Psychogeriatr. 2007;19(2):307–21.
24. Shulman KI. Clock-drawing: is it the ideal cognitive screening test? Int J Geriatr Psychiatry. 2000;15(6):548–61.
25. Strauss E, Sherman EMS, Spreen O. A compendium of neuropsychological tests. Administration, norms, and commentary. 3rd ed. New York (NY): Oxford University Press; 2006.
26. Yesavage JA, Rose T, Lum O, Huang V, Adey M, Leirer V. Development and validation of a geriatric depression screening scale: a preliminary report. J Psychiatr Res. 1983;17:37–49.

E. Israel

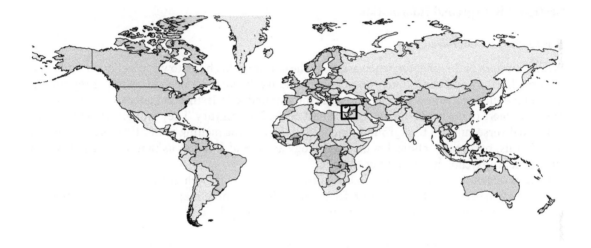

27 Cultural Diversity and Clinical Neuropsychology in Israel

Neuropsychological Rehabilitation within a Cultural, Religious, and Political Melting Pot

Dan Hoofien and Eli Vakil

Section I: Background Information

Perspective and Overview

We, the authors of this chapter, when asked by the editor of this book to write a chapter on Israel's cultural diversity and clinical neuropsychology, did not have to dig deep in search of representations of the subject. Our own nuclear families immigrated to Palestine and later to Israel from two remote corners of the world during the first half of the 20th century. They brought with them their rich and diverse cultural backgrounds and added them to the melting pot of Israel's evolving culture. For us, personally, clinical neuropsychology acted and still acts as that melting pot. Israeli clinical neuropsychology brought us together.

Israel is one of the smallest states in the world, with a long and rich history of cultural diversity, affecting all aspects of life. Here we refer to the following three major aspects of the impact of Israel's cultural diversity on the practice of clinical neuropsychology:

a Cultural and religious diversity and geopolitical tension as integral parts of Israel's social DNA.
b Israel's welfare policy and the ethics of social solidarity.
c The consideration of the above aspects and the strong emphasis on treatment and rehabilitation rather than assessment in the development of clinical neuropsychology in Israel.

We then continue by describing four neuropsychological rehabilitation cases that, in our minds, demonstrate the effects of these characteristics on the practice of clinical neuropsychology in Israel. The first two cases demonstrate how the ethic of social solidarity within the patients' specific communities (A Kibbutz and a governmental security agency) assisted their rehabilitation. The other two cases demonstrate how the involvement of spiritual believes and religion (in the Hasidic and in the Jewish Yemenite communities) were harnessed to enhance the process of treatment.

Geography/Geopolitics

The state of Israel, the declared homeland of the Jewish people, and the holy land for all three monotheistic religions measures 22,100 km², approximately a quarter of the size of the larger New York metropolitan area. Of Israel's 9 million citizens, 75% are Jews, 20% are Arabs, and 5% are of other origins.[1] Located on the eastern shores of the Mediterranean Sea, Israel is surrounded

DOI: 10.4324/9781003051862-55

by Arab countries, many of them still object its legitimate existence. Hence, the area has suffered decades of political tensions, conflicts, terror, and wars.

Geopolitical tension is "the name of the game" in Israel, affecting all aspects of life, including clinical neuropsychology's strong emphasis on the rehabilitation of brain-injured army veterans and civilians. However, political and cultural conflicts are not new to this area.

History

During the long period between 1500 BC and the mid-20th century, the area of Biblical Canaan and later Palestine was conquered by at least 14 empires. Each of these transitions left its cultural fingerprints on the land. Hence, cultural diversity is rooted in Israel's DNA.

During this long history, the Israelites and later the Jews were forcefully deported three times. The last deportation (1st century AD) lasted approximately 2000 years, during which the Jews were integrated in Western and Eastern countries all around the world. Only during the second half of the 19th century, with the establishment of the Zionist movement, and especially in the aftermath of the WWII Holocaust, did Jews start to reinhabit their sacred homeland, bringing with them a diversity of Western and Eastern cultural influences from the diaspora. The current Israeli cultural melting pot is the direct result of the waves of Jewish immigration to Zion (as the region was called prior to official statehood in 1948) and later to the state of Israel until the present day. In 1948, the year of its establishment, the state was inhabited by close to 800,000 citizens. Seventy years later, this number has multiplied to approximately 9.1 million citizens, a growth largely accounted for by Jewish immigration.

People

Among the Jewish population, 43% define themselves as secular, 33% as partly observant, 11% as observant, and 10% as Orthodox, which, among themselves, are divided into approximately a dozen different subgroups.[2] For country of origin, 10% of the Jews emigrated from Asia (mainly from Iraq, Yemen, and Iran); 13% from Africa (mainly from Morocco, Tunisia, Algeria, and Ethiopia); 13% from Russia and the former USSR; and 15% from Europe and America (mainly from the United States, Poland, Romania, and France). The remaining 49% were born in Israel.[3] Among the Arab population, approximately 85% are Muslims, 7.5% are Christians, and 7.5% are Druses. Israel's past and current cultural diversity affects all aspects of life, including the focus and quality of clinical neuropsychology services.

Language and Therapy in a Culturally Diversified Society

For approximately 50% of Israel's population, Hebrew, the formal language of the state of Israel, is not their native language. Various dialects of Arabic, Russian, Amharic, Yiddish, English, and French are commonly used. As will be detailed later in this chapter, this has strongly affected, and not positively, the use of assessment tools in general and of neuropsychological tests in particular.

Israel's clinical neuropsychologists are educated and trained to pay special attention to cultural and ethnic habits, sensitivities, and customs (e.g., a female therapist should not close her office door when treating an Orthodox Jewish patient or shake his hand. Among persons of Ethiopian origin, especially females, eye contact is regarded as impolite. A lack of eye contact is not a sign of anxiety or shyness as it would usually be referred to). In fact, many neuropsychologists specialize in the treatment of individuals from specific cultural communities compatible with their own origins and backgrounds. Non-Hebrew-speaking Arab-Israelis and newcomers from the former

USSR are usually treated by psychologists of the same origin. There are no formal interpretation services for other non-Hebrew-speaking patients.

Socioeconomics

Another important feature of the state of Israel to be considered in the context of this chapter is Israel's welfare policy. Since its establishment, the state has emphasized social solidarity in principle and in its laws. Education is free up to the 12th grade. The average year of education is 13 years, with a little less than 2% of illiteracy; an obligatory progressive social security tax covers various kinds of benefits and compensations, including retirement, disability, rehabilitation, and more.

Within this frame of reference, special consideration is given to the armed forces. Service in the Israel Defense Forces (IDF) for two-and-a-half years, and later in reserve units, is obligatory for men and women aged 18. Since the establishment of its armed forces, the state has declared its utmost responsibility in cases of disability due to service. As part of that, the rehabilitation services of the defense ministry have made tremendous contributions to the development of local clinical and neuropsychological rehabilitation services, strongly emphasizing the development of neuropsychological rehabilitation programs and methods.

Health Status

Excellent public medical services are available for all Israeli citizens for a relatively cheap obligatory medical insurance tax. Both physical and mental health services are delivered by four public health services which are regulated by law in terms of type and extent of eligibility. Long-term neuropsychological rehabilitation services are fully covered by the Social Security or by the Defense Ministry's rehabilitation department.

Neuropsychological Approach

The development of clinical neuropsychology in Israel since the early 1970s has been influenced to a large degree by the three aspects described in the previous sections: the state's prolonged existence under the pressures of geopolitical violence, its existence as a cultural melting pot, and its welfare and social solidarity policies, especially regarding army veterans. In two previous articles,[4,5] we described in detail how these aspects affected Israeli neuropsychology.

Compared with clinical neuropsychologists in other Western countries, Israeli clinical neuropsychologists specialize much more in treatment and rehabilitation than in assessment. Most of the professionals in this field are licensed rehabilitation psychologists (or interns) who specialize in the treatment of patients with pediatric and adult traumatic brain injuries (TBIs) and various other neurological disabilities. Based on a professional survey we conducted in our 2016 papers,[4,5] we reported that only 8% of Israeli clinical neuropsychologists are primarily involved in clinical or forensic assessments. As mentioned above, rehabilitation and disability compensations are fully covered by various state agencies. Thus, compensation claims and neuropsychological assessments as part of them are less needed, relative to what is common in nonwelfare countries. This trend is also manifested in the four cases we present later—they are all rehabilitation case studies rather than assessments. The strong emphasis on neuropsychological treatment and rehabilitation rather than assessment is probably one of the reasons why the development of locally adapted assessment tools has been underdeveloped. Some Intelligence, memory and executive functions assessment batteries have been wholly or partly translated but only a few of them were adequately validated. The relative lack of local norms in Hebrew, Arabic, and other local languages raises questions about their clinical applications. The Appendix includes a short list of the tests that have been translated or psychometrically validated for local use in Hebrew.

Section II: Case Presentations

Note: Possible identifying information and several aspects of history and presentation have been changed to protect patient identity and privacy.

The Case of BR—Communal Social Solidarity and Neuropsychological Rehabilitation in a Kibbutz Community (Therapist EV)

A kibbutz is a type of settlement that is unique to Israel. It is a collective community (the word kibbutz means "gathering"). The residents of the community share everything and work as members of a collective. Kibbutzim were founded in the 1920s on the ideology of combined socialism/communism and Zionism. Currently, approximately 100,000 people live in 270 kibbutzim in Israel (approximately 1.1% of the population). The principles of equality and solidarity are taken extremely seriously, and they are expressed in the principle of "give what you can, take what you need." Only in this context can the rehabilitation process of BR, a kibbutz member, be understood.

BR was born and raised in a kibbutz in the northern part of Israel. BR served as an officer in the IDF and then returned to the kibbutz. Although kibbutz occupations were traditionally based on agriculture, his kibbutz, like many other kibbutzim, branched out into industry. More specifically, the kibbutz built a large plastic factory that produces all kinds of plastic pipes. About a year after returning from the army, BR asked the kibbutz to allow him to study mechanical engineering (and to pay his tuition). The kibbutz approved his application under the condition that when BR graduated as an engineer, he would join the kibbutz's factory. At the age of 28, BR graduated from a very prestigious institute of technology in Israel as a mechanical engineer, and as planned, he started to work at the kibbutz's factory. He did very well in the factory and was consistently promoted, up to the level of a manager in one of the factory's wings. He got married in the kibbutz and has three children, two boys and a girl.

At the age of 52, BR was hospitalized after suffering from a severe cerebrovascular accident (CVA) affecting some parts of his right temporal and parietal lobes. After two weeks in a general hospital, he was transferred to a rehabilitation center where he was hospitalized for approximately three months. During these months, he received primarily physical and occupational therapy. The medical report issued upon his discharge indicated that BR had a weak left arm. From a cognitive perspective, based on previous neuropsychological assessment, there were no language problems, but he had impaired spatial orientation, visual memory, and some attentional difficulties. In terms of his behavior, he was described as impatient and tending toward impulsivity. After approximately a month of medical leave he insisted on going back to his previous job in the factory. His intact language was apparently very misleading regarding his abilities, so he returned to his job. However, very soon, it was apparent that the job was beyond his capabilities, and his performance at the factory was described by one of his colleagues as a disaster.

BR was referred to me at the age of 54, approximately two years after his discharge from the hospital. I met with him on a weekly basis; he came to my clinic in the center of Israel from his kibbutz (almost an hour and a half each direction). He was always escorted by a kibbutz member who drove him in a kibbutz car. At the first visit, he arrived with the kibbutz's financial manager, who assured me that the kibbutz was committed to BR's rehabilitation and that they were willing to do what it took to get him better. It was clear on the one hand that BR lacked awareness of the full consequences of his injury and, on the other hand, that he was still mourning the losses he was experiencing, although he did not always have a clear, understanding as to what they were. Thus, the first sessions were dedicated to addressing these issues, supporting him in the mourning process, and helping him accept what he had lost but at the same time recognize what was preserved.

In the next phase, I felt that we were ready to deal with the issue of his occupation. I asked his permission to visit the kibbutz and the factory and meet with his colleagues which is acceptable among kibbutz members. During the visit, he explained to me exactly what his job involved. In addition, I met with some of his coworkers in an attempt to understand what BR's difficulties were in resuming his job. The conclusions we reached were that his technical skills were well preserved and that he could make good decisions regarding specific professional issues. However, there were more problems at the managerial and interpersonal levels. BR's coworkers described him as being impatient and impulsive and as having difficulties listening to others. He had difficulties prioritizing the tasks at hand. He was not successful at assigning the right people to the right tasks.

Following these sessions, it became clear to BR that if he wanted to succeed, he could not return to his job as a manager. He agreed to work under the supervision of a colleague with whom he felt there was mutual respect. The supervisor/colleague and BR were asked to discuss difficulties encountered with BR and me possible solutions. With time, BR showed gradual adjustment to the new position. The frequency of our meetings was reduced gradually until the meetings ended approximately a year later. Occasionally BR called me to ask for advice, but that too gradually stopped, which indicated to me that BR finally accepted his new situation.

The take-home message is as follows: this case report demonstrated the pivotal role of BR's kibbutz in his rehabilitation process, which was expressed by the declaration of the kibbutz's financial manager in committing that the kibbutz was willing to do whatever it took to help BR get better. This commitment was expressed financially by choosing the therapist they wanted even if it was far from the kibbutz and driving BR to the meetings with the kibbutz's car. Second, it was expressed by their involvement in BR's work placement and their willingness to make the needed adjustments to enable his success, including assignment of a colleague to supervise him. However, above all, the readiness of the kibbutz representatives to collaborate with the therapist enabled the success of the rehabilitation process for BR. Thus, this case presentation exemplified how the value of civil social solidarity was applied to its extreme in the kibbutz community.

The Case of GV—Social Solidarity within the Armed and Security Forces (Therapist EV)

Due to its complicated security situation, Israel has developed several highly specialized security and intelligence agencies in addition to the IDF. Men and women are employed by these organizations in intense life-long careers that form and foster an "institutional family" atmosphere with a very strong emphasis on interorganizational solidarity.

GV was born in Tel Aviv to parents who had immigrated to Israel from one of the Arab countries three years earlier. His native language was Arabic. In high school, he studied Arabic as a second language. He served as an officer in one of the IDF's intelligence units for six years. Upon discharge, he went to school and graduated with a degree in Middle East studies. At the age of 27, he was recruited to one of Israel's intelligence agencies. He was very successful in his job as an interrogator and was rapidly promoted. At the age of 49, he suffered a severe CVA to his left temporal and frontal lobes, including to the Broca area. The major consequence of the stroke was expressive aphasia. The neuropsychological evaluation upon his discharge two months later indicated that GV had above-average intelligence and that his spatial and perceptual skills were well preserved. Expressive aphasia was his most pronounced impairment following his stroke, but it was emphasized that GV's receptive language was intact. In addition, the report indicated mild attentional difficulties, a low frustration threshold and a tendency toward impulsivity.

Despite GV's enthusiasm to return to the intelligence agency, he realized he could not return to his previous position as an interrogator because of his severe language deficit. The agency was committed to its employees and decided not to lay off GV and gave him a paid leave of absence for a year with the hope that GV's condition would improve. During this year, his friends from work visited him on a regular basis, and he also visited his workplace (a classified complex) several times but was also very frustrated with his condition. Speech therapy was the major therapy he received that year in addition to sporadic meetings with the agency's social worker. He refused to receive psychotherapy because he did not feel that he had emotional problems.

Toward the end of the year, the agency's social worker contacted me to consult about rehabilitation options for GV. At first, I was very skeptical about whether I would be able to communicate with a person with such an expressive language deficit. The social worker made it clear that the agency was dedicated to helping GV through his rehabilitation process. The agency was willing to accept him back into the agency in any job that he could perform or helping him find a job outside of the agency if necessary. The agency was also committed to paying for all the necessary expenses, including the therapy. After several meetings, it was clear to me that GV understood well what we discussed, and with the help of his wife, I was able to obtain meaningful responses from GV, which was very encouraging. The most frequent feeling expressed by GV was frustration with the fact that he could not return to his previous position. Thus, the next phase of the therapy was to help him through his mourning phase, i.e., help him accept that he was unable to pick up where he left off because of his injury. It was a very slow and painful process for him to give up a role that had in many ways defined him for the last four decades. My working assumptions were that GV had the potential to be employed, he was very motivated to go out and work, and obtaining employment would be a critical move in his rehabilitation process. The goal in the next step was to try and identify preserved skills that could be utilized in a new, gratifying occupation. I received an indication of GV's preserved skills from his wife's description of him as a talented handyman at home. At that stage, I asked the social worker whether there was a maintenance job in their classified complex that could be suitable for GV. The option to work in maintenance was immediately rejected by the social worker as being inadequate for a person with his status in such a hierarchal organization. I was convinced that GV's only chance to succeed in a new job at the agency was to find a job with workers at his level of clearance, which would reflect the status to which he belonged. The next step was asking the social worker to share with me the various jobs that people with his clearance rank were doing other than interrogations. One of the possible options was for GV to work in the photo laboratory, in which photos and videos were processed and analyzed. GV was very enthusiastic to join the laboratory, as he knew most people there and they knew him. In addition, he felt that his experience in looking for the right information could serve him well in his new job. I recommended appointing a senior colleague to mentor GV. We had a joint meeting with his mentor to discuss potential difficulties that might arise, such as frustration learning new skills at his advanced stage of his career. I continued to meet with GV once a week for a few months, and gradually, we reduced the frequency of the meetings. When necessary, his mentor asked to join the sessions (with GV's approval) to raise and discuss some issues that came up at work and for which he needed guidance on handling. The sessions ended approximately a year later, when GV seemed very satisfied and rewarded by his new job. His wife, who joined us occasionally, reported how his mood and behavior had significantly improved since he went back to work.

The take-home message is as follows: this rehabilitation process would not have been successful without the dedication and support of the agency GV came from. The role of the agency's social worker as the liaison between the agency, GV, and me was critical. She was authorized to choose the therapist and act upon my recommendation. The agency's commitment to GV was evident when it declared that it was willing to reemploy him when he was ready. The agency showed great flexibility and the willingness to adjust the workplace according to GV's needs.

The Case of SK—The Effect of Extreme Hasidic Religious Obedience on Neuropsychological Rehabilitation (Therapist DH)

Hasidic Judaism arose as a spiritual movement during the 18th century in Eastern Europe. Today, most Hasidic groups live in Israel and the United States, and their members account for approximately 140,000 households and are regarded as ultraorthodox Jews. The Hasidim are organized in many "courts," each spiritually led by a "Rebbe" to whom members adhere and bond to gain optimal closeness to God. Hasidic courts differ in religious practices, customs, family and personal habits, and even dress. The affiliation to a specific court is hereditary.

SK was one of my first patients at the neuropsychological rehabilitation day center. The center was a therapeutic-milieu group program for patients with TBI.

SK was a big, heavy man in his mid-30s. He and his family were members of an orthodox Hasidic group. Their spiritual leader lived in the United States and was admired by his followers for being able to foresee the future. His blessings were believed to determine personal fates. SK, his wife, and their five children lived in a small community of his congregation in the northern part of the country. In addition to his orthodox education, SK acquired a license in accounting and served in the Israeli army as a clerk. At the age of 18, he married YK, who maintained their household and took care of their children until late night while SK worked and observed his orthodox practice. Life seemed to flow smoothly except that from time to time, mainly in the springtime, SK suffered from manic attacks. He spent excessive amounts of money and was extremely restless. He was never violent toward his wife, but their relations were never warm.

During the *Yom Kippur War (1973)*, SK was drafted to his reserve unit. A week later, he was involved in a car accident as a passenger. He suffered a mild-moderate TBI confined to the right prefrontal lobe, with no significant motor, language, or intellectual deficiencies. Upon his release from the hospital, he returned home and tried to resume his work but was released due to minor errors he made. Close to that time, he was referred to our clinic to help him regain his professional abilities. He was more restless than usual and had difficulties falling asleep but somehow managed his daily routines and religious practice, although with less enthusiasm.

In spring, chaos ensued (i.e., a vicious comorbid combination of mania and orbitofrontal lobe syndrome). SK became extremely agitated both physically and emotionally. In group sessions, he could not sit down for more than a few minutes and burst into uncontrolled and unrelated attacks of laughter and tears. In group and individual sessions, he repeatedly quoted religious commandments, beliefs, and sayings, supposedly quoting his Hasidic Rebbe. His wife told us that SK had become verbally and physically violent, mainly toward her but also toward his elder children. When confronted during treatment with the worsening of his condition, he developed a negativistic attitude, repeatedly quoting religious commandments that he supposedly obeyed. To my bewilderment when I tried to confront him about his violent behavior toward his wife, he said, "You know that unlike you (secular) guys, we respect our mothers and wives as queens... You'll never be able to understand that ..." For a couple of weeks, we tried to calm him down through relaxation and behavioral techniques and finally through psychiatric treatment, which he refused, claiming that "... it's all in the hands of the Lord ..." We were very close to dismissing him from the program, as his behavior became a serious nuisance for other patients. As a final step, we decided, with his permission, to consult his local Rebbe, who was unaware of the situation and was very eager to cooperate. We invited him to a staff meeting with SK. In came a tall, respectful-looking young man wearing an elegant business suit. In the presence of his Rebbe, SK underwent a complete transformation. He sat quietly and participated seriously in the discussion. At the end of the meeting, the Rebbe faced SK and said, "Listen very carefully ... from now on these good guys are my delegates ... everything they advise you to do is my command, and you know very well that my command is our Rebbe's command ... I need you to take full responsibility for your misdoings, especially at home and here at the program ... I urge you to do so as there is no other way I or our Rebbe will be able to help you."

As expected, SK's frontal lobe syndrome was not resolved solely by persuasion. It took us another couple of months to stabilize SK's behavior and teach him to overcome his impulsive urges to react physically or violently. What made the change occur was his willingness to take responsibility, which left us with the mission to teach him how to do that. From time to time, we kept in touch with the Rebbe, who ultimately helped us integrate SK into a part-time clerical job at one of his community's offices and took care of SK's family.

The take-home messages are as follows: the case of SK demonstrates how consideration of cultural/religious diversity may significantly affect the outcomes of neuropsychological rehabilitation. If we had not involved SK's Rebbe in the rehabilitation process, we never would have been able to manage the vicious combination of premorbid manic tendencies and frontal lobe syndrome that precluded SK's cooperation at the beginning of the treatment. Spiritual leaders have tremendous powers of persuasion that may be harnessed as an integral part of treatment. SK overcame his negativistic attitude not through psychological change, but through religious obedience. These are different mental processes; the result is the same.

The Case of YE—Religious and Cultural Jewish-Yemenite Practices as an Existential \Solution in Neuropsychological Rehabilitation (Therapist DH)

Yemenite Jews are Jews who immigrated to Israel during the early 1950s from Yemen. At the time, they were unique (and many of them still are) in religious and cultural practices, in mentality, in look (complexion), and in dress (Eastern). All of them were originally observant or orthodox but adopted more secular practices once integrated in the then-dominant Ashkenazi culture, which considered them to be culturally inferior. They are considered hard workers and scholars.

At the age of 28, YE was a junior commander in the northern border police corps when his car was hit by a truck on a foggy winter morning as he was on the way to his base. He suffered from a mild left frontotemporal injury, which left him with moderate attention and verbal memory deficits. He tried to resume his commanding position but failed and was ultimately released from the police corps to his deep frustration. At that time, he was referred to our center. In addition to his cognitive impairments, we observed that he was severely depressed and suffering from post-traumatic reactions in the form of restlessness, avoidant behavior, zoophobia (especially of pets and insects), and even mild paranoid ideation. These were accompanied by physical symptoms of irritable bowel and sleep disturbances.

YE is the fourth of six siblings. His parents were born in a small village in Yemen, married there and immigrated to Israel in the late 1940s. The family settled in a small village in the south desert zone of the country. Traditionally, Jewish-Yemen families were patriarchal. With much resentment, YE described his father as rigid, authoritative, and at times even rude. However, his father was apparently very smart, as he managed to develop a very successful agriculture services business, which made them wealthy and enabled all his children except for YE to be employed in the family business. YE described his mother as naïve. From a very young age, YE was designated by his father to be the family's bridge to the Israeli mainstream. He was the only child who was sent to study at the "heder" (room), a Yemenite system of advanced language and tradition studies for toddlers and young children. Indeed, YE had perfect linguistic abilities and deep knowledge of biblical and religious literature. He was the only child who graduated high school and was then drafted to a prestigious police unit where he successfully finished the combat officers' course and served as a commander. YE described himself as a very successful and charismatic commander, admired by his soldiers and highly appreciated by his superiors. His father's aspirations for him were to be realized. YE's postinjury deep depression and posttraumatic reactions could be understood in this context. As the designated and successful "ambassador" of his family to the Israeli mainstream, he developed narcissistic perceptions of himself, which deprived him of the ability to cope with personal hardships and failure. There was no way he could cope with the breakdown of his dream or with his father's and family's disappointment.

The beginning of the treatment was impacted by YE's emotional and psychosomatic reactions. Most of the time, he stayed in his place—a mobile caravan attached to his parents' home—entirely preoccupied by anxieties and pain. He rarely left his room, except to have meals with his family, which he resented. A combination of supportive psychotherapy, psychoeducation, and psychiatric treatment was employed to ease and "normalize" his reactions and inspire hope in his ability to overcome the hardships. Indeed, within a couple of months, his depression and fears eased, replaced by boredom and a sense of worthlessness. We then searched for focuses of personal interest that could potentially fill the current void in his life. YE decided to virtually "go back" to the "heder." With my support and encouragement, he decided to relearn by heart all the prayers and biblical chapters that are read in synagogues during Sabbath ceremonies. According to the Yemenite tradition, there are two versions of these chapters, so he rehearsed both. He also decided to publish the two versions for local use. YE approached the mission with typical scholastic motivation and diligence. He used his excellent preserved executive functions to plan his work through daily missions and progress reports for the months ahead. Rehearsing was organized in a repetitive order (e.g., learn chapter A, rehearse chapter A, learn chapter B, rehearse chapters A and B, and so on). He published the booklets and even managed to sell a couple of them. Within a year from the beginning of treatment, his mood improved, and he overcame most of the posttraumatic anxieties. Having achieved that, the next phase of the treatment focused on work reentry and age-related social involvement. His father pressed hard for YE to join the family business. Knowing his father's personality, YE refused and intended to start a business of his own in the food industry, producing traditional Yemenite food. He took two academic courses in economics but lost interest and decided to approach the mission more practically. YE's personal strengths were his good social relations, charm, and financial wit. I suggested that we employ these assets by examining his ability as a salesman. With the help of our center's vocational counselor, YE started to work as a salesman in an electrical appliances store and succeeded. However, YE was very lonely. He was still feeling socially inferior and like less of a "man" than he felt before. At the same time, he was especially attracted to young female foreign workers from Russia and Eastern Europe who were employed in Israel as caretakers for elderly people. However, the language barrier prevented any attempt to realize his desires. Therefore, YE decided to learn the Russian language by himself. For this purpose, he harnessed the same typical "Jewish-Yemenite" scholastic aptitudes and exceptional linguistic aptitudes that he harnessed for learning the two versions of the Sabbath prayers. Within less than a year, he acquired a good command of the Russian language. He managed to have a couple of relationships in which conversations were held in Russian, but unfortunately, neither of them developed into a serious, long-term relationship. YE is most likely the only Jewish-Yemenite man who has good command of the Russian language.

The take-home message is as follows: the case of YE demonstrates how his deep involvement in his ethnical sub-culture was harnessed to existentially fill the void in his life and induce meaning and control of his fate. Religious practices and interests were adopted, in this case, less for their spiritual influence than for their "organizing" effect. Indeed, we have met many young men and women who in the face of a disastrous brain injury began to practice strict religious commands for the commands' organizing effects on their lives in addition to the commands' spiritual effects.

Section III: Lessons Learned

There are three lessons to be learned from our experience as neuropsychologists in Israel:

- **Cultural diversity and neuropsychological rehabilitation:** Approximately 50% of Israel's Jewish citizens are not native to Israel, originating from more than a dozen different cultures from all parts of the world. Thus, as a clinical neuropsychologist, one can expect that one of every two patients will come from a different origin and culture, not to mention the large community of Arab citizens. Israeli neuropsychologists are educated to be especially attentive to cultural differences. Cultural traditions and religious customs are frequently embraced to improve the effects of treatment.
- **Social solidarity and neuropsychological rehabilitation:** With more than 2000 years of living in the diaspora in small segregated communities, and the horrific effects of the holocaust at their historical background, Israelis put a strong emphasis on social solidarity. As part of it, health and medical services in general and neuropsychological rehabilitation in particular, are fully covered by several state-agencies. In addition, social and professional sub-communities tend to take responsibility of their members in the face of personal disasters, a trend that is frequently harnessed to enhance vocational and social reintegration of our patients.
- **Clinical neuropsychology in a regional conflict zone:** In face of constant regional conflicts, wars, and terror attacks, Israeli clinical neuropsychologists are primarily involved in treatment and rehabilitation of patients with various kinds of brain injuries, less so in forensic and clinical assessment. This is probably the reason for the paucity of locally and culturally adapted assessment tools in Hebrew and especially in Arabic.

References

1. Religion and Self-Definition of Extent of Religiosity Selected Data from the Society in Israel (2018) *Report No. 10*. Central Bureau of Statistics, Israel.
2. Wodziński, M. (2018) Historical atlas of Hasidism. Princeton University Press; Princeton New Jersey. p. 192–6.
3. *Israel Central Bureau of Statistics report No. 71* (2020). Jews, by country of origin and age. Chap. 2.8. Jerusalem, Israel.
4. Vakil, E., Hoofien, D. (2016) The history of clinical neuropsychology in Israel. In: Barr W, Bielauslas LA, editors. The Oxford Handbook of the history of clinical neuropsychology. New-York (NY). Oxford University Press.
5. Vakil, E; Hoofien, D. Clinical Neuropsychology in Israel. International Perspectives on Training and Practice in Clinical Neuropsychology—Special Issue of Clin Neuropsychol. 2016;30(8):1267–77.

F. Latin America and the Caribbean

Overview

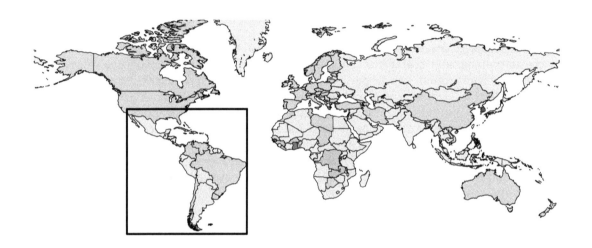

28 Neuropsychology in Latin America and the Caribbean

*Paula Karina Pérez Delgadillo, Daniela Ramos Usuga,
Laiene Olabarrieta Landa, Gloria M. Morel Valdés,
and Juan Carlos Arango Lasprilla*

Introduction

Latin America and the Caribbean (LAC) is a region of the American continent made up of 33 countries in Central America, South America, and the Caribbean. This region stretches about 22,222,000 km[2], from Mexico to Cape Horn in Chile, and includes several Caribbean islands whose inhabitants speak a Romance language (e.g., Spanish, Portuguese, or French). According to the World Bank,[1] the LAC population amounted to 646,430,841 inhabitants in 2019. This chapter aims to capture the most salient demographics and cultural aspects of this region and its inhabitants. Given the inherent diversity of the LAC population and local governments, the history and development of neuropsychology in this region has been heterogeneous, resulting in varying degrees of clinical and research advancement.

About LAC

Migration

LAC has had a linear increase in its population since the 1960s[1] due to the migration flow patterns. On the one hand, international migration has been characteristically bidirectional in the last two centuries with the arrival of Japanese and other Asians in Peru and Brazil at the end of the 19th century, and Mexican and South American migration to the United States and Spain in the 20th and 21st centuries. On the other hand, there has also been an increase in intraregional migration in recent years. Chile is one of the leading destinations for Haitian and Venezuelan migrants and cross-border migration in Mexico, Paraguay, and Colombia yields 80% of immigrants from neighboring countries. Notably, Venezuela's serious economic and social crisis for the last two decades has resulted in almost 5 million Venezuelans leaving their homeland in search of opportunities and better living conditions in countries like Colombia and Chile.[2]

Language

The term *LAC* emerged in the 19th century to identify parts of the American territory whose languages derived from Latin (Spanish, Portuguese, and to a lesser extent, French) as a result of colonization carried out by the Spanish and Portuguese.[3] Understanding the LAC population and its development over time requires a closer look at various aspects that have significantly shaped its culture. One important component of this process is the interaction between language and all aspects of society. This is known as *sociolinguistics* and examines how groups of people have used language and linguistic differences to form identity and establish differentiation.[4]

DOI: 10.4324/9781003051862-57

Spanish is the official language in most LAC countries, followed by Portuguese, spoken by more than 211 million people in Brazil.[5] Although scarcer, English and French are still spoken in many countries (e.g., Guyana), while as many as 420 other indigenous languages (e.g., Quechua, Aymara, Guaraní) are recognized as official languages.[6]

There is the heterogeneity of Spanish in LAC, which reflects the great cultural wealth that defines this region. Original dialects were introduced to the Americas by European colonizers, along with linguistic interactions with various indigenous linguistic groups. This resulted in a great diversity of Spanish dialects and accents across the region. For instance, *LAC* Spanish differentiates from *European* Spanish in its pronunciation, intonation, and vocabulary.

It is worth noting that although Spanish speakers can generally understand each other with minimal effort, individuals from Central America may speak and use completely different nouns and verbs as those used by South American or Caribbean people. Within countries, unique linguistic differences are closely related to other important factors, including geographic location, population migration, literacy, and education. It is therefore not surprising to find areas in LAC with very specific Spanish dialects. For instance, *Rioplatense* Spanish is primarily spoken in Argentina and Uruguay, and predominantly in the River Basin region that divides both countries. This version of Spanish is known for its distinctive pronunciation features of the letters "*y*" and "*ll*."[7] There is also *Caribbean* Spanish, which is predominantly spoken in Caribbean countries like Cuba, Puerto Rico, and the Dominican Republic as well as some coastal regions of Central America and northern South America. To this day, this variation of Spanish maintains many lexical borrowings from African and Amerindian languages.[8]

Ethnicity

Language and communication in LAC are greatly influenced by the diversity of ethnic backgrounds that characterize this region. People from LAC tend to express great pride in their country's local dialects and generally self-identify in terms of their specific country of origin rather than in a general LAC identity.[9] For instance, people from LAC may identify with European, Middle Eastern, African, or Indigenous ethnic backgrounds. The majority of the 133 million Afro-Latin Americans in LAC[10] descend from slaves brought by European merchants from the West African coast.[11] In addition, according to Freire et al.,[12] Mexico, Guatemala, Peru, and Bolivia are home to over 80% of the 42 million indigenous people in LAC. There are 780 indigenous groups and over 560 indigenous languages that share co-official status with Spanish in LAC (e.g., Colombia, Bolivia, and Mexico). Many indigenous languages may be used for formal education (e.g., Brazil, Chile, Honduras, Panama) and official regional purposes (e.g., Nicaragua and Ecuador), while others receive no recognition (e.g., Belize).

It is worth noting that despite the presence of indigenous peoples in LAC, spoken indigenous languages are increasingly uncommon. This could be attributed, in part, to systemic issues involving poverty, social and political segregation, and acculturation at the expense of language and other salient aspects of their culture. There are important ongoing initiatives such as "The United Nations Declaration on the Rights of Indigenous Peoples"[13] and "The Sociolinguistic Atlas of Indigenous Peoples in LAC"[14] that attempt to protect the rights and cultural identity of indigenous people residing in LAC.

Education and Literacy

Literacy rates in LAC have been marginally improving across age groups in the last decade. As of 2019, the literacy rate of adult females (15 years and older) was 94.8% when compared to the

94.7% literacy rate of their adult male counterparts.[15] Similarly, the gender parity index (GPI) in this region has remained steady between 1.004 and 1.008 since 2005, suggesting a parity rate that marginally favors females in the last years.[16] According to the World Bank,[12] children between ages 6 and 11 report school attendance rates of 83% in Brazil, 96% in Ecuador, 92% in Panama, and 93% in Peru.

Not surprisingly, a gap in school attendance persists between indigenous and non-indigenous children, particularly in countries with smaller and more scattered indigenous populations. Educational attainment of indigenous groups also varies significantly across the region, with a large portion of members of these communities having completed less than primary school (55%–76%), primary school (17%–34%), secondary school (1%–14%), and only less than 2% having obtained a college degree.[12]

Similarly, the Afro-Latin American population in most LAC countries has significantly lower levels of educational attainment. On average, about 64% of Afro-Latin Americans complete primary education, 30% secondary education, and only 5% have achieved tertiary education or higher. Disparities in academic attainment among the Afro-Latin American and indigenous communities might be related to multiple factors including gender roles, access to education, and lower socio-economic status.[10]

An important aspect of education access is *intergenerational mobility*, broadly defined as the changes in the socio-economic status of parents and children across generations. While younger generations have better access to education than their parents in most world regions, LAC children continue to fall behind in relative intergenerational mobility. In other words, children born in the least educated households are significantly more prone to become the least educated in their generations.[17] The impact of intergenerational mobility on the LAC region extends beyond educational access and completion. The Program for International Student Assessment (PISA), an international test of education quality collected by the Organization for Economic Co-operation and Development (OECD), consistently finds that when compared to other regions, LAC students underperform across all tested subject areas, particularly in reading, suggesting that intergenerational mobility may also have an impact on the quality of education received by individuals from this region.[17]

Poverty

Poverty is a major problem that continues to affect LAC. While the region does not have the largest number of poor people in the world, it has the most unequal income distribution.[18] Recent data estimated that nearly 45 million more Latin Americans will be forced into poverty, with tens of millions facing extreme poverty as a result of the COVID-19 pandemic.[19] Additionally, more than one-third of the population will face unemployment resulting in food insecurity,[19] increased risk of illness, and earlier disability.

Healthcare Systems in LAC

Prior to the middle of the 20th century, healthcare coverage in LAC was offered only to employed individuals in the formal labor market through public health insurance plans and contributions made by employers, workers, and the government. The rest of the population received limited assistance from their local health department, church, charitable organizations, or universities.[20] Undoubtedly, the underpinning principles of this healthcare model provided more access to wealthier individuals, with restricted or no access to the poor. The 1960s brought a wave of transition to the region from traditional healthcare into a more unified model, first led by Cuba, followed by Costa Rica in the 1970s, and Brazil in the 1980s.

The 1990s welcomed the extension of healthcare coverage to urban and poor neighborhoods, inspired by the 1978 Alma-Ata Declaration and the World Health Assembly strategy "Health for all in the Year 2000" in 1979. Two opposed models of reform have been implemented in the region: The Universal Health Coverage (UHC) model and the Single Universal Health System model. The UHC depends on the payer/provider split, free choice, and pre-priced health service plans. In this framework, insurance (public or private) is critical to assure market solvency. Conversely, the Single Universal Health System is a public health model funded by tax revenue that provides access to healthcare to every individual free of charge. Today, the UHS is considered the dominant healthcare model in LAC, with Argentina, Brazil, Cuba, Chile, Colombia, Ecuador, Mexico, Peru, Trinidad and Tobago, Uruguay, and Venezuela making adequate implementations.[21]

However, the UHS is far from perfect. According to Laurell and Giovanella,[21] the UHC model increases bias in access, generates administrative barriers for timely access, and does not provide financial protection for its members. Conversely, the Single Universal Health System has increased health access to millions in the region. Nonetheless, private health insurance has also increased among unionized employees and those in the upper-middle class.

Health Conditions and Social Disparities

Despite significant improvement in access to healthcare that has been observed in recent decades, and that life expectancy has improved by almost four years from 2000 to 2017, LAC still has some of the most persistent social and health inequalities worldwide.

At the social level, it should be noted that historically racial/ethnic minorities have had limited access to healthcare services, in part due to geographical locations, socio-economic status, and cultural factors (e.g., communication barriers, prejudice, stereotypes).[11] Regarding health, there is a lack of access to physicians and physical resources that prevents an effective response to the population's healthcare needs. As tabulated by the World Bank and OECD,[22] there is an average of two doctors and less than three nurses available per 1000 individuals, falling below OECD standards (3.5 and almost 9, respectively). There is also an average of 2.1 available hospital beds per 1000 individuals. Similarly, the availability of medical technologies, as well as effective treatments for some diseases is also very limited.[22] For instance, there is only 55% coverage for antiretroviral drug treatment among people living with human immunodeficiency virus (HIV).[22]

On the other hand, according to the World Bank and OECD,[22] there are several risk factors for poor health in LAC, including smoking, drinking alcohol, and being overweight; the latter is considered one of the most salient risk factors for poor health in children under age 5 (8%), adolescents (28%), and adults (men, over 53%; women, 61%). Sanitation is another health-related concern for people living in rural (1 out of 4, on average) and urban (1 out of 8, on average) areas, with some countries reporting less than 50% sanitation in the same areas.[22]

In addition to the aforementioned social and health disparities, LAC faces another challenge with non-communicable diseases (NCD) (e.g., cardiovascular disease, most cancers, diabetes, chronic respiratory diseases, Alzheimer's disease (AD), and Parkinson's disease (PD), which were the leading cause of death between 2000 and 2015.[23]

Psychiatric Disorders in LAC

There is a scarcity of available mental health professionals in LAC,[22] with 1.6 psychiatrists, 2.7 psychiatric nurses, 2.8 psychologists, and 1.9 social workers per 100,000 population.[23] Nonetheless, this region has seen significant advances in mental healthcare in the last two decades. According to Rodriguez,[24] between 2005 and 2011, the region reported the highest percentage of countries providing psychosocial interventions (64%) and follow-up community care (35%). Since the Caracas declaration, 39% of LAC have created or revised their mental health legislations, and after 2001, significant steps were taken to integrate international to national regulations on human rights.

Despite substantial improvements, the field of mental health continues to face many challenges. According to the PAHO and WHO,[25] psychiatric and neurological disorders account for 22% of the total burden of disease (measured in disability-adjusted life years, DALYs). The most common neuropsychiatric disorders are unipolar depressive disorders (13.2%) and alcohol use disorders (6.9%). Despite the significant burden of mental health disorders, the treatment gap is astounding. The region reports a 4.9 prevalence for major depressive disorder, persistent depressive disorder (dysthymia) (1.7, 59%), non-affective psychosis (1, 37%), bipolar disorder (0.8, 64%), anxiety disorder (3.4, 63%), panic disorder (1.0, 53%), obsessive-compulsive disorder (1.4, 60%), and alcohol use disorders and harmful alcohol use (5.7, 71%). In practical terms, this means that only a minority of those needing mental healthcare receive it. Moreover, an estimated 65,000 individuals die from suicide every year, an age-adjusted mortality rate of 7.3 per 100,000 populations between 2005 and 2009. Consistent with global trends, suicide rates remain higher in males, accounting for 79% of all suicide deaths. The majority of deaths from suicide occurred in individuals ages 25 to 44 (37%) and 45 to 59 (26%), while only 20% occurred in individuals aged 60 and over, and 12% in those aged 70 and older.[25]

There is a scarcity of epidemiological studies looking into psychiatric and mental health disorders of LAC children and adolescents, making understanding prevalence rates problematic. A study conducted in a pediatric hospital in Colombia established that the most prevalent conditions in this population were impaired learning, attention deficit hyperactivity disorder (ADHD), depression and suicide associated disorders, anxiety, eating disorders, substance use, psychotic disorders, conduct disorders, and pervasive developmental disorders or autism spectrum disorder (ASD).[26] According to Oschilewsky et al.,[27] several LAC countries are home to some of the highest at-risk children population with mental health disorders (e.g., Brazil, Mexico), with abandoned children at a higher risk of engaging in criminal behavior or substance use as survival strategies. Another study conducted in northern Chile found differences by sex in depression, anxiety, and behavioral disorders, demonstrating the female population to be the most affected, with a high probability of carrying these disorders into adulthood.[28]

Neurological Conditions in LAC

In terms of neurological diseases, dementia is one of LAC's major health and social challenges; however, it is continuously neglected by the government and policymakers. Accurate dementia estimates have been difficult to establish, mainly due to low disease awareness and diagnostic accuracy.[29] From 2015 to 2050, the number of people living with dementia in LAC is predicted to increase fourfold.[25] In 2020, an estimated 89.28 million people in LAC lived with dementia, with Argentina, Brazil, Chile, Costa Rica, Cuba, Colombia, Dominican Republic, Ecuador, Mexico, Peru, Uruguay, and Venezuela experiencing the highest dementia rates.[26] According to the 2015 Alzheimer's Disease International (ADI) report, LAC has the highest worldwide prevalence of dementia (8.4%) in people age 60 and older, with incidence rates as high as 13.8 (per 10,000 people) for individuals 65 years and older.[30] AD is the most common cause of dementia in LAC (56.3%), followed by a mixed etiology (AD and vascular dementia [VD, 15.5%]) and VD (8.7%).[30] The literature is limited on frontotemporal dementia (FTD), with prevalence and incidence rates largely unknown. Similarly, prevalence estimates of Huntington's disease in LAC are challenging due to misdiagnosis. Reported estimates range from 0.5% (Venezuela) to 4% (Mexico City).[31] Moreover, LAC provides access to unique populations, including the world's largest familial AD (Colombia),

Huntington disease (Venezuela), ataxia (Cuba), and high late-onset dementia incidence in the Caribbean.[29] Overall, dementia is considered the largest cause of disability for countries such as Cuba, Dominican Republic, Mexico, and Peru,[32] with higher deaths (hospital settings) occurring in Cuba (41.4%), Dominican Republic (29.1%), Peru (urban, 31%, rural, 83.3%), and Mexico (31.3%)[33] making hospitalizations the leading healthcare cost.[29]

Stroke is the second leading cause of death and disability in LAC countries. In 2017, more than 5.5 million stroke survivors, 0.60 million new cases, and more than 0.26 million deaths were reported in this region. In particular, Paraguay has the highest incidence rate (128 cases per 100,000) and mortality (67 cases per 100,000), while the prevalence is higher in Brazil (1,133 cases per 100,000) and Uruguay (1,120 cases per 100,000). On the contrary, Colombia and Peru are the countries with the lowest incidence (85–87 cases per 100,000), prevalence (790–812 cases per 100,000), and mortality (25–29 cases per 100,000). The main types of stroke in this population are intracerebral hemorrhage and subarachnoid hemorrhage.[34]

The incidence of traumatic brain injury (TBI) is also high in LAC. According to the 1998 WHO data,[35] the incidence of TBI secondary to road accidents and violence was 163 per 100,000 and 67 per 100,000, respectively, the highest in the world. The prevalence has likely increased in recent years; however, the scarcity of epidemiological studies on TBI in LAC countries has limited obtaining updated data. Regarding mortality, a recent study evidenced that 37% of patients in LAC died due to TBI, and of the surviving patients, 44% were left with mild-moderate disability.[36] The situation is even more dramatic if one considers that public rehabilitation services are scarce, if not non-existent, in some countries. The majority of the population lacks sufficient socio-economic status to afford private services. Furthermore, it has been estimated that only 1% of people living with disabilities in rural areas benefit from rehabilitation following a TBI and other brain-related injuries.[37,38]

In terms of epilepsy, approximately five million individuals live with the disorder in LAC, with a prevalence of 17.8%, and without significant group differences (e.g., age, sex). Epilepsy mortality in LAC is 1.04%, a figure considered higher than the rate of the United States and Canada (0.50).[39]

Regarding the epidemiology of multiple sclerosis (MS) in LAC, a recent systematic review[40] reported an incidence between 0.15 and 3 cases per 100,000 from 1995 to 2016. On the other hand, the prevalence of this disease varied throughout countries, with the highest rates in Brazil and Argentina (12 to 38.2 cases per 100,000), and lowest rates in Ecuador, Colombia, and Panama (0.75 to 6.5 cases per 100,000). It is important to note that the incidence and prevalence of MS in LAC is considerably lower than in developed countries, such as Europe and North America. In fact, Caucasians are more vulnerable to suffering from this disease than mestizos, which supports the genetic and environmental influence on the development of the disease.[41]

Finally, although epidemiological studies on PD are really scarce, a recent study on the worldwide burden of this disease reported that between the period 1990 and 2016, Chile was the Latin American country that experienced the greatest increase in the prevalence of PD (19.9%), followed by Paraguay (19.4%), El Salvador (18.6%), Honduras (18.4%), and Guatemala (18%). Regarding the number of deaths attributed to PD, Paraguay (23.4%) tops the list, followed by Haiti (21.7%), Bolivia (21.1%), Honduras (19.8%), and Chile (16.5%). This increase has been attributed to the increase in life expectancy, as well as to other environmental factors such as industrialization.[42]

Toward a Better Health System

Overall, healthcare inequalities have precluded millions of Latin Americans from receiving adequate access to healthcare, leading to unnecessary suffering, disabilities, deaths, and thus impacting the region's economy. Subsequently, recent initiatives have been created with the sole purpose of improving healthcare in LAC. In 2016, the Director of the Pan American Sanitary Bureau

(PASB, or the Bureau) established the Commission on Equity and Health Inequalities in the Americas, delegating it with promoting actions to reduce inequities and inequalities in the region. This is the first large-scale initiative developed to gather evidence on health disparities in LAC. The commission comprises 12 regional experts from different countries geared to focus on specific areas, including gender, equity, human rights, and ethnicity.[43] Overall, this initiative is promising, given the opportunity of reducing inequality and improving health-related outcomes across LAC.

History of Neuropsychology in LAC

The beginnings of neuropsychology in LAC date back to the period between 1950 and 1970. Pioneers at that time included Alberto Leónidas Merani and Juan Enrique Azcoaga in Argentina and Carlos Mendilaharsu in Uruguay.[44] Their efforts focused primarily on the study of language and linguistic alterations. At the same time, their research interests and clinical practice were unequivocally influenced by French-speaking authors, including Henri Hécaen and Julián de Ajuriaguerra, and Soviet authors Iván Pavlov, Lev Vygotsky, and Alexander Luria. The influence of Luria is particularly evident in the evolution of LAC neuropsychology as many of his works were translated to Spanish, and many pioneers from this era spent time in the Soviet Union.[45] At the same time, several groups dedicated to studying the brain were forming in Mexico.[46] In contrast, very few efforts were observed in the field in Central and South America during this time, except for René Calderón de Soria in Bolivia, who is regarded as a pioneer of neuropsychology, and who is responsible for the underpinnings of neuropsychiatry in this country.[47]

Between 1970 and 1999, neuropsychology in Colombia and Mexico advanced considerably, due in great part to the work of Dr. Alfredo Ardila, though it remained at the beginning stages in other countries. Additionally, LAC neuropsychology began to expand its horizons and feed on North American authors and researchers. During this period, numerous organizations were formed, including the Neuropsychological Society of Argentina, the Chilean Neuropsychological Society, the Mexican Society of Neuropsychology, the Colombian Association of Neuropsychology, and the Brazilian Society of Neuropsychology, among others. In addition to country-specific organizations, two other organizations brought LAC neuropsychology professionals together: The LAC Association of Neuropsychology (ALAN) and the LAC Society of Neuropsychology (SLAN). It is also during this era when the first congresses and symposiums of the region emerged, such as the SLAN and ALAN congresses, as well as the selection of LAC countries to host relevant international congresses (e.g., The International Neuropsychological Society congress in Mexico City in 1983).[44]

Other countries started to become involved in the field of neuropsychology during this period. Ernesto Vela and José Luis Henríquez introduced neuropsychology into El Salvador, Lucio Balarezo into Ecuador, Ricardo de Obaldía into Panamá, José Luis Henríquez and Tedd Judd into Nicaragua, Eduardo Cairo into Cuba, Otto Lima Gómez into Venezuela, and Artidoro Cáceres Velásquez into Peru. However, other countries of the region faced a delay in the field as a result of dictatorships. Such was the case of Chile (1973–1990), Argentina (1976–1983), and Uruguay (1973–1985) under civil-military dictatorship, and Brazil under military dictatorship (1964–1985).[44]

The field of neuropsychology began to solidify in the 2000s with the creation of graduate programs in the field (e.g., Master in Neuropsychology in Bolivia and Mexico) and the introduction of requirements for obtaining specialty in neuropsychology (e.g., Brazil). LAC specific journals began to be published (e.g., Iberoamerican Journal of Neuropsychology, Argentinian Journal of Neuropsychology, and the Chilean Journal of Neuropsychology) along with more neuropsychology books ("Fundamentos de Neuropsicología Clínica" by Jorge Lorenzo Otero and Luis Fontán Scheitler, "Tratado de Neuropsicología Clínica" by Edith Labos, "Rehabilitación Neuropsicológica" by Juan Carlos Arango-Lasprilla, among others).[44] Neuropsychological measures also began to be developed (e.g., Batería Neuropsicológica Neuropsi, batería ECOFON, Evaluación de la Conciencia Fonológica, batería ENI, Evaluación Neuropsicológica Infantil) and new neuropsychology organizations grew (Venezuelan Society of Neuropsychology, Colombian Society of Neuropsychology).

Numerous scientific events have taken place in the last decade. In 2011, the XII SLAN Congress was celebrated in Santiago, Chile, and in 2012 and 2013, Colombia was selected to host the VII and VIII Cerebro y Mente SLAN congresses. In 2016, the 1st Iberoamerican Neuropsychology Congress was organized in Bilbao, Spain, by its president, Juan Carlos Arango-Lasprilla, to advance the field of neuropsychology in Spanish and Portuguese countries. Subsequently, this congress was celebrated in 2018 in Almería, Spain, and in 2019 in Cali, Colombia. Finally, and given the current situation as a result of the pandemic due to the SARS-CoV-2, the IV Iberoamerican Congress of Neuropsychology was held as a virtual conference in May, 2021 witn 1806 participants from 43 countries.[44]

Nevertheless, interested readers should note that it is difficult to fully understand the state of the literature and history of neuropsychology in several LAC countries such as Belize, Haiti, and the Dominican Republic, given the lack of literature on the subject. For more detailed information on the history of neuropsychology in LAC, readers are invited to review Arango-Lasprilla et al.[44]

Neuropsychology in LAC: State of the Art

The development of neuropsychology in LAC and its current state of the art is known to the world, in part, thanks to Juan Carlos Arango-Lasprilla and his research team's goals. More specifically, two important research studies in neuropsychology were conducted in LAC, and the details are further discussed below.

The first study[48] which was the first record about the state of the literature of LAC neuropsychology, involved a survey of 808 neuropsychologists from 16 LAC countries (Argentina, Bolivia, Brazil, Chile, Colombia, Cuba, Ecuador, Guatemala, Honduras, Mexico, Panama, Paraguay, Peru, Puerto Rico, Uruguay, and Venezuela). The majority of the professionals who participated in the survey completed training in neuropsychology during graduate school and worked part-time (44%) in private practice (25%). Interestingly, participants identified lack of academic training programs (47%), clinical training (45%), and collaboration among professionals (36%) as the main obstacles to the growth of the field of neuropsychology in LAC. In terms of neuropsychological evaluations, an alarming 52% of participants reported using normative data from other countries. Similarly, the lack of normative data for their country (62%) and cultural adaptation (54%) were two of the main challenges identified by participants regarding neuropsychological tests. The most common reason for referrals included ADHD (35%), learning disorders (33%), intellectual disability (26%), and dementia (24%), which were typically referred by neurology (67%), psychology (63%), and the school system (54%) to obtain a diagnosis (77%).

Furthermore, the percentage of professionals who provided neuropsychological rehabilitation was lower (61%) when compared to those who completed neuropsychological evaluations (81%). For the most part, individuals engaged in individual neuropsychological rehabilitation (78%) focused mainly on attention and concentration (87%), memory (80%), and executive function (79%). A lower percentage (46%) of individuals noted being involved in teaching at private institutions (53.8%) and primarily at the undergraduate level (70.8%). About 62% of the participants indicated being involved in research in the last year, though only 90% of them reported obtaining Institutional Review Board (IRB) approval prior to conducting research. In addition, 60% of the participants reported not having sufficient resources to conduct research projects, while 61% of participants had never obtained financial support.

The second study[49] focused on the state of the literature of pediatric neuropsychology in LAC and Spain. A total of 409 neuropsychologists from 12 LAC countries participated, including Argentina, Bolivia, Colombia, Costa Rica, Cuba, Ecuador, Guatemala, Honduras, Mexico, Paraguay, Peru as well as Puerto Rico and Spain. Interestingly, 61% of participants indicated having completed graduate studies in pediatric neuropsychology. Surprisingly, while 53% indicated not completing graduate-level studies in pediatric neuropsychology, they self-identified as pediatric neuropsychologists. The majority of participants worked full time (53%). Lack of academic training programs (42%), clinical training (41%), and financial resources (36%) were identified as the three main obstacles to the development of pediatric neuropsychology in LAC.

Participants in this study worked primarily with children with ADHD (87%), learning disorders (85%), and intellectual disability (72%) between ages 6 and 11 (89%) who were referred by teachers (76%), parents (61%), and neurologists (60%), mainly to obtain a diagnosis (86%). Further, professionals surveyed in the latter study indicated working with a multidisciplinary team, specifically with child psychologists (61%), speech and language pathologists (61%), and neurologists (61%). Approximately 74% of participants reported working in a forensic setting to determine the premorbid cognitive, social, and emotional functioning as well as the neuropsychological sequelae and level of disability of children in this setting. The elevated cost was reportedly the principal problem with neuropsychological tests (61%). In addition, challenges with the lack of normative data for each country (56%) and cultural adaptation of tests (45%) were also reported. Similarly, the principal barriers to complete neuropsychological evaluations included limited neuropsychological positions in hospitals (48.4%), followed by the high cost of neuropsychological evaluations (43%) and small selection of neuropsychological measures with normative data in their country (42%).

Similar to the previous study, the percentage of participants who provided neuropsychological rehabilitation (78%) was smaller when compared to individuals conducting neuropsychological evaluations (96%), and the treatment model included family intervention (75%) followed by adaptive functioning (69%), and behavioral-emotional intervention (69%). For participants, the greatest limitation of providing rehabilitation was the limited number of rehabilitation programs available for children (45%). Fifty-one percent of the faculty focused on undergraduate teaching (39%), while 43% were involved in research. Once again, only 84% indicated obtaining IRB approval. Interestingly, while 97% of participants noted obtaining only informed consent from parents, only 68.1% requested consent or assent from the minor.

Country-Specific Normative Data and Culturally Appropriate Instruments

In the aforementioned studies, the state of the literature in LAC neuropsychology evidenced the lack of normative data for different countries in the region. The studies conducted until then (2013) are characterized by (1) focusing on the Colombian, Argentine, and Mexican population, (2) being outdated (as majority were published prior to 2009), and (3) generating normative data that utilizes traditional methodologies based on mean scores and standard deviations, and the limitations associated with this method[50] (see Appendix for a list of available tests).

These limitations motivated Juan Carlos Arango-Lasprilla and his research team to conduct two research projects to generate normative data for neuropsychological measures in Spanish-speaking countries. The first study started in 2013 by developing normative data for the most frequently used neuropsychological measures with the LAC adult population (based on the study about the state of the literature of LAC neuropsychology[48] including Rey-Osterrieth Complex Figure test (ROCF), Stroop Color-Word Interference Test, Modified Wisconsin Card Sorting Test (M-WCST), Trail Making Test (TMT), Brief Test of Attention (BTA), Phonological and Semantic

Verbal Fluency Test (VFT), Boston Naming Test (BNT), Symbol Digit Modalities Test (SDMT), Hopkins Verbal Learning Test–Revised (HVLT-R), and the Test of Memory Malingering (TOMM). The study included 5,402 healthy adults from Argentina, Bolivia, Chile, Colombia, Cuba, El Salvador, Guatemala, Honduras, Mexico, Paraguay, Peru, and Puerto Rico. Normative data for the Colombian population ($n = 1425$) were published in the book "Neuropsicología en Colombia: Datos normativos, estado actual y retos a future."[51] Normative data for the remaining countries were published in the monograph "Commonly used Neuropsychological Tests for Spanish Speakers: Normative Data from LAC."[52–62]

The second normative study, which began in 2016, focused on the pediatric population of 10 LAC countries, including Chile, Colombia, Cuba, Ecuador, Guatemala, Honduras, Mexico, Paraguay, Pere, Puerto Rico, and Spain. A total of 6,030 children ages 6 to 17 were evaluated using a fixed battery that included the following tests: ROCF, Stroop Color-Word Interference Test, M-WCST, TMT, SDMT, a shortened version of Token Test, Concentration Endurance Test (d2), VFT, Peabody Picture Vocabulary Test-III (PPVT-III) and the Learning and Verbal Memory Test (TAMV-I). Normative data of the study were published in the monograph "Normative Data for Spanish-Language Neuropsychological Tests: A Step Forward in the Assessment of Pediatric Populations."[50,62–71] As with normative data for Colombian adults, results from this study were published in the textbook "Neuropsicología infantil."[72]

Given that LAC is one of the world regions with higher rates of illiteracy, Juan Carlos Arango-Lasprilla and his research team decided to generate normative data for this population in nine LAC countries, including Bolivia, Colombia, Ecuador, El Salvador, Guatemala, Honduras, Mexico, Pere, and Puerto Rico. The total sample included 402 adult participants ages 18–93. Normative data for the ROCF, M-WCST, BTA, VFT, BNT, SDMT, and HVLT-R tests were published in the textbook "Neuropsicología y analfabetismo."[73]

Other important initiatives have been carried out to adapt existing neuropsychological measures, and even more importantly, to develop new measures for Spanish-speakers. For example, Olabarrieta-Landa et al.[56,67] published an administration and scoring guide of verbal phonemic, semantic, and action fluency, taking into consideration the general characteristics of the Spanish language. In addition, Rivera et al.[74] developed the TAMV-I; a new measure to assess the learning and memory of LAC children ages 6–17. The stimuli selection was carefully performed while other important factors, such as categories previously normed, the degree of adaptation to the target population, interference with existing measures (e.g., semantic fluency), and its cultural adaptation to LAC countries, including Spain, were considered.

Juan Carlos Arango-Lasprilla and his team made further efforts to advance appropriate neuropsychological evaluations of LAC people by exploring the frequency of low scores in the general population when administered a battery of cognitive tests.[75] They found that low scores are common when multiple neuropsychological outcomes (tests and/or scores) are evaluated in healthy individuals, the higher the number of tests, the greater the probability of obtaining one or more low scores that are not necessarily indicative of cognitive impairment.[76]

It was with this in mind that several studies with adults, children, and adolescents were published, showing that approximately 30% of the clinical sample obtained at least one or more low scores below the 16th percentile on different cognitive batteries including language, learning and memory,[77] and executive function.[74–76] Furthermore, it has been demonstrated that the number of low scores obtained by LAC individuals when using norms for non-Hispanic White individuals is higher when compared to when normative data for the LAC population are used.[75] Therefore, it is essential to use norms that have been adequately adapted to the population being tested as well as consider the percentage of clinically healthy individuals who commonly obtain low scores at this percentile to avoid false positives and misdiagnosis.

Training/Educational Challenges

It has become apparent that neuropsychology has advanced significantly in LAC during the last decade. Depending on how this field develops over time, professionals could face challenges that would vary considerably across countries. Nonetheless, LAC countries face similar challenges in their efforts to advance and consolidate the discipline in this region as well as to make the health system and general population acknowledge the need and contribution of the discipline to the field. Below we focus on neuropsychology training challenges in LAC.[44,78]

1   At the undergraduate level, students receive basic training (e.g., neuropsychology-focused coursework and practicum externships). Those students who are interested in furthering their neuropsychology knowledge have limited training programs at the master's level, while options for academic training at the doctorate and postdoctoral level are even scarcer. As a result, only those who can afford it receive training outside LAC. Additionally, students who leave to pursue training abroad generally stay overseas and never return to practice in their home country, resulting in a high number of young, qualified LAC professionals not getting involved with initiatives to advance neuropsychology in this region.
2   Graduate education is generally private and expensive in LAC, making it harder for many individuals to enroll in these programs. Some institutions take advantage of this situation by offering shortened and expensive graduate programs (often brief and intense courses) at the expense of quality.
3   The scientific and academic literature in Spanish is minimal. Considering that most research in this field is conducted and published in English and that most LAC individuals lack English proficiency, the capacity of faculty and students to become familiar with the latest research in the field is limited.
4   There are limited academic and training programs in pediatric neuropsychology, neuropsychological rehabilitation, experimental neuropsychology, and forensic neuropsychology. Currently, the majority of programs offered in this region focus on adult clinical neuropsychology.
5   Most training programs focus on clinical practice, limiting opportunities for teaching as related to research methodology, data analysis, and scientific writing. Hence, while many professionals generate exciting data, they lack the know-how of publishing in academic journals and often publish in local journals in Spanish, which results in research from this region not getting disseminated to the rest of the world.
6   The possibility of training clinically is limited due to the lack of qualified professionals in the region who can provide adequate training for students in their places of employment.
7   A common limitation of LAC countries, except Brazil, is the lack of guidelines regulating the profession. Without shared criteria of minimum standards of practice, any individual who completes graduate studies (or without graduate studies, as demonstrated by the study on the state of the literature of pediatric neuropsychology) can identify as a neuropsychologist. Moreover, the lack of uniform guidelines governing the profession furthers the gap of qualified professionals working in institutions who can, in turn, train the future neuropsychologists of the region.

Conclusions

LAC extends over 33 countries and is home to millions of individuals from diverse ethnic and cultural backgrounds. LAC neuropsychology remains an emerging discipline that has advanced greatly in the last several decades. The progress of neuropsychology in this region has been gradual. During its initial stages, psychologists of the time were highly influenced by European theorists and researchers who pioneered in the field. A new era emerged with creating academic programs that helped further the field by providing opportunities for specialized training and skill set development. More recently, efforts to expand the field have resulted in the development of major norming studies designed to capture the cultural differences of the LAC population to generate normative data that is appropriate, valid, and reliable to meet the clinical needs of the people from this region. Like other areas of the world, cultural, social, and governmental aspects have played a salient role in advancing the field in this region, including a limited number of neuropsychology academic and training programs and competent clinicians who can provide pre-and postdoctoral instruction across the region.

Equally, there are significant differences across LAC countries, including language, psychosocial factors, and national healthcare structure that further complicate the establishment of neuropsychology as a uniform discipline. These differences further highlight the need for culturally appropriate test measures and norms that incorporate and reflect the intricacies and diversity of the population from this region. While recent norming efforts have aimed to close the gap, research on the different cultural and ethnic backgrounds is warranted to further expand, solidify, make neuropsychological services available to underserved populations in this region.

References

1. Population, total—Latin America & Caribbean [Internet]. World Bank. 2019. Available from: https://data.worldbank.org/indicator/SP.POP.TOTL?locations=ZJ
2. World Bank. Latin American and the Caribbean [Internet]. 2019. Available from: www.worldbank.org/en/region/lac/overview
3. Kittleson RA, Bushnell D, Lockhart J. History of Latin America [Internet]. 2019. Available from: https://www.britannica.com/place/Latin-America
4. Bayley R, Cameron R, Lucas C. The Oxford handbook of sociolinguistics. New York (NY): Oxford University Press; 2013.
5. Data for ZJ, Brazil [Internet]. World Bank. 2020. Available from: https://data.worldbank.org/?locations=%20ZJ-BR
6. Physical & Human Geography of Latin America [Internet]. Study.com. 2016. Available from: https://study.com/academy/lesson/physical-human-geography-of-latin-america.html
7. Staggs C. A perception study of Rioplatense Spanish. McNair Sch Res J. [Internet]. 2019;14(1). Available from: https://scholarworks.boisestate.edu/mcnair_journal/vol14/iss1/11
8. Escobar AM. Bilingualism in Latin America. In: Bhatia TK, Ritchie WC, editors. The Handbook of bilingualism and multilingualism. 2nd ed. Chichester, West Sussex (UK) ; Malden (MA): Wiley-Blackwell; 2013. p. 725–44.
9. Albert R, McKay-Semmler K. Communication modes, Latin American/Latino. In: The international encyclopedia of intercultural communication. John Wiley & Sons, Inc; 2017. DOI:10.1002/9781118783665.ieicc0144
10. World Bank. Afro-Descendants in Latin America: towards a framework of inclusion. [Internet]. 2018. Available from: https://openknowledge.worldbank.org/handle/10986/30201
11. Giuffrida A. Racial and ethnic disparities in Latin America and the Caribbean: a literature review. Divers Equal Health Care. 2010;7:115–28.
12. Freire G, Schwartz Orellana SD, Zumaeta Aurazo M, Costa DC, Lundvall JM, Viveros Mendoza MC, et al. Indigenous Latin America in the twenty-first century [Internet]. Washington (DC): World Bank; 2015. Available from: http://documents.worldbank.org/curated/en/145891467991974540/Indigenous-Latin-America-in-the-twenty-first-century-the-first-decade
13. Assembly UG. United Nations declaration on the rights of indigenous peoples [Internet]. 2007. Available from: https://www.un.org/esa/socdev/unpfii/documents/DRIPS_es.pdf

14. Atlas sociolingüística de los pueblos indígenas en América Latina [Internet]. UNICEF. 2009. Available from: https://atlaspueblosindigenas.wordpress.com/

15. Literacy rate—Latin America & Caribbean [Internet]. World Bank. 2019. Available from: https://data.worldbank.org/indicator/SE.ADT.LITR.FE.ZS?locations=ZJ

16. Ratio of boys to girls in primary, secondary, and tertiary education [Internet]. United Nations Education, Scientific and Cultural Organization. 2019. Available from: https://unstats.un.org/unsd/mdg/Metadata.aspx?IndicatorId=9

17. Poverty and Inequality: Monitoring Latin American and the Caribbean [Internet]. World Bank. 2017. Available from: http://documents1.worldbank.org/curated/en/540231508162105763/pdf/120437-REVISED-Intergenerational-mobility-in-LAC-October-16-2017.pdf

18. Lustig N. Most unequal on Earth [Internet]. International Monetary Fund. 2015. Available from: http://www.imf.org/external/pubs/ft/fandd/2015/09/lustig.htm

19. Political and social compacts for equality and sustainable development in Latin America and the Caribbean in the post-COVID-19 recovery [Internet]. Economic Commission for Latin America and the Caribbean. 2020. Report No.: 8. Available from: https://www.cepal.org/en/publications/46146-political-and-social-compacts-equality-and-sustainable-development-latin-america

20. Cotlear D, Gómez-Dantés O, Knaul F, Atun R, Barreto ICHC, Cetrángolo O, et al. Overcoming social segregation in health care in Latin America. The Lancet. 2015 Mar;385(9974):1248–59.

21. Laurell AC, Giovanella L. Health policies and systems in Latin America. In: Oxford research encyclopedia of global public health [Internet]. Oxford University Press; 2018 [cited 2020 Dec 11]. Available from: https://oxfordre.com/publichealth/view/10.1093/acrefore/9780190632366.001.0001/acrefore-9780190632366-e-60

22. OECD, The World Bank. Health at a Glance: Latin America and the Caribbean 2020 [Internet]. 2020 [cited 2020 Dec 14]. Available from: https://www.oecd-ilibrary.org/social-issues-migration-health/health-at-a-glance-latin-america-and-the-caribbean-2020_6089164f-en

23. Alarcón RD. Mental health and mental health care in Latin America. World Psychiatry. 2003 Feb;2(1):54–6.

24. Rodríguez JJ. Mental health care systems in Latin America and the Caribbean. Int Rev Psychiatry. 2010 Aug;22(4):317–24.

25. Strategy for universal access to health and universal health coverage. [Internet]. Pan American Health Organization. 2014. Available from: https://www.paho.org/en/documents/brochure-strategy-universal-access-health-and-universal-health-coverage-toward-consensus

26. Rohde LA, Celia S, Berganza C. Systems of care in South America. In: Remschmidt M, Belfer M, Gooyer I, editors. Facilitating pathways, care, treatment and prevention in child and adolescent mental health. Heidelberg, Germany: Spring Verlag; 2004. p. 42–51.

27. Oschilewsky RC, Gómez CM, Belfort E. Child psychiatry and mental health in Latin America. Int Rev Psychiatry. 2010 Aug;22(4):355–62.

28. Caqueo-Urízar A, Flores J, Escobar C, Urzúa A, Irarrázaval M. Psychiatric disorders in children and adolescents in a middle-income Latin American country. BMC Psychiatry. 2020 Dec;20(1):104.

29. Parra MA, Baez S, Allegri R, Nitrini R, Lopera F, Slachevsky A, et al. Dementia in Latin America: assessing the present and envisioning the future. Neurology. 2018 Jan 30;90(5):222–31.

30. Custodio N, Wheelock A, Thumala D, Slachevsky A. Dementia in Latin America: epidemiological evidence and implications for public policy. Front Aging Neurosci. 2017 Jul 13;9:221.

31. Walker RH, Gatto EM, Bustamante ML, Bernal-Pacheco O, Cardoso F, Castilhos RM, et al. Huntington's disease-like disorders in Latin America and the Caribbean. Parkinsonism Relat Disord. 2018 Aug;53:10–20.

32. Sousa RM, Ferri CP, Acosta D, Albanese E, Guerra M, Huang Y, et al. Contribution of chronic diseases to disability in elderly people in countries with low and middle incomes: a 10/66 Dementia Research Group population-based survey. Lancet. 2009 Nov;374(9704):1821–30.

33. Prince M, Bryce R, Albanese E, Wimo A, Ribeiro W, Ferri CP. The global prevalence of dementia: a systematic review and metaanalysis. Alzheimers Dement. 2013 Jan;9(1):63–75.e2.

34. Ouriques Martins SC, Sacks C, Hacke W, Brainin M, de Assis Figueiredo F, Marques Pontes-Neto O, et al. Priorities to reduce the burden of stroke in Latin American countries. Lancet Neurol. 2019 Jul;18(7):674–83.

35. Murray CJ, Lopez AD. The global burden of disease: a comprehensive assessment of mortality and disability from diseases, injuries, and risk factors in 1990 and projected to 2020: summary. Boston: Harvard School of Public Health on behalf of the World Health Organization; 1996.

36. Bonow RH, Barber J, Temkin NR, Videtta W, Rondina C, Petroni G, et al. The outcome of severe traumatic brain injury in Latin America. World Neurosurg. 2018 Mar;111:e82–e90.

37. de Ferranti D, Perry G, Ferreira F, Walton M. Inequality in Latin America. Washington (DC): The World Bank; 2014.

38. Dudzik P, Elwan A, Metts R. Disability policies, statistics, and strategies in Latin America and the Caribbean: a review. Washington (DC): The World Bank; 2002.

39. The management of epilepsy in the public health sector [Internet]. Pan American Health Organization. 2018. Available from: https://iris.paho.org/handle/10665.2/49509

40. Cristiano E, Rojas JI. Multiple sclerosis epidemiology in Latin America: an updated survey. Mult Scler J. 2017 Jun;3(2): doi: 10.1177/2055217317715050.

41. Rivera VM. Multiple sclerosis in Latin Americans: genetic aspects. Curr Neurol Neurosci Rep. 2017 Aug;17(8):57.

42. GBD 2016 Parkinson's Disease Collaborators. Global, regional, and national burden of Parkinson's disease, 1990–2016: a systematic analysis for the Global Burden of Disease Study 2016. Lancet Neurol. 2018 Nov;17(11):939–53.

43. Strategic plan of the Pan American Health Organization [Internet]. Pan American Health Organization. 2018. Available from: https://www.paho.org/hq/index.php?option=com_content&view=article&id=9774:2014-53rd-directing-council&Itemid=40507&lang=en

44. Arango Lasprilla JC, Olabarrieta-Landa L, Gonzalez I, Leal G, Álvarez Alcántara JE, Rivera D. History of neuropsychology in Latin America. In: Barr WB, Bieliauskas LA, editors. The Oxford handbook of history of clinical neuropsychology. New York, NY: Oxford University Press; 2019.

45. Ardila A. Spanish applications of Luria's assessment methods. Neuropsychol Rev. 1999;9(2):63–9.

46. Ostrosky-Solis F, Matute Duran E. La Neuropsicología en México. Rev Neuropsicol Neuropsiquiatría Neurocienc. 2009;9(2):85–98.

47. Ocampo-Barba N. René Calderón. Rev Neuropsicol Neuropsiquiatría Neurocienc. 2017;21(1):17–25.

48. Arango-Lasprilla JC, Stevens L, Morlett Paredes A, Ardila A, Rivera D. Profession of neuropsychology in Latin America. Appl Neuropsychol Adult. 2017 Jul 4;24(4):318–30.

49. Oliveras-Rentas RE, Romero-García I, Benito-Sánchez I, Ramos-Usuga D, Arango-Lasprilla JC. The practice of child neuropsychology in Spanish-speaking countries: what we've learned and where to go from here. Dev Neuropsychol. 2020 May 18;45(4):169–88.

50. Rivera D, Arango-Lasprilla JC. Methodology for the development of normative data for Spanish-speaking pediatric populations. NeuroRehabilitation. 2017 Oct 24;41(3):581–92.

51. Arango Lasprilla JC, Rivera D. Neuropsicología en Colombia: datos normativos, estado actual y retos a futuro. Manizales, Colombia: UAM, Universidad Autónoma de Manizales; 2015. p. 287 (Colección Ciencias de la salud. Investigación).

52. Arango-Lasprilla JC, Rivera D, Longoni M, Saracho CP, Garza MT, Aliaga A, et al. Modified Wisconsin Card Sorting Test (M-WCST): normative data for the Latin American Spanish speaking adult population. NeurorRehabilitation. 2015 Nov 26;37(4):563–90.

53. Arango-Lasprilla JC, Rivera D, Aguayo A, Rodríguez W, Garza MT, Saracho CP, et al. Trail Making Test: normative data for the Latin American Spanish speaking adult population. NeuroRehabilitation. 2015 Nov 26;37(4):639–61.

54. Arango-Lasprilla JC, Rivera D, Garza MT, Saracho CP, Rodríguez W, Rodríguez-Agudelo Y, et al. Hopkins Verbal Learning Test–revised: normative data for the Latin American Spanish speaking adult population. NeuroRehabilitation. 2015 Nov 26;37(4):699–718.

55. Guàrdia-Olmos J, Peró-Cebollero M, Rivera D, Arango-Lasprilla JC. Methodology for the development of normative data for ten Spanish-language neuropsychological tests in eleven Latin American countries. NeuroRehabilitation. 2015 Nov 9;37(4):493–9.

56. Olabarrieta-Landa L, Rivera D, Galarza-del-Angel J, Garza M, Saracho C, Rodríguez W, et al. Verbal fluency tests: normative data for the Latin American Spanish speaking adult population. NeuroRehabilitation. 2015 Apr 25;37(4):515–61.

57. Olabarrieta-Landa L, Rivera D, Morlett-Paredes A, Jaimes-Bautista A, Garza MT, Galarza-del-Angel J, et al. Standard form of the Boston Naming Test: normative data for the Latin American Spanish speaking adult population. NeuroRehabilitation. 2015 Nov 26;37(4):501–13.

58. Rivera D, Perrin PB, Morlett-Paredes A, Galarza-del-Angel J, Martínez C, Garza MT, et al. Rey–Osterrieth complex figure—copy and immediate recall: normative data for the Latin American Spanish speaking adult population. NeuroRehabilitation. 2015 Nov 28;37(4):677–98.

59. Rivera D, Perrin PB, Stevens LF, Garza MT, Weil C, Saracho CP, et al. Stroop Color-Word Interference Test: normative data for the Latin American Spanish speaking adult population. NeuroRehabilitation. 2015 Nov 28;37(4):591–624.

60. Rivera D, Perrin PB, Aliaga A, Garza MT, Saracho CP, Rodríguez W, et al. Brief Test of Attention: normative data for the Latin American Spanish speaking adult population. NeuroRehabilitation. 2015 Nov 25;37(4):663–76.

61. Rivera D, Perrin PB, Weiler G, Ocampo-Barba N, Aliaga A, Rodríguez W, et al. Test of Memory Malingering (TOMM): normative data for the Latin American Spanish speaking adult population. NeuroRehabilitation. 2015 Nov 26;37(4):719–35.

62. Arango-Lasprilla JC, Rivera D, Trapp S, Jiménez-Pérez C, Hernández Carrillo CL, Pohlenz Amador S, et al. Symbol Digit Modalities Test: normative data for Spanish-speaking pediatric population. NeuroRehabilitation. 2017 Oct 24;41(3):639–47.

63. Arango-Lasprilla JC, Rivera D, Ramos-Usuga D, Vergara-Moragues E, Montero-López E, Adana Díaz LA, et al. Trail Making Test: normative data for the Latin American Spanish-speaking pediatric population. NeuroRehabilitation. 2017 Oct 24;41(3):627–37.

64. Arango-Lasprilla JC, Rivera D, Nicholls E, Aguayo Arelis A, García de la Cadena C, Peñalver Guia AI, et al. Modified Wisconsin Card Sorting Test (M-WCST): normative data for Spanish-speaking pediatric population. NeuroRehabilitation. 2017 Oct 24;41(3):617–26.

65. Arango-Lasprilla JC, Rivera D, Ertl MM, Muñoz Mancilla JM, García-Guerrero CE, Rodriguez-Irizarry W, et al. Rey–Osterrieth Complex Figure—copy and immediate recall (3 minutes): normative data for Spanish-speaking pediatric populations. NeuroRehabilitation. 2017 Oct 24;41(3):593–603.

66. Olabarrieta-Landa L, Rivera D, Rodríguez-Lorenzana A, Pohlenz Amador S, García-Guerrero CE, Padilla-López A, et al. Shortened Version of the Token Test: normative data for Spanish-speaking pediatric population. NeuroRehabilitation. 2017 Oct 24;41(3):649–59.

67. Olabarrieta-Landa L, Rivera D, Lara L, Rute-Pérez S, Rodríguez-Lorenzana A, Galarza-del-Angel J, et al. Verbal fluency tests: normative data for Spanish-speaking pediatric population. NeuroRehabilitation. 2017 Oct 24;41(3):673–86.

68. Olabarrieta-Landa L, Rivera D, Ibáñez-Alfonso JA, Albaladejo-Blázquez N, Martín-Lobo P, Delgado-Mejía ID, et al. Peabody Picture Vocabulary Test-III: normative data for Spanish-speaking pediatric population. NeuroRehabilitation. 2017 Oct 24;41(3):687–94.

69. Rivera D, Folleco J, Benito Sánchez I, Acosta Barreto M, Riaño Garzón M, Herrera Bravo C, et al. Datos normativos para el test de aprendizaje Verbal (TAMV-I) en población de 6 a 17 años de edad en Colombia. In: Arango-Lasprilla JC, Rivera D, Olabarrieta Landa L, editors. Neuropsicologia Infantil. Bogota DC, Colombia: Manual Moderno; 2017. p. 339–49.

70. Rivera D, Salinas C, Ramos-Usuga D, Delgado-Mejía ID, Vasallo Key Y, Hernández Agurcia GP, et al. Concentration Endurance Test (d2): normative data for Spanish-speaking pediatric population. NeuroRehabilitation. 2017 Oct 24;41(3):661–71.

71. Rivera D, Olabarrieta-Landa L, Rabago Barajas BV, Irías Escher MJ, Saracostti Schwartzman M, Ferrer-Cascales R, et al. Newly developed Learning and Verbal Memory Test (TAMV-I): normative data for Spanish-speaking pediatric population. NeuroRehabilitation. 2017 Oct 24;41(3):695–706.

72. Arango Lasprilla JC, Olabarrieta Landa L, Rivera D. Neuropsicología Infantil. Bogota DC, Colombia: Manual Moderno; 2017.

73. Rivera D, Morlett A, Arango-Lasprilla JC. Neuropsicología y analfabetismo. Bogota DC, Colombia: Manual Moderno; 2019.

74. Rivera D, Olabarrieta-Landa L, Brooks BL, Ertl MM, Benito-Sánchez I, Quijano MC, et al. Multivariate base rates of low scores on tests of learning and memory among Latino adult populations. J Int Neuropsychol Soc. 2019 Sep;25(08):834–44.

75. Rivera D, Mascialino G, Brooks BL, Olabarrieta-Landa L, Longoni M, Galarza-Del-Angel J, et al. Multivariate base rates of low scores on tests of executive functions in a multi-country Latin American sample. Dev Neuropsychol. 2021 Jan 2;46(1):1–15.

76. Benito-Sánchez I, Gonzalez I, Oliveras-Rentas RE, Ferrer-Cascales R, Romero-García I, Restrepo Botero JC, et al. Prevalence of low scores on executive functions tests in a Spanish-speaking pediatric population from 10 Latin American countries and Spain. Dev Neuropsychol. 2020 May 18;45(4):200–10.

77. Olabarrieta-Landa L, Ramos Usuga D, Rivera D, Leal G, Bailey KC, Calderón Chagualá A, et al. Prevalence of low scores on language tests as a potential factor in misdiagnosis of cognitive impairment in a Spanish-speaking adult population. Appl Neuropsychol Adult. 2019 Dec 27;1–12.

78. Arango-Lasprilla JC, Olabarrieta Landa L, Diaz-Victoria AR, Pereira AP, Labos E, De los Reyes Aragón C. Historia de la rehabilitación neuropsicológica en Latinoamérica. Neuropsicol Neuropsiquiatría Neurocienc. 2016;16(1):1–24.

Brazilian

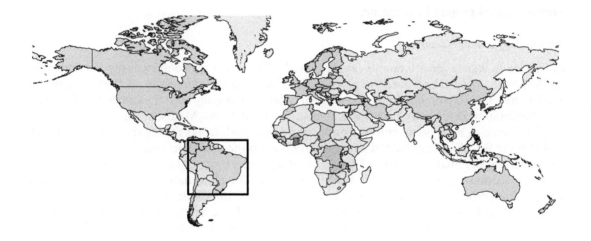

29 Support with Autonomy

Untangling the Family Role in Neuropsychological Rehabilitation in Brazil

Ana Paula Almeida de Pereira

Section I: Background Information

Terminology and Perspective

I was born in Rio de Janeiro but my family moved a lot around the country as my father worked for the Brazilian Navy. I got my BS in psychology in São Paulo, the largest city in South America. I lived in the United States for almost ten years in order to obtain my master's and doctoral degrees in Rehabilitation Psychology from the University of Wisconsin—Madison. This experience was crucial to making me a better culture-conscious professional. It was during that time that I realized that my Brazilian background gave me a different professional perspective compared to my American and Brazilian colleagues. I had to adapt my future practice to Brazilian culture as some of the procedures I learned in the United States would not be adequate in Brazil. I am currently a psychology professor at a federal university in Curitiba, the capital of the state of Paraná in Southern Brazil. Let me try to explain how this life experience has affected my perspective as a neuropsychologist by presenting some important information about Brazil and Brazilians.

Geography

Brazil is the largest country in South America, spanning 8,514,215 km², bordering the Atlantic Ocean and with a population of over 211 million. Brazil's 26 states and the Federal District are divided into five regions (North, Northeast, Southeast, South, and Center-West), each region with specific characteristics. Due to its continental size, Brazil has six ecosystems: the Amazon Basin (a tropical rain forest in the north); the Pantanal (a tropical wetland in the west); the Cerrado (a savanna system that covers the center of the country); the Caatinga (a scrubland region in the northeast); the Atlantic Forest that extends along the entire coast; and the Pampas (lowland plains in the south). The country's diverse ecosystems contributed to important economic and demographic differences among its regions. Ninety percent of Brazil presents a tropical climate.

The history of population settlement also varied widely among regions. The North and the Center-West have lower population density compared to the other parts of the country and farming is the major economic activity. In 1960, the Brazilian federal government moved to a planned city called Brasilia. This shift of the decision-making center to the country's central region increased the development of this part of Brazil. The Northeast, though it was historically one of the first areas to be colonized, presents the lowest living standards and human development index compared to the rest of the country. The Southeast has a dense urban network with high levels of industrial activities and contains the largest cities in the country, such as Rio de Janeiro and São Paulo. The South also has a large population density and enjoys relatively high living standards.

DOI: 10.4324/9781003051862-59

In sum, regional differences impact the cultural, economic, and social environment, and a range of ways of life can be observed among Brazilians as a result.

History and Language

Brazil was a Portuguese colony for several centuries and independence was achieved in 1822. It is the only Latin American country where Portuguese is spoken and considered the official language. However, we have states with co-official languages that are taught at some public schools such as in the state of Amazonas, where several indigenous traditions are observed. Brazilians use Portuguese for common communication, but bilingualism is common in certain regions where indigenous populations and immigrants are settled. The school system (private and public) teaches Portuguese in all levels of education and English or Spanish as a second language in most high schools. Brazil's economic history was based on agriculture (sugarcane and coffee, mainly) and cattle farming, with slavery being abolished only in 1888. Structural transformations began in the 1930s with political and economic changes leading to the industrialization of the southern regions. Racial issues related to indigenous groups and descendants of African slaves remain an important struggle today.

Immigration and Relocation

Brazil has a long history of immigration, especially from Europe, the Middle East, and Japan. Brazil has foreign-born people legally living in its territory from across all continents and immigration from neighboring countries is frequent. Therefore, Brazil is a very ethnically diverse country, with cultural influences from all over the world.

Since the severe economic crisis of the 1980s, Brazilians have initiated an emigration flow to the United States, Paraguay, Japan, and European countries that previously had large numbers of immigrants settling in Brazil, such as Portugal, Spain, and Italy. Brazilians differ from other Latin American immigrants as they tend to present a higher level of education when they move abroad. In the United States, the most frequent destination, cities like Boston and Atlanta have a large Brazilian community. Paraguay is the second most frequent destination, as this country offers several incentives for farmers to immigrate. Japan is another popular country, especially for Japanese descendants up to third generation, who can get a working visa according to this country's law. Moreover, several European countries also permit children and grandchildren of past immigrants to obtain passports. Many Brazilian descendants of European immigrants are allowed to reside and work in such countries and in the European Union generally.

People

Brazilians are considered hospitable and friendly people who approach life in a positive way and with a sense of humor. Family life is a major aspect of our culture. It is very common to keep close contact with one's extended family and social gatherings are frequent among families. Most Brazilians work 45 hours a week and, if regularly employed, they have 30 days of paid vacation. As we have a large coast, family leisure time in coastal cities and communities usually is related to beach sports and activities. Families living in small cities away from the coast enjoy fishing in our several rivers, hiking, and picnics in the park. Soccer is the greatest Brazilian passion, regardless of social class and educational level. Brazilians celebrate many traditional dates, most of them linked to Catholic traditions. The most well-known celebration is Carnival, a popular holiday with street parties, costumes, and songs. Christmas and New Year's Eve are other occasions largely celebrated by Brazilians.

Communication

Brazilians, in general, have an informal communication style. The use of first names to refer to people socially, including in work environments, is frequent. Most Brazilians include non-verbal gestures and facial expressions to enhance or focus on a specific part of the content communicated. Therefore, observing *how* the Brazilian client communicates and not only *what* is said can be an important source of information. Communication within family and friends usually includes affectionate nicknames and some body contact. So, it is not uncommon to observe Brazilians hugging and kissing on the cheek when greeting. Gender boundaries vary considerably according to social and educational background. Handshaking is common in a professional environment, especially in the initial contact. After the COVID-19 pandemic, this practice might become more restricted but the average Brazilian enjoys social contact and physical proximity as a demonstration of affection and friendship.

There are some remarkable generational differences concerning professional and public communication. Brazilians over 45 years of age tend to be more formal, respectful, and indirect when communicating with authority figures (boss, medical staff, and teachers). Sometimes to avoid confrontation, they would not answer with a "no" as it could be interpreted as harsh and unpolite, so Brazilians would prefer more vague responses (e.g., "I am not sure…"). However, young generations from urban environments can show a more direct communication style and not adopt formal titles (e.g., Dr., Sir/Madam, Mr./Mrs). Neither age group would argue with a health professional nor seek additional understanding about a recommendation or prescription and, after the consultation, they would simply not follow up on these recommendations. To facilitate that Brazilian clients be more open about their disagreements and concerns, I ask them what they understood from the conversation and what they think about my ideas. This can open a more direct conversation as I show I am concerned about the client's opinion and understanding.

Portuguese spoken in Brazil has different accents, vocabulary, and expressions compared to the language spoken in Portugal or other former colonies. When using an interpreter or translator, it would be better to make sure this issue is clear.

Education

Brazil has an extensive public education system and it is mandatory to attend school until the child is 17 years old, though this is not regularly reinforced. Dropout rates tend to rise during high school. In 2019, it was estimated that 46.6% of people 25 years old and over had completed middle school, 27.4% had finished high school and only 17.4% graduated from a university.[1] Most Brazilian immigrants have at least high school degrees, but it is important to investigate not only the number of years in formal education but also if it was accomplished in public or private schools.

The United Nations' 2019 Human Development report indicated that in 2018, the country's expected years of schooling was 15.4 and the mean years of schooling was 7.8 years.[2] As neuropsychological assessment tests require that the educational level be considered while choosing an adequate test battery, clinical neuropsychology practice within the public health and educational systems tends to use instruments that require lower educational levels when compared to the instruments available to use in private practice.

There is a considerable qualitative difference between the public and private school systems in Brazil. When considering basic education up to high school levels, private schools are thought to offer better education standards, but when analyzing higher education, public universities (provided free of charge by the federation or states) generally offer better conditions. The Brazilian federal government organizes every year a nationwide exam, called ENEM, for high school graduates interested in entering university programs. Every university has its own selection process but all of them use the ENEM scores somehow. Though Brazilians value education very much and the job market pays better wages for people who graduated, higher education is pursued mainly by the higher-income classes and not easily accessed by low-income students. Over the past decade, a few "affirmative action" educational policies have been implemented to address this issue and facilitate the inclusion of different students (e.g., racial minorities and lower socio-economic classes) at universities.

Frequently, Brazilian immigrants might give up their previous careers and accept any job available when abroad, expecting to change to better jobs later, but such change seldom occurs. Also, some Brazilians plan to spend a few years abroad and then return to Brazil to open their own business. It would be important to investigate the acculturation process and the initial plan of clients, as the emotional consequences and the changes in the socio-economic status can impact the neuropsychological intervention.

Literacy

In 2019, 6.6% (about 11 million) Brazilians 15 years old or more were illiterate and in the northeast region, these rates were even higher (13.9%).[3] Poverty and illiteracy in the northern part of Brazil are systemic in rural areas and represent a challenge to different political projects. Several adult education programs have been introduced in the public system. In urban areas, illiterate people participate in the country's large informal economy, finding jobs linked to recycling different materials, domestic work, and selling trinkets on the streets.

Since the beginning of the century, the government has implemented a welfare plan to help families with children of school age: each qualifying family receives an amount for each child registered in the school system. This program also has courses and projects to improve parents' professional qualifications.

One important challenge neuropsychologists face in Brazil is to design suitable assessments for this group, as most standard psychological instruments require some basic reading skills. Moreover, due to disparities in formal education levels among states, just considering the number of years of formal education is not enough to identify functional illiterate groups. Especially when working within the public education and health systems, we have to screen literacy skills before planning assessment. A helpful way to identify the actual literacy level would be to ask about reading and writing habits, investigating if the client reads the news, when was the last time a magazine or book was read, and how often the person had to write or read (e.g., a note, a message, a text for work).

Technology literacy or the individual's ability to assess, acquire, and communicate information in a fully digital environment is one potential issue after the pandemic outbreak. Brazilian society is relying more and more on technology. Banks, stores, and the government are investing in digital processes. Brazil has a huge number of mobile phones throughout all social classes. But formal education has not introduced this topic as part of the curriculum in public schools, which leads to a struggle to access reliable ways to learn how to use different technologies. This situation limits access to social participation when considering services, information, and opportunities. Moreover, regarding Brazil's size and the long distances, one has to cover to find health and educational services, telemedicine, and remote education have been an issue even before the COVID-19 pandemic crisis, but these initiatives are still finding a lack of infrastructure (such as internet coverage) that would allow them to reach all regions.

Socio-Economic Status

Brazil's economy has been among the ten largest in the world since the 1990s and it is first in Latin America according to the World Monetary Fund. Brazil has a strong agricultural sector and a growing industry. However, the COVID-19 pandemic represented an enormous challenge to the Brazilian economy as it was still recovering from the 2015/2016 recession. The health policy required to deal with the pandemic and the decline in the external demand of trade partners showed a record contraction. The government has adopted emergency social assistance to protect vulnerable groups, but the impact of lower tax revenues and rise in government expenses weakened the economy and increased the primary deficit. In 2020, the unemployment rate reached the highest rate in the last few years. Currently, the economy is slowly recovering but the services sector, which traditionally has a great number of workers, remains in recession.

In the past 40 years, the Brazilian economy has developed considerably. However, inequalities are still observed. There is still a significant economic gap between northern and southern regions. Inequality in human development is not only about disparities in income and wealth. According to the United Nations' 2019 Human Development report, Brazil's Human Development Index (HDI) value for 2018 was 0.76. This number puts the country in the high human development category by positioning it at 79 out of 189 countries and territories considered in the report.[2] The HDI is considered a measure for evaluating progress in three basic dimensions of human development: a long and healthy life, access to knowledge, and a decent standard of living.

The disparities between rich and poor have increased during the pandemic. We have many people living in slums, both in small and large communities. Sanitation levels are extremely low in the North and Northeast regions. And the Sistema Único de Saúde(SUS), our universal health system, cannot provide efficient basic preventive medical attention to more isolated rural areas in these regions. However, important goals were achieved in the 20th century: vaccination policies were successfully implemented and several diseases were eradicated, infants' mortality rates decreased considerably, and HIV treatment and control policies showed high efficacy.

The public school system provides free meals for all students, but such support might not be enough to prevent malnutrition in preschool and school-aged children. The Brazilian diet is based on rice, beans, and meat or fish (for people who live near the coast or by a river). The investigation of dietary conditions along child development might be an important issue to cover with clients as malnutrition or unhealthy diets can contribute to hypertension and diabetes.

When working with Brazilian clients, regardless of their age, I always investigate their place of birth (country region, rural/urban, etc.), access to the public medical system during childhood, living conditions, and diet. These factors may have affected neurological development, general mental and physical health, and cognitive reserve in different ways. For example, several Brazilians decided to immigrate due to the increasing urban violence in the major cities, growing up in an unsafe environment and having family and friends injured or killed in this type of conflict might influence copying skills and emotional well-being conditions.

Values and Customs

Brazilian culture is diverse and rich in many aspects, but the dominant values are based on Western Christian values and customs (e.g., respect, hospitality, generosity, peace, liberalism, social pluralism, and rationality) due to the influence of European colonization. Particularly, the importance of family support and relationships through different stages of life can reflect on how a successful intervention should be designed. Protocols to include families during assessment and rehabilitation are needed as families usually have a crucial role in clients' quality of life. Regardless of the client's age (children and adults, equally), families should be integrated into as many phases of the intervention as possible. Family psychoeducation is an essential part of the process as it can prevent further social isolation and decrease misconceptions about clients' potentials and limitations. I adopt a "Negotiation Model"[4] that proposes families should learn to adopt a partnership role with the clinician and feel empowered to actively participate in the decision-making process of the treatment and in electing priorities.

Brazilians might offer small gifts to the medical staff to show appreciation and gratitude and it could be considered snobbish not to accept. Especially if the clinician assists the client over a long period of time, such gifts are frequently given on special dates, for example, on Christmas and Easter.

Another issue that could be relevant is the meaning the client and/or the family give to the neuropsychological deficits or disease. The interpretations they create are based on their values (religious, social, and ethical) and usually impact, positively or negatively, the rehabilitation process, so it would be helpful to inquire about this issue. For example, families can interpret a patient's apathy, a well-known sequelae of brain injury, as laziness or lack of interest.

Understanding the different family structures and roles is also helpful. It is not uncommon that the traditional family structure (mother, father, and children) is not present in the Brazilian client's everyday routine. Grandparents, uncles and aunts, cousins or stepparents and siblings can live in the same house. Particularly when the client has immigrated, different social bonds can be built (close friendships and neighbors) and greatly influence the implementation of rehabilitation strategies and procedures in the client's routine, both by enhancing such interventions or sabotaging them. Sometimes the key agents to be included in the intervention planning are not relatives. Therefore, always ask about significant others and people that the patient trusts and don't assume that relatives are the best people to be included in the intervention plan.

As in many other cultures, Brazilians tend to have a different approach to time than people from the United States and the United Kingdom. This might surface during the assessment, as timed tests and activities are viewed as anxiety-provoking and can lead to lower scores. Brazilian culture does not emphasize quick performance as much as precision. At school or at work, delivering tasks quickly is not always a priority. Arriving early in a meeting or appointment can be seen as anxiety, while a ten-minute delay is not something frequently reproachable. Use timed activities only after a good rapport has been established and explain why it would be necessary to study how the client's performance is affected by time restrictions.

Gender and Sexuality

Brazil still is mainly a patriarchal society. Gender roles within families tend to reveal that an adult man is responsible for providing economically for the family, while the woman is the main caretaker. Currently, however, women are getting more years of education and better work positions, several media campaigns have raised the topic of gender equality of rights and opportunities. A few social policies and nongovernmental agencies have promoted some changes in the attitudes, but we have a long way to achieve effective change.

Recently, the Brazilian LGBTQ+ community has made several advances such as same-sex marriage and the inclusion of medical procedures to address specific needs of this group as part of the public health system. Additionally, affirmative actions were implemented in the legislative and justice systems. Political changes and social tolerance also vary greatly across Brazil and depending on families' values and attitudes.

Brazilians tend to display behaviors showing affection and physical connection in public, especially young couples. Sex education is taught in some high schools as a means to prevent discrimination and bullying toward LGBTQ+, sexually transmitted diseases, and adolescent pregnancy. Currently, however, there has been a political movement to review this topic at public schools.

People with several neurological and psychiatric conditions are at risk of having their sexual life disrupted. As a clinical neuropsychologist, I include questions about possible relationship conflicts and sexual life during the initial interview, as this issue directly interferes with quality of life. If I notice that the person is shy to answer the questions, I explain the importance of the rehabilitation plan to understand these aspects but always leave the option to talk about it on a later occasion.

Spirituality and Religion

Religion has a major role in Brazilian history as the Catholic Church actively contributed to political, educational, and social relations since colonial times. Brazil has the largest Catholic population in Latin America and over 80% of the population follows Christian traditions. However, centuries of slavery in Brazil promoted the expansion of African-based religions as part of several states' traditions. Today, they influence behavior, gastronomy, celebrations, and values, and reveal the common religious syncretism among Brazilians.

As Brazil has immigrants from several ethnic backgrounds in different regions, other religions are found depending on where you live. Nevertheless, Brazil has no recent history of large-scale conflicts triggered by religion and as it is illegal to discriminate, people of different religions tend to live together in peace.

The client's religious community might occupy the role of a support system and facilitate social interactions. As social isolation and anxiety are so often found in patients and represent barriers to rehabilitation and quality of life, the clinician should pay close attention to the religious background. The religious community might be a safe environment for building social skills and finding social activities. When adapting to a foreign country, immigrants might find in their religious community networking conditions that improve their acculturation process and, in these cases, including religious activities in the rehabilitation plan or inviting religious leaders to participate in the educational program might be an effective action.

Acculturation and Systemic Barriers

As we consider Brazilian culture and the experience of Brazilian immigration to different countries around the world, it is important to point out that adaptation to the new country is a long-term process that is not limited to objective variables such as speaking a new language correctly, acquiring all the legal papers, finding a job and rebuilding a financial history. This important life transition encompasses nuances of the relation between the native and the host country that might be a barrier for acculturation such as perceived discrimination, cultural identity, intercultural strategies, and emotional coping style.[5] Moreover, immigration often leads to significant changes within family systems, values, and life goals.

Brazilians can be perceived differently around the world; some countries might emphasize the Brazilian festive and extroverted cultural aspects, others might consider the soccer traditions and love for outdoor sports and leisure, and others might focus on the socio-economical and political difficulties in our country often shown by the media. It is crucial that the clinician realize what is their own conception of the Brazilian and consider how it might affect the therapeutic alliance.

I suggest that the clinician first understand the reasons that led to the decision to migrate, what steps were taken to organize the change of countries, the expectations and goals involved in the initial adaptation to the new country, the first experiences and negotiations needed to adapt, and networking strategies. This understanding by itself can give crucial information on the client's social (coworkers, friends, and family), cognitive (organization, planning, self-monitoring, and flexibility), and emotional (anger and frustration, anxiety, depression, and loneliness) profiles. There are some intervention models such as the Holistic Rehabilitation Model and the Ecological Assessment Principles that facilitate the exploration of acculturation aspects and cultural identity.[6]

Health Status

Chronic non-transmissible diseases are responsible for 70% of deaths in Brazil. High cholesterol, hypertension, diabetes, Parkinson's disease, and Alzheimer's disease are among the most frequent causes of death in Brazil. Brazil Public Health System created a program to distribute medication to control diabetes and hypertension free of charge that has succeeded in decreasing hospitalizations and improving the quality of life of low-income elderly people. Since the beginning of this century, Brazil began to prepare new health policies to address the aging of the population with hospitals and preventive programs specifically for people 60 years old and above.

A large number of adolescents' and young adults' deaths in Brazil are related to interpersonal violence and motor vehicle accidents (MVAs). Traumatic brain injuries due to these growing problems are frequently found in this group. Only recently, a protocol was published by the ministry of health with medical guidelines and a registration system to build a database. This fact might improve the epidemiological data in Brazil, and consequently, influence more efficient health policies. Different aspects of urban violence in large Brazilian cities have become a public health problem difficult to solve as it involves several variables.

Brazil has a large road system around the country as well as a considerable number of motor vehicles. An alarming number of MVAs with drivers and pedestrians being injured every year is observed. As in other countries, improvements in emergency medical procedures have increased the survival rates of patients after traumatic brain injury. After hospitalization, however, there is a paucity of community services to follow these patients needing assistance to return to their previous activities such as work and school. Usually, such rehabilitation services are found only in the private sector in Brazil or at public university hospitals in one of the country's major cities.

Mental Health Views

Since the end of the 20th century, mental health public services in Brazil have gradually turned to a community-based approach with small ambulatory units with multi-disciplinary professional staff where patients can have a variety of services including brief psychotherapy and support groups, but a neuropsychologist seldom is part of the team. Mental health services are still scarce and expensive in general and frequently, when patients seek out psychological or psychiatric services, they are already in severe mental distress.

There is a considerable number of "alternative" mental health services provided by people with exoteric traditions and little training, if any. It is almost impossible to restrict this type of services as some of them are deeply linked to cultural traditions and religious beliefs.

Professional associations and certification boards every year design campaigns to disseminate information about important mental health issues like suicide, anxiety, and drug abuse. However, their impact on the general population is difficult to measure. One important issue that the federal health system has consistently tried to solve is rampant self-medication, currently pharmacies have designed a more efficient control over sales of drugs, including psychoactive drugs, and prescriptions are demanded more consistently. "Alternative" medicine and self-medication are so common in Brazil; I explore this topic systematically with clients to understand how they view them and what they have already tried doing before to cope with reported symptoms.

Approach to Neuropsychological Evaluations

Brazilian neuropsychology started in clinical settings such as university hospitals and research laboratories in the 1970s. Several fields contributed to spreading the knowledge of this discipline, but only a few formal training programs existed until the beginning of this century in Brazil. Only in 2004, a national psychology association responsible for giving licenses needed for professional practice recognized neuropsychology as a specialized service in psychology, and only a few professionals have proper training in clinical neuropsychology in Brazil. There still is a paucity of professional training programs. Because such training requires a long period of studies, supervised practice, and more financial resources, the number of qualified neuropsychologists is insufficient.

The national health system does not regularly offer neuropsychological services and only the specialized (neurology and psychiatric) private clinics and hospitals might have neuropsychologists as part of their staff. Usually, when the client is referred to a neuropsychological evaluation, an explanation about the aims and the procedures of such evaluation can improve participation and motivate clients as they expect to have feedback by the end of the process.

Lately, several cognitive assessment and training tools using different equipment and technology have been translated and published in Brazil; nevertheless, many of these tools have not been properly culturally adapted and investigated in their psychometric characteristics and efficacy in our cultural context. So before using any electronic tool, it would be advised to make sure the clients use that type of technology in their daily life.

Psychologists have to observe some restrictions while using neuropsychological testing as the professional has to choose from a list of certified tests. This online list, called SATEPSI, has been published and updated by the national professional association according to the test's psychometric characteristics.[7] This was an initiative to facilitate that psychologists use only validated and normed tests and, consequently, improve assessment interpretations and ethical practice. Several research endeavors to develop and to adapt neuropsychological tests and activities appropriate to Brazilian culture and to develop normative data to guide interpretation have been published, but there are still limited tests from which to choose and sometimes we have to rely on clinical judgment only.

Section II: Case Study — "How Can I Say Thanks for My Family Support While Telling Them Goodbye?"

The following case is an example of a 31-year-old single man who sought services after a traumatic brain injury (TBI) following a motorcycle accident and received services from both private practices and a public university service. The client's family sought neuropsychological assistance in order to outline the client's cognitive and emotional functioning for the purpose of starting a rehabilitation program one year after the accident. After initial hospitalization, Mr. Silva (pseudonym) was treated at the Center for Rehabilitation and Interdisciplinary Studies of the Federal University of Paraná (CEREI-UFPR). Treatment consisted of participation in cognitive rehabilitation groups, psychotherapy, and systematic family orientations. Other health services such as occupational therapy, physical education, and neurology were received from private practice elsewhere. Cognitive rehabilitation focused on the functions of attention, perception, memory, and executive function, and intended to introduce compensatory strategies in the client's daily life. In the initial interview, the patient's mother and one of his sisters, who was a physician, were the major source of information about the accident and the long hospitalization process that followed. The following information was gathered during the intake assessment interviews both with family members and the patient as he presented a severe memory problem at that time.

Behavioral Observations

Mr. Silva arrived on time for all assessment sessions and was very cooperative. He showed a high level of dependency on his family while answering the questions and trying to remember major life facts such as the name of his last employer, his current address, and details about his routine.

At times, he would present superficial awareness of his dependence and frustration by often complaining about his cognitive limitations and self-deprecating about his performance. He was always very polite and we built good rapport from the beginning. His major expectation was to return to work in the same position as before the accident. I explained how the rehabilitation process works and the aim of the initial neuropsychological assessment as well as how difficult it would be to make predictions during its initial stages as there were many factors involved in the process. It is very important to prepare the patient for the usually long rehabilitation period while acknowledging his expectations and goals as sources of motivation. During the testing sessions, he reported that he was used to participating in evaluations and testing and very knowledgeable in computerized and mobile phone resources. We had to keep assessment sessions shorter than usual as he reported mental fatigue after 40 minutes of cognitive testing. He was very engaged with the tasks and seemed to like the challenge offered by some of them, particularly the executive functions instruments.

Main Concerns

Initially, Mr. Silva only had a vague idea of the major changes in his life since his TBI and could not give examples of the activities in which he had difficulties or the strategies he had developed to deal with such difficulties. At that point, I considered the family's concerns as starting points to investigate the client's thoughts and emotions toward them. The family reported several attentional and memory deficits, some communication difficulties, and perseverative behaviors. I informally would ask Mr. Silva about a situation reported by his mother, for example, and waited to have his impressions. It soon became clear that he did not realize how deeply affected his mother, his major caregiver, was by his current limitations. I hypothesized that the family members actively tried to minimize his difficulties to spare him of further distress. This is a common reaction of Brazilian families and, though in the first months just after a brain injury, it could be a good strategy to diminish patient's anxiety, as the recovery progresses, a patient's awareness of his/her neuropsychological problems enhances rehabilitation program participation. Therefore, I began periodical family sessions to guide when and how these feedback could be provided to Mr. Silva.

Daily Functioning

Mr. Silva has lived independently in his own apartment since graduation. In Brazilian families, it is common that children just leave their parents' house after getting married. Brazilian men seldom know basic house chores, such as cooking and cleaning, independently of social class. Mr. Silva, before the accident, used to live alone and did all housekeeping tasks, however, after the accident, he moved to his parents' apartment. Both parents would "take care of everything": from getting him a glass of water to helping with his financial organization. During family orientation, the need to let the client try to do daily activities and regain some organizational skills with gradual independence was introduced as a first goal. A workbook teaching how to introduce and guide step-by-step house chores and a plan were developed with the assistance of an occupational therapist and were given to the client and his family.

Health History

Mr. Silva was a young and healthy man who did not smoke nor reported any health concern before the motorcycle accident. He sustained a severe left frontotemporal injury, a diffuse axonal injury was also diagnosed, and the emergency rescue reported a score of 3/15 at the Glasgow Coma Scale. The accident happened when he was working abroad. He was hospitalized for two months and presented with post-traumatic amnesia when he awoke from coma. His family in Brazil was informed about the accident and, immediately, traveled to the foreign country. His parents stayed the entire hospitalization time with him and when the patient was well enough to travel, they moved back to Brazil for the long-term treatment.

His accident happened when he was going to work and he was sober. In Brazil, the majority of MVAs are related to alcohol and drug abuse, so it is always advisable to include questions about this topic to understand precisely what the client's habits are. Mr. Silva did report frequently drinking at weekend parties. At the time of the initial interviews, his friends would invite him to go out, but as he knew he could not drink, he preferred to stay home.

During the initial interview, he reported sleeping eight to nine hours daily. After TBI, he had one convulsive epileptic episode and anti-convulsant medication was introduced. Moreover, he had visual problems that led to double vision and some reduced acuity which were surgically corrected after the first year in CEREI. Visual limitations should be considered when choosing assessment tools. He had a personal trainer to guide regular physical activities.

Work and Educational History

Mr. Silva reported an impeccable educational history: he was always one of the best students in his class and entered university without difficulties. He had a master's degree in science when he got his first job. He learned English as a second language during his teenage years, which allowed him to work for multinational corporations. Mr. Silva was a successful professional in his field and had worked in several foreign countries. At the time of the accident, he was working in an English-speaking country for two years. He was a team supervisor and his position required field and administrative tasks.

Language Proficiency

Portuguese was Mr. Silva's native language, but he was fluent in English. As part of his work, he wrote reports and documents in English frequently. During one of the final sessions of the assessment, I tried to have an English conversation with Mr. Silva, and he seemed able to understand part of the instructions but did not respond orally to any question. This suggested that only some aspects of these previously fluent language skills remained.

On the other hand, according to Mr. Silva's family, he was still able to speak, to write, and to read Portuguese correctly. I observed that he had problems maintaining a dialog when the topic required to deepen the information and build arguments. For example, I asked him to describe any of his work routines or even to give his opinion about a well-discussed topic such as minimum wages, but he could not elaborate even after reading a text about these topics. Moreover, there were times that he had difficulties answering objective questions, attending to details, and being tangential.

Brazil does not have standardized tests in several specific areas, including certain language domains. The clinician should often create tasks and questions linked to the client's history and interests to check skills and use clinical observation skills. Due to his pre-morbid high educational level and foreign language knowledge, I included a series of activities to address Portuguese languages' abilities (a diary, read news sites daily and write a summary).

Cultural History

Mr. Silva was the family's only male child; he had two adult married sisters and had small children. At the time of the accident, he was living in a foreign country, and the family arranged for

Mr. Silva to return home to his native city in the south of Brazil as soon as he was able to travel. His sister, who was a physician, helped the communication with hospital staff and the treatment decision-making process.

His family was the second generation of Italian immigrants and his parents valued education and expected all children to graduate from a university. They were a middle-class family; his father worked for the government and his mother a homemaker. His father and sisters helped with specific treatment recommendations, but as it is common in Brazil, his mother was his main caregiver. His mother recognized that sometimes she could not avoid treating him as a teenager, and frequently, she would struggle to find a balance between taking care of her own needs and her son's.

While working abroad, Mr. Silva would return to Brazil three to four times a year on special occasions but he reported that his family did not know much about his daily life. When he visited, he would go out with old friends to celebrate but he considered himself a tourist in his own country. After the MVA, he returned to live with his parents. They re-established a similar relationship to the one they had when Mr. Silva was still at the university. His parents would control and have strict rules. Mr. Silva was grateful for his parents' assistance and dedication but had difficulties creating clear boundaries and showing responsibility, partly because he was afraid to offend his parents by gaining his independence again and partly because he was insecure about his actual abilities and autonomy. This is a common situation within Brazilian families as they feel obligated to participate in the rehabilitation process and, seldom, hire a professional caretaker. Patients as well as family members often find themselves in a challenging predicament of knowing when and how to gradually reduce supports and to facilitate a patient's independence again. Neuropsychologists could have a primary role in pointing out these moments of dependency and assist in establishing greater independence and in generating social participation without exposing the patient to embarrassing situations.

Emotional Functioning

According to his parents, as soon as Mr. Silva started to recover some level of self-awareness about his physical and cognitive functioning, he began to have outbursts where he "reacted irritably and with tantrums." Emotional turbulence is frequently reported, and anxiety and depressive symptoms as well as anger and aggressive outbursts are common. As Brazilians are used to showing their feelings freely, family and friends are tolerant toward these feelings initially and, usually, very reluctant to search for psychological or psychiatric assistance. In the present case, as soon as the client showed better awareness of his emotional instability while in CEREI, he began a psychotherapeutic intervention which included anger management strategies. In terms of personality after injury, Mr. Silva usually presented himself as a friendly and funny person, always striving to be as cordial and appropriate as possible, a characteristic observed through his contact and interaction with staff and patients working group.

Preliminary Formulation

In summary, initial sessions with family and the client indicated that the client had a severe TBI with many cognitive, emotional, and social consequences. Cognitively, the major complaints related to attentional and memory skills. Emotionally, the family would recognize some anger outbursts, lower self-esteem issues, and I also observed certain dependency issues facilitated by the family relations. Socially, Mr. Silva had an extensive social network with family and friends willing to participate in his recovery, but he had difficulty to sharing his needs and limitations and the necessary changes after TBI.

Test and Norm Selection

I adopt an ecological assessment approach that recommends the evaluation of the client's behavior and skills in different contexts and always includes the perspectives of significant others. So besides extensive interviews with the client and his family, I gave them questionnaires about the client's cognitive and emotional aspects to be filled and discussed during interviews. The test battery consisted of tests adapted and standardized to Brazilian Portuguese. I administered the following tests:

1 WAIS III—Escala de Inteligência Wechsler para Adultos.[8]
2 Rey Auditory Verbal Learning Test.[9]
3 Rey Complex Figure Test.[10]
4 Trail Making Test.[11]
5 Five Digits Test[12]
6 Verbal Fluency Test.[13]
7 Category Fluency Test.[14]
8 Attention Psychological Battery—Bateria Psicológica da Atenção—BPA.[15]
9 Wisconsin Card Sort Test.[16]
10 Beck Depression Scale.[17]
11 Beck Anxiety Scale.[18]
12 Patient Competency Rating Scale.[19]

Test Results and Impressions

The data presented below are derived from clinical observation during consultations, interviews with the client's mother, main caregiver, a battery of neuropsychological tests and questionnaires.

The client was cooperative during all the evaluation sessions and seemed committed to carrying out the tasks presented. Mr. Silva has an intellectual level within the average range when compared to his age group. On measures of attention (selective, sustained, alternating, and divided), he presented scores below two standard deviations according to Brazilian norms. This score indicated that the client had severe difficulties performing attentional tasks. In a visual perception task, the client presented adequate performance both in visual scanning and in the formation of gestalts.

Visual and verbal memory and learning were significantly reduced. In visual memory tasks, he was able to retain about 50% of the relevant details of a figure after a delay. On a verbal memory test, the client retained 10% of the information presented verbally after a long-term delay. The client required several repetitions to improve learning and distracting stimuli interfered considerably with its performance.

It was observed that working memory performance was within the average range. Information processing speed and fine motor coordination were deficient. His cognitive flexibility was within the average range. The client required a long period of time to make decisions and implement behavioral changes in the face of new circumstances. Other components of his executive functions, such as his ability to organize and monitor his actions were preserved. Mr. Silva seemed to become increasingly aware of his deficits and difficulties during the assessment.

His behavior reflected a certain emotional dependence and insecurity, especially when compared to his pre-morbid characteristics when he already had complete independence from his family and an extensive social life. Another important factor that probably interfered with his cognitive performance was his level of anxiety, which proved to be high. It would be possible to conjecture that emotional factors are negatively affecting his ability to solve social problems and face situations of frustration, however, there was no trend toward social isolation or socially inappropriate behavior.

Feedback Session and Follow-Up

Feedback sessions and a written report were provided for the client and then to his family. I initially asked their impressions about the assessment process and explored if there were any changes in their perceptions. Later, I explained the major findings. Attentional and memory functions were his major difficulties within the neuropsychological domains. Considering Mr. Silva's academic background and professional experience, there was a serious impairment of his cognitive functions and emotional instability with difficulties in dealing with situations of frustration. Although cognitive and behavioral gains were observed by the client's team and family, returning to pre-morbid work and the social activities were not possible at that time. I introduced the idea of cognitive reserve and pointed out that Mr. Silva could build compensatory strategies and successfully regain independence after rehabilitation. But at that time, it was important to begin his neuropsychological rehabilitation process even if he still had physical issues to deal with such as his visual and balance problems.

After explaining the neuropsychological test results, priorities and a few rehabilitation goals were established in collaboration with Mr. Silva and his family. The long-term goal remained to return to work adequate to his new condition but we agreed that such job position should be in Brazil. Then we established smaller steps to be achieved along the first year of rehabilitation. I referred him to an occupational therapist and a speech and language therapist to assist with some of the difficulties observed. After that feedback session, family orientation sessions were held and Mr. Silva started his participation in the neuropsychological rehabilitation group. Every semester, we met to review his goals and evaluate possible changes in the plan.

Section III: Lessons Learned

- Brazil is the only Latin American country that speaks Portuguese, and this fact led to a unique cultural situation in the continent despite its rich immigration history.
- Brazilian immigrants usually have high school degrees and some work history but after moving to foreign countries, they usually are forced to take jobs that demand lower educational levels.
- It is very common that Brazilians plan to return to Brazil after a few years with improved financial resources to open their own business. That initial plan is often postponed and this can be a source of frustration and sometimes even shame.
- Brazilians value social relationships and taking time to establish a strong rapport based on trust in the clinician professional training and willingness to help is essential to facilitate treatment participation and long-term interventions.
- Portuguese is spoken in different countries, so it is important that the interpreter/translator knows Brazilian Portuguese to avoid misunderstandings.
- Literacy level and familiarity with technology should be carefully assessed as usually only knowing the number of years of formal education is not enough to evaluate these skills.
- As Brazil has a continental dimension with a variety of cultural traditions, it is always suggested that this information be explored as a source of socio-economic information and developmental issues.
- Brazilians usually value a family-centered lifestyle and hospitality. Including family in the rehabilitation, planning can be a central pillar of a successful process.

- A relaxed sense of time and informal relationship rules are common.
- Assessment of immigration history and their plans and expectations might give some insight on the meaning of current facts and life situations.
- As neuropsychologists are rare in Brazil, information about services and their possible benefits can promote client's engagement. Family should always be included in assessment and rehabilitation.
- Explanations about medical conditions and possible treatments in a simple language have a central role in promoting family and client active participation. Validation of their feelings and assessing their fears can increase their trust in professional abilities and avoid misunderstandings.
- When making referrals, first present a work frame/case formulation and then articulate the reasons for including other professionals or treatments.
- There is a paucity of reliable neuropsychological tests published, and the SATEPSI list is the best resource to find them. But clinical observations and a functional perspective can be crucial while planning assessment sessions.

References

1. Organisation for Economic Co-operation and Development—OECD [Internet]. 2021. Available from: https://gpseducation.oecd.org/CountryProfile?primaryCountry=BRA&treshold=10&topic=EO [Accessed 8th January 2021].
2. World Health Organization. Country Cooperation Strategy [Internet]. Available from: https://www.who.int/publications/i/item/WHO-CCO-18.02-Brazil [Accessed 8th January 2021].
3. Empresa Brasileira de Comunicação [Internet]. 2020. Available from: https://agenciabrasil.ebc.com.br/en/educacao/noticia/2020-07/brazil-illiteracy-wane-11-mi-still-cannot-read-or-write [Accessed 8th January 2021].
4. Dale N. Working with families of children with special needs. 1st ed. New York (NY): Routledge; 1996.
5. Neto J, Oliveira EM, Neto F. Acculturation, adaptation and loneliness among Brazilian migrants living in Portugal [Internet]. IntechOpen; 2017. Available from: https://www.intechopen.com/chapters/52690
6. Pereira AP, Fish J, Maley D, Bateman A. The importance of culture in holistic neuropsychological rehabilitation: suggestions for improving cultural competence. In: Wilson BA, Winegardner J, Van Heugten CM, Ownsworth T, editors. Neuropsychological rehabilitation: International Handbook. 1st ed. New York (NY): Routledge; 2017.
7. Conselho Federal de Psicologia. SATEPSI [Internet]. Available from: https://satepsi.cfp.org.br/ [Accessed 8th January 2021].
8. Nascimento E. Escala de Inteligência Wechsler para Adultos—WAIS. São Paulo: Pearson; 1997.
9. Malloy-Diz LF, de Paula JJ. Teste de Aprendizagem Auditivo-Verbal de Rey (Rey Auditory Verbal Learning Test). São Paulo: Vetor; 2019.
10. Oliveira MS, Rigoni MS. Teste de Cópia e de Reprodução de Memória de Figuras Geométricas Complexas (Rey Complex Figure Test). São Paulo: Vetor; 2010.
11. Zimmermann N, Cardoso CO, Kristensen CH, Fonseca RP. Brazilian norms and effects of age and education on the Hayling and Trail Making Tests. Trends Psychiatry Psychother [Internet]. 2017;39(3):188–95. Available from: http://dx.doi.org/10.1590/2237-6089-2016-0082
12. Sedó M, de Paula JJ, Malloy-Diniz LF. Teste dos Cinco Digitos (Five Digit Test). São Paulo: Hogrefe; 2015.
13. Rodrigues AB, Yamashita ET, Chiappetta ALML. Teste de Fluência Verbal no Adulto e no Idoso: Verificação da Aprendizagem Verbal (Verbal Fluency Test in adult and elderly: verification of verbal learning). Rev CEFAC, São Paulo. 2008 out–dez;10(4):443–51.
14. Passos VMA, Giatti L, Barreto SM, Figueiredo RC, Caramelli P, Benseñor I et al. Article Verbal fluency tests reliability in a Brazilian multicentric study, ELSA-Brasil; Arq Neuropsiquiatr. 2011;69(5):814–6.

15. Rueda FJM. Bateria Psicológica para Avaliação da Atenção—BPA. São Paulo: Vetor; 2013.
16. Cunha JA, Trentini CM, Argimon IL, Oliveira MS, Werlang BG, Prieb RG. Testes de Wisconsin de Classificação de Cartas (Wisconsin Card Sorting Test). São Paulo: Caso do Psicólogo; 2005.
17. Werlang BSG, Gorenstein C, Argimon IIL, Wang YP. Escala de Depressão de Beck (Beck Depression Scale). São Paulo: CASAPSI; 2010.
18. Quintao S, Delgado AR, Prieto, G. Validity study of the Beck Anxiety Inventory (Portuguese version) by the Rasch Rating Scale model. Psicol. Reflex. Crit [Internet]. 2013;26(2):305–10. Available from: https://doi.org/10.1590/S0102-79722013000200010
19. Zimmermann N, Pereira APA, Fonseca, RP. Brazilian Portuguese version of the Patient Competency Rating Scale (PCRS-R-BR): semantic adaptation and validity. Trends Psychiatry Psychother [Internet]. 2014;36(1):40–51. Available from: http://dx.doi.org/10.1590/2237-6089-2013-0021

Colombian

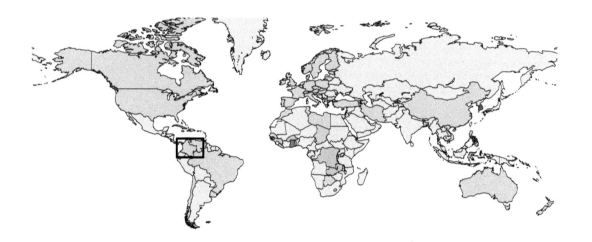

30 Diagnostic Challenges in Remote Communities from Colombia

A Case Study of a Patient with CADASIL

Lina Velilla-Jiménez, Dorothee Schoemaker, Diana Múnera, Joseph Arboleda-Velásquez, Francisco Lopera, and Yakeel T. Quiroz

Section I: Background Information

Terminology and Perspective

People from Colombia are referred to as Colombian, while Colombians who were born and raised in the Departments of Antioquia, Caldas, and Quindío are called Paisas. We will use the words Paisa and Colombian throughout to describe cultural, social, and historical perspectives of the Paisa culture and their relationships to clinical neuropsychology in the region of Antioquia in Colombia.

The first and senior authors are Paisa neuropsychologists trained in Colombia and the United States. The first author currently conducts clinical research and neuropsychological assessments of patients with neurodegenerative diseases at the Group of Neuroscience of Antioquia (GNA) in Colombia. The senior author leads a longitudinal biomarker study of paisa families with familial Alzheimer's disease in Boston, Massachusetts.

In this chapter, we will share the story of Roberto,[1] originally from the mountains of Antioquia, Colombia. He first showed behavioral changes at age 40 including loss of motivation and sadness. He referred to himself as "a plague" to express feelings of inferiority and low self-esteem in the context of neuropsychiatric symptoms for which he was diagnosed with bipolar disorder (BD). After five years into treatment for those behavioral and mood changes, Roberto and his wife did not observe significant improvements and the differential diagnosis began to include multiple sclerosis (MS). Ultimately, cerebral autosomal-dominant arteriopathy with subcortical infarcts and leukoencephalopathy (CADASIL) was diagnosed. Through Roberto's case, we will highlight the link between relevant clinical/cognitive and cultural/historic aspects uniquely inherent in the Antiochian culture, which can make a difference in the approach used to determine accurate differential diagnoses.

Geography

The Republic of Colombia is a northwestern South American country. It is bordered by Panama, Venezuela, Brazil, Ecuador, and Peru. The Department of Antioquia is located in northwestern Colombia, in South America, with coastal areas stretching to both the Atlantic and Pacific Oceans. Its landscape is characterized by a mix of valleys and mountains, with altitudes reaching up to 4,000 meters. The territory of Antioquia presents a great diversity of ecosystems, from coastal plains, dry and deep forests, and Andean forests, to the high mountains of the central and Western mountain ranges. A network of rivers irrigates these ecosystems connecting the highlands and lowlands. The geological changes implicated in the evolution of the Antioquia ecosystem led to a concentration

DOI: 10.4324/9781003051862-61

of gold. The geographical features of Antioquia's territory are deeply connected to the mining tradition and social, economic, and cultural aspects.[2] Antioquia encompasses both urban and rural communities, with nearly a quarter of the population living in rural or remote areas.[1]

History

The term "Paisa culture" has been widely used in Colombia to refer to the values, customs, and history of Antioqueños.[1] Colombia is a diverse country with each region and sub-region within the country having different customs, ethnicities, accents, and cultural anchors. The characteristic diversity of Colombia is rooted in its history of Spanish colonizing missions. These were decisive in the socio-geographic divisions of the country and because of them some sub-regions experienced stronger racial segregation while others had greater ethnic and racial admixture with subsequently different processes of socioeconomic development.[2] Specifically, during the first decade of the XVI century, Antioquia faced invasive colonization by Spanish conquerors and during the 16th and 17th centuries, the Antioquia population grew by the admixture of Antioquia natives and Spanish colonists. Since its population is mainly expanded by internal growth, Antioquia is considered genetically isolated and presents a relatively high prevalence of genetic diseases.[3] In addition, since the Antioquia population especially experienced greater isolation and a movement toward internal colonization, this also impacted the configuration of the political and economic history of the entire country.[4] The ethnic segregation that happened during the colonization helps to understand the highly genetically based components of neuropsychiatric clinical conditions prevalent in Antioquia and highlights the importance of paying attention to family history and genealogy in clinical conditions in those from Antioquia.

People

When evaluating behavioral and emotional changes among Colombians, Paisas, and Latinos is always important to account for unique cultural backgrounds. Frequently, behavioral scales are designed from Western cultural standards, which might not fit into Latin American socially accepted behaviors. Even more, it is not possible to have a homogenous cultural code or standard among Colombians due to each geographic region in the country having unique cultural parameters and characteristics.[5]

In our case, we will observe how Roberto initially started to present himself as someone very concerned about cleaning and became quieter and more reluctant to socially share. These behaviors can be concerning for someone who used to be socially engaged and belongs to a cultural region generally known for being very social, open, talkative, and welcoming.[4] This highlights the importance of performing deep clinical interviews together with administering behavioral scales to compare personality changes against pre-morbid personality traits and in the context of generally accepted social standards.[6]

Language and Communication

Colombians have Spanish as the main and official language.[7] The remaining indigenous communities in Colombia are bilingual and can communicate fluently in both Spanish and their dialect. It is worth knowing that Colombia is known for its extensive diversity of idioms according to the geographical region. Thus, it is necessary for a neuropsychologist evaluating Colombians to be aware that there are many different words available to name things. For example, when patients perform semantic fluency tests (fruits and animal), it is suggested to perform an exhaustive search using a thesaurus to ensure correct scoring. Rural patients, in particular, are likely to use frequent expositions to elements of nature and produce lots of names of animals and fruits that may be unknown to an urban neuropsychologist.[8,9] Similarly, it is important to pay attention to the need to allow a range of words on naming tests due to the large number of different words that can be used to name objects across regions in Colombia.[10] On the other hand, when evaluating phonemic fluency using F, A, S letters, it is important to consider that this may introduce bias among Spanish-speaking populations since those particular letters are based on the frequency of words in English.[11]

Education and Socioeconomic Status

The Colombian education system includes elementary, secondary (including high school), and graduate schooling. Elementary education consists of five years, and secondary education takes an additional six years.[12] When someone from Colombia completes basic education (elementary and secondary), that person has a total of 11 years of education. Regarding economics, Colombia is classified as an upper-middle-income country. However, a considerable proportion (i.e., 14%) of Antioquia's population lives below the poverty line and reports unsatisfied basic needs. Most of the underserved people in Antioquia live in rural areas or segregated areas of urban centers.[13]

Education and socioeconomic background are important considerations for cognitive evaluations and behavioral analysis. The clinical case we are sharing was evaluated using norms according to the patient's education, and exploration of his neuropsychiatric symptoms was oriented to his socio-cultural background. These are important considerations when evaluating people from Colombia since socially accepted behaviors, habits, and customs may change according to socioeconomic influences.

Health Status

Patients in Antioquia face significant geopolitical and socioeconomic barriers to the diagnosis and treatment of neurological and neurocognitive disorders. This includes reduced access to differentiated healthcare services, long wait times, limited follow-ups, incomplete medical records, unreliable disease coding systems, and others.[14] We will see those conditions reflected in Roberto's case since he spent several years without an accurate diagnosis and received suboptimal medical treatment.

As noted, Antioquia has a genetic kindred of neurodegenerative and psychiatrist diseases including the biggest family groups in the world with early-onset Alzheimer's disease,[15] a family group with CADASIL,[16] a family cluster of BD[17] and attention deficit hyperactivity disorder.[18] Therefore, within the context of Antioquia's history, it is very important to perform a complete genealogy when a patient complains about cognitive, behavioral, and emotional disturbances. We will show later in the case how the family history of our patient was key to elucidate the differential diagnosis.

Approach to Neuropsychological Evaluations

The neuropsychological evaluation of Paisas comes with its challenges. Spanish translations of neuropsychological tests are not always available or adapted to the linguistic and cultural characteristics of Antioquia's population. Due to socioeconomic constraints and scarce resources for funding, it has been widely difficult in Latin American to conduct research to validate and culturally adapt cognitive tools. The scarcity of normative data and validated cognitive tools in Latin America often leads researchers to use normative data derived from other Spanish-speaking countries. However, this may not appropriately reflect the sociodemographic features of specific regions, including different levels of educational and occupational attainment.

Recognizing the importance of culturally appropriate cognitive assessment, our group has engaged in efforts to adapt and validate common neuropsychological tests for the evaluation of neurocognitive disorders in Antioquia's patient population. This has included tests from the Consortium to Establish a Registry for Alzheimer's Disease (CERAD) neuropsychological battery[19] and the Face-Name Associative Memory Exam (FNAME).[20] We also recently published comprehensive population-based normative data stratified by age and education for specific use in Colombian patients, thereby significantly improving our abilities to interpret results from neuropsychological tests in patients from Colombia.[21]

In addition, for more than 30 years, the Group of Neuroscience of Antioquia (GNA) has followed large extended families with genetic mutations leading to neurodegenerative diseases. The GNA is a multidisciplinary team that includes neurologists, psychiatrists, family medicine physicians, nurses, gerontologists, speech therapists, clinical psychologists, and neuropsychologists. From the beginning, the GNA has sent clinical and research teams to rural areas in Antioquia to facilitate access to evaluation, diagnosis, and research participation for individuals living in remote areas.

Over the years, the GNA has established a registry of these extended families with genetic mutations leading to neurodegenerative diseases. Our registry regroups individuals presenting with and without cognitive or neurological symptoms. Upon enrollment, every patient completes a comprehensive evaluation of their family history. The investigation of family history and family trees is especially relevant in this context to assist with the identification of possible inheritance patterns among relatives across generations. Patients also undergo comprehensive neurological and neuropsychological evaluations. After the initial evaluation, members of our team meet to discuss findings, propose a probable diagnosis, and establish a treatment plan. The longitudinal follow-up of patients enrolled in the registry is another important aspect of the GNA's framework. This allows the careful monitoring of disease progression and appropriate adjustment of the clinical management plan. In addition to building a rich dataset for clinical research, enrollment in this program provides families with access to annual medical and cognitive evaluations. Since most members of these families live in rural areas of Antioquia, these services would otherwise often not be available to them.

One of the cohorts we have been following at the GNA includes individuals from large families with mutations in the *NOTCH3* gene leading to a neurodegenerative condition known as (CADASIL).[22] We have identified and enrolled over 200 subjects with CADASIL, due to R1031C, C455R, and R141C mutations in the *NOTCH3* gene, in our registry.[23] Individuals with CADASIL develop cerebral small vessel disease at a young age and are prone to suffer from recurrent ischemic strokes and vascular dementia at a young age.[24] CADASIL is a low prevalence syndrome and a rare disease, leading to frequent misdiagnosis, especially in non-specialized settings.[25]

Section II: Case Study — "When the Clinical History Is Bewildering, the Family History Enlightens"

Roberto was a 49-year-old man who was born and raised in Antioquia, Colombia. He was married with no children and lived with his wife in the city of Medellin-Antioquia. He completed 11 years of formal education, which is the equivalent of a high school degree in Colombia. His developmental history was unremarkable, and he showed no evidence of learning difficulties. He held different occupations throughout his life, such as taxi driver, security guard, and bicycle mechanic, but had been retired since 2015. In Colombia, the typical retirement age is 57 for women and 62 for men. However, a person that is disabled due to a job injury or a chronic medical condition can qualify for retirement at a younger age.

Roberto was first seen at the GNA in 2017, accompanied by his wife, because of a history of progressing behavioral changes. He was seen again approximately two years later, in early 2020, for a follow-up neuropsychological evaluation. Since the GNA follows the population for several years, it is often possible to have a detailed history of disease evolution from baseline until the last outcomes. However, this is not true more broadly in Colombia or Latin America, where due to difficulties accessing health care and specialized medical providers, it is hard for patients to receive longer-term follow-ups.

History of Presenting Symptoms

A detailed interview with Roberto and his wife, together with a review of his medical chart, suggested that initial behavioral changes occurred approximately eight years ago (2009) when he was 41, and consisted of mainly significant mood disturbances. He started presenting with emotional lability (uncontrollable crying), auditory hallucinations (hearing voices encouraging him to hit someone or throw himself off the window), increased irritability, and aggressiveness toward himself and others. His wife further reported compulsion with cleaning and explained that he cleans the house up to three times a day. She described an episode during which her husband was found cleaning the bathroom at a friend's house during a visit. These symptoms were a marked departure from his pre-morbid status. After consulting with a private psychiatrist, he was diagnosed with BD and started to receive treatment with a mood stabilizer (Lithium) and antidepressants (sertraline, and later escitalopram).

In 2014, despite remission of psychotic symptoms, there was no significant improvement in psychoactive symptoms, and he showed increasing irritability, impulsivity, and anhedonia. His wife also noticed that he was experiencing difficulties in handling financial transactions and was becoming increasingly forgetful. She described her husband as forgetting to pay bills and important dates. Examination by a private neurologist, together with an MRI showed signs of white matter lesions which led to an additional diagnosis of MS. Treatment with betaferon (interferon beta-1b) was initiated in early 2015. The patient's wife explained that no improvements were observed with this new medication over the following two years. Instead, she noticed a progression of symptoms, including the onset of ptosis, loss of sensation in his limbs, loss of strength in lower limbs, unusual lip/mouth movements considered to be Bell's palsy, frequent falls, and sensory hallucinations (i.e., the patient would say that he has "animals in his face and ears"). However, because of limitations associated with Roberto's medical insurance, he had irregular access to medical follow-up with his psychiatrist and neurologist, and no further medical investigations were pursued at the time.

Initial Clinical Interview

During the initial medical interview at the GNA, Roberto came accompanied by his wife and was cooperative. He reported a sedentary lifestyle and denied smoking tobacco, drinking alcohol, or taking recreational drugs. At the time of the interview, he complained about a heavy global oppressive headache and a global sense of fatigue. He further endorsed current symptoms of depression, including a sense of worthlessness and passive suicidal ideation. Sleep disturbances and a lack of appetite were also reported. He however felt that the sleep disorder was likely a consequence of intermittent sleep patterns he had to adapt over the last two decades because of his prior work as a security guard and taxi driver. He reported taking quetiapine nightly for management of sleep difficulties. The clinical interview further highlighted memory and word-finding difficulties, as well as disorientation to time and space.

At the beginning of symptoms, Roberto presented irritability, motor restlessness, aggressiveness, auditory hallucinations, and obsession with cleaning. At the clinical interview, his wife said that they stopped visiting friends and engaging socially due to his husband's behavioral changes, she explained that they felt embarrassed for the situation and experienced loneliness and isolation.

This situation is not exceptional since, in Antioquia, it is still needed to raise awareness about mental disease stigma and education in the community to improve social support for people with mental diseases. Roberto and his wife were advised by the GNA psychologist about strategies to cope with mood disturbance and to improve their socialization.

The medical history further highlighted the frequent occurrence of pulsatile, insidious frontal region headaches, without aura, for the past three years, which usually improved with acetaminophen. He did not have a history of hypertension, diabetes, or dyslipidemia. Examination of his family history revealed that his father had a history of dementia, his brother and niece had a history of stroke (age 39 and 22, respectively), and his half-sister had been diagnosed with CADASIL. Taking this information into consideration, suspicion for a potential diagnosis of CADASIL was raised by the GNA neurologist, and genotyping for NOTCH3 mutations known to be present in the region of Antioquia was recommended. A neuropsychological evaluation was also performed to characterize the nature and severity of cognitive symptoms.

Baseline Neuropsychological Evaluation

The baseline neuropsychological evaluation was administered by a neuropsychologist at the GNA. Since Roberto is Spanish monolingual and does not speak any indigenous language, the evaluation was administered in Spanish using questionnaires and cognitive measures previously adapted and validated for use in patients from Antioquia. Since Roberto had completed secondary school, we used normative data for 11 years of education. In concordance with the clinical interview, the patient's score on a depression questionnaire[26] revealed the presence of moderate to severe depressive symptoms. His score on a Global Deterioration Scale[27] confirmed the presence of cognitive deficits and suggested a significant decline in cognition from his estimated pre-morbid level of functioning. However, he was still able to perform most Instrumental Activities of Daily Living (IADL) independently. To obtain an objective and unbiased estimation of Roberto's cognitive performance, his scores were standardized based on normative data recently published by our group and derived from 2,673 cognitively unimpaired individuals from Colombia.[28] The standardized neuropsychological test data for his baseline and follow-up evaluation data are summarized in Table 30.1.

The results of this evaluation highlighted a significant impairment in global cognitive status, with an MMSE score of 22/30. While performance on a confrontational naming task was in the superior range, his performance in semantic fluency (i.e., animal naming) was in the borderline range. Performance on verbal free and cued delayed recall was in the borderline range, suggesting difficulties with verbal episodic memory. Performance on visual free delayed recall was less affected and in the low average range. Performance on tasks assessing processing speed and attention was in the low average range. Finally, performance on tasks assessing executive function and visuoconstructional praxis were unaffected and in the average range. In summary, the initial neuropsychological evaluation revealed a wide range of performance across cognitive domains, ranging from superior to extremely low, with predominant impairments observed on tasks of semantic fluency and memory, tasks commonly linked to dysfunction of temporal lobes systems.

Initial Clinical Impressions

The review of the family history by the GNA's neurologist was key in this case, as it shed light on a family history of CADASIL, strokes at an early age, and dementia. The occurrence of frequent headaches, the presence of cognitive impairment, and the family history led to initial suspicions for an alternative diagnosis of CADASIL and a referral to genetic analysis of the *NOTCH3* gene. Genotyping was performed shortly after the initial clinical interview at the GNA and confirmed

Table 30.1 Summary of cognitive performance

	Baseline Z-score (qualitative range)	Follow-up Z-score (qualitative range)	Changes in performance Δ Z-score
Global Cognitive Functioning[19,28]			
MMSE	−3.66 (extremely low)	−3.66 (extremely low)	**0.00**
CERAD Total Score	−1.46 (borderline)	−1.56 (borderline)	**−0.10**
Language/Semantics[19,28]			
Boston Naming Test—15 items	1.37 (superior)	1.37 (superior)	**0.00**
Semantic Fluency (Animals)	−1.45 (borderline)	−1.83 (borderline)	**−0.38**
Memory[19,28,29,30]			
Word List Learning—Total Immediate Recall	−2.04 (borderline)	−1.27 (low average)	**0.77**
Word List Learning— Delayed Recall	−1.85 (borderline)	−1.27 (low average)	**0.58**
Word List Learning—Recognition	−1.52 (borderline)	−0.50 (average)	**1.02**
Constructional Praxis—Recall	−0.78 (low average)	−1.52 (borderline)	**−0.74**
ROCFT—Recall	−0.77 (low average)	−1.05 (low average)	**−0.38**
Processing Speed/Attention[30,31]			
Trail Making Test A	−1.22 (low average)	−2.58 (extremely low)	**−1.36**
Digit-Symbol Coding (WAIS-III)	−1.30 (low average)	−1.54 (borderline)	**−0.24**
Executive Function[32,33]			
Phonemic Fluency (F-A-S)	2.64 (very superior)	3.07 (very superior)	**0.33**
WCST—Perseveration	0.35 (average)	−0.06 (average)	**−0.41**
Visuoconstructional Praxis[19,29,30]			
Constructional Praxis—Copy	0.75 (average)	−1.09 (low average)	**−1.84**
ROCFT—Copy	−0.21 (average)	−2.57 (extremely low)	**−2.36**

Presented values are Z-scores normalized for age and education (qualitative range of performance), using previously published normative data derived from a Colombian sample.[28] MMSE—Mini-Mental State Examination; CERAD—Consortium to Establish a Registry for Alzheimer's Disease neuropsychological battery; WAIS-III—Third Edition of the Wechsler Adult Intelligence Scale; WCST—Wisconsin Card Sorting Test; ROCT—Rey-Osterrieth Complex Figure Test. Qualitative range of performance was determined as such: ≤1 percentile rank = extremely low; 2–9 percentile rank = borderline; 9–24 percentile rank = low average; 25–74 percentile rank = average; 75–90 percentile rank = high average; 91–97 percentile rank = superior; ≥98 percentile rank = very superior.

the presence of an R141C mutation on the NOTCH3 gene. After an interdisciplinary team meeting including neurologist experts in demyelinating diseases, a comorbid diagnosis of MS was judged unlikely. Roberto was given a diagnosis of CADASIL and treatment with betaferon was discontinued. Roberto and his family were invited to follow-up evaluations to characterize the progression of his clinical and cognitive symptoms.

Follow-Up Neuropsychological Evaluation

Roberto, now diagnosed with CADASIL, was seen again by the GNA team after two years. His wife described increasing memory difficulties and spatial disorientation in familiar settings. He reported a lack of appetite and weight loss. There was new onset of slurred speech, which appeared approximately four months before the evaluation. He also complained of numbness in his right arm and weakness in his inferior limbs. He reported mood disturbance, characterized by a general feeling of sadness, frequent unmotivated crying episodes, and passive suicidal ideation. His score on the GDS-15 corroborated the presence of moderate to severe depressive symptoms. He described feeling like a burden to his wife and being worried that she was going to leave him. He also reported auditory hallucinations in the form of "voices telling him to do bad things."

Roberto also now required assistance with instrumental activities of daily living, including selecting his clothes and dressing. He had difficulty using familiar objects, including utensils and the telephone, and needed reminders related to personal hygiene (i.e., taking a shower). His score on the Global Deterioration Scale corroborated the severity of cognitive decline, and now suggested the presence of dementia. Over the past years, there were also issues with accessing medications prescribed for the management of his affective and behavioral symptoms due to limitations associated with their insurance policy. His wife described a sense of exhaustion due to caregiver burden, which was exacerbated by a lack of social support.

To objectively characterize the pattern of cognitive decline over time, Roberto completed the same neuropsychological evaluation battery as during his initial visit (see Table 30.1). The neuropsychological evaluation revealed a mix of both preserved and declining cognitive functions over the last two years. The MMSE score remained unchanged, at 22/30. Congruently, global cognitive functioning estimated with the CERAD total score was stable and in the borderline range. Performance on tests assessing language/semantics and executive function also remained relatively stable when compared to performance at the baseline evaluation. In contrast, a decline in performance was noted on tasks involving visuoconstructional praxis. Performance on both the copy of the Rey-Osterrieth Complex Figure Test (ROCT) and the CERAD Constructional Praxis, which was in the average range at the baseline visit, now dropped to the low average to extremely low range. There was also a notable reduction in performance on the Trail Making Test A, suggesting progressive impairment in visuospatial attention and processing speed. Interestingly, scores for verbal memory improved in comparison to the previous evaluation. On the other hand, his score on nonverbal memory tasks showed a trend toward a reduction in performance, possibly secondary to impairments in visuoconstructional praxis.

Follow-Up Clinical Impressions

After two years, Roberto, now with a diagnosis of CADASIL, was seen by members of the GNA for a follow-up evaluation highlighting the onset of new physical symptoms, including slurred speech, weakness in inferior limbs, and numbness in the right arm. He was depressed and anxious and experienced auditory hallucinations. He was increasingly dependent on his wife for daily life activities, needed assistance to dress, and had difficulties using familiar objects, indicating a progression of dementia syndrome. On objective cognitive testing, he displayed a prominent decline in visuoconstructional abilities. The GNA team concluded that the pattern of physical and cognitive deterioration was likely associated with the progression of cerebrovascular changes linked to CADASIL, and consistent with the presence of vascular dementia. Unfortunately, because of limited resources in this setting, we did not have access to neuroimaging data to explore potential neurological correlates of this decline.

Discussion

CADASIL is a genetic disorder leading to the early and progressive onset of cerebral small vessel disease. Patients with CADASIL often suffer from recurrent ischemic strokes and develop vascular cognitive impairment at a young age, typically in the absence of conventional cardiovascular risk factors. CADASIL is a rare disease, with large-scale longitudinal European studies estimating a prevalence ranging from 4 to 15 cases per 100,000 individuals.[34] CADASIL is still underrecognized in the medical community, with common misdiagnosis including MS (most common), dementia, encephalitis, or migraines.[35]

Further contributing to its diagnostic complexity, CADASIL has a highly heterogeneous clinical presentation. The age of onset, nature, severity, and progression of clinical symptoms in CADASIL is variable, even within members of the same family. The genotype, sex, and environmental factors (e.g., cardiovascular risk) have been discussed as potential factors influencing the disease presentation and trajectory in CADASIL. However, factors surrounding the phenotypic heterogeneity of CADASIL are still poorly understood and require further investigation. CADASIL can be accompanied by diverse neurological symptoms, including migraines with aura, seizures, or gait disturbances. Psychiatric disturbances are also highly prevalent in CADASIL, affecting an estimated 20 to 40% of patients and having a deleterious impact on their quality of life.[24,36] Some of the most prevalent psychiatric symptoms in CADASIL include major depression, mania, BDs, and apathy.

The described case is therefore not unique in its presentation, and multiple reports have described cases of CADASIL with a clinical picture consistent with BD.[37,38] The occurrence of psychotic symptoms and hallucinations has also been described, albeit fewer frequently.[39,40] Interestingly, it has been demonstrated that psychiatric disturbances represent the initial presenting symptom in as much as 15% of cases and that CADASIL might be underdiagnosed in late-onset psychiatric patients.[41]

CADASIL should be considered as a possible differential diagnosis whenever the MRI confirms the presence of white matter lesion, especially when observed at a relatively young age and in the absence of cardiovascular risk factors or comorbidities. A family history suggestive of an autosomal dominant mode of inheritance, stroke, dementia, and migraine with aura would further support this hypothesis. In this case, genotypic analysis for NOTCH 3 should be considered.

This case study illustrates challenges associated with the diagnosis of complex neurological syndromes in Antioquia, Colombia. This case study is a fitting illustration, as CADASIL is a rare and under-recognized disorder with a heterogeneous clinical presentation. The patient presented in this case study was misdiagnosed for eight years and prescribed various ineffective medications that are costly, have potential side effects, and are not always available due to limitations associated with medical insurance. The restricted access to regular follow-up, specialists, and advanced diagnostic tools (e.g., MRI) in this setting are important barriers to appropriate diagnosis and clinical management, particularly when confronted with complex cases.

Section III: Lessons Learned

- It is important to carefully review family histories in clinical interviews. Family history is particularly relevant in Antioquia, a location that is associated with a relatively high frequency of hereditary diseases. In CADASIL, the investigation of family history should expand beyond premature stroke and target other cardinal features of the disease, including migraines with aura and neurocognitive impairment. An incomplete investigation of family history can lead to misdiagnosis.[35]
- Genealogy is essential to establish since the approach to paisas patients with neuropsychiatric and motor symptoms requires remembering that this ethnic group comes from a history made up of large family groups where genetic pathologies have been identified.
- Social norms and cultural practices vary in Colombia, and it is important to evaluate behavioral and emotional changes from the perspective of the patient and the family rather than against socially accepted standards.
- It is important to consider linguistic aspects specific to the patient's sociodemographic background when administering and scoring cognitive tests to avoid misinterpretation due to accents or prototypical use of idioms and language (e.g., number of different words used to name things in Paisa communities).
- The development of regionally relevant normative data can improve diagnostic precision in specific cultural communities that may have distinct features even within the same country.
- The use of a multidisciplinary, culturally relevant framework with longitudinal follow-up can improve the diagnostic accuracy of neurological disorders and facilitate access to medical care for underserved populations.

References

1. Larraín González A, Madrid Garcés PJ. Aproximaciones al discurso de lo paisa en Colombia. Revista de Antropología y Sociología: Virajes. 2020;22(2):185–209.
2. Londoño, J. El modelo de colonización antioqueña de James Parsons. Un balance historiográfico. Fronteras de la Historia. 2002;7:187–226.
3. Carvajal-Carmona LG, Ophoff R, Service S, Hartiala J, Molina J, Leon P et al. Genetic demography of Antioquia (Colombia) and the Central Valley of Costa Rica. Hum Genet. 2003 May;112(5–6):534–41.
4. Antioquia GD, Uribe de Hincapié MT, Patiño B, Mejía-Restrepo H. Paisas memoria de un pueblo: la colonizacion Antioqueña. Paisas Memoria De Un Pueblo. Medellin: Gobernacion De Antioquia. Idea ed. Colombia; 2006.
5. Arango, J. Literature and culture in Antioquia: between stories and accounts. In Williams R, editor. A history of Colombian literature. Cambridge: Cambridge University Press; 2016. p. 269–86. doi:10.1017/CBO9781139963060.015
6. Archer N, Brown RG, Reeves SJ, Boothby H, Nicholas H, Foy C, Williams J, Lovestone S. Premorbid personality and behavioral and psychological symptoms in probable Alzheimer disease. Am J Geriatr Psychiatry. 2007 Mar;15(3):202–13. doi:10.1097/01.JGP.0000232510.77213.10
7. Kaufman T. Language history in South America: what we know and how to know more. In: Payne DL, editor. Amazonian linguistics: studies in Lowland South American languages. University of Texas Press; Austin, Texas, United States: 1990. p. 13–67.
8. Da Silva CG, Petersson KM, Faísca L, Ingvar M, Reis A. The effects of literacy and education on the quantitative and qualitative aspects of semantic verbal fluency. J Clin Exp Neuropsychol. 2004 Apr;26(2):266–77.
9. Brucki SM, Rocha MS. Category fluency test: effects of age, gender and education on total scores, clustering and switching in Brazilian Portuguese-speaking subjects. Braz J Med Biol Res. 2004 Dec;37(12):1771–7.
10. Lasprilla, JCA, Rivera, D, editors. Neuropsicología en Colombia: Datos normativos, estado actual y retos a futuro. Universidad Autonoma de Manizalez; Manizales, Caldas, Colombia: 2015.
11. Peña-Casanova J, Quiñones-Ubeda S, Gramunt-Fombuena N, Quintana-Aparicio M, Aguilar M, Badenes D. NEURONORMA Study Team. Spanish Multicenter Normative Studies (NEURONORMA Project): norms for verbal fluency tests. Arch Clin Neuropsychol. 2009 Jun;24(4):395–411.
12. La education es de todos [Internet]. Available in: https://www.mineducacion.gov.co/1759/articles-84243_recurso_8.pdf
13. Brunner JJ, Gacel-Avilà J, Laverde M, et al. Higher Education in Regional and City Development Antioquia, Colombia; 2016.
14. Garcia-Subirats I, Vargas I, Mogollón-Pérez AS, De Paepe P, Ferreira da Silva MR, Unger JP, Vázquez ML. Barriers in access to healthcare in countries with different health systems. A cross-sectional study in municipalities of central Colombia and north-eastern Brazil. Soc Sci Med. 2014;106:204–13.
15. Lalli MA, Cox HC, Arcila ML, Cadavid L, Moreno S, Garcia G. Origin of the PSEN1 E280A mutation causing early-onset Alzheimer's disease. Alzheimers Dement. 2014; 10(5 Suppl):S277–S283.e10.
16. Zuluaga-Castaño Y, Montoya-Arenas DA, Velilla L, Ospina C, Arboleda-Velasquez JF, Quiroz YT. Cognitive performance in asymptomatic carriers of mutations R1031C and R141C in CADASIL. Int J Psychol Res (Medellin). 2018;11(2):46–55. doi:10.21500/20112084.3373
17. Kremeyer B, García J, Müller H, Burley MW, Herzberg I, Parra MV. Genome-wide linkage scan of bipolar disorder in a Colombian population isolate replicates Loci on chromosomes 7p21-22, 1p31, 16p12 and 21q21-22 and identifies a novel locus on chromosome 12q. Hum Hered. 2010;70(4):255–68. doi:10.1159/000320914
18. Pineda DA, Lopera F, Puerta IC, Trujillo-Orrego N, Aguirre-Acevedo DC, Hincapié-Henao L. Potential cognitive endophenotypes in multigenerational families: segregating ADHD from a genetic isolate. Atten Defic Hyperact Disord. 2011;3(3):291–9. doi:10.1007/s12402-011-0061-3
19. Aguirre-Acevedo D, Gomez R, Moreno S, Arboleda-Henao E, Motta M, Muñoz C. Validity and reliability of the CERAD-Col neuropsychological battery. Revista de neurologia. 2007;45:655–60.

20. Vila-Castelar C, Papp KV, Amariglio RE, et al. Validation of the Latin American Spanish version of the face-name associative memory exam in a Colombian Sample. Clin Neuropsychol. 2020;34(Suppl 1):1–12.
21. Torres VL, Vila-Castelar C, Bocanegra Y, Baena A, Guzmán-Vélez E, Aguirre-Acevedo DC et al. Normative data stratified by age and education for a Spanish neuropsychological test battery: results from the Colombian Alzheimer's prevention initiative registry. Appl Neuropsychol Adult. 2021 Mar–Apr;28(2):230–44.
22. Joutel A, Corpechot C, Ducros A, Vahedi K, Chabriat H, Mouton P. Notch3 mutations in CADASIL, a hereditary adult-onset condition causing stroke and dementia. Nature. 1996;383:707–10.
23. Henao-Arboleda E, Aguirre-Acevedo D, Pacheco C, Yamile-Bocanegra O, Lopera F. Seguimiento de las características cognitivas en una población con enfermedad cerebrovascular hereditaria (CADASIL) en Colombia. Rev Neurol. 2007;45:729–33.
24. Chabriat H, Joutel A, Dichgans M, Tournier-Lasserve E, Bousser M-G. Cadasil. Lancet Neurol. 2009;8:643–53.
25. Papakonstantinou E, Bacopoulou F, Brouzas D, Megalooikonomou V, D'Elia D, Bongcam-Rudloff E. NOTCH3 and CADASIL syndrome: a genetic and structural overview. EMBnet j. 2019;24.
26. Campo-Arias A, Mendoza YU, Morales TS, Pino AJV, Cogollo Z. Consistencia interna, estructura factorial y confiabilidad del constructo de la Escala de Yesavage para depresión geriátrica (GDS-15) en Cartagena (Colombia). Salud Uninorte. 2008;24:1–9.
27. Reisberg B, Ferris S, de Leon M, Crook T. Global Deterioration Scale (GDS). Psychopharmacol Bull. 1988;24:661–3.
28. Torres VL, Vila-Castelar C, Bocanegra Y, Baena A, Guzmán-Vélez E, Aguirre-Acevedo DC. Normative data stratified by age and education for a Spanish neuropsychological test battery: results from the Colombian Alzheimer's prevention initiative registry. Appl Neuropsychol Adult. 2021;28(2):230–44.
29. Welsh KA, Butters N, Mohs RC, Beekly D, Edland S, Fillenbaum G. The Consortium to Establish a Registry for Alzheimer's Disease (CERAD). Part V. A normative study of the neuropsychological battery Neurology. 1994;44(4):609–14.
30. Osterrieth PA. Le test de copie d'une figure complexe; contribution a l'etude de la perception et de la memoire [Test of copying a complex figure; contribution to the study of perception and memory]. Archives de psychologie. 1944;30:206–356.
31. Reitan RM. Validity of the Trail Making Test as an indicator of organic brain damage. Percept Mot Skills. 1958;8:271–6.
32. Tombaugh TN, Kozak J, Rees L. Normative data stratified by age and education for two measures of verbal fluency: FAS and animal naming. Arch Clin Neuropsychol. 1999;14:167–77.
33. Berg EA. A simple objective technique for measuring flexibility in thinking. J Gen Psychol. 1948;39:15–22.
34. Razvi S, Davidson R, Bone I, Muir K. The prevalence of cerebral autosomal dominant arteriopathy with subcortical infarcts and leucoencephalopathy (CADASIL) in the west of Scotland. J Neurol Neurosurg Psychiatry. 2005;76:739–41.
35. Razvi S, Davidson R, Bone I, Muir K. Is inadequate family history a barrier to diagnosis in CADASIL? Acta Neurol Scand. 2005;112:323–6.
36. Valenti R, Poggesi A, Pescini F, Inzitari D, Pantoni L. Psychiatric disturbances in CADASIL: a brief review. Acta Neurol Scand. 2008;118:291–5.
37. Chabriat H, Vahedi K, Bousser M, et al. Clinical spectrum of CADASIL: a study of 7 families. Lancet. 1995;346:934–9.
38. Park S, Park B, Koh MK, Joo YH. Case report: bipolar disorder as the first manifestation of CADASIL. BMC Psychiatry. 2014;14:175.
39. Dichgans M, Mayer M, Uttner I, Brüning R, Müller-Höcker J, Rungger G. The phenotypic spectrum of CADASIL: clinical findings in 102 cases. Ann Neurol. 1998;44:731–9.
40. Pentti A. Schizophrenia in a patient with cerebral autosomally dominant arteriopathy with subcortical infarcts and leucoencephalopathy (CADASIL disease). Nord J Psychiatry. 2001;55:41–2.
41. Leyhe T, Wiendl H, Buchkremer G, Wormstall H. CADASIL: underdiagnosed in psychiatric patients? Acta Psychiatr Scand. 2005;111:392.

Cuban

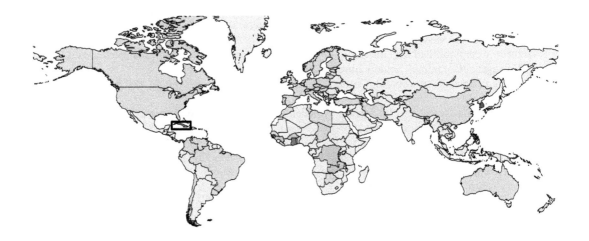

31   A Cultural Approach to the Development of Neuropsychology in Cuba

Ana M Rodriguez-Salgado, Ana I Peñalver-Guía, and Jorge J Llibre-Guerra

Section I: Background Information

Terminology and Perspective

Neuropsychology practice is highly influenced by population characteristics typically related to the diversity of ethnicity, language, educational level, values, socio-economic status (SES), and population health.[1] In our perspective, in order to address neuropsychology practice, each of those factors needs to be taken into consideration to understand that higher mental functions are based on a complex dynamic system with a social origin.[2] In this chapter, we address current neuropsychology practices in the Cuban population by sharing our perspective as neuropsychologists and neurologists practicing in Cuba.

Geography

Cuba is a Caribbean Island located in the northern Caribbean Sea at the confluence of the Gulf of Mexico and the Atlantic Ocean. It constitutes the largest island in the Caribbean and is the 17th largest island in the world by land area. The local climate is warm, tropical, and moderated by northeasterly trade winds that blow year-round. Cuba's population is currently 11,193,470 habitants, with the highest population density in the capital city of Havana, with a total of 2928.1 habitants per km.[3]

History and Ethnography

The Cuban population is very diverse in its origin and is made up of various ethnic groups. Population ancestry includes European and African and to a lesser extent (<3%) other populations such as Native Americans and Asians.[4] Self-identified races include whites, blacks, and **mulatos**, where the latter group is described as the result of mixture of the first two population groups.

Population diversity in Cuba was shaped by Spanish colonization. Due to the systematic disappearance of the native Cuban population as a result of slavery, African origin populations were introduced to Cuba by Spanish *Conquistadores* to increase the workforce and expedite exploits for the Crown. African populations and Spanish conquistadores were also ethnically diverse. Africans in Cuba were originally from the west coast of Africa, the Gulf of Guinea, and southern Angola. A small proportion were brought from the central region of the African continent.[5,6] Spanish settlers came from Valencia, the Canary Islands, Asturias, Galicia, Andalusia, Catalonia, and Castile. This process resulted in a great mixture amongst the people and the creation of a multicultural and multi-ethnic population.

DOI: 10.4324/9781003051862-63

According to the last census carried out in Cuba in 2012, the Cuban population was anthropologically classified as white (64.0%), black (9.3%), and *mestizo*, the vast majority, *mulatto* (26.6%), and Asians 1.0%.[3,4] This admixture process created a very strong transculturation process that shaped the Cuban culture, with influences from exchanges with and between multiple cultures. Modern Cuban culture is therefore the result of an active transition between the confluent of Iberian European (white), Central West African (black) components, with influences from other Chinese cultures. This cultural influence is manifested above all in a diversity of music (danzon, chachacha, salsa, jazz, rumba), dance (Spanish dance, casino or Cuban salsa, ballet, folklore), and food with a variety of flavors. The influence of the admixture process in the culture also shapes the personological characteristics of the Cuban population to be more supportive, happy, affective, sociable, and uninhibited during social interactions. These idiosyncratic characteristics may create confusion for professionals from other cultures who may see these traits as part of a Behavioral Psychological Symptom of the disease (e.g., disinhibition in frontotemporal dementia.)

Immigration and Relocation

Immigration has played a unique role in the island, experiencing extensive diasporas in the last century, especially in the United States, and establishing well-known and large communities, in Miami, New Jersey, and Texas.[7,8] Migrants are often young, and their departure has re-shaped the population structure, and as a result, the age structure of the population has changed significantly.

Language

Spanish is the official language of Cuba. Although there are no local dialects, the island's diverse ethnic groups have influenced speech patterns. Africans, in particular, have greatly enriched the vocabulary and contributed the soft, somewhat nasal accent and rhythmic intonation that distinguish contemporary Cuban speech. Some words are of native Indian origin, and a few of these—such as hamaca ("hammock")—have passed into other languages. Many practitioners of the Santería religion also speak Lucumí, a "secret" Yoruboid language of the Niger-Congo family.[9] Also, we have expressions that are typical of our popular slang and we use them to refer to certain things. These are used by most Cubans regardless of educational level or social class.

Religion

Cuba is recognized as a predominantly Catholic country (60%), but the mixture of cultures from different origins has given rise to an authentic religious syncretism where, especially, African religions are mixed with Catholicism, giving rise to the well-known Santeria religion.[10] Other religions include Protestants (5%), Jehovah's Witnesses, Methodists, Anglicans, Seventh-day Adventists, among many others, as well as Muslims, Jews, and Buddhists. Although there is great diversity in religions, to the best of our knowledge and clinical experience, there is little to no interference with the medical practice since regardless of religion, the Cuban population seeks medical attention and follows therapeutic recommendations from their physicians. The educational efforts and the expansion of free medical care to all the population, coupled with the existence of community doctors, have created a "medical culture" in the population that favors the absence of antagonistic relations between medical practice and religion. At the same time, health care providers are trained to recognize and accept the religions and cultural beliefs without exercising opposition to those. Cuban populations who practice Afro-Cuban religions will also seek advice from local healers to dispel **"el mal de ojo"** or some diseases but will also seek medical attention.

Education and Literacy

Educational level and cognitive enrichment early during life are associated with greater levels of cognitive functioning.[11–14] Therefore, this is a crucial factor when trying to assess neuropsychological performances in our population. Educational levels in Cuba are relatively high compared to other countries in Latin America.[15] This has been influenced by a few factors. In 1961, the Cuban government incited a country-wide literacy campaign, "Campaña de Alfabetización Nacional," which allowed a quantitative and qualitative change in educational level. By the year 1962, Cuba had become the first illiteracy-free territory in Latin America.[16] Education in Cuba is free at any level (including university and postgraduate studies) and is compulsory until middle school.[3] In relation to university studies, there are different education modalities, including regular daytime education and nighttime courses for workers.[3] Other types of educational programs such as technical and professional teaching are also available, with many trade schools available to facilitate the inclusion in society of those who could be trained to gain pre-university or technical education level. The National Population and Housing Census of Cuba (2019) reported a population of 11.17 million inhabitants, of which 712, 672 (6.9%) are university graduates. Of those aged 30 to 59, 11.6% completed university studies and 52.1% are women. Within the general population, 46.1% have reached at least one higher education degree, 77.6% completed middle school, and 99.6% have completed primary education, of whom 52.1% are women.[17,18] Compared to other Latin American countries/Hispanic populations, the higher educational level in the Cuban population plays a relevant role when assessing Cuban origin populations as this will required adjustment on the normative references to be used.

Socio-Economic Status

A growing body of cognitive research shows causal connections between SES and cognitive outcomes.[19] Brain development involves different processes at different stages, and SES may shape this development and influence cognitive performance and within-population differences.

Although Cuba is a low- and middle-income country (LMIC), since 1990, Cuba has developed in the biotechnology and medical services industries. The export of biotechnology and medical services represents one of the major sources of income for the Cuban economy. Biotechnology productions also allow the substitution of imports to supply Cuban pharmacies and hospitals. In addition, the export of medical services and health tourism has grown and become the most dynamic activity in the Cuban economy, representing 75% of its GDP. Cuba also provides health services to several countries in need by sending over 130,000 medical personnel on aid missions to developing nations, primarily in the Global South.[20]

Despite Cuban success in health care, it is important to note that due to the United States' embargo on Cuba, there are severe limitations on Cuba's access to international supplies of medicines and medical equipment. Furthermore, the expansion of US pharmaceutical companies over the last three decades has limited the number of companies that can export their products to Cuba without exposing themselves to penalties from the US government. The Helms-Burton Act penalizes businesses and citizens trading with Cuba.[21] In the healthcare sector, in particular, the Cuban population is denied the latest generation of equipment and medicines, available in some cases only from US companies or only to a few with prohibitively high prices.

These restrictions have affected the practice of neuropsychology since many neuropsychological tests that we have in Cuba are donated by other professionals or obtained through collaboration projects with other countries. Despite this, there is a shortage of psychological tests accessible to Cuban neuropsychologists. Limited tests are not available in all departments of psychology, and if available, there is either only one original copy or incomplete test materials.

Values and Customs

Being generous and hospitable is highly valued among Cubans. The Cuban population considers it rude not to greet all men with a handshake and all women with a kiss on the cheek. In addition, compared to other Central and South American cultures, Cubans tend to have louder conversations, especially with hand gestures, are more expressive, and are very passionate. In addition, Cubans consider direct eye contact as a sign of respect, and it is much more preferred than indirect or fleeting eye contact. These are important considerations during behavioral assessments, and these manifestations should be considered as a display of affection and do not have a sexual connotation nor evidence of disinhibition.

Health Status

Like education, health care in Cuba is free. The Cuban government operates a national health system and assumes fiscal and administrative responsibility for all its citizens' health care. Medical care is available to the entire population, without distinction of race, social origin, or ideological affiliation. There is a state, universal, and free character. Health is assumed from a procedural, integrative, and active view of the human being. Promotion and prevention actions aimed at reaching higher levels in the population's quality of life are emphasized. Close interrelation of research, teaching, and assistance, that is multisectoral, international, and collaborative, constitutes guiding principles of work.[3] The number of doctors per inhabitant in Cuba in 2019 was 1 doctor for every 116 inhabitants. The maternal mortality rate per 100,000 live births is 37.4, with an infant mortality rate of 5 per 1,000 live births. The three leading causes of death in the country are cardiovascular diseases, malignant tumors, and cerebrovascular diseases.[4]

History of Neuropsychology in Cuba

The development of neuropsychology in Cuba had a marked influence from the former Soviet Union. Its roots date back to the late 1960s, when Cuban psychologists were trained at Alexander R. Luria's lab at the University Lomonosov of Moscow. Dr. Eduardo Cairo Valcárcel, Dr. Luis Oliva Ruiz, and Dr. Clemente Trujillo Matienzo, mentored by Alexander R. Luria, were the first Cuban psychologists to receive training in the field. Upon return to Cuba, they used Luria's approach in their clinical and research activities.

Dr. Eduardo Cairo, professor at the Faculty of Psychology of the University of Havana, extended neuropsychological research in Cuba and wrote several books on neuropsychology. Furthermore, he implemented psychology training at the University of Havana. Dr. Luis Oliva Ruiz and Dr. Clemente Trujillo were tasked to develop clinical neuropsychology in Cuba. Dr. Oliva Ruiz and Trujillo founded the Neuropsychology Department at the National Institute of Neurology and Neurosurgery (INN) and started sub-specialty training at the INN. For the first time, neuropsychologists and neurologists worked together to assess neurological disorders in the national Cuban health system. Since the creation of the neuropsychology department, the neuropsychology group has worked continuously at the frontline of the institution in several areas including research, training, and clinical assessment. This group was formally created in January 1971 by psychologist Dr. Clemente Trujillo, who continued the work initiated by Dr. Oliva guided by Luria's teachings. Dr. Trujillo has trained several specialists from all over the country and is currently continuing his work at the Institute of Neurology. For their work and contributions to neuropsychology in Cuba, Drs. Luis Oliva Ruiz Clemente Trujillo and Eduardo Cairo are considered the founding fathers of the field in Cuba.[22]

Despite the development of neuropsychology in Cuba, there are still several challenges that must be addressed in order to advance the field and the profession further. These include increasing training options and a greater need for standardized and normalized neuropsychological tests for the Cuban population.

Neuropsychology Training in Cuba

All Cuban psychologists study basic courses in neuropsychology, including specific courses within undergraduate psychology training such as "Biological Bases of Behavior 'and' Cognitive Psychology." However, this is still insufficient for those who decide to dedicate their career to this branch of psychology. As a result, most Cuban neuropsychology specialists are trained abroad or receive theoretical-practical training from more experienced neuropsychologists. There are no postgraduate doctorate studies focused on this sub-specialty in Cuba. For years, Cuban neuropsychology has been enriched by exchanges with foreign institutions and professors through courses and research collaborations. In addition, some of our neuropsychologists complete master's degrees or other diploma courses abroad.

The master's degree is the usual level of educational attainment for those who wish to practice clinical neuropsychology, and there is not a board certification process in neuropsychology, although there is one in clinical psychology. Recent efforts to increase Cuba's training options include a master's degree program created in 2004 by the Center for Neurosciences. Although the program's scope is mainly focused on Neurosciences, there are several courses on Neuropsychology, Cognitive Neurosciences, and Infant Neurodevelopment available.

Currently, neuropsychology is practiced in several healthcare centers throughout our country. Centers like the Institute of Neurology and Neurosurgery, the International Center for Neurological Restoration, and the Hermanos Amejeiras Hospital stand out for research and training. In the Cuban health system, neuropsychology services are especially tasked with determining the presence, severity, and location of brain disorders and supporting dementia and depression diagnoses in particular. Neuropsychology services are also regularly sought for pre- and post-neurosurgical interventions and play a relevant role during neurological rehabilitation. Yet, establishing neuropsychology-specific training and practice standards at the provincial or national level is still needed.

Neuropsychology Assessments in Cuba

Neuropsychological test validations in Spanish-speaking populations are relatively scarce in Latin America. Cuba does not have enough normative data for neurocognitive tests to evaluate the pediatric or adult population. There is a lack of neuropsychological batteries designed to evaluate cognitive functions that can identify the different etiologies of dementia syndrome and its cognitive decline.

Currently, neuropsychological tests that are more widely used in Cuba include Luria's assessment[2] and the Brief Neuropsychological Evaluation in Spanish (NEUROPSI),[23] Trail-Making Test,[24] Digit Retention,[25] Boston Naming Test,[26] Wisconsin Card Sorting Test,[25] and Category Formation tests among others. Intelligence tests, used with a relatively high frequency, include the Raven's Progressive Matrices[27] and the Wechsler Adult Intelligence Scale,[28] although the latter is not available in all the centers.

Recent efforts to improve population-based measures in assessing cognitive complaints include the development of the 10/66 studies in the Cuban population. The 10/66 dementia diagnosis protocol has been validated and widely implemented in Cuba. The 10/66 protocols encompass a new method to dementia research in LMICs intended to develop a novel approach to diagnosing dementia (the 10/66 Dementia Diagnosis) and addressing difficulties in making diagnoses among older people with little or no education and the use of standardized protocols across all sites. Therefore, it is well suited to be used in our population. Further details of the 10/66 studies have been described elsewhere.[29,30]

More recently, the Cuban Alzheimer Research collaboration with researchers from the National Institute of Neurology introduced and validated tablet-based cognitive screening measures known as the Brain Health Assessment (BHA) to improve early diagnosis of mild cognitive impairment and dementia in primary care settings.[31] The BHA is a short tablet-based cognitive battery developed at UCSF Memory and Aging Center by neuropsychologist Katherine Possin.[32] The BHA was translated and adapted into Cuban Spanish by a multidisciplinary team of four language experts and later validated in the Cuban population.[31]

Furthermore, there are ongoing efforts to validate and introduce a structured neuropsychological battery aimed at secondary and tertiary levels of care for cognitive complaints. A newly developed neuropsychological battery is based on the UCSF Memory and Aging Center Bedside neuropsychological screening (Spanish version). This battery allows assessment of cognitive functions in older adults to facilitate the diagnosis and early identification of dementia, with rapid and reliable evaluation of episodic memory, working memory, executive functions, verbal fluency, naming, visuospatial functions, and abstract thinking. The test generally requires 45 minutes to complete.

Finally, in collaboration with international groups, we have developed a multicenter study to establish normative data for Latin American adult populations. The methodology for the development of normative data in ten Spanish-language neuropsychological tests in Latin American countries has been described elsewhere.[33]

The Role of Neuropsychology on Prevention and Community Care

In Cuba, mental health and well-being are a national priority of the Ministry of Public Health. In 1995, all mental health services were re-oriented to implement practices at a community level.[34] Easy and accessible mental health services in a community are key aspects to better understand and assess patients' concerns; also the easy access can prompt early consultation.

Health professionals, including neuropsychologists, psychologists, neurologists, psychiatrists, and social workers, practice in a coordinated effort throughout a network of specialized services (from primary care to third level of care) to addresses the population's care in all stages of life. There are currently more than 170 mental health departments and 421 outpatient mental health facilities available in the country that constitute the cornerstone of community care, and 3.5% of those are specialized services for children and adolescents.[34] Most of the mental health services are located in the community and linked to primary health care (PHC) with the existence of Mental Health Services (SSM) within polyclinics, which are the care units of this level of care and cover a health area with a population that ranges between 20,000 and 35,000 inhabitants. The SSM multidisciplinary teams develop a comprehensive approach with a particular focus on promoting healthy, preventive, educational, and rehabilitation lifestyles and establishing a direct link between the primary care level with the second and third levels of care.

The training of human resources to address this area of health is done through the careers of medicine, with the specialty of psychiatry, bachelor's degrees in psychology, nursing, health technology in the specialties of social work and occupational therapy as well as education, postgraduate in master's degrees and diplomas in community mental health, health psychology, natural and traditional medicine, sexuality, among others related. In this field, a Master in

Community Mental Health is being developed, which already has 9 editions and 227 graduates from all over the country.[34]

Section II: Case Study — "… My Life Changed from One Day to the Next"

History of Present Illness

Mrs. PM is a 54-year-old right-handed woman, born and raised in Havana city. She had nine years of formal education, which is considered a low educational level in Cuba since only 24% of the population have nine or less years of education, according to data reported by the population and housing census of 2012. This educational level is consistent with her employment at the time of symptom of onset; she worked as an operator in a factory, which is a job typically held by individuals with similar educational levels. Other common activities in groups with similar educational levels include cleaning services and food processing centers, among others.

Mrs. PM has a history of controlled arterial hypertension and does not report any pathological family history of interest. Her husband indicates that at age 50, she received an ophthalmology consultation because his wife started to present vision difficulties where she skipped lines when reading. A visual exam completed by an ophthalmologist revealed no relevant visual defects. On a follow-up consultation with neurology, Mrs. PM showed evidence of mild cognitive impairment and visuospatial alterations. As a result, she was referred to the neuropsychology service for evaluation of possible posterior cortical atrophy.

In the interview with her husband, he reported that his wife began showing problems related to spatial disorientation and visual disturbances approximately three years prior to neuropsychological evaluation. She also got lost on the way to work, and as a result, he began accompanying her to work every day. Difficulties were also evident in managing her finances. For example, she could not make the payments or purchases that were previously routine and had issues managing money. At the age of 53, three years after visuospatial and executive symptoms began, she began with memory decline where she forgot to season her food, lost things, and put her clothes on backward. On one occasion, she went out to the street, half-dressed. However, the husband says that the memory problems were not as significant or disabling as her visuospatial disturbance. The impact of her neuropsychological difficulties is most evident in Mrs. PM's employment. She works as a factory operator but can no longer assemble the boxes she used to assemble before and cannot pack the products properly.

During the neuropsychological evaluation, Mrs. PM was anxious when performing the tests, especially those requiring greater cognitive demand. Mrs. PM reported that she feels depressed because she depends on her husband to carry out daily life's instrumental activities. In general, the presence of depression referred by the patient is quite common and expected in these cases. Despite significant advances in gender equality over the past decades, the historical influence of "machismo" remains present in the Cuban culture, especially related to gender-specific roles in domestic activities. Women are expected to maintain the role of homemaker and perform household tasks such as cleaning, cooking, washing, and scrubbing. Therefore, the loss of her independence to carry out household tasks successfully may create depression and anxiety, even in the presence of strong family support.

Her neurocognitive evaluation cognitive included several tests administered in Spanish by a trained psychologist. Of note, some of these tests, including the Trail Making Test, Stroop Color Word Interference Test, Hopkins Verbal Learning Test, Boston Naming Test, and the Controlled Oral Word Association Test, have normative data collected in Cuban populations as part of a multi-site project in Latin American countries (see Guardia-Olmos et al., 2015[35] for methodology). Details of the neurocognitive evaluation are presented below.

Test and Norm Selection

1 Hopkins Verbal Learning Test-Revised form 5HVLT-R.[36]
2 Rey–Osterrieth Complex Figure—copy and immediate recall.[37]
3 Verbal Fluency Tests.[38]
4 Montreal Cognitive Assessment (MoCA).[39]
5 Subtest of digits in progression and regression.[40]
6 Visual Perception of Objects in VOSP Space.[41]
7 Design Fluency Test.[42]
8 Trail Making Test part A and B.[24]
9 Boston Naming Test.[26]
10 Facial Recognition Test.[43]
11 Discrimination of superimposed images from the Barcelona Test.[44]
12 Stroop Color Word Interference Test.[45]
13 Beck's Depression Inventory.[46]

Review of Cognitive, Visuospatial, and Behavioral Systems

On the MoCA, she scored 20/30 points, failing especially on visuospatial/executive processes. She did not manage to draw the three-dimensional cube properly. In the clock test, she drew the circle well; however, she placed the numbers outside the circle in a disaggregated way. She also failed in attention and calculation, especially in the consecutive subtraction "100-7" (0/3 points)

Orientation

Mrs. PM was oriented in time, space and person.

Memory

On the Hopkins Verbal Learning Test, Mrs. PM presented discrete alterations in the delayed recall; she managed to evoke (6/12) previously learned words, so she was in the 30th percentile. In late recognition, she improved discretely (7/12). This result has been discreetly diminished than expected according to their age and school level. In visual memory, her memory was compromised; she could not evoke visual material due to alterations in visual processing (0/36 points) (Rey's complex figure). In Benton's Facial Recognition Test, she showed moderate difficulties in recognizing faces.

Language

Expressive language (prosody and speech production) was without alteration at the time of evaluation. The functions of naming and repetition of sentences were affected due to their amnesic and attention problems. Sometimes she had verbal and literal paraphasias. Semantic Verbal Fluency (six words) and phonological fluency had decreased, especially the latter where she only managed to evoke two words in a minute.

Visuospatial Skills

In the superimposed image discrimination test, she presented simultagnosia. In the copy of Rey's complex figure, visuoconstructive apraxia (4/36 points) was found; she could not integrate the elements of the figure, incurred in intrusions of elements and incorrect spatial locations. Dress apraxia and ideational apraxia were also appreciated. She presented difficulties in visual tracking. In Ruff's design fluency test, Mrs. PM showed difficulties in visual-motor programming.

Working Memory and Executive Functions

In the attention processes, she presented difficulties in selective and sustained simple sequential attention. Executive and auditory attention and working memory were greatly diminished. Digit Span Backward 1/8 and Digit Span Forward 4/9 also showed very little attentional control, which is verified in the Stroop test. In the reading-writing processes, alexia and agraphia are appreciated. In the calculation subtest, acalculia was found. A great affectation in the representation and mental execution of simple calculation operations is appreciated in the executive functions. She fails to establish common links between elements of the same semantic category, denoting little abstraction and generalization. She was unable to sequence an alternating pattern of symbols (Trail Making Test-B).

Psychiatric Symptoms

In the affective sphere, we found moderate depression (Beck's Depression Inventory—23 points), the indicators of failure, feeling of guilt, social isolation, and inability to work stand out. It is important to note that the development of disease-related symptoms will significantly influence Mrs. PM's emotional state and social impact. Mrs. PM has always been linked to work, providing her contribution to the community, and she will no longer be able to do it; as we mentioned earlier in the chapter, Cubans are outgoing, hospitable, and value a sense of community, with the development of disease. Mrs. PM's social interaction will be limited due to word-finding difficulties and special disorientation.

At the end of the evaluation, she expressed feeling frustrated for not complying with the demands of the tests carried out. This may be expected, especially with Cuban populations, given the importance of healthcare and the need for positive social interactions that underlie Cuban identity.

To reassure Mrs. PM, we asked her to attend an upcoming appointment to provide strategies to improve her cognitive and functional functioning to improve her quality of life.

Recommendations and Follow-Up

Mrs. PM attended the appointment accompanied by her husband. She expressed to us feeling many doubts and concerns related to her health; the husband told us that it was also a bit complicated because he did not know what he should do to be able to help her adequately in her illness.

We began by telling him that although there is no curative treatment for her condition, there are other alternatives for disease management not limited to the use of medications, including joining a cognitive stimulation workshop at our center twice a week, with the aim of delaying the loss of both cognitive and functional skills and reducing the presence of emotional and/or behavioral problems and family support groups for the family and caregivers. These support groups may play an important role in the Cuban culture, especially because of the sense of community.

We explained that the intervention would be focused in the first place on the visual-perceptual processes that are mainly affecting their quality of life, and later we would address other functions or neuropsychological skills such as praxis, calculation, and reading-writing, always trying to favor her performance and independence in her daily activities. We suggested to the husband some tips for the home so that it would be a safe place for Mrs. PM, taking into account the visuospatial alterations, for example, the distribution of the furniture in the house, the adequate lighting in all the rooms, as well as the organization of her belongings to facilitate an easy visual search for her.

We appreciated in the consultation that Mrs. PM had improved her mood, and she expressed her desire, to begin with, the cognitive rehabilitation sessions.

Section III: Lessons Learned

- The Cuban society is very cheerful, expressive, supportive, and affective. They do not need to know someone to help them, they like to share without expecting anything in return, and they are excellent hosts. Cubans have a very good sense of humor and are always making jokes about the bad things that happen in society and in their lives.
- They feel a lot of trust and admiration for their doctors and see them as people close to them. On Latin American Medicine Day, it is common for patients to give gifts to their doctors as a token of appreciation. This relationship is reciprocal, and doctors often share their phone numbers with patients so they can call you in case they have any questions about treatment or an emergency arises.
- The Cuban society has extensive knowledge on medical issues. For years, they have tried to educate the population in this regard. There are many programs on national television with sessions dedicated to health and disease where top-level professionals are invited to explain topics of this type and share their wisdom.
- There is great diversity in the Cuban culture, especially related to religion; however, religion, medical science, and neuropsychology co-exist without antagonism.
- The high educational level in the Cuban populations should be taken into consideration during neuropsychological assessments and proper normative data should be applied.
- Neuropsychological tests can cause the patient some anxiety due to fear of failure, so it is very important to explain the characteristics of the evaluation to the patient so that they feel more confident and relaxed at the time of performing the tests.
- In the clinical or psychological interview, it is common for Cuban patients to give extensive answers and provide additional details that might not be of interest or relevant to the case, so the doctor or psychologist must be very skilled to redirect the interview and lead them to answer the question.
- There are standardized neuropsychological measures for Cuban patients; however, more validation studies are needed to generate more normative data. Meanwhile, standardized norms for similar populations in Latin America (e.g., Puerto Rico, Chile, Argentina) might be useful.

Glossary

Mulatos. A racial classification to refer to people of mixed black African and white European ancestry. The term is used as an ethnic/racial category in Cuba.

El mal de ojo. A superstitious curse or legend, believed to be cast by a malevolent glare, usually given to a person when one is unaware.

References

1. Manly JJ. Critical issues in cultural neuropsychology: profit from diversity. Neuropsychol Rev. 2008;18(3):179.
2. Kotik-Friedgut B, Ardila A. A.R. Luria's cultural neuropsychology in the 21st century. Cult Psychol. 2020 Jun;26(2):274–86.

3. Anuario Estadístico de Cuba. Oficina Nacional de Estadística e Información, Sitio en Actualización. 2021.
4. Censo de Población y Viviendas. Oficina Nacional de Estadística e Información, Sitio en Actualización. 2012.
5. Centro Nacional de Informacion y Estadistica. El Color de la Piel según el Censo de Población y Viviendas. 2012.
6. Catalino R, Ustariz Garcia Morera Barrios C. Origen y composición genética de la población cubana. Rev Cubana Hematol Inmunol Hemoter. 2011 Jul;27(3):273–82.
7. Moya JC. A continent of immigrants: postcolonial shifts in the Western Hemisphere. Hisp Am Hist Rev. 2006;86:1–28.
8. Rumbaut RG. The making of a people [Internet]. 2006 [cited 2020 Aug 19]. Available from: https://www.ncbi.nlm.nih.gov/books/NBK19896/
9. Chomsky A, Carr B, Prieto A, Smorkaloff PM. The Cuba reader. History, culture, politics [Internet]. 2nd ed. Vol. 1. [cited 2021 May 2]. p. 774. 2019. Available from: https://www.dukeupress.edu/the-cuba-reader-second-edition
10. Pérez-Brignoli H. Aculturación, transculturación, mestizaje: Metáforas y espejos en la historiografía latinoamericana. Cuad Lit. 2017 Jan;21(41):96–113.
11. Albert MS, Jones K, Savage CR, Berkman L, Seeman T, Blazer D et al. Predictors of cognitive change in older persons: MacArthur studies of successful aging. Psychol Aging. 1995;10(4):578–89.
12. Lyketsos CG, Chen LS, Anthony JC. Cognitive decline in adulthood: an 11.5-year follow-up of the Baltimore Epidemiologic Catchment Area study. Am J Psychiatry. 1999 Jan;156(1):58–65.
13. Tucker-Drob EM, Johnson KE, Jones RN. The cognitive reserve hypothesis: a longitudinal examination of age-associated declines in reasoning and processing speed. Dev Psychol. 2009 Mar;45(2):431–46.
14. Wilson RS, Hebert LE, Scherr PA, Barnes LL, De Leon CFM, Evans DA. Educational attainment and cognitive decline in old age. Neurology. 2009 Feb;72(5):460–5.
15. Noda Hernandez M. Informe Nacional: Cuba. Educación Superior en Iberoamérica—Informe; 2016.
16. Gonzalez Gonzalez JP, Reyes Velazquez R. Desarrollo de la Educación en Cuba después del año 1959. Revista Complutense de Educacion. 2010;21(1):13–35.
17. Santiago DV. Métodos y desafíos en la medición de desigualdades sociales en salud de Cuba Methods and challenges in the measurement of social inequalities in health of. 2020;46(1):1–19.
18. Sinesio C, Gutiérrez S, López Segrera F. Revolución cubana y educación superior. Avaliacao (Campinas). 2008 June;13(2):391–424.
19. Duncan GJ, Magnuson K. Socioeconomic status and cognitive functioning: moving from correlation to causation. Wiley Interdiscip Rev Cogn Sci. 2012;3:377–86.
20. Kirk JM, Walker C. Cuban medical internationalism: the Ebola campaign of 2014–15. Int J Cuba Stud. 2016;8(1):9.
21. Amnistia Internacional. El Embargo EStadounidense contra Cuba.Su Impacto en los Derechos Económicos y Sociales. Amnesty International Publications. Madrid, Espana: 2009.
22. Bringas Vega ML, Fernandez Garcia Y, Garcia Navarro ME. La Neuropsicologia en Cuba. Revista Neuropsicologia, Neuropsiquiatria y Neurociencias. 2009 Octubre;9(2):53–76.
23. Ardila A, Ostrosky F. Guía para el diagnóstico neuropsicológico. Rev Int Segur Soc [Internet]. 2009;62(4):127–9. Available from: http://doi.wiley.com/10.1111/j.1752-1734.2009.01350.x
24. Tombaugh TN. Trail Making Test A and B: normative data stratified by age and education. Arch Clin Neuropsychol. 2004 Mar 1;19(2):203–14.
25. Mitrushina MN. Handbook of normative data for neuropsychological assessment. New York (NY): Oxford University Press; 2005.
26. Segal O, Goodglass H, Kaplan E, Weintraub S. Boston Naming Test. Philadelphia (PA): Lea & Febiger; 1983.
27. Raven J. The Raven's progressive matrices: change and stability over culture and time. Cogn Psychol. [Internet]. 2000 [cited 2021 May 2];41(1):1–48. Available from: https://pubmed.ncbi.nlm.nih.gov/10945921/
28. Elwood RW. The Wechsler Memory Scale-Revised: psychometric characteristics and clinical application. Neuropsychol Rev [Internet]. 1991 Jun [cited 2020 Jun 22];2(2):179–201. Available from: https://link.springer.com/article/10.1007/BF01109053

29. Prina AM, Acosta D, Acostas I, Guerra M, Huang Y, Jotheeswaran AT et al. Cohort Profile: The 10/66 study. Int J Epidemiol. [Internet]. 2016 May 6 [cited 2018 Jun 14];46(2):dyw056. Available from: https://academic.oup.com/ije/article-lookup/doi/10.1093/ije/dyw056

30. Prina AM, Mayston R, Wu Y-T, Prince M. A review of the 10/66 dementia research group. Soc Psychiatry Psychiatr Epidemiol. [Internet]. 2018 Nov 22 [cited 2018 Nov 27];1–10. Available from: http://link.springer.com/10.1007/s00127-018-1626-7

31. Rodríguez-Salgado AM, Llibre-Guerra JJ, Tsoy E, Peñalver-Guia AI, Bringas G, Erlhoff SJ et al. A brief digital cognitive assessment for detection of cognitive impairment in Cuban older adults. J Alzheimer's Dis. [Internet]. 2020 Nov 20 [cited 2021 Jan 18];79(1):85–94. Available from: https://pubmed.ncbi.nlm.nih.gov/33216033/

32. Possin KL, Moskowitz T, Erlhoff SJ, Rogers KM, Johnson ET, Steele NZR et al. The brain health assessment for detecting and diagnosing neurocognitive disorders. J Am Geriatr Soc. 2018 Jan 1;66(1):150–6.

33. Arango-Lasprilla JC, Rivera D, Ramos-Usuga D, Vergara-Moragues E, Montero-López E, Adana Díaz LA et al. Trail Making Test: normative data for the Latin American Spanish-speaking pediatric population. NeuroRehabilitation. 2017;41(3):627–637. doi: 10.3233/NRE-172247.

34. Gorry C, Añé E. Servicios comunitarios de salud mental en Cuba. MEDICC Review, October 2013, Vol 15, No 4. http://mediccreview.org/wp-content/uploads/2018/04/mr_323.pdf.

35. Guàrdia, Joan & Cebollero, Maribel & Rivera, Daniel & Arango-Lasprilla, Juan. (2015). Methodology for the development of normative data for ten Spanish-language neuropsychological tests in eleven Latin American countries. NeuroRehabilitation. 37. 10.3233/NRE-151277.

36. Benedict RHB, Schretlen D, Groninger L, Brandt J. Hopkins verbal learning test—Revised: normative data and analysis of inter-form and test-retest reliability. Clin Neuropsychol. [Internet]. 1998 [cited 2021 May 25];12(1):43–55. Available from: https://www.tandfonline.com/doi/abs/10.1076/clin.12.1.43.1726

37. Shin M-S, Park S-Y, Park S-R, Seol S-H, Kwon JS. Clinical and empirical applications of the Rey–Osterrieth Complex Figure Test. Nat Protoc. [Internet]. 2006 Aug 27 [cited 2019 Sep 20];1(2):892–9. Available from: http://www.ncbi.nlm.nih.gov/pubmed/17406322

38. Delis DC, Kaplan E, Kramer JH. Delis-Kaplan Executive Function System (DKEFS): examiner's manual. San Antonio (TX): Psychol Corp; 2001.

39. Aguilar-Navarro SG, Mimenza-Alvarado AJ, Palacios-García AA, Samudio-Cruz A, Gutiérrez-Gutiérrez LA, Ávila-Funes JA. Validity and Reliability of the Spanish Version of the Montreal Cognitive Assessment (MoCA) for the detection of cognitive impairment in Mexico. Rev Colomb Psiquiatr. [Internet]. 2018 Oct 1 [cited 2018 Oct 17];47(4):237–43. Available from: https://www.sciencedirect.com/science/article/pii/S0034745017300598

40. Dumont R, Willis JO, Veizel K, Zibulsky J. Wechsler Adult Intelligence Scale. 4th ed. In: Encyclopedia of special education [Internet]. Hoboken (NJ): John Wiley & Sons, Inc.; 2014 [cited 2019 Sep 20]. Available from: http://doi.wiley.com/10.1002/9781118660584.ese2520

41. Warrington EK, James M. The visual object and space perception battery : VOSP. Queen Square, London: Pearson; 1991.

42. Kramer JH, Jurik J, Sha SJ, Rankin KP, Rosen HJ, Johnson JK et al. Distinctive neuropsychological patterns in frontotemporal dementia, semantic dementia, and Alzheimer disease. Cogn Behav Neurol. 2003;16(4):211–8.

43. Benton AL, Van Allen MW. Impairment in facial recognition in patients with cerebral disease. Trans Am Neurol Assoc. 1968 Dec 1;93(4):38–42.

44. Quintana M, Peña-Casanova J, Sánchez-Benavides G, Langohr K, Manero RM, Aguilar M et al. Spanish multicenter normative studies (neuronorma project): norms for the abbreviated Barcelona test. Arch Clin Neuropsychol. [Internet]. 2011 Mar 1 [cited 2021 May 25];26(2):144–57. Available from: https://academic.oup.com/acn/article/26/2/144/4024

45. Stroop JR. Studies of interference in serial verbal reactions. J Exp Psychol. [Internet]. 1935 [cited 2018 Jun 17];18(6):643–62. Available from: http://content.apa.org/journals/xge/18/6/643

46. Beck AT, Ward CH, Mendelson M, Mock J, Erbaugh J. An inventory for measuring depression. Arch Gen Psychiatry. [Internet]. 1961 [cited 2021 May 25];4(6):561–71. Available from: https://pubmed.ncbi.nlm.nih.gov/13688369/

Guatemala

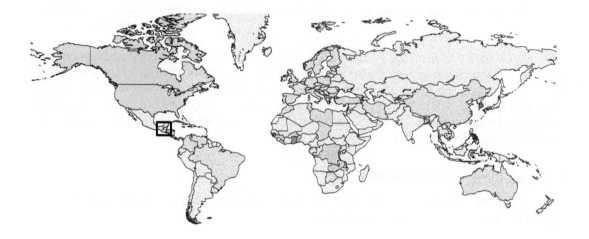

32 Neuropsychology in Guatemala

The Eyes Don't See What the Mind Does Not Understand

Beatriz MacDonald, Tedd Judd, Claudia García de la Cadena, and Isis Yahaira Marroquin Jerez de Cifuentes

> *Los ojos no ven lo que la mente no entiende.* (The eyes don't see what the mind does not understand.)
> (Dr. Henry Berrisford Stokes)

The late Guatemalan neurologist, Dr. Stokes, championed neuropsychology in Guatemala for decades. He observed that neurologists and other medical providers often do not appreciate what neuropsychology contributes until they witness it firsthand. Similarly, when we do not see and learn about our client's culture, we do not appreciate it and apply it to their care. This chapter is dedicated to the memory of our elders and mentors, Dr. Stokes and the great Colombian neuropsychologist, Alfredo Ardila.

Section I: Background Information

Throughout this chapter, we share general information about Guatemala with a focus on the Mam Mayan community to support the case study.

Terminology and Perspective

People from Guatemala are referred to as Guatemalans, Central Americans, Latin-Americans, Hispanics, or Latinos(as)/Latinx/Latine, and, colloquially, *Chapines*. The preferred terminology is Guatemalan.

This chapter depicts the contributions and knowledge of four authors from different geographical locations. We partnered together to present how neuropsychology has developed in Guatemala and how each one of us has contributed to this process.

I, Dr. Beatriz MacDonald, was raised in Guatemala and moved to the United States to complete college. I left Guatemala with the hope of studying neuropsychology in another country since the field did not exist in my home country. After almost 20 years, I relish the excitement of teaching as invited faculty at the Universidad del Valle de Guatemala (UVG) for the Master's Program in Clinical Neuropsychology. I am eternally grateful to my dear colleagues and visionaries, Drs. García de la Cadena and Judd, who solidified the field of neuropsychology in Guatemala.

I, Dr. Tedd Judd, was raised in the United States. I began learning Spanish through immersion in Guatemala at age 24 (1977). Since 1986, I have regularly traveled to teach neuropsychology in Latin America, especially Nicaragua, Costa Rica, and Guatemala. I am delighted that we are fulfilling my long-time dream of a Master's Program in Clinical Neuropsychology for Central America. In the United States, I am the past president of the Hispanic Neuropsychological Society, and I have a multicultural specialty private practice, working with clinical, forensic, immigration, and social issues.

DOI: 10.4324/9781003051862-65

I, Dra. Claudia García de la Cadena was born in Mexico City, and my professional training was carried out at the National Autonomous University of Mexico and at the University of La Laguna in Spain. Since 2002, I have worked at the Universidad del Valle de Guatemala as a professor and director. After an unexpected encounter with Dr. Tedd Judd, we began to design a Master's Program in Neuropsychology in Guatemala. This project took almost seven years to consolidate, and in 2015, we started with the first group of students. Now, we are enrolling the fifth cohort with students from Central American countries.

I, Lcda. Isis Yahaira Marroquin Jerez de Cifuentes, am a graduate student completing my last semester of the Master Program in Clinical Neuropsychology at UVG. My title of Lcda means *licenciada* or "licensed" (psychologist). I was born in Puerto Barrios, Izabal, on the Caribbean coast of Guatemala, and belong to the Afro-descendant community. I trained with a pioneer of neurosciences and neuropsychology, Dr. Henry Stokes, who opened the doors to the field. He instilled in me continuous learning and love for the most important organ of our body, "the brain," which led me to become interested in the Master's Program in Clinical Neuropsychology.

All four authors have different degrees of language fluency and proficiency in English. Much of this paper is translated from Spanish, intentionally preserving the nuances of the Spanish language and writing style and illustrating the richness of the Guatemalan culture. This undertaking has been particularly broad in its cultural diversity: an Afrodescendent Guatemalan, a Mexican-Guatemalan, a Guatemalan-American, and a gringo working with Mayans. Multiculturalism is typical of Guatemalan neuropsychological encounters.

Geography

The Republic of Guatemala is home to 17 million and located in Central America, the isthmus that connects North and South America. Guatemala borders with Mexico, Belize, El Salvador, Honduras, and the Pacific and Atlantic oceans. While divided into twenty departments (*departamentos* in Spanish; equivalent to states), Guatemala contains mountains, beach, tropical rain forest, desert, and valleys. We have 37 volcanoes, three of which are active.

History and People

The indigenous community in Guatemala is the direct descendant of the ancient Mayan civilization. They erected pyramids for polytheistic ceremonial rituals, wrote hieroglyphics, developed an advanced calendar system, and traded goods (e.g., cacao). Major lowland regions and cities (e.g., Tikal) were abandoned around 1,100 years ago, possibly due to drought, deforestation, and climate change. All major features of the civilization continued in the highlands until the Spanish conquest.

The Spanish *conquistadores* (conquerors) arrived in 1524, bringing diseases and military conquest that decimated the Mayan civilization and population. Guatemala was part of the Spanish Captaincy General of Guatemala (colonial government) for nearly 330 years. The Spanish established feudal patterns of land ownership. European elites ruled with the assistance of *ladinos(as)*, a label identifying non-indigenous Guatemalans. *Mestizos* or biracial Indigenous-European people were next in the social hierarchy and the bottom rank belonged to the Mayan community, who were stripped of their community life.[1] Such demarcation of status marked a divide that continues to drive the economy and social life in Guatemala.

The current distribution by ethnic self-identification is as follows: 56% Ladino, 41.7% Maya, 1.8% Xinka, 0.1% Garífuna, 0.2% Afro-descendant/Creole/Afromestizo and 0.2% foreigners. Ethnic self-identification is complex and influenced by half a millennium of repression and racism that persist to the present.[2] Based on the census in 2017, 33.4% of the population were between

1 and 14 years of age, 61.0% were between 15 and 64 years of age, and only 5.6% were older than 65 years of age.[3]

Guatemala became independent of Spain in 1821 and a fully independent nation in 1841. A popular uprising in 1944 led to a ten-year revolution and a US-backed coup in 1954 with an installed military dictatorship. From 1960 to 1996, we lived a civil war with human rights violations and a genocide of the indigenous Maya. Many Mayans sought asylum in Mexico; for example, the Mam used to be one of the larger groups but were forced to migrate and spread to different areas in Guatemala and the United States. The 1996 Peace Treaty reestablished a representative democracy and established indigenous rights, which are poorly enforced due to high crime and government corruption.[4]

The Mayan diaspora during the civil war from 1960 to 1996 initiated major relocation struggles for the Mayan population, who sought asylum in Mexico and the United States and moved to different parts of the country to avoid persecution and genocide. Prior to this, each Mayan community mainly interacted within their respective members and had unique typical handwoven clothing language and territory. However, displacement prompted Mayan communities to interact with each other, learn how to communicate with each other, and exchange goods and, clothing with profound impact on Mayan community identities. In addition, as of 2017, there were 1,444,000 Guatemalans in the United States, with the largest populations in California, Florida, and Texas. Diaspora communities tend to cluster, for example, there are Mam communities in East Oakland, CA, Forks, WA, and Lynn, MA.[5]

Language

Twenty-four languages are spoken in Guatemala. The majority (93%) of citizens speak Spanish as either their first or second language. Twenty-one Mayan languages (completely unrelated to Spanish) are heard and used throughout the country as a musical melody. The most used are K'iche' (1 million speakers), Q'eqchi', Kaqchikel, and Mam, while some are endangered.[6] Most of these have multiple dialects that may not be fully mutually intelligible, important in selecting interpreters. Mam has 686,000 speakers in southeastern Guatemala. The order of the sentence is usually verb, subject, and object. There are no independent pronouns. Numbers above 20 are rarely known or used.[7] Communities in three departments speak two additional non-Mayan languages, Garífuna (an Afro-Caribbean creole) and Xincan.

Communication

Forms of address are more complex in Spanish than in English. When speaking English, we use either first names (e.g., Mary) for informal close relationships or titles for formal relationships (Ms., Dr., or Rev). In-groups will sometimes use "brother" and "sister" metaphorically, but these would rarely be used in a mainstream clinical context or cross-culturally. Spanish has these options and, additionally, has Don (male) and Doña (female) titles for respected elders. In addition, "tío" (uncle), "tía" (aunt), "abuelo" (grandfather), and "abuela" (grandmother) may be used in the same metaphorical ways. Guatemalan clinical relationships with a psychologist can progress to being more informal and could include such terms. In the United States, we typically use "señora" or "señor" as a sign of deference with Guatemalan families and clients. However, in Guatemala, it may be considered a sign of poor rapport to address a client overly formally.

Personal disclosure helps to build an alliance. Guatemalans value *personalismo*—personal relationship—and psychologists are expected to disclose about themselves, for example, sharing where one is from and one's knowledge about Guatemala. Guatemalans have a deep respect for the medical community and as a sign of deference, they typically do not question physicians or psychologists. Therefore, we have to be mindful to ensure that clients and families understand the purpose, results, impressions, and recommendations of an assessment.

Professional interpreter training for Mayan languages is not well developed in Guatemala, the United States, or elsewhere and few trained interpreters are available. Briefing and debriefing the interpreter and explaining the use of an interpreter during an assessment are instrumental. In diaspora communities, the language community may be small, and interpreters may have dual relationships with the clients. Therefore, providers need to navigate these considerations carefully. Many Mayans are bilingual in their Mayan language and Spanish. Even when Spanish is not their better language, it is sometimes the most pragmatic language for portions of the evaluation.

Translation of words is a nuanced process and providers need to be aware of the subtle differences. For example, *demencia*, in Spanish, is understood as "crazy," with much more stigma than "dementia" in English. Additionally, the Spanish second person has three forms—informal "tu," colloquial informal "vos" (similar to English "thou"), and formal "usted." These also have cultural and political implications beyond the scope of this chapter. When an English speaker says "you," the interpreter has to choose which form to use. This introduces the potential for misunderstanding the English speaker's intentions about the nature of the relationship.

Education

The educational system in Guatemala perpetuates vast disparities based on socioeconomic access. There is an abyss between public and private education that perpetuates differences in educational experience and quality. Public education rarely offers English or other foreign languages. Special education in Guatemala started in 1940 for vision impairment. Disability accommodations and special education laws and policies were enacted in the 1990s and early 2000s, but implementation is lagging due to lack of resources and funding.[8]

Mayan language preservation and education was a promise of the 1996 peace accords, still only partially fulfilled. Recently, UNICEF and the Ministry of Intercultural Bilingual Education have constructed curricula by towns, codified Intercultural Bilingual schools (Spanish and the local Mayan language), and promulgated educational policies to strengthen the National Education System. The program has also contributed to the evaluation of language, culture, the participation of parents, and the generation of community education experiences. Mayan community colleges are emerging.

Literacy

The Guatemalan literacy rate had steadily increased from 64.2% in 1994 to 81.3% in 2014. Of the literate population, only 5% of women report more than seven years of schooling. Literacy over age 65 was 46.8% in 2015. Indigenous populations register higher percentages of illiteracy.[3] Mayan languages are mostly oral, but a written literature is developing, especially in K'iche', Q'eqchi', Kaqchikel, and Mam.

Socioeconomic Status

Living conditions in rural and urban areas are impoverished. A small percentage of the population holds most of the wealth. About 59% of households have running water, 56% have indoor toilets, 88% have electricity, 54% cook with firewood, and 44% buy propane gas. In rural communities, many homes are made of metal roof panels with dirt floors.[3]

Values and Customs

The folklore of Guatemala is rooted in colorful clothing, delicious food, strong beliefs, and rich traditions. Guatemalans value a collective community, with customs and traditions centered on family.

Gender and Sexuality

Machismo (strong or aggressive masculine pride and family responsibility) and *marianismo,* (female submissiveness, self-sacrifice for family, chastity, religiosity) continue to be part of relationships that permeate all social spaces, including social policy, employment, educational choices, and family life.[9,10]

Homosexual activity became legal in 1871, but sexual orientation and the LGBTQIA+ community are still largely taboo topics.[11] In January 2018, the Inter-American Court of Human Rights (IACHR) ruled that the American Convention on Human Rights requires the recognition of same-sex marriage, but this is not recognized in Guatemala. Guatemalan laws do not safeguard the LGBTQIA+ community and there is no prohibition against discrimination in housing, education, healthcare, employment, banking, etc.

Spirituality and Religion

Mayan religious practices are syncretic or blended. Preconquest Mayans practiced polytheism. Spaniards imposed Catholicism. Mayan communities blended both, often blending specific Catholic saints with Mayan gods and blending rituals. Some traditions endure, such as patron saints/Gods and festival days for each village or pueblo. In recent decades, there has been a shift toward evangelical Christianity.[1]

Acculturation and Systemic Barriers

Guatemala has entrenched systemic barriers to access to power, wealth, justice, health care, etc., due to governmental corruption and socioeconomic class divides dating back to the conquest. Rural-urban acculturation is a major change for rural Mayans who move to Guatemala City to work as housekeepers, construction workers, etc. They confront entirely different languages, beliefs, institutions, technologies, clothing, and food.

Health and Mental Health Views

When speaking with families and clients, information gathering is often difficult because of different conceptualizations of medical conditions and medications. Our strategies for gathering information include asking for pictures of medication bottles, calling more knowledgeable family members, asking in several different ways, and familiarity with idioms of symptoms. The coordination of medical records and medications among providers is poor. Additionally, medication adherence is impacted by an understanding of how to take the medication. For example, "I was feeling depressed yesterday, so I took one of my antidepressants."

Malnutrition is a fundamental health problem among Mayan communities, affecting all other neurological risks. The majority of Mayan children show growth stunting due to malnutrition, which impairs cognitive development, and increases susceptibility to diseases including infections, hypertension, diabetes, and stroke.[12,13] Vascular disease is prevalent and medical treatment and prevention are poorly understood and followed by the public. Neurologically important infectious diseases include cysticercosis, HIV, Zika, COVID-19, dengue, and malaria. Pesticide toxicity and drug and alcohol abuse are widespread.

Many Mam believe that diseases have supernatural causes or are due to moral transgressions. Traditional healers are very important in the community, with political and religious functions. They attend to illnesses of the spirit, such as strong emotions, anger, sadness, and shame. Anger is seen as an emotion that upsets the body's balance and leads to headaches, stomachaches, fatigue, and chronic illness. *Nervios* (nerves) is a disease due to experiencing strong emotions, particularly anxiety, pain, and sadness. Other examples of Mayan conceptualization of emotional/physical/social disorders with their K'iche names are listed in Table 32.1.

Table 32.1 Mayan conceptualization of emotional/physical/social disorders with their K'iche names

Disorder	Description
Q'ij Alaxik	The discomfort of not knowing oneself. If one does not know or ignores the vocation that is destined to follow from birth, an imbalance arises in the health and life circles of the person.
X'ibiliril	Loss of spirit (jaleb') arises due to a violent or traumatic event affecting the normal balance of the human body.
Pakq'ab Chuch Tat	Health effects due to traditional ethical transgressions, especially from a level of authority.
Moxrik	Physical and mental discomfort due to assimilation to a foreign culture, especially for personal reasons.
Molem Yab'il	Psychosomatic consequences from the dissatisfaction of basic needs of food, land, housing, health, and education.

The most frequent diseases in the Mam community are parasites and respiratory infections.[14] Diseases are generally cured by herbalists, who are often also midwives. Health depends on the blood as it is perceived as "the seat of physical strength and sensory perceptions." Traditional medicine has over a thousand treatments derived from local flora and fauna.

Approach to Neuropsychological or Psychological Evaluations

The development of neuropsychology in Central America has a long history.[15] The Master's Program in Clinical Neuropsychology was born from collaborative work among Dr. Judd, Dr. García de la Cadena, and Guatemalan psychologists. The program began in 2015 with a student cohort of psychologists, neurologists, a psychiatrist, and a criminologist. The subsequent four cohorts have been psychologists. The program offers two years of training with 21 courses, 500 hours of practical experience, a portfolio of 20 cases, and a final project. (https://www.uvg.edu.gt/uvgmaster/neuropsicologia-clinica/). The design of monthly, three-day intensive courses in Guatemala City has drawn students from rural parts of Guatemala and from Honduras, El Salvador, and Costa Rica, as well as professors from Colombia, Mexico, Spain, Brazil, and the United States. These courses became virtual during the COVID-19 pandemic, which improved geographic and disability access and broader teaching and clinical experiences. While this training is modest compared to North America, Europe, and other Latin American neuropsychology master's programs, it has established recognition of the profession and field. The Master's Program has a truly Guatemalan and Central American identity, with instruction entirely in Spanish, and a strong focus on local cultures, languages, needs, and conditions.

Supervised practice is adapted to available instruments, limited resources, illiteracy, low formal education, and single session assessments. The Department of Neuropsychology at UVG has researched the adaptation of neuropsychological tests in adult and pediatric Guatemalan populations.

The program has been able to address some of the country's greatest needs through practice sites in the two main public health national hospitals, the Roosevelt Hospital and the San Juan de

Dios Hospital. Other programs include the Military Hospital, the Social Security health system, and the university clinic CIPA (Centro Integral de Psicología Aplicada) at UVG, which offers care at low cost for low-income populations.

The case study we selected is a portfolio case for Lcda. Marroquin Jerez de Cifuentes under the supervision of Dr. García de la Cadena. Presenting this case highlights not only neuropsychology in Guatemala but also the training achieved through the Master's Program in Clinical Neuropsychology.

Section II: Case Study — "The Eyes Don't See What the Mind Does Not Understand"

Note: Possible identifying information and several aspects of history and presentation have been changed to protect client identity and privacy.

The client is a 72-year-old female from the Mam community who speaks Mam and Spanish. Per the request of a provider in the rural areas of Guatemala, the Chief for External Consults coordinated the referral for an evaluation due to concerns with memory and changes in behavior. She was seen at the San Juan de Dios Public Health Hospital in the Department of Neuropsychology. The hospital is in Guatemala City, a 4-hour bus ride from her home village. The information below was reported by Sra. Milagro, her granddaughter, and daughter.

The examiner contacted multiple providers in the hospital for access to Sra. Milagro's medical records. However, since these are not electronic, access is limited, and she was unable to obtain imaging records. In general, access to medical care in rural regions in Guatemala is extremely limited, and urban medical healthcare has systemic barriers in place.

Presenting Concerns

Sra. Milagro reported distress because her eldest son decreased the frequency of visits and calls. This change in the relationship, according to Sra. Milagro, was because she told her son that his wife (Sra. Milagro's daughter-in-law) was cheating on him with a man, who reportedly was also in love with Sra. Milagro. Sra. Milagro's daughter and granddaughter shared that the existence of this man and infidelity was not true, and part of Sra. Milagro's imagination. The family also indicated that Sra. Milagro's eldest son was upset because Sra. Milagro shared the supposed infidelity with the whole family causing problems in his marriage. Also, she had been saying sexually disinhibited statements to men in the street and hugging everyone, so that her family no longer let her go out alone.

The family's greatest concern was that Sra. Milagro's independence had declined. Several times she left home and got lost. Once she got off a bus and did not recognize where she was, even though it was a place she frequented. She had decreased motivation to clean the house. In the past, Sra. Milagro was a highly active woman, who took care of her home and family.

Daily Functioning

Sra. Milagro indicated that she started working as a child with her father in agriculture. From a very young age, she worked at home doing domestic work. After moving in with her partner and father of her children, Sra. Milagro started working in her village's market selling meat and vegetables. She continued selling produce until her family recently asked her to stop because she was giving away the merchandise without payment. According to her daughter, Sra. Milagro started struggling with business transactions, such as charging another amount or giving the wrong change back to clients. Sra. Milagro also started accusing others of stealing because she misplaced the money or had lost it. Consequently, Sra. Milagro's daughter and other family members were managing Sra. Milagro's finances because she was giving away money. Her daughter added that "[Sra. Milagro] is a person who likes to share, but now she gives everything away."

Sra. Milagro reported feeling sad because of the changes in her daily life. She no longer interacted with the people who worked in the market and whom she had known for many years and had a lot of affection for them. Consequently, at home, she was unmotivated to complete housework. Most recently, she helped in the kitchen when her daughter asked her. She described feeling bore, as well as getting upset with the noise of her grandchildren playing, the chickens, and of people passing the house at night. She expressed frustration because her family did not allow her to take the bus or go outside alone. Sra. Milagro shared that she used her daughter's cell phone to communicate with her children. Her children were aware of changes in personal hygiene and the cleanliness of her clothes.

Health History

Sra. Milagro described visual alterations in both eyes. She was diagnosed with hyperthyroidism six years ago that was managed with medication. Her family noted that three years previously she had been admitted to a hospital in Retalhuleu (a nearby town) for a cerebrovascular event producing memory and language difficulties. She recovered leaving sequelae in her memory. Since that time, she had taken medication for hypertension. She reported frequent headaches that made her irritable, which she treated with over-the-counter medication. Her daughter reported that Sra. Milagro may have tremors, but they were not often, and she struggled to describe them. Because her father died of alcoholism, Sra. Milagro learned that alcohol is not good, so she did not have a history of alcohol or cigarette use. At home, she and her family ate tortillas, herbs, and vegetables, with very little animal protein. She reported that her sleep time had decreased, she woke up very early and it was difficult for her to fall asleep. On two occasions at the beginning of a dream, she woke up screaming because, according to Sra. Milagro, her grandson, let a person enter the house to have sex with her. This bothered her and she was angry with her grandson. According to her daughter, this was part of her imagination because when they got up and did not find the man either inside or outside the house. From what the family described, both Sra. Milagro's mother and uncle passed away from vascular events. She had also told her sister that she saw a man in the marketplace who was of normal size, but as he came toward her, he shrank until he disappeared.

Educational History

Sra. Milagro's parents did not enroll her in school when she was a child because she was a girl and had to take care of her younger siblings. She did not read, but she learned to count on her own and through her work, it became increasingly easier for her. However, she now had difficulty performing basic mathematical operations.

Language Proficiency

Sra. Milagro's mother tongue was Mam. She reported speaking and understanding Mam very well compared to Spanish. She noted that in Spanish, she struggled with pronouncing certain words. She learned most of her Spanish vocabulary while working in the village. Sra. Milagro spoke Mam with her siblings, children, family, and acquaintances in her village, and used Spanish to communicate with her grandchildren and acquaintances. According to her family, there had been no changes in language functioning at the time of the assessment.

Sra. Milagro's dominant language was clearly Mam. Given limitations in available measures, her Spanish skills were determined to be adequate to evaluate her in Spanish and administer neuropsychological tests. However, this significantly limited the evaluation.

Cultural History

Sra. Milagro was the first daughter of two boys and two girls. She was born and continued to reside in a small village in the *departmento* of Retalhuleu in southwestern Guatemala. Guatemalans navigating rural and urban spaces, as well as crossing ethnic and Mayan communities, engage in identity processes. Sra. Milagro rarely visited urban spaces.

Sra. Milagro's family worked in agriculture, growing corn and vegetables for the home and for sale. Her mother was a homemaker. Sra. Milagro recalled that as a child, she helped her mother at home to take care of her younger siblings and in the afternoons, she played with the children in the community. When Sra. Milagro was eight years old, her mother died of a cerebral vascular event. Sra. Milagro, her father, and siblings then dedicated themselves to working the land. They left home to go sowing before dawn, which taught her to be a hard-working woman. From eight years of age, Sra. Milagro worked the fields, tended the home, and took care of her younger siblings, a burden made harder by her father's alcoholism. She knew that in her community, young women were offered to older men and in return they received financial help for the bride's family. She said that when her father wanted to give her to a man, she ran away from home, which led her to look for work in a home where she was subjected to sexual abuse. She became pregnant with her first child at the age of 12, and a year later, she became pregnant with her second child. At age 16, she was together as a couple with the man with whom she lived for 34 years until he died. With her partner, they procreated eight children—she was the mother of seven living children and one died in an accident.

Emotional Functioning

Sra. Milagro communicated her sadness by describing the activities that changed due to being sad versus stating she felt sad. She reported that she could not go out alone and could not work or see her friends in the market or her relatives. Consequently, she was not motivated to do housework and was bored. Her grandchildren's noise irritated her, and she did not like her children telling her what to do.

Behavioral Observations

Sra. Milagro came to the neuropsychology clinic for the first time accompanied by her granddaughter who was the only relative who could accompany her that day. They left at dawn for the 4-hour, 140-km interurban bus ride to be at the hospital early. She started the session by expressing relief and saying, "it's good that it's early because I have to go home." Sra. Milagro was alert. Sra. Milagro appeared disoriented but was smiling, polite, and greeted the examiner with a hug, as if she knew her. She was wearing the traditional Mayan clothing of her region with purple güipil (handwoven blouse) with a colorful handwoven skirt. She appeared to have taken little interest in her hygiene.

During the interview, Sra. Milagro spoke in Spanish with some grammatical errors and her Spanish was coherent but somewhat disorganized. She consented for the evaluation to be in

Spanish. Her facial expression was generally consistent with what she was sharing. She constantly called on her granddaughter to answer for her when she did not remember some general information. It also became evident that Sra. Milagro wanted to express herself alone. Her granddaughter was asked to wait outside, allowing Sra. Milagro to describe the event that most concerned her at that time, building a relationship of trust with the examiner. As the interview progressed, Sra. Milagro appeared worried, so the evaluator asked her why. She explained that she was hungry and wanted to return home early. Therefore, the first portion of the evaluation was completed, with the recommendation to return to the next appointment accompanied by a person she lived with to provide the necessary data for the history. Instructions also included to sleep well and eat before the next appointment. Sra. Milagro said goodbye with several hugs, smiling, and gratitude.

After the information and data gathered during the first session, the examiner was extremely concerned about Sra. Milagro' neurological well-being and requested a consult with neurology. Consequently, Sra. Milagro's neurologist started her on Fulcrum (https://www.eurofarma.com.gt/produtos/fulcrum), which is the combination of the benzodiazepine, *chlordiazepoxide*, together with the tricyclic antidepressant, *amitriptyline*. She started taking this medication before the second session.

For the second session, seven weeks later, Sra. Milagro greeted the examiner with a loving hug. She maintained a sense of good humor for a long period of time, as well as told several stories of her life. Sometimes Sra. Milagro had to be asked the same question several times and in different ways to ensure her understanding. In this session, her daughter corroborated and elaborated on previous information.

Sra. Milagro was not comfortable with testing and constantly tried to tell stories to avoid it. She did not like to wear glasses and did not bring them to the sessions, making visual tests impractical. Additionally, she refused reading and writing activities, justifying her illiteracy by saying that in their culture, women "should take care of others and do things around the house."

Test and Norm Selection

Tests were selected considering age, no schooling and illiteracy, visual limitations, commute to the evaluation, socioeconomic conditions, and relevant data that were obtained in the interview.

Session 1: Montreal Cognitive Assessment (MoCA)—Basic in Spanish.

Session 2: Evaluación Neuropsicológica Estandarizada—Adulto (ENE-A; Standard Neuropsychological Evaluation for Hospitalized Adults)[16]: orientation, attention and concentration (digits forward and successive series), working memory (digits backward), processing speed (coding), verbal memory, executive functioning, praxias, visual-verbal name memory, verbal fluency, and verbal abstract reasoning (similarities). The Depresión Geriátrica Escala abreviada de Yesavage (Abbreviated Geriatric Depression Scale; GDS)[17] in Spanish, which was read to her. The Actividades Básicas del Indice Barthel de Vida Diaria (Barthel Index of Basic activities Daily Life).[18]

Test Results

Sra. Milagro did not know her age, the name of her *departamento*, or the day, month, or year. She could not distinguish left from right. These limitations in her conventional orientation to space were all potentially culturally congruent. However, she also had difficulty remembering the names of her children and other family members, which is atypical.

On the MoCA Sra. Milagro scored in the moderate impairment range. On the ENE-A, she evidenced abilities within normal limits (average or low average) in verbal memory recall and recognition, motor functioning, working memory, understanding of directions, confrontational naming, semantic fluency, sentence repetition, and tactile perception. She demonstrated mild deficits in verbal auditory attention, learning rote-verbal information, and phonemic fluency. Her conversational language in Spanish was notable for reduced fluency, repeating the same phrases, not conjugating verbs correctly, semantic paraphasias, and disorganized sentences, which is often observed in individuals who Spanish is their second language. Due to the limitation of not using an interpreter, language data need to be broadly examined. In making compromises, the ethical standard of *do no harm* is central. On the questionnaires (orally administered), Sra. Milagro scored in the mildly depressed range. Her family rated her as independent in basic activities of daily living.

Impressions and Case Conceptualization

Overall, there were marked changes in Sra. Milagro's behavior, including disinhibition, as well as forgetfulness and reduced independence in the completion of activities of daily living. Table 32.2 documents the delusions that Sra. Milagro and her family described. These fit within Nomura and colleagues'[19] cross-cultural dementia delusion classification system. It balances the relativism (cultural variations) and universality of the construct of dementia, highlighting the universality of delusions, such as phantom boarder, infidelity, and theft. Applying this approach allowed the family to understand Sra. Milagro's symptoms and provide reassurance that the delusions were due to her illness. This helped mend the rupture in the relationship between Sra. Milagro and her son and daughter-in-law.

When working with individuals from culturally and linguistically diverse backgrounds, the triangulation of clinical observation, family data, and testing results is critical. Testing data carry less weight in case conceptualization. For this case, clinical information and observations indicated memory decline impacting functioning and emotional well-being, as well as delusions and prior history of a vascular event. During the evaluation, Sra. Milagro's disinhibited behaviors were concerning. Although Guatemalans are warm by nature, greeting a medical provider with a

Table 32.2 Applied classification of delusions

Classification of delusions	Sra. Milagro's symptomatology
Factor 1 • Belief that her house is not her house • Phantom boarder • Delusion of abandonment • Belief that others are no who they claim to be	Sra. Milagro reports that her grandson lets a man come into the house at night (phantom boarder).
Factor 2 • Delusion relating to the TV • Delusion of persecution	None
Factor 3 • Delusion of abandonment • Delusional jealousy	Sra. Milagro reports that her daughter-in-law cheated on her son with Sra. Milagro's imaginary boyfriend.
Other symptoms • Delusion of theft	Sra. Milagro hides her belongings and believes others have stolen them when she cannot find them.

Source: Material taken and adapted from Nomura.[19]

hug at the first meeting is not customary, and this fits her family's description of her changed and atypical behavior in her village.

When considering what type of neurological event, dementia, or neurocognitive disorder to diagnose, there are limitations to consider. First, the neuropsychological battery was administered in Spanish and not Mam, and the normative data were based on the Mexican population. However, testing results were average for verbal comprehension, memory recognition, and semantic fluency, allowing us to interpret these results and rule out the possibility of an Alzheimer's dementia diagnosis. Without brain imaging, it was difficult with certainty to rule out frontal dementia or vascular dementia, so we hypothesized that it was mixed given her history. Since neuroimaging was not readily available, the focus then shifted from a specific diagnosis to symptomatology and treatment planning. The importance to differentiate between these two dementias would be the medication to be prescribed. Additionally, Sra. Milagro presented with depressive symptoms and the prescribed medication (Fulcrum) needed to be taken daily. Yet, medication adherence is a cultural aspect to integrate. If the client does not feel well or has side effects, the client may stop taking the medication without consulting the doctor. Therefore, emphasizing the importance of medication adherence to family was necessary.

Feedback Session and Follow-Up

Feedback to Sra. Milagro and her family was impacted by the COVID-19 pandemic and follow-up was provided over the phone over the course of two sessions. Technological limitations prevented videoconferencing.

The examiner explained validation therapy (https://vfvalidation.org/get-started/what-is-validation/) to Sra. Milagro's daughter as a strategy to accept Sra. Milagro's reality and not argue with her. The examiner emphasized the importance of understanding, respecting, and valuing Sra. Milagro's experience by recognizing that her behavior was due to an illness. The feedback included mutual problem solving regarding safely managing Sra. Milagro's problematic behavior while increasing her access to friends and household participation. Additionally, medication adherence and increased behavioral activities were emphasized to support Sra. Milagro's emotional well-being. As part of follow-up, the examiner recommended speaking with each family member and sharing the results to support their acceptance.

We recognize that this was an extremely limited neuropsychological service. Challenges of language, culture, access, transportation, tests, and other resources greatly limited conventional testing and diagnosis. Nevertheless, a respectful and caring attitude and a neuropsychological perspective allowed our student to provide this family with a better understanding of their loved elder and mitigated family conflicts.

Section III: Lessons Learned

The lessons learned from this case study are unique because of where the authors live, practice, and supervise. In the United States, the first and second authors deliver clinical services to Guatemalans, who may or may not be Mayan, and remotely supervise trainees who are enrolled in the graduate program in Guatemala. In Guatemala, the third author teaches and supervises, and the fourth author is completing her graduate training. Our diverse experiences coupled with our deep commitment to the emerging field of neuropsychology in Guatemala creates a multifaceted approach on how to practice. Therefore, we hope that the lessons learned we share can be applied when assessing individuals living not only in Guatemala but also in other countries. As a result of writing this book chapter, we also reflected on possible next steps in the development of Mayan Neuropsychology (see Section below on "How Can We Develop Mayan Neuropsychology?").

What to consider and learn when delivering neuropsychological care to Guatemalans?

- **Diversity**—Guatemala is comprised of a multitude of diverse languages and cultures. Neuropsychologists can thoughtfully research the cultural background of potential clients to be proactively prepared and practice socially responsible neuropsychology. Unless providers take the time to learn about the richness of Guatemala's diversity, we will not know what to ask—*"the eyes don't see what the mind does not understand."*
- **Culture**—Acculturation, assimilation, and enculturation occur not only for immigrants leaving Guatemala but also for individuals living in Guatemala, especially Mayan rural-to-urban migration.
- **Epidemiology**—Guatemalans may be exposed to malnutrition, infectious diseases, and toxins uncommon in the United States.
- **Access**—Guatemalans often face significant barriers to access healthcare in Guatemala and the United States.[20] It is the provider's responsibility to understand these barriers as systemic health disparities and not attribute them to the client's character. One step further is, as providers, to tackle these barriers, drive social justice change, and increase access to services.
- **Collective Community**—As members of a collective, family-based community, individuals with dementia rarely seek help because families compensate for behaviors and offer protections and supports. Families may finally seek help once symptoms are fairly advanced. This can also happen with developmental and other progressive diseases/disorders (e.g., autism spectrum disorder and multiple sclerosis), as well as intermittent ones, such as epilepsy.
- **Collateral Information**—As part of the assessment, providers often cannot access all the necessary medical records and clinical history to inform case conceptualization. For example, we may receive a diagnosis of intellectual disability on a prescription pad or not have neurodiagnostic information for a client with a history of a stroke. This happens in Guatemala, the United States, and other countries. Barriers that perpetuate these limitations are resources, beliefs about medical care, and geographic access. Additionally, clients and their family members are often not knowledgeable to provide such information. One can say that oftentimes, providers are both clinicians and detectives in trying to acquire all of the necessary data.
- **Language**—It is of great importance to inquire about language usage, bilingualism, and level of language skills in each language. Having this knowledge prior to the assessment is ideal, but often we do not know it until the appointment. An advance phone call may help determine languages of interview, interpreter needs, and test selection. A detailed language use interview and testing may be needed to determine whether language difficulties reflect impairment or fluency, as well as provide documentation and resources in the appropriate language. This is most often best done with an informed clinical interview.
- **Interpreters**—Ideally, we ethically strive to use professionally trained interpreters and complete assessments in the client's dominant language. However, Mayan language interpreter training and resources are limited,[21] so we make necessary compromises, on a case-by-case basis, to serve the best needs of the client.
- **Communication**—Guatemalans and Mayan communities may describe symptomatology differently (e.g., physical pain instead of sadness) and define diseases differently. Forms of address and of physical contact in greeting are culturally complex in Guatemala. Practitioners need to be aware of the range of responses and follow the client's lead. It is safest to start with *usted* with adults and to switch to *tu* or *vos* if they do, and to be aware of this when working with

interpreters. Acceptable greetings may range from no physical contact and little eye contact to handshakes, single "air kisses," or hugs.

- **Family Involvement**—For effective continuation of care, it is best for the client's family to be involved from the outset to understand the client's context, roles, resources, barriers, aspirations, etc.

- **Alliance**—Establishing rapport to facilitate disclosure and trust to conduct an assessment are the cornerstones for non-Mayan providers working with Mayan communities. Families will not share information if they do not trust the provider. Practitioners may need to share about themselves more and take time to connect with the client and family before starting an interview. Guatemalans love to joke and have a great sense of humor, so sharing a laugh is a safe icebreaker.

- **Cultural Practices**—When conceptualizing a case, we thoughtfully determine if the behavioral presentation and changes of a client may be a cultural practice or an atypical presentation; this is especially important cross-culturally. For example, this case study highlighted mental health stigma, social isolation, and family dynamics.

- **Cultural Healing Practices**—Mayan cultural healing practices are particularly important in mobilizing community in support of those in need. It is prudent for neuropsychologists to be aware of such practices and to view them as complementary when possible, so that conceptualizations and interventions support one another rather than compete.

- **Medications**—Medications vary around the globe in their type, names, and availability. Internet searches may be needed to determine what someone is or was taking.

- **Measurements and Normative Data**—There are many neuropsychological measures in Spanish, but quality and norms are very varied. Dr. García de la Cadena and colleagues have developed normative data in Guatemala for specific adult and pediatric measures.[22,23]

- **Feedback and Recommendations**—Collaborative follow-up with other professionals, creates an emerging network of consultation. Sharing our findings with professionals, family, and the community is especially important and harder to put in a cultural context since neuropsychology is barely known, even by professionals in Guatemala. We can add more value in doing psychoeducation in a cultural context and address the need to increase disability rights and access, practice inclusion, reducing overprotection, and fostering independence. As a growing field in Guatemala, neuropsychology has the responsibility to educate the community about mental and behavioral health. Explaining relationships between quality of life and well-being, and its connection to the brain could foster preventative care. We can increase awareness of the value of taking care of the brain and how it relates to the quality of life.

- **Impressions**—Evaluating is a dance concerning how it will be received by the client and family—not only to find out what they see but how they will process the resource.

- **Training Challenges**—Clinical cases in public hospitals are of great educational value in neuropsychology for trainees. For supervisors, the perspective shifts when providing supervision for clinical cases in Guatemalan public hospitals. These cases are significantly more challenging for trainees and supervisors due to the limited armamentarium of appropriate neuropsychological measures and norms. Often trainees have only pieces of information to determine the level of functionality of the client and to make a diagnosis. Supervisors need to model a modified conceptualization process that mainly focuses on symptomatology and clinical history so the trainees can develop a refined, culturally informed neuropsychological approach.

- **Improvements**—As we reflect on this case, there are certain things we could have done differently. We would have tested odor identification as a dementia marker. Teleneuropsychology may have allowed us to deal with the distance, interview more family members who were more knowledgeable about the patient, and have follow-up over time. We might have attempted more advocacy with local primary care and other community resources.

- **COVID-19 Pandemic**—Our case study and the completion of the assessment were impacted by the COVID-19 pandemic. In Guatemala, public hospitals have closed outpatient services, so the evaluation could not be completed. However, telephone was used to provide feedback to the family for the continuation of care.
- **Mayan Neuropsychology**—As per this case, it seems to us that neuropsychology currently is only marginally able to contribute to the well-being of Mayans. Cases such as this one give us direction on how to continue to develop as a field in Guatemala.

How Can We Develop Mayan Neuropsychology?

This case is an illustration of what we regard as the current state of Mayan neuropsychology within Guatemala. Developing a viable service of neuropsychology is a long social process and we believe that we are barely at the point of being able to offer something of value to Mayans. Among the needs for and barriers to such services, as seen in this case, are:

- Mayan community knowledge about neuropsychological problems
- Mayan community access to professionals who would refer them to our services
- Confidence in and willingness to seek professional help for such problems
- Confidence in and willingness to complain to professionals about neuropsychological problems when they have them
- Understanding that such problems can be treated
- Asking for an evaluation and treatment for these problems
- Professionals who know about and have confidence in our services
- Professionals who will make the referral
- Timely referrals with adequate information
- Follow-through to make sure it happens
- Adequate payment system
- Neuropsychologists available
- Adequate transportation and communication
- Availability of informed family members
- Neuropsychologists with cultural knowledge and skill
- Availability of interpreters
- Adequate tests and norms
- A clinical process that is satisfactory to the family
- Recommendations that are viable in the context of the community resources and belief systems
- Follow-through on recommendations

Many of these considerations are involved in the development of neuropsychology services more generally in Guatemala. Many concern issues of poverty and infrastructure development that are well beyond the direct reach of the neuropsychologist and neuropsychology community. But an important component also involves neuropsychological public health. The World Health Organization's Community Based Rehabilitation program was developed as a community economic development strategy. When neuropsychology can contribute to vocational rehabilitation for those affected by brain disabilities and to reducing caregiver burden, then this is also a contribution to community economic development.

Certainly, it is possible to look at each of the barriers mentioned above and propose a solution to it. For example, conducting public health education in Mayan languages and communities about neurodisabilities and available services, education of referral sources, improving health and transportation infrastructure, training culturally competent neuropsychologists, developing and researching tests, and the list goes on. Perhaps, many of these solutions are appropriate. However, framing them up that way maybe externally imposed, paternalistic solutions that may fail. If we are to approach this process with cultural humility not only at the level of the client but also at the level of the system, then, we will want to engage Mayan communities in the process of deciding if we, as neuropsychologists, have anything of value to offer them, to prioritize what we offer, and to shape how it is offered. We cannot even be certain how to approach such engagement since we will want to do so in a way that establishes trust and is congruent with Mayan community decision-making systems. We can hope for future indications from models of community-based health care, mental health care, rehabilitation, and research.[24]

Acknowledgments

First and foremost, we would like to express our most sincere gratitude to the client of the case study and her family, whose story continues to inspire us to do better every day. All authors are proud to be members of the Guatemalan community and we greatly appreciate the people of Guatemala and their rich diversity and Mayan history. Establishing the neuropsychology field in Guatemala has been possible due to the sponsorship of the Universidad del Valle de Guatemala, the eagerness of the trainees, and the generosity of the faculty of the Master's Program in Clinical Neuropsychology faculty—¡Muchísimas gracias! We would like to highlight Dr. Orlando Sanchez and his foundational coursework on Clinical Competencies, Multiculturalism, and Ethics. Finally, the fourth author is a representative of the San Juan de Dios Hospital, Neurosciences Department, and the Section of Neuropsychology, where the burgeoning field of neuropsychology is celebrated and welcomed.

References

1. Grandin G, Oglesby E. Guatemala reader: history, culture, politics. London: Duke University Press; 2011. p. 688.
2. Soto-Quiros, R. Reflexiones sobre el mestizaje y la identidad nacional en Centroamérica: de la colonia a las Républicas liberales [Internet]. France: AFEHC; 2008 Oct [cited 2021 Mar 28]. Available from: https://www.afehc-historia-centroamericana.org/_articles/portada_afehc_articulos29.pdf
3. Instituto Nacional de Estadística. República de Guatemala: XII censo nacional de población y VII de vivienda [Internet]. GUA: INE; 2019. Available from: https://www.ine.gob.gt/ine/poblacion-menu/
4. United Nations Development Programme. Más allá del conflict, luchas por el bienestar Informe Nacional de Desarrollo Humano 2015/2016 [Internet]. GUA: UNDP; 2016 Oct 10 [cited 2021 May 25]. Available from: https://www.gt.undp.org/content/guatemala/es/home/library/poverty/informes-nacionales-de-desarrollo-humano.html
5. Loucky J, Moors MM. Maya diaspora: Guatemalan roots, new American lives. Philadelphia (PA): Temple University Press; 2000. p. 283.
6. Promotora Española de Lingüística. Presentation [Internet]. Madrid: PROEL; 2013 [cited 25 May 2021]. Available from: http://www.proel.org/index.php
7. Wikipedia. Mam language [Internet]. [place unknown]: Wikipedia; 2003 Nov 2 [updated 2021 May 11; cited 2021 Jan 5]. Available from: https://en.wikipedia.org/wiki/Mam_language
8. Rodriguez D, Luterbach KJ, de Gaitan RE. Special education international perspectives: practices across the globe. Adv Spec Ed [Internet]. 2014 Sep 16;28:ii. Available from: https://doi.org/10.1108/S0270-401320140000028007

9. Hallman K, Peracca S, Catino J, Ruiz MJ. Assessing the multiple disadvantages of Mayan girls: the effects of gender, ethnicity, poverty, and residence on education in Guatemala. Pov Gend Youth [Internet]. 2007;16. Available from: https://knowledgecommons.popcouncil.org/departments_sbsr-pgy/814/

10. Lainez Z. La democracia también comienza en casa [Internet]. GUAT: Plaza Publica; 2013 Oct 18 [cited 2021 May 25]. Available from: https://www.plazapublica.com.gt/content/la-democracia-tambien-comienza-en-casa

11. Research Directorate, Immigration and Refugee Board of Canada, Ottawa. Guatemala: Treatment of gay, lesbian, bisexual and transgendered/transsexual individuals and availability of state protection; police attitudes towards same-sex domestic violence and state protection available to victims [Internet]. [place unknown]: Immigration and Refugee Board of Canada; 26 Oct 2006 [cited 2020 December 8]. Available from: https://www.refworld.org/docid/45f1473e11.html

12. Chomat AM, Solomons NW, Montenegro G, Crowley C, Bermudez OI. Maternal health and health-seeking behaviors among indigenous Mam mothers from Quetzaltenango, Guatemala. Rev Panam Salud Publica [Internet]. 2014 Feb [cited 2021 May 25];35(2):113–20.

13. Wehr H, Chary A, Webb MF, Rohloff P. Implications of gender and household roles in Indigenous Maya communities in Guatemala for child nutrition interventions. Int J Indig Health [Internet]. 2014 Dec 19 [cited 2021 May 25];10(1):100–13. Available from: https://doi.org/10.18357/ijih.101201513196

14. Gragnolati M, Marini A. Health and poverty in Guatemala. World Bank policy research working papers [Internet]. 2003 Jan [cited 2021 May 25];2966. Available from: https://openknowledge.worldbank.org/handle/10986/9

15. García de la Cadena C, Henríquez JL, Sequeira E, Cortés-Ojeda AL, De Obaldía R, Judd T. La neuropsicología en América Central. Revista Neuropsicología, Neuropsiquiatría y Neurociencias 2009 Oct [cited 2021 May 25];9(2):1–19.

16. Matute VE, Rosselli M, Ardila AA, López ER, López CM, Ontiveros A et al. Evaluación neuropsicológica estándar para adultos hospitalizados, ENE-A. México: Departamento de neurociencias, hospital civil de Guadalajara; [date unknown].

17. Gomez-Angulo C, Campo-Arias A. Escala de Yesavage para Depresión Geriátrica (GDS-15 y GDS-5): Estudio de la consistencia interna y estructura factorial. Univ Psych [Internet]. 2011 [cited 2021 May 25];10(3):735–43.

18. Solis C, Garcia S, Manzano A. Índice de Barthel (IB): Un instrumento esencial para la evaluación funcional y la rehabilitación. Plast Restaur Neuro. 2005;4(1–2):81–5.

19. Nomura, K., Kazui, H., Wada, T., Sugiyama, H., Yamamoto, D., Yoshiyama, K., Shimosegawa, E., Hatazawa, J., & Takeda, M. (2012). Classification of delusions in Alzheimer's disease and their neural correlates. Psychogeriatrics: the official journal of the Japanese Psychogeriatric Society, 12(3), 200–210. https://doi.org/10.1111/j.1479-8301.2012.00427.

20. Becerril-Montekio V, López-Dávila L. Sistema de salud de Guatemala. Salud pública de México [Internet]. 2011 April 24 [cited 2021 May 25];53:s197.

21. Medina-Cadena M. Oakland-raised Maya are bridging the Mam language gap in local courts [Internet]. San Francisco (CA): KALW; 2019 Apr 9 [cited 2021 May 25]. Available from: https://www.kalw.org/post/oakland-raised-maya-are-bridging-the-mam-language-gap-local-courts#stream/0

22. Guàrdia-Olmos J, Peró-Cebollero M, Rivera D, Arango-Lasprilla JC. Methodology for the development of normative data for ten Spanish-language neuropsychological tests in eleven Latin American countries. NeuroRehab [Internet]. 2015;37(4):493–9. Available from: https://doi.org/10.3233/NRE-151277

23. Rivera D, Arango-Lasprilla JC. Methodology for the development of normative data for Spanish-speaking pediatric populations. NeuroRehab [Internet]. 2017;41(3):581–92. Available from: https://doi.org/10.3233/NRE-172275

24. Gould, B., MacQuarrie, C., O'Connell, M. E., & Bourassa, C. (2021). Mental wellness needs of two Indigenous communities: Bases for culturally competent clinical services. Canadian Psychology/Psychologie canadienne, 62(3), 213–226. https://doi.org/10.1037/cap0000247

Mexico

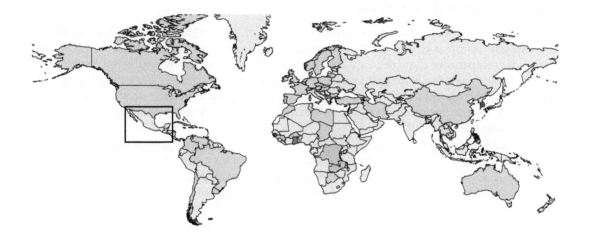

33 Mexican Origin Communities and Neurodegenerative Conditions

Adriana M. Strutt, Ana Linda Diaz Santos,
Adriana Puente Calzada, and Orlando Sánchez

Section I: Background Information

In this chapter, we present cultural profiles for two of the largest demographics in Mexico (i.e., *dominant-culture Mexican* or *Mestizo and Indigenous* or *Amerindian*). However, before proceeding, it is imperative that we pause to recognize that Mexico is ethnically and linguistically diverse.[1] Several complex historical factors such as census shortcomings, including the fact that prior to 2015, Mexico did not collect data on ethnicity[2] perpetuate inaccurate views of the population. Thus, despite misconceptions about Mexican homogeneity, it is important that the reader appreciate Mexico's diversity.

Briefly, dominant-culture Mexicans or *Mestizos* (mixed Spanish/indigenous ancestry) comprise the largest demographic followed by Amerindians/Indigenous people.[2] It is worth noting that, within the Americas, Mexico houses the largest indigenous population with 78 distinct ethnic groups and 68 distinct languages from 11 language families including 364 recognized dialects.[1,3,4] Other ethnic groups, to name a few, include African Mexicans[5,6] and Mexicans of Asian descent,[7] both brought to Mexico as slaves, and Mexicans of Arab descent who immigrated to Mexico as early as the 19th century.[8]

Thus, considering the aforementioned, what does it mean to be *Mexican, dominant-culture Mexican, Amerindian*, **Mexican American**, **Hispanic**, **Chicano**, **Latinos**, or of **Mexican descent**? Where does this terminology come from, why do we use it, and, perhaps more importantly, does it matter? Without a doubt! A delicate exploration of our patient's cultural background has profound implications for our work as psychologists/neuropsychologists. In this chapter, we utilize select terminology (see Glossary), cultural characteristics, and a case illustration to weave this complex discussion. However, we caution the reader against the human tendency to view others in terms of broad ethnic/cultural categories. We rely on cultural profiles as the backdrop for a deeper discussion concerning the importance of understanding our patient's unique experiences and perspectives.

Terminology

Language is not only a unique human ability but a powerful mechanism of cultural transmission relying on symbols, categories, and labels, including specialized terminology.[9] Thus, language is "intrinsic to the expression of culture," including our sense of self.[10] As such, rather than reviewing a menu of terminology ascribed to individuals from Mexico or of Mexican ancestry, it is vastly more important to discuss the origins of said terminology as well as the function and limitations of its use.

Two constructs borrowed from linguists are particularly relevant to our discussion: etic—an outsider's perspective/worldview; emic—perspective/worldview stemming from within the culture or context of interest.[11] There is an array of terms available to describe individuals from

DOI: 10.4324/9781003051862-67

Mexico or those of Mexican ancestry (e.g., Hispanic, Latino/a/x, Mexican American). What we must recognize is that the vast majority of our terminology reflects the US culture and its institutions. In fact, many are US census labels or the result of US-based sociopolitical movements. If we delve in deeper, what we are, in fact doing is relying on these etic terms to extrapolate information about the other's presumed worldview—identity, behavior, values, beliefs, etc. When we preoccupy ourselves exclusively with such US-based terminology/perspective, we risk failing to incorporate our patient's unique experience and perspective.

With respect to Mexicans, the emic perspective must consider complex Mexican historical and sociopolitical factors that shape(d) their unique worldview. One such factor is the *Mestizo ideology*, which should not to be confused with *Mestizo* the ethnic self-identification denoting mixed Spanish/indigenous ancestry. Briefly, the *Mestizo ideology* can be summarized as a concerted effort in Mexico to eliminate racial/ethnic distinctions in favor of a national identity.[12-14] Consequently, to many Mexicans, "ethnic identity" is an unfamiliar concept and, as such, an imposed etic from Euro-American cultures. Thus, when we ask patients from other cultures to self-identify, many are perplexed by this concept (i.e., unsure how to respond). Thus, in Mexico (all through Latin America, in fact), with respect to identity, people coalesce around a national rather than an ethnic/racial identity.

So, what bearing does this have on the clinical encounter? Though we juxtapose both perspectives here (etic vs. emic), our intention is not merely to simplify these into a false dichotomy and/or suggest that one takes precedence over the other. Our point is that, when working with individuals whose cultural background is different than ourselves, the shared experience requires awareness and integration of both cultural perspectives. Psychologists/neuropsychologists must be aware of the unique cultural/subcultural perspective they bring into the encounter and, simultaneously, explore and integrate the patients' internalized characteristics on health/illness. Through this process, a unique working alliance is created with opportunities for optimal assessment/treatment.

Author Perspective

I (AMS) consider myself a Mexican American female, highlighting my status as a first-generation American with deep-rooted Mexican traditions/lifestyle practices. My upbringing in a predominant Mexican neighborhood in Southern California depicted primarily Spanish-speaking, working-class families who valued Mexican culture and had minimal interaction with the English-speaking community. A neighborhood composed of small bungalows and apartment complexes, my boundaries consisted of landmarks: a small park to the west, my English-based-majority White religious school to the east, the *panaderia* (bakery) to the south, and the north was off limits as that is where the *cholos* (gangsters) lived. After leaving this neighborhood as a pre-adolescent, I learned about the "questionable safety" of the area, a stark contrast to my fond childhood memories. I can picture our small apartment and my neighborhood friends (with cute Spanish nicknames like Albondiga (Meatball). I did not suffer materialistic needs; I was not even aware of what I did not have until later in life. I had everyone I needed and truly enjoyed life on 56th street, a place where cultural practices were valued and respected, where weekends were filled with music and the small materialistic gains that each family accomplished were acknowledged. This neighborhood also introduced me to White, English-based school structures, where as the only Latina, many of my core values were not the norm. I remember what it was like to be different: unfamiliar with Westernized practices, limited English mastery, and lower socio-economic standing. It is these childhood experiences that molded me into the clinician I am today and that remind me of the importance of culturally informed, patient-centered care.

I (ALDS) identify as a Puerto Rican female, born and raised in the mountains of the island surrounded by family and friends, speaking only Spanish until I attended graduate school on the mainland. Picking fruits and vegetables from the garden and feeding the chickens, rabbits, and horses were my primary chores after school. We enjoyed family gatherings to celebrate everything! Everyone coming to *abuela's* (grandmother's) house for dinner was a serious tradition. We shared a close relationship among family members, always available to help one another. After my immediate family immigrated to Florida following better employment opportunities, my process of acculturation to the mainstream American culture began. It was not a shock as I was surrounded by **Latinos** from the Caribbean and South America. Throughout my training, I have been taught the importance of being human first. The compilation of my upbringing, my "immigration" experience, acquisition of English and my training have shaped the clinician I am today. That is, aware of the need to provide individualized, quality care to all.

Born and raised in Mexico City, I (AP) have engaged and enjoyed the different traditions of my parents' families. My father was from Durango (north of Mexico) and my mother is from Mexico City. This interplay of traditions and my exposure to American culture sparked my interest in learning about and appreciating different cultural lifestyle practices.

My perspective (OS) is that of a *Ñuu Savi (Mixteco)* immigrant neuropsychologist born in southern Mexico with professional and research interests in multicultural education and training, "cultural competency," and health disparities.

Geography

Knowing your patient's exact origin (specific city/town) prior to the clinical encounter may help generate hypotheses about their potentially distinctive characteristics (e.g., Amerindian vs. dominant-culture Mexican, bilingualism, socio-economic status, and implications for dietary deficiencies known to impact cognition). The uniqueness of each community will vary according to the specific geographical location. Of note, individuals from Mexico may often indicate that they are from "*un rancho/ranchito*" (ranch, little ranch), which generally implies that the individual is from a rural area and/or an indigenous village.

History

As articulated in Mexico's Constitution (1917, Article 2), at the heart of the Mexican nation, lies its Amerindian roots.[15–18] It is estimated that, upon the first encounter with Europeans, between 50 and 100 million people already inhabited the Americas.[19] In the centuries that followed, these numbers declined considerably as a function of disease and wars provoked and/or exacerbated by Europeans.[20,21] The conquest (1521) also brought new social structures, including a racial caste system that favored White European descent.[22–24] To this day, White European features continue to be associated with positive attributes while indigenous or African features are viewed negatively.[13,14,23]

The Mexican War of Independence from Spain (1810–1821) was followed by the Mexican Revolution (1910–1920), which largely disenfranchised indigenous people. Following the Mexican Revolution, there was an official government endorsement of "*mestizaje*" (i.e., mixed Spanish/indigenous ancestry) as *the* national identity whereby delegitimizing all other identities and cultures. As a result, the government did not recognize racial/ethnic self-identification until 2015.[2] At this juncture; it is important to clarify that "*mestizaje*" is a socially constructed reality with complex historical-sociopolitical implications.[12,25–27] Suffice it to say that, among other things, "*mestizaje*" (the ideology) obfuscated the indigenous and Afro-Mexican identity in Mexico and, in many ways, facilitated unchecked racism, discrimination, and oppression that persists to this day.[13,14,23]

While the Mexican Revolution sought to address social inequality, the wealth gap in the 21st century remains a major problem in Mexico, with many citizens living in deep poverty (44% of dominant-culture Mexicans and 78% of Amerindians).[28-30] Overall, Mexico remains crippled by "poor governance in critical domains of public policy, high impunity and corruption rates, weak rule of law and protection of civil liberties and rights, entrenched marginalization, ... growing inequality, and low public confidence in political officials and institutions."[31] In the absence of healthy governance, over the past three decades, drug cartel-related crime and flagrant violence have engulfed Mexico. Thus, it is no wonder that Mexicans eagerly risk everything for a opportunity at the "American dream."

Immigration and Relocation

Since 1980, Mexicans have represented the largest immigrant group within the United States.[32-34] However, after four decades of burgeoning Mexican immigration, this surge plateaued in 2014 and has steadily declined since. Nevertheless, despite this decline, Mexicans remain the largest foreign-born group in the nation, accounting for 25% of all immigrants.[32,34] Though the aforementioned statistics largely pertain to dominant-culture Mexicans, it is important to highlight that, since at least the 1960s, Amerindians have likewise been immigrating to the United States in large numbers with rapid population growth since the 1980s.[35,36-39] The Amerindian presence in the United States has grown large enough that, as of 2010, the US census has endeavored to capture the racial/ethnic heterogeneity reflective of Mexico as well as the broader Native American population.[40] According to recent data, Amerindians from Mexico comprise the fourth largest indigenous population within the United States (Cherokee, Navajo, and Choctaw are largest, respectively).[40]

Language

Considering the heterogeneity of the Mexican population, including its large presence in the United States, clinicians should be mindful of their Mexican patient's language proficiency and fluency, particularly with respect to Spanish, Amerindian language(s), and/or English. Bi or multilingualism will be an important factor to consider as Mexican individuals may speak said languages at various levels of proficiency, fluency, and literacy. Consequently, it is important that the reader not assume that Amerindian patients are fluent in Spanish. Ignoring these elements may greatly impact the evaluation, with potentially significant negative consequences for the patient.

Communication

Mexican culture, as it pertains to *Mestizo* individuals, is considered a "high-context culture."[41] Accordingly, communication is less direct and points are made in a more diplomatic, subtle, and less confrontational manner.[41,42] American linguist Robert Kaplan described the Romance languages' communication style as "an arrow that makes sharp turns before getting to its destination."[42] As such, communication often "digresses" or moves away from the main point.[43] However, following the flow of the conversation is considered integral to the point. In contrast, European Americans might find this style to be "disorganized or intellectually weak" as it deviates from the Eurocentric "direct or linear" form of communication.[42] Meaning is conveyed via non-verbal cues and less direct verbal messages. For instance, a "no" would be conveyed with a "maybe" or a "we'll see" in order to avoid causing disappointment or offense to the inquiring party. Given such practices, dominant-culture Mexicans may find the English-speaker to be aggressive/intimidating. Conversely, the English-speaker may perceive the dominant-culture Spanish-speaker as timid or taciturn.[42]

Interpersonally, the focus is placed on relationship building; thus, the timing allotted to this aspect of the professional relationship is imperative. In clinical practice, it is important to establish rapport, providing the patient with an explanation of standardized practices (including the expectation of minimal interpersonal conversations during testing) to aid the examiner in respectfully engaging/disengaging the patient. Timing is considered *flexible, relaxed, and circular* within the dominant Mexican culture. The concept of *ahorita* (right now) or *mañana* (tomorrow) is utilized within the dominant Mexican culture to denote *later* (in some cases due to perceived lack of urgency).[41] The lax concept of time and the stress on relationship building must be considered when managing clinical procedures. In regard to personal space, dominant-culture Mexicans normalize less spacing between people in a group. The typical "2–3" feet European/American social standard may be considered distant/indifferent to dominant-culture Mexican patients.[42] Tying in with the relationship-building aspect, dominant Mexican culture focuses on collectivism. Direct eye contact with individuals in authority may be viewed as disrespectful for some.[42] Hence, the European American norm of maintaining eye contact while communicating might not be reciprocated. Lastly, both the initial and closing greeting toward the professional from the patient/family may include a hug and/or kiss on the cheek. This might not occur on the first session but can be part of the relationship that develops over time. The provider should be aware of this cultural interaction which should not be considered a boundary violation.

While Amerindians may also exhibit aspects of the aforementioned communication and interpersonal style, by virtue of their distinctive history, language, and culture, their characteristics are different from that of dominant-culture Mexicans. Broadly speaking, the characteristics detailed above *can* be observed within Amerindians but to greater degrees (e.g., more "disorganized" in communication; time as more flexible). Given shared commonalities with US Native Americans, Mexican indigenous people exhibit aspects resembling that of indigenous people of the United States. For example, given their semi-autonomous governments and history with chronic racism/discrimination, Amerindians are highly interdependent and may be more distrusting of others and reluctant to identify as indigenous to non-indigenous individuals. Clinicians should be aware of the cultural tendency to prefer politeness and less direct modes of communication, as this might result in a patient ostensibly abiding by the clinical recommendations provided without adherence.

Education

Mexico's education system (see Table 33.1), established in 1917, is not only enormous but incredibly complex, marked by pervasive social inequality, corruption, and poor educational outcomes.[44,45] Succinctly, this system was initially overseen by the federal government under the Secretariat of Public Education.[46] However, in pursuit of quality and equity in education, in 1992, the federal government decentralized this system to Mexico's 32 federal states, including the National Teachers Union (SNTE).[46] Unfortunately, while the system slowly evolved over several decades with the SNTE increasingly accumulating power, the goal for quality and equity was lost.

Today, with respect to quality, national and international data consistently reveal disappointing results. For example, according to the National Plan for the Evaluation of Learning (PLANEA), more than 30% of all students in 2017 scored at the lowest level in Spanish. In other words, these students experienced difficulty comprehending or interpreting texts considered to be of medium complexity.[45,47] Similarly, only approximately 8% of students could analyze complex arguments.[45,47] By international standards, Mexico consistently ranks poorly in literacy, math, and science.[45] Overall, 1 in 2 Mexican students lack the necessary knowledge required to obtain higher education, to confront the challenges of modern life, and/or to solve complex social/environmental problems.[48]

With respect to equity, poverty is a major factor impacting the education system in Mexico, with Amerindian communities, the poorest of the poor, being disproportionally impacted. Amerindians face unique challenges including poverty and racism/discrimination that contribute to disproportionate access to education and have the highest dropout rates along with the highest rates of illiteracy in Mexico.[1,49] At the opposite end of the spectrum, private institutions are available for the select elite with such programs offering multilingual curriculums, some teaching in English and a second foreign language with no Spanish components.

Overall, careful exploration of the quantity and quality of education is of paramount importance in an evaluation. Simply inquiring about the highest level of education completed does not begin to capture the complexity described above. Furthermore, it is important to explore the age the individual initiated schooling, consistency of attendance and available academic resources. Other factors worth exploring include grade failure/retention and reading skill, specifically in terms of reading comprehension.

It is also worth cautioning the reader with respect to the possible assumption that premorbid functioning can be estimated as easily as with a native English speaker (i.e., reading test). Unlike English (opaque language with many irregular words), Spanish is considered a transparent language where simple, rudimentary phonetic skills are enough to decode college-level words.[50]

Table 33.1 Structure of the Mexican education system

Mexico's education law defines three main levels of education. Each level of education is further subdivided as follows:

- ***Educación Basica (Basic Education)***

  1 *Educación Preescolar* (early childhood education): Ages 3–6
  2 *Educación Primaria* (elementary education): Grades 1–6
  3 *Educación Secundaria* (lower-secondary education): Grades 7–9

- ***Educación Média Superior* (Upper Secondary Education)**: Typically grades 10–12

  1 Bachillerato General (general academic)
  2 Bachillerato Tecnológico (technological education)
  3 Profesional Técnico (vocational and technical education)

- ***Educación Superior (Higher Education)***

  1 *Técnico Superior* (post-secondary/associate/diploma)
  2 *Licenciatura* (undergraduate and first professional degrees)
  3 *Postgrado* (graduate/postgraduate education)

Socio-Economic Status

As previously discussed, poverty and wealth inequality in Mexico are major challenges for Mexican citizens. While some improve their situation by immigrating to the United States, others continue to face challenges even within their host country. Within the United States, these individuals live in poor conditions (~20% live at or below the poverty line),[51,52] lack health insurance,[53] and face disproportionate rates of chronic health conditions including obesity, diabetes, and heart disease.[54,55] Many factors contribute to the aforementioned situation including English language proficiency,[34] discrimination,[56,57] low education,[58,59] and limited employment opportunities.[60–62]

Values and Customs

Knowledge about commonly held values and customs (i.e., religious, spiritual, patriotic, and rite of passage customs or celebrations) in Mexican communities can support rapport building and help provide thoughtful/culturally informed services. Nonetheless, as emphasized throughout, clinicians should also recognize the heterogeneity inherent in the Mexican population and consider possible variability in individual values and customs.

Health Status/Health Providers

In addition to marked social inequality, Mexico's complex history and cultural diversity characterize its formal/informal health care system. Perspective on health and illness, including etiology of diseases, diagnosis, and approach to treatment reflect an amalgamation of Amerindian, Greek, and modern Euro-American medical practices.[63,64] Mexico's medical system is primarily composed of Amerindian traditional healing practices that exist parallel to, but separate from, modern medical practices (e.g. **Curanderos/Medicos Brujos**).[64] Overall, traditional Amerindian practices are poorly understood and, as such, devalued by formal/modern medical institutions and providers. Consequently, efforts to integrate both models have consistently failed.[65,66] While these may not be formally integrated to the average dominant-culture *Mestizo;* both medical perspectives are complementary. However, for economic reasons, *Mestizos* regularly access traditional healers. Consequently, in some respects, traditional practices such as herbology may be preferred over modern pharmacotherapy.[67-71] Perceived etiology of ailments includes spiritual/supernatural, physical/natural, or both. Thus, treatment must match the perceived etiology for optimal results examples of traditional diseases include *empacho, mal de ojo, caida de mollera,* and *susto/espanto.*

Gender and Sexuality

Gender inequality and violence is a major problem in Mexico. Sources indicate that violence against women is experienced across age, social, economic, and cultural spheres.[72-74] Data suggests that more than 65% of Mexican women will experience at least one incident of emotional, physical, or sexual violence in their lifetime.[71] Unfortunately, sociocultural attitudes and government/legal enforcement apathy contribute to this epidemic. While laws exist, these are rarely honored and most women are reluctant to press charges. Given systemic apathy, acculturation factors are likely to influence outcomes in such situations, particularly among young Mexican women growing up in the United States who are caught between a home culture that potentially values **marianismo** *(virgin moral purity)* and a host culture that is perceived as more "liberal", leading to high acculturation stress *(acculturation gap)*.[75,76] Additionally, research has revealed how immigration and context challenges gendered and culturally bound depictions of marriage.[77]

Gender inequality is also observed across social domains, such as education; for example, females are more likely to drop out of school by age 12 due to domestic demands.[49] Consequently, they are less likely to graduate high school and attend higher education, whereby limiting economic opportunities as well as upward social mobility. In addition, Mexican women are likely to marry young and, as a result, terminate their education.[49] Overall, Amerindian women have the highest rates of illiteracy, school dropout, domestic violence, health complications, and considerably less job opportunities.

Spirituality and Religion

Currently, more than 80% of individuals living in Mexico identify as Catholic.[78] However, unlike Catholicism elsewhere, Mexican practices incorporate pre-colonial perspectives. Approximately half of Mexicans (44%) endorse a "medium" to "high" level of engagement with Amerindian beliefs and practices, such that 45% believe in "evil eye," 39% believe in witchcraft, sorcery, and magic, and 31% believe that one can communicate with spirits.[79] With respect to Mexicans living in the United States, 61% identify as Catholic, 39% believe in "evil eye," 44% believe in witchcraft, sorcery, and magic, and 57% believe in spiritual possessions.[80]

The Virgin Mary, the most revered religious icon in Mexico, is a good example of how Catholicism incorporated indigenous people without integrating their worldview. In this example, inclusion of the indigenous community is only via the Virgin's origin story, appearing to Juan Diego, an indigenous figure who served as her envoy. Mainstream Catholicism does not incorporate the indigenous cosmovision and/or spirituality. Thus, if the aforementioned is conceptualized as "syncretism" it is on the light end. Mexican Catholicism is unique from other forms of Catholicism practiced outside of Mexico and religion or "Catholicism" practiced by indigenous people is marked with differences, depending on the particular indigenous group, geographic location, and level of community acculturation.

Acculturation and Systemic Barriers

Within the United States, Mexican immigrants, on average, have better health compared to US-born Mexicans and non-Hispanic Whites despite significant risk factors such as low[81–83] socio-economic status. However, the health of Mexican immigrants declines the longer they remain within the United States.[82,84,85] Though it is hypothesized that unique aspects of acculturation contribute to sharp declines in health, specific pathways have yet to be identified; nevertheless, hypotheses include discrimination and the erosion of cultural protective factors such as *familismo*. This phenomenon is most commonly referred to as the *Hispanic/Latino immigrant paradox*.[86]

Overall, compared to other foreign-born immigrants in the United States, Mexican immigrants, on average—are more likely to be Limited English Proficient (LEP), report lower levels of education, face poverty, and have inadequate health insurance.[34] This is particularly true of Amerindians who, additionally, encounter racism/discrimination from both dominant-culture Mexicans as well as US nationals. Although second-generation immigrants may have higher rates of assimilation, acculturative stressors encumbered should be examined. Models of acculturation are particularly relevant here as they allow us to understand the unique acculturation strategies of Mexicans, as not all espouse the same strategy.[87–90] Some employ a *separation* strategy of acculturation and retain a strong Mexican national identity aiming to preserve their home culture and language, while others espouse an *assimilation* strategy, striving to fully incorporate themselves into mainstream US society and, consequently, may take offense to any assumptions about their presumed cultural identity, including assumptions about their use, ability, and/or willingness to speak Spanish. These are the emic factors that clinicians must carefully explore as they not only influence the working alliance but inform the assessment process.

Mental Health Views

Overall, mental health services in Mexico are largely non-existent and significantly underdeveloped. According to national studies, few Mexicans access psychiatric care, and half of those who access care receive only minimally adequate services.[91] In addition, three decades of drug cartel-related violence have increased the need for psychological/psychiatric care. Though not as disheartening as the situation in Mexico, Mexicans living in the United States also face challenges with access to psychiatric care due to multiple barriers including language, poverty and lack of health insurance, legal status, acculturation, stigma, and lack of culturally competent providers.[92] Given how underdeveloped psychological and neuropsychological services are in Mexico, the reader should anticipate that Mexican individuals may likely be unfamiliar with the "rules of engagement" with respect to mental health care. Thus, at the outset (after exchanging pleasantries, building rapport, and displaying **pesonalismo**), it is wise to offer education with respect to the clinical enterprise—what a psychologist/neuropsychologist is, nature of and reason for the evaluation/referral, mode of interaction, boundaries/confidentiality, expectations, testing, etc.

Approach to Neuropsychological Evaluations

Neuropsychological services in Mexico are fairly new. Nevertheless, current efforts in improving and formalizing specialized training in clinical neuropsychology are being prioritized. Current services are similar to those offered in the United States including assessment, diagnosis, and cognitive rehabilitation. However, it is important to note that historically, neuropsychological services in Mexico have been rendered primarily to children with neurodevelopmental disorders and it was not until the recent decades that services extended to adults.

Research has shown that Latinos may view cognitive changes, specifically memory loss and even a diagnosis of dementia as an unavoidable part of the natural aging process.[93] Should patient/family share such perspective; providers should utilize this opportunity to reduce health outcome disparities by focusing on modifiable host factors that would otherwise prevent patients/families from seeking disease-modifying therapies. Health literacy regarding the process of normal aging and the impact of mental and physical health on brain health should be shared in a respectful and holistic manner, embracing the patient's worldview.

Psychological and neuropsychological services are practically non-existent for Amerindians (both in Mexico as well as the United States). Nevertheless, a handful of studies suggest that Amerindians have unique cognitive profiles as a function of their unique sociocultural environments.[94] Available data suggests that Amerindians have lower performances on working and verbal memory tasks but higher performances on visuospatial tasks compared to non-indigenous individuals. Overall, two factors have surfaced as particularly relevant, education (quantity/quality) and cultural relevance (test naiveté); some tasks are simply meaningless to indigenous people, therefore, impossible to comprehend and/or perform.[95–98]

Section II: Case Study — "No Estoy Demente Sólo Vieja/I am Not Demented Just Old"

Our approach to neuropsychological services with Latino patients is one that takes into account the sociocultural/economic context of the individual. Patients are always welcomed in Spanish with **respeto** and *personalismo*, as the initial step toward the successful establishment of rapport. Patients are asked about their understanding of what will take place during their visit followed by psychoeducation regarding the expected process.

Presenting Concerns

Ms. Reynosa is a 76-year-old right handed, married female referred for declines in short-term memory as well as an increase in depression and anxiety. Family assists with finances and medication management.

Social History

Ms. Reynosa, of Meztizo dominant culture, was born and raised in a remote town in Mexico where she had to walk long distances to attend school. She completed eight years of education and denied academic difficulties. She described terminating her education due to safety concerns; her family felt she was at risk for violence due to her lengthy commute to and from school, and they also needed her assistance with the family farm and household obligations. She immigrated to the United States in 1984 following her husband, who had immigrated seeking employment. She lived with her husband and worked in housekeeping until 2018, when she became his full-time caregiver.

Cultural History

Ms. Reynosa identified as bilingual (Spanish/English) and reported English as her dominant language. She resides in a "Mexican community" in the greater Houston area, and social interactions and media use are mainly conducted in Spanish. She identified as catholic and described stressors as tests of faith from God. Although she follows up with her doctor annually, she reported increased trust in community healers, given her past results. Ms. Reynosa described being inclined to take herbal supplements over prescription drugs and described distrust in medications. When inquired further, she described remembering how her mother used to care for her and her siblings with natural remedies without the need for doctors. Her current insurance plan covered neuropsychological assessment but did not approve neuroimaging studies requested by her referring doctor.

Medical History

Diagnosed conditions include diabetes, polyneuropathy, kidney disease, hyperlipidemia, hyperkalemia, hypertension, and GERD. She denied a history of seizures, head injury, or TIA/stroke. Medical records reveal poor diet compliance (coffee with peanut cookies for breakfast, a glycemic-control shake for lunch, and a shake with peanut cookies for dinner). Familial medical history is significant for Alzheimer's disease, although she stated that memory problems are part of aging given her experience of memory problems in older family members.

Psychiatric history is significant for depression and anxiety, initially attributed to "un nido vacio" (empty nest) and recently exacerbated by her husband's health status. She was started on an antidepressant one month ago but discontinued due to side effects and her report of lack of benefit. Familial psychiatric history is noncontributory. She denied a remote history and current use of alcohol, tobacco, or illicit drugs.

Behavioral Observations

Ms. Reynosa was tested in Spanish by a bilingual examiner. She was fully oriented. General appearance was neat and clean. Motor behavior was normal. Her mood was pleasant, albeit apprehensive at the beginning. Affect was mood-congruent. After a short conversation regarding the purpose of the evaluation and the process of testing, Ms. Reynosa was visibly more comfortable. She smiled and engaged actively. Conversational speech was coherent and goal-directed. She occasionally needed repetition of directions and lost place intermittently during complex set-tasks. She exhibited cooperative test-taking behavior. Attitude was appropriate and friendly. She expressed feeling comfortable with the examiner, as if with one of her granddaughters. The following results were considered a valid estimate of her current functioning.

Ms. Reynosa had identified English as her primary language (reporting a higher level of English mastery can be common among first-generation Mexican immigrants given experiences of discrimination). However, during the clinical interview, it was apparent that English was not her dominant language. Thus, acculturation and language[99] were examined and results were interpreted immediately for Ms. Reynosa with the goal of highlighting the impact of language and culture on standardized neurocognitive testing and encouraging her to accept a Spanish (bilingual where needed) testing session.

Examiners working with Mexican monolingual and bilingual patients should be aware that inquiring about language dominance/mastery can be a difficult process, depending on the life experiences of the examinee. The use of standardized measures in determining language dominance is suggested (i.e., acculturation measure and Language Dominance Index,[99] as this objective data can help the patient understand the examiner's reason for encouraging testing be conducted in one language over the other. We have experienced a variety of reactions in our initial patient/family interaction with our monolingual and bilingual patients/families. While some have been appreciative of receiving clinical services in Spanish, others have been offended at the time of the initial Spanish greeting or when inquiry has been made regarding their dominant language. Moreover, hesitancy in receiving services in Spanish has been evident and discussed by patients/families as individuals can feel a sense of guilt/shame when provided with the option of receiving services in Spanish (especially if they have resided in the United States for many years), while others have questioned whether Spanish evaluations reflect a lower quality of care or a "less than" attribution in reference to the examiner's skill set.

Test and Norm Selection

Measures and normative data that generalized to her sociodemographics were selected (see Table 33.2 in the Appendix).

Test Results and Impressions

Ms. Reynosa's profile exhibited global impairments. With regard to memory, she displayed a pattern of rapid forgetting. Findings met the criteria for a diagnosis of Major Neurocognitive Disorder secondary to probable Alzheimer's disease. Impacting social and environmental factors included acculturation difficulties (Z60.3) and exclusion and isolation (Z60.4). The impact of her poor mood was also considered.

Feedback Session and Follow-Up

Presenting complaints and testing procedures were reviewed. This practice highlights personal attention and psychoeducation assists the patient in understanding the process, which can be perceived as sterile/distant. Presentation of cognitive profile and diagnosis was the focus versus detailed findings by domain given global impairments. Examples of functional declines secondary to cognitive skills were helpful in highlighting a neurodegenerative process versus healthy aging. Psychoeducation (i.e., medication adherence) was provided.

Recommendations for Patient/Family

1 Dietary changes (i.e. MIND: Mediterranean-DASH Intervention for Neurodegenerative Delay Diet)
2 Psychiatric care to monitor and treat psychological symptoms and possible neurobehavioral changes
3 Psychological counseling for patient/family to discuss current and future care needs
4 Compensatory strategies (i.e., "memory station" where she would consistently place personal items; external memory aids such as shopping lists, calendars, pill reminders)
5 Intellectual stimulation: reading, jigsaw puzzles, familiar games (e.g., loteria)
6 Daily/weekly activities for physical and cognitive stimulation. Nostalgia-oriented materials for recreational purposes (e.g., old movies and music) are recommended over new materials.

7 Health literacy materials (a list of Spanish websites and reading materials for family and caregivers)

8 Community resources (a list of Spanish programming near the patient's home)

9 Maintain or increase her current level of intellectual and physical stimulation to help improve stamina, buoy her mood, and maintain her current level of quality of life

Section III: Lessons Learned

- Each Mexican immigrant brings unique experiences in terms of language and cultural preference. Formal language assessment should be conducted to identify the dominant language for testing purposes and level of acculturation should be considered.
- Findings need to be interpreted in context with the individual's sociocultural/economic circumstances to appropriately interpret data and tailor recommendations.
- Services with ethnically diverse individuals may include a higher level of advocacy on behalf of the patient given language mastery and other sociodemographic variables, particularly if the provider speaks the same language as the patient. When available, recommendations should include providers who can speak the patient's language or provide interpreter services.
- The use of a certified medical interpreter is highly encouraged. It is typical for older patients to be "excluded" from their care as family (proficient in English with varying levels of education, acculturation and Spanish language mastery) may take the lead and communicate with the medical provider. Thus, speaking directly to the patient is imperative.
- Mexican immigrants have vast disparities in educational backgrounds and levels of literacy. Understanding their educational experience is critical given the known impact of education on neuropsychological outcomes. Feedback sessions are vital. Information should be provided at the patient's level. General brain health psychoeducation (importance of optimal management of comorbidities, impact of diet, sleep, and psychiatric factors, etc.) and promotion of treatment adherence should be included.
- Little is available in terms of measures, normative data, and cognitive profiles of the *Indigenous/Amerindian* population. Materials available for the dominant Mexican culture may not be appropriate, depending on Spanish language mastery, cultural/lifestyle practices, education, and life experiences.

Acknowledgments

We would like to thank our Latino/a patients who trust us with their care as we work toward improving the cultural competence and humility of our specialty field.

Glossary

Chicano. More popular in the west coast area of the U.S., refers primarily to those of Mexican origin. Initially derogatory, but later adopted by civil rights activists to demonstrate solidarity. May be used by those who grew up in the civil rights era and can also be used in terms of gang affiliations.

Curanderos/Medicos Brujos. Healers who use traditional curing procedures, rituals, and medicinal plants to treat disease/illness, physical and psychological symptoms.

Educado. A cultural value in reference to appropriate social and moral behaviors and not academic standing (*educated* is literal translation). Variations of this socio-emotional construct may vary across socio-economic classes.

Espiritistas.   Spiritualists who consider themselves religious practitioners first and alternative health providers second.

Familismo.   A central Latin cultural value involves dedication, commitment, and loyalty to family. Regularly spending time with one's immediate and extended family is part of *familismo*. It also involves seeking the family's advice and involvement in important decisions.

Fatalismo.   Fatalism, belief that the course of fate cannot be changed and that life events are beyond one's control. In the health literature, fatalism usually is conceptualized as a set of pessimistic and negative beliefs and attitudes regarding health-seeking behaviors, screening practices, and illness.[99] Some will use a religious perspective, leaving their burdens in the hands of God.

Hispanic.   Refers to people who share an ethnic background in a Latin American or Spanish-speaking country. The term implies an association with Spain, which might produce negative reactions as Spain decimated the indigenous populations of Central/South America during colonization.

Latinos/as.   Used to describe people with origins in Latin America including Brazil or whose native language is Spanish. The term signifies solidarity between ethnically and culturally diverse individuals who might not necessarily share the same country of origin within the Americas or Europe (e.g., Spain).

Latinx.   A gender-neutral or non-binary term referring to people of Latin American origin or descent residing in the United States.

Machismo.   Social behaviors which evidence a sense of masculine pride. From the negative connotation of an untouchable/unwavering position of authority as the head of household (strong or overbearing attitude to anyone perceived as inferior; demanding of complete subservience), highlighting aggressiveness, physical strength, emotional insensitivity, and womanizing to positive traits of valor, a caring/involved, responsible, decisive, strong temperament/character, family protector.[100]

Marianismo.   An idealized traditional feminine gender role characterized by submissiveness, selflessness, chastity, hyperfemininity, and acceptance of machismo in males. Although clearly derived from the traditional ideal of the Virgin Mary, *marianismo* is not to be confused with a specific religious practice of the Roman Catholic Church.

Mexican American.   Refers to those whose families emigrated from Mexico to the United States sans implication concerning generational status. The term could be considered politically divisive since it is not inclusive of other Latin countries.

Mexican descent.   Denotes individuals whose parents or grandparents emigrated from Mexico. It is preferred by some who wish to eliminate the ambiguity of *Mexican-American*.

Parteras.   Provider who specializes in childbirth. Historically, these individuals did not offer prenatal care; however, current practices are evolving.

Personalismo.   Often defined as "formal friendliness," refers to the tendency to place great emphasis on personal relationships by Latinos. Latin culture is both people-oriented and collectivist, meaning that Latinos generally value personal relationships ("charisma") over status, material gain, and institutional relationships.

Respeto.   Considered a cultural value including deference to authority, setting clear boundaries, and knowing the level of courtesy required in a given situation in relation to the other person or a particular age, gender, or social status.

Sobadores.   Practitioners who use *sobada* (massage) to care for pulled muscles and injured joints, as well as to stimulate internal organs.[101]

Yerbero.   Herbalists, experts in plants/herbs/natural ingredients used to treat symptoms/ailments.

References

1. International Work Group for Indigenous Affairs (IWGIA) [Internet]. 2020. Retrieved 17 December 2020, from: https://www.iwgia.org/en/mexico.html
2. Morrison J, Ratzlaff A, Rojas M, Jaramillo M, Lins C, Peña MO. Counting ethnicity and race: harmonizing race and ethnicity data in Latin America (2000–2016). Washington, DC: Inter-American Development Bank; 2017.
3. United Nations Economic Commission on Latin America and the Caribbean (ECLAC). The millennium development goals. A Latin American and Caribbean perspective. Santiago, Chile: United Nations Publications; 2005.
4. Instituto Nacional de Estadística y Geografía (INEGI) [Internet]. Retrieved 21 December 2020, from: https://www.inegi.org.mx/
5. Richmond D. The legacy of African slavery in colonial Mexico, 1519–1810. J Pop Cult [Internet]. 2001;35(2):1–16. Available from: https://doi.org/10.1111/j.0022-3840.2001.00001.x
6. Hass A. La historia de los afrodescendientes en México: visibilizando un pasado común. En Revista Mexicana de Política Exterior. 2019;116:1–18.
7. Seijas T. Asian slaves in colonial Mexico. New York: Cambridge University Press; 2015.
8. Marin-Guzman R, Zeraoui Z. Arab immigration in Mexico in the nineteenth and twentieth centuries: assimilation and Arab heritage (Monterrey, Mexico and Austin, Texas: Instituto Tecnológico de Monterrey and Augustine Press; 2003. p. 212). Int J Middle East Stud [Internet]. 2003;37(2):266–69. Available from: https://doi.org/10.1017/s0020743805232063
9. Gelman S, Roberts S. How language shapes the cultural inheritance of categories. Proc Natl Acad Sci [Internet]. 2017;114(30):7900–07. Available from: https://doi.org/10.1073/pnas.1621073114
10. Banham V. Language: an important social and cultural marker of identity. Paper presented at the Language and Social Justice Issues Conference, held on 26 November 2014, at Edith Conway University, Perth, Australia; 2014.
11. Hahn C, Jorgenson J, Leeds-Hurwitz W. "A Curious Mixture of Passion and Reserve": understanding the etic/emic distinction. Éducation Et Didactique [Internet]. 2011;5(3):145–54. Available from: https://doi.org/10.4000/educationdidactique.1167
12. Manrique L. Dreaming of a cosmic race: José Vasconcelos and the politics of race in Mexico, 1920s–1930s. Cogent Arts Humanit [Internet]. 2016;3(1):1218316. Available from: https://doi.org/10.1080/23311983.2016.1218316
13. Moreno Figueroa MG. Distributed intensities: whiteness, mestizaje and the logics of Mexican racism. Ethnicities. 2010;10(3):387–401.
14. Moreno Figueroa MG. El archivo del estudio del racismo en México. Desacatos. 2016;51:92–107.
15. International Language Services, I. Not just Spanish—a look at the language of Mexico [Internet]. 2019. Retrieved from: https://www.ilstranslations.com/blog/language-of-mexico/
16. Coe MD, Koontz R. Mexico: from the Olmecs to the Aztecs. Thames & Hudson; 2013. Available from: https://www.thamesandhudsonusa.com/books/mexico-from-the-olmecs-to-the-aztecs-softcover-7th-edition
17. Demarest AA. The political, economic, and cultural correlates of late preclassic southern highland material culture. In Love M, Kaplan J, editors. The southern Maya in the late preclassic: The rise and fall of an early Mesoamerican Civilization. University Press of Colorado; 2011. pp. 345–86.
18. Gibson C. The hidden life of the ancient Maya: revelations from a mysterious world. Saraband; 2010. https://www.bibliovault.org/BV.book.epl?ISBN=9781607320920.
19. Taylor A. American colonies: the settling of North America (the Penguin history of the United States, Volume 1). Penguin; 2002.
20. Rossi A. Two cultures meet: native American and European. National Geographic Society; 2002.
21. Koch A, Brierley C, Maslin MM, Lewis SL. Earth system impacts of the European arrival and Great Dying in the Americas after 1492. Quat Sci Rev [Internet]. 2019;207:13–36. Available from: https://doi.org/10.1016/j.quascirev.2018.12.004
22. Chavez-Dueñas NY, Adames HY, Organista KC. Skin-color prejudice and within-group racial discrimination: historical and current impact on Latino/a populations. Hisp J Behav Sci [Internet]. 2014;36(1):3–26. Available from: https://doi.org/10.1177/0739986313511306

510

23. Telles E, Flores R. Not just color: whiteness, nation, status, in Latin America. Hisp Am Hist Rev [Internet]. 2013;93(3):411–49. Available from: https://doi.org/10.1215/00182168-2210858

24. Vinson B. III. Before Mestizaje: the frontiers of race and caste in colonial Mexico. New York: Cambridge University Press; 2018.

25. Mallon F. Constructing Meztizaje in Latin America: authenticity, marginality, and gender in claiming of ethnic identities. J Lat Am Anthropol. 1996;2(1):170–81.

26. Martínez-Echazábal L. Mestizaje and the discourse of national/cultural identity in Latin America, 1845–1959. Lat Am Perspect [Internet]. 1998;25(3):21–37. Available from: https://doi.org/10.1177/00945 82X9802500302

27. Telles E. Pigmentocracies: ethnicity, race, and color in Latin America. The University of North Carolina Press; 2014.

28. Organización Mundial de la Salud (OMS). México. Resumen: estrategia de cooperación [Internet]. 2018. Available from: http://apps.who.int/iris/bitstream/handle/10665/250865/ccsbrief_mex_es.pdf?sequence=1; fecha de consulta: 5 de Junio de 2018.

29. Moreno-Brid JC, Garry S, Krozer A. Minimum wages and inequality in Mexico: a Latin American perspective. Revista de Economía Mundial. 2016;43:113–29.

30. Reyes M, Teruel G, López M. Measuring true income inequality in Mexico. Lat Am Policy. 2017;8(1):127–48.

31. Felbab-Brown V. The ills and cures of Mexico's democracy [Internet]. Washington, DC: The Brookings Institution; 2019 [March]. Available from: https://www.brookings.edu/research/the-ills-and-cures-of-mexicos-democracy/GoogleScholar

32. Radford J. *Key findings about U.S. immigrants.* (Online report) [Internet]. Washington, DC: Pew Research Center; 2019. Retrieved from: https://www.pewresearch.org/fact-tank/2019/06/17/key-findings-about-u-s-immigrants/#:~:text=Mexico%20is%20the%20top%20origin,and%20El%20Salvador%20(3%25)

33. Zong J, Batalova J. Mexican immigrants in the United States in 2013. The Online Journal of the Migration Policy Institute [Internet]. 2014. Available from: https://www.migrationpolicy.org/article/mexican-immigrants-united-states-2013#:~:text=Immigration%20from%20Mexico%20to%20the,1900%20to%20624%2C400%20in%201930

34. Zong J, Batalova, J. Mexican immigrants in the United States. The Online Journal of the Migration Policy Institute. 2018. August 19, 2020.

35. Adler RH. Yucatecans in the "big D": an ethnography of migrant agendas and transnationalism (Doctoral dissertation). Retrieved from Arizona State University; 2000.

36. Adler RH. Yucatecans in Dallas. Texas: Breaching the border, bridging the distance. New York, NY: Routledge; 2004.

37. Fox J. Reframing Mexican migration as a multi-ethnic process. Lat Stud [Internet]. 2006;4:39–61. Available from: https://doi.org/10.1057/palgrave.lst.8600173

38. Nagengast C, Kearney M. Mixtec ethnicity: social identity, political consciousness, and political activism. Lat Am Res Rev. 1990;25(2):61–91.

39. Anuario de Migración y Remesas México [Internet]. 2020. Available from: https://www.bbvaresearch.com/publicaciones/anuario-de-migracion-y-remesas-mexico-2020/

40. Norris T, Vines PL, Hoeffel EM. The American Indian and Alaskan native population: 2010. Washington, DC: U.S. Department of Commerce Economics and Statistics Administration; 2012.

41. Durio S. The Mexican business culture: what to know about doing business in Mexico [Internet]. 2018. Retrieved from: https://www.worldwideerc.org/news/the-mexican-business-culture-what-to-know-about-doing-business-in-mexico#:~:text=%E2%80%9CIn%20Mexico's%20high%2Dcontext%20culture,%2C%E2%80%9D%20notes%20Mexico%20Business%20Associates

42. Elliott CE. Cross-cultural communication styles, pre-publication Master's thesis [Internet]. 1999. Available from: http://www.awesomelibrary.org/multiculturaltoolkit-patterns.html

43. Kaplan RB. Cultural thought patterns in intercultural education. Lang Learn. 1966;16:1–20.

44. OECD. Strong foundations for quality and equity in Mexican schools, implementing education policies [Internet]. Paris: OECD Publishing; 2019. Available from: https://doi.org/10.1787/9789264312548-en

45. Roach E. Education in Mexico [Internet]. 2020. Retrieved 27 December 2020, from: https://wenr.wes. org/2019/05/education-in-mexico-2
46. Bonilla-Rius E. Education truly matters: key Lessons from Mexico's educational reform for educating the whole child. In: F. Reimers, editor. Audacious education purposes: How governments transform the role of education systems. Cham: Springer; 2020. pp. 105–52.
47. INEE. El aprendizaje de los alumnos de tercero de secundaria en México. Informe de resultados. PLANEA 2017. Lenguaje y Comunicación, y Matemáticas [Internet]. Mexico City, Mexico: INEE; 2019. Available from: https://www.inee.edu.mx/publicaciones/informe-de-resultados-planea-ems-2017-el-aprendizaje-de-los-alumnos-de-educacion-media-superior-en-mexico-lenguaje-y-comunicacion-matematicas/. Accessed 10 December 2020.
48. Aguayo-Téllez E, Martínez-Rodríguez F. Early school entrance and middle-run academic performance in Mexico: evidence for 15-year-old students from the PISA test. Large-Scale Assess Educ, 2020;8(1). doi:10.1186/s40536-020-00089-8
49. International Community Foundation. (ICF) [Internet]. 2020. Retrieved 27 December 2020, from: https://icfdn.org/barriers-quality-education-mexico/
50. Del Pino R, Peña J, Ibarretxe-Bilbao N, Schretlen DJ, Ojeda N. Demographically calibrated norms for two premorbid intelligence measures: the word accentuation test and pseudo-words reading subtest. Front Psychol 2018;9:1950. [PMC free article] [PubMed] [Google Scholar].
51. Creamer J. Inequalities persist despite decline in poverty for all major race and Hispanic origin groups [Internet]. 2020 Sept 15. Available from: https://www.census.gov/library/stories/2020/09/poverty-rates-for-blacks-and-hispanics-reached-historic-lows-in-2019.html
52. Pew Research Center, 2017. https://www.pewresearch.org/hispanic/fact-sheet/u-s-hispanics-facts-on-mexican-origin-latinos/#poverty-status.
53. Brown ER, Ojeda VD, Wyn R, Levan R. Racial and ethnic disparities in access to health insurance and healthcare. Los Angeles, CA: UCLA Center for Health Policy Research and The Henry J. Kaiser Family Foundation; 2000.
54. Velasco-Mondragon E, Jimenez A, Palladino-Davis AG, Davis D, Escarmilla-Cejudo JA. Hispanic health in the USA: a scoping review of the literature. Public Health Rev. 2016;37:31–58.
55. Smedley BD, Stith AY, Nelson AR. Unequal treatment: confronting racial and ethnic disparities in health care. Washington: National Academies Press; 2002.
56. Flores E, Tschann JM, Dimas JM, Bachen EA, Pasch LA, de Groat CL. Perceived discrimination, perceived stress, and mental and physical health among Mexican origin adults. Hisp J Behav Sci. 2008;30(4), 401–24. doi:10.1177/0739986308323056
57. Williams DR, Neighbors HW, Jackson JS. Racial/ethnic discrimination and health: findings from community studies. Am J Public Health. 2003;93(2), 200–08. doi:10.2105/AJPH.93.2.200
58. Murphey D, Guzman L, Torres A. America's Hispanic children: gaining ground, looking forward. Bethesda, MD: Child Trends Hispanic Institute; 2014. Retrieved from: http://www.childtrends.org/wp-content/uploads/2014/09/2014-38AmericaHispanicChildren.pdf
59. Zhou M, Lee J, Vallejo JA, Tafoya-Estrada R, Xiong YS. Success attained, deterred, and denied: divergent pathways to social mobility in Los Angeles's second generation. Ann Am Acad Pol Soc Sci. 2008;620:37–61.
60. Gonzalez N, Consoli MLM. The aftermath of deportation: effects on the family. Revista Interamericana de Psicología. 2012;46(3):425–34.
61. Howard G, Peace F, Howard VJ. The contributions of selected diseases to disparities in death rates and years of life lost for racial/ethnic minorities in the United States, 1999–2010. Prev Chronic Dis. 2014;11:E129.
62. U.S. Census Bureau. Table 11: Employed persons by detailed occupation, sex, race, and Hispanic or Latino ethnicity [Internet]. 2016. Labor Force Statistics from the Current Population Survey Retrieved December 11 2020, from: http://www.bls.gov/cps/cpsaat11.htm
63. Smith AB. Hispanic/Latino [Internet]. 2020. Retrieved 27 December 2020, from: https://ethnomed. org/culture/hispanic-latino/
64. Geck MS, Cristians S, Berger-González M, Casu L, Heinrich M, Leonti M. Traditional herbal medicine in Mesoamerica: toward its evidence base for improving universal health coverage. Front. Pharmacol. 2020;11:1160. doi:10.3389/fphar.2020.01160

65. Bye R, Linares E. Perspectives on ethnopharmacology in Mexico. In: Heinrich M, Jäger AK, editors. Ethnopharmacology. West Sussex, Chichester: John Wiley & Sons, Ltd; 2015. pp. 393–404.

66. Colon-Gonzalez M.C, El Rayess F, Guevara S, Anandarajah G. Successes, challenges and needs regarding rural health medical education in continental Central America: a literature review and narrative synthesis. Rural Remote Health. 2015;15:3361.

67. Brown MT, Bussell JK. Medication adherence: WHO cares? Mayo Clin Proc. 2011;86(4):304–14. doi:10.4065/mcp.2010.0575

68. Lora CM, Gordon EJ, Sharp LK, Fischer MJ, Gerber BS, Lash JP. Progression of CKD in Hispanics: potential roles of health literacy, acculturation, and social support. Am J Kidney Dis. 2011;58(2):282–90. doi:10.1053/j.ajkd.2011.05.004

69. Villagran M, Hajek C, Zhao X, Peterson E, Wittenberg-Lyles E. Communication and culture: predictors of treatment adherence among Mexican immigrant patients. J Health Psychol. 2011;17(3):443–52.

70. Zagaar M. Medication nonadherence in the Latino population: a challenge and an opportunity for specialized services [Internet]. 2017. Retrieved from: https://www.pharmacytimes.com/news/medication-adherence-in-the-latino-population

71. INEGI. Encuesta Nacional sobre la Dinámica de las Relaciones en los Hogares (ENDIREH) [Internet]. 2016. Retrieved 13 October 2020, from: https://www.inegi.org.mx/programas/endireh/2016/

72. Essayag S. From commitment to action: policies to end violence against women in Latin America and the Caribbean. Regional Analysis Document. UNDP, UN Women. Panamá; 2017.

73. Hsu Y, Kovacevic M. *Violence against women: Unacceptable and unmeasured | Human Development Reports* [Internet]. United Nations development programme, Human Development Reports. 2020. Retrieved 13 October 2020, from: http://hdr.undp.org/en/content/violence-against-women-unacceptable-and-unmeasured

74. WOLA. *Hidden in Plain Sight: Violence against Women in Mexico and Guatemala—WOLA* [Internet]. 2020. Available from: https://www.wola.org/analysis/hidden-in-plain-sight-violence-against-women-in-mexico-and-guatemala/. Accessed 28 December 2020.

75. Marsiglia FF, Nagoshi JL, Parsai M, Booth JM, Castro FG. The parent–child acculturation gap, parental monitoring, and substance use in Mexican heritage adolescents in Mexican neighborhoods of the Southwest U.S. J Community Psychol. 2014 Jul 1;42(5):530–543. doi: 10.1002/jcop.21635.

76. Estadísticas a propósito del día internacional de la eliminación de la violencia contra la mujer Comunicado de Prensa Numero 568/20; 23 Noviembre 2020; [Internet]. Available from: https://www.inegi.org.mx/contenidos/saladeprensa/aproposito/2020/Violencia2020_Nal.pdf

77. Wood CA, Helms HM, Supple AJ, Perlman D. Gender-typed attributes and marital satisfaction among Mexican immigrant couples: a latent profile approach. J Fam Psychol. 2015;29(3):321.

78. Pasquali M. *Religion Affiliations In Mexico | Statista.* [Internet]. 2020. Available from: https://www.statista.com/statistics/275436/religious-affiliation-in-mexico/. Accessed 28 December 2020.

79. Pew Research Center's Religion & Public Life Project. *Latin American Religious Beliefs.* [Internet]. 2020a. Available from: https://www.pewforum.org/2014/11/13/chapter-3-religious-beliefs/. Accessed 29 December 2020.

80. Pew Research Center. *On Religion, Mexicans Are More Catholic and Often More Traditional Than Mexican Americans.* [Internet] 2020b. Available from: https://www.pewresearch.org/fact-tank/2014/12/08/on-religion-mexicans-are-more-catholic-and-often-more-traditional-than-mexican-americans/. Accessed 29 December 2020.

81. Burnam MA, Hough RL, Escobar JI, Karno M, Timbers DM, Telles CA, Locke BZ. Six-month prevalence of specific psychiatric disorders among Mexican Americans and non-Hispanic whites in Los Angeles. Arch Gen Psychiatry. 1987;44(8):687–94.

82. Cook B, Alegría M, Lin JY, Guo J. Pathways and correlates connecting Latinos' mental health with exposure to the United States. Am J Public Health. 2009;99(12):2247–54. doi:10.2105/AJPH.2008.137091

83. Ortega AN, Rosenheck R, Alegría M, Desai RA. Acculturation and the lifetime risk of psychiatric and substance use disorders among Hispanics. J Nerv Ment Dis. 2000;188(11), 728–35. doi:10.1097/00005053-200011000-00002

84. Vega WA, Alderete E, Kolody B, Aguilar-Gaxiola S. Illicit drug use among Mexicans and Mexican Americans in California: the effects of gender and acculturation. Addiction (Abingdon, England). 1998a;93(12):1839–50.

85. Vega WA, Kolody B, Aguilar-Gaxiola S, Alderete E, Catalano R, Caraveo-Anduaga J. Lifetime prevalence of DSM-III-R psychiatric disorders among urban and rural Mexican Americans in California. Arch Gen Psychiatry. 1998b;55(9):771–8.

86. Taningco MTV. Revisiting the Latino health paradox [Internet]. Los Angeles: The Tomas Rivera Policy Institute; 2007. Available from: http://www.trpi.org/PDFs/LatinoParadoxAug2007PDF.pdf

87. Berry JW. Contexts of acculturation. In: Sam DL, Berry, JW, editors. The Cambridge handbook of acculturation psychology. New York, NY: Cambridge University Press; 2006. pp. 27–42.

88. Berry JW. Conceptual approaches to acculturation. In: Chun KM, Organista PB, Marin G, editors. Acculturation: advances in theory, measurement, and applied research. Washington, DC: American Psychological Association; 2003. pp. 17–37. doi:10.1037/10472-004

89. Berry JW, Kim U, Minde T, Mok D. Comparative studies of acculturative stress. Int Migr Rev. 1987;21:491–511.

90. Berry JW. Acculturation as varieties of adaptation. In: Padilla AM, editor. Acculturation: theory, models, and some new findings. Boulder, CO: Westview; 1980. pp. 9–25.

91. Medina-Mora ME, Borges G, Muñoz CL, Benjet C, Jaimes JB, Fleiz Bautista C, et al. Prevalencia de trastornos mentales y uso de servicios: resultados de la Encuesta Nacional de Epidemiología Psiquiátrica en México. Salud Mental. 2003;26(4):1–16.

92. NAMI. *Hispanic/Latinx | NAMI: National Alliance on Mental Illness* [Internet]. 2020. Available from: https://www.nami.org/Your-Journey/Identity-and-Cultural-Dimensions/Hispanic-Latinx. Accessed 29 December 2020.

93. Mahoney DF, Cloutterbuck J, Neary S, Zhan L. African American, Chinese, and Latino family caregivers' impressions of the onset and diagnosis of dementia: cross-cultural similarities and differences. Gerontologist. 2005 Dec;45(6):783–92. doi: 10.1093/geront/45.6.783.

94. Ostrosky-Solís F, Ramírez M, Lozano A, Picasso H, Vélez A. Culture or education? Neuropsychological test performance of a Maya indigenous population. Int J Psychol. 2004;39(1):36–46.

95. Ostrosky-Solis F, Ramirez M, Ardila A. Effects of culture and education on neuropsychological testing: a preliminary study with indigenous and nonindigenous population. Appl Neuropsychol. 2004;11(4):186–93.

96. Pontius AA. Color and spatial errors in Block Design in stone-age Auca Indians: ecological underuse of occipital parietal system in men and of frontal lobes in women. Brain Lang. 1989;10:54–71.

97. Pontius AA. In similarity judgements hunter-gatherers prefer shapes over spatial relations in contrast to literate groups. Percept Mot Ski. 1995;81:1027–41.

98. Ardila A, Moreno S. Neuropsychological test performance in Aruaco Indians: An exploratory study. J Int Neuropsychol Soc. 2001;7(4):510–15.

99. Abraído-Lanza AF, Viladrich A, Flórez KR, Céspedes A, Aguirre AN, De La Cruz AA. Commentary: Fatalismo reconsidered: A cautionary note for health-related research and practice with Latino populations. Ethn Dis. 2007;17(1):153.

Puerto Rican

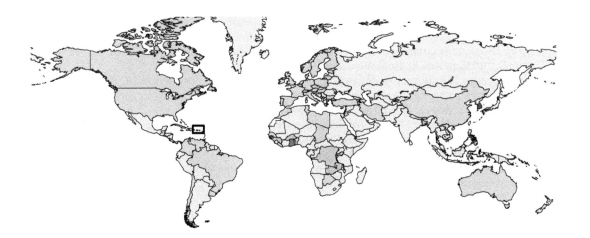

34 Neuropsychology and Access to Services in Puerto Rico

A Family's Journey with Autism Spectrum Disorder

Rafael E. Oliveras-Rentas, Mairim Vega-Carrero, and Walter Rodríguez-Irizarry

Section I: Background Information

Terminology and Perspective

People from Puerto Rico are referred as *puertorriqueño* (or *puertorriqueña* for feminine gender classification in Spanish Language) o *puertorricense*. Other terminologies are also used, including the terms *boricua, borinqueño* and *borincano* (or *borinqueña* and *borincana,* respectively), stemming from the name that our native Taíno people had originally given the Island: *Borikén.* Our preferred terminology is *puertorriqueños* or, in English, Puerto Ricans, which we will use throughout this chapter.

We will present the following content from the perspective of three Puerto Rican neuropsychologists. All of us completed doctoral degrees in Puerto Rico, and two of us circulated to the United States for the completion of post-doctoral fellowships in Neuropsychology. We are all bilingual (Spanish/English) and currently work in both academic settings and private practice in Puerto Rico.

Geography

Puerto Rico is the smallest of the Greater Antilles in the Caribbean, located between Hispaniola and the Virgin Islands. Puerto Rico itself is a small archipelago surrounded to the north by the Atlantic Ocean and to the south by the Caribbean Sea. Its geographical extension is approximately 100 × 35 miles.

Puerto Rico has a warm tropical climate throughout the year that provides a very colorful natural landscape. The shores of Puerto Rico have beautiful beaches and the center of the Island is mountainous with several rain forests and diverse vegetation. This climate is considered decisive in the culture, in the economy, and in the formation of the cheerful, communicative, and spontaneous characteristics of the people.[1]

However, its tropical climate and geographical location expose the Island to the passage of frequent storms and hurricanes. In addition, Puerto Rico is surrounded by several geological faults that have been recently active on the southwestern part of the Island.

History

Puerto Rico was identified in 1493 by Christopher Columbus and colonized by Spain by 1508. At that time, the Island was populated by native Taíno culture, described as a tribal society. That culture rapidly diminished due to diseases and forced labor to retrieve gold for the colonizers.[2]

DOI: 10.4324/9781003051862-69

However, cultural and racial traits from Taínos are still present throughout our vocabulary, art, folklore, and food.

From the 17th century, the Spanish introduced enslaved and displaced individuals from Africa to work in agriculture, considerably increasing the Afro-descendant population on the Island. This practice was abolished in 1873. However, the African influence has been a significant determining factor in our national identity. This heritage extends to our vocabulary, food, arts, music, religion, and physical features. Overall, we consider ourselves mainly a racial mix of the native Taínos, Africans, and Europeans originating mostly from Spain.

The uniquely Puerto Rican identity can be traced to the 19th century, when national awareness grew out of independent and autonomous movements from the Spanish metropolis. Puerto Rico was able to obtain regional autonomy from Spain only months before the North American invasion in 1898, during the Spanish–American war. After the war, Puerto Rico was ceded to the United States along with Cuba and other Pacific Islands. Puerto Rico is still an unincorporated territorial possession and is considered the world's oldest colony.

The change of sovereignty implied an attempt of transculturation, substituting the Hispanic culture for the Anglo-Saxon one. Military bases were quickly installed, and the US currency was established. Since 1917, Puerto Ricans have been citizens of the United States, allowing them to enlist in its armed forces and travel freely to and from the United States. Since 1952, Puerto Rico established a relationship with the United States known as the Commonwealth of Puerto Rico. This allowed for a government with greater "autonomy." This political formula quickly transformed Puerto Rico from an agricultural to an industrial economy, producing a cultural breakdown with problems reconfiguring a new set of values.[3] Because it is still a colony, Puerto Ricans do not control their borders. Federal laws overcome local laws. Economy is also controlled by the United States, along with their cabotage laws. Puerto Ricans living in Puerto Rico are not allowed to vote in US elections, despite being US citizens.

Today's Puerto Rican culture integrates much of the *American Way of Life*, but without abandoning the Hispanic heritage. The Spanish of Puerto Rico is full of Anglicisms and many of our behaviors (eating habits, business organization, and residential developments) emulate the American middle class. Likewise, our institutions are a mixture of Anglo-Saxon and Hispanic traditions. For example, the educational system follows the North American culture, but our justice system maintains both civil law as well as common law. Also, Puerto Rico also has established communities of North American, Latin American, Caribbean, and even Asian cultures.

People

Puerto Rico is known as the Island of Enchantment for the beauty of its landscapes and for the hospitality of its people. Puerto Ricans are distinguished by their optimistic attitude, their good sense of humor, and a great sense of solidarity. For Puerto Ricans, family is the most important value.[4] This caring attitude, along with the strong family support system, is present in many families that we see.

The sense of group and familiarity is also seen in our teamwork. We all met within the Clinical Psychology doctoral program at the same university. We are all currently colleagues, but we have in the past worked in a supervisor-trainee and/or professor-student relationship. The case that we will present was initially referred by a family friend, and throughout the years, the family kept frequent communication with us.

Migration or "Circulation"

Puerto Rico is one of the countries with the highest migration rates in the world.[3] Currently, 5.5 million Puerto Ricans live in the United States, which represents 61% of our population.[5]

Large migratory waves to US agricultural and industrial centers started in the last century due to government policies and the convenience of having American citizenship. Most recently, new migratory waves are seen from families looking for better educational, health, and employment opportunities, particularly after recent natural disasters. This has resulted in a population decline of –3.5% on the Island.[6] Those Puerto Ricans in the United States maintain their culture, as well as social and family ties. That is why, instead of migration, many families experience a "circulation" between Puerto Rico and the United States.[3]

Language

As a Hispanic country, 95% of Puerto Rican communities use Spanish in daily activities. Our Spanish has a rich and diverse vocabulary from Taíno, African, and English dialect influences. Public school systems include English as part of the regular curriculum for all grades, which means all Puerto Ricans obtain some level of English instruction. Many private schools provide bilingual education. There are some people that perceive that the English language is better taught in private schools. In technical and industrial contexts, and in certain academic fields, English can be frequently used. Universities maintain Spanish as the main language but often require some courses in English. In specialty courses, the textbooks and other references are often in English, even when the classes are taught in Spanish. This is also our case as neuropsychologists: many of our training, continuing education, and the references we use are from scientific literature are written in English. Puerto Ricans are also very exposed to English through television, radio, the press, and most recently, through social media and the internet. However, it is estimated that less than 20 percent of the Island's population speaks English at an advanced level.

Education

The education system of Puerto Rico follows the North American model from preschool to university level. By constitutional law, the Puerto Rico government currently provides education to 424,000 children in 1,464 public schools. Of these, around 29% participate in the Special Education Program (SEP), according to the Individuals with Disabilities Education Improvement Act.[7] This is a US law that guarantees from the government free and appropriate public education to all students with disabilities, as defined in different categories of mental, health, or physical impairments. The private educational system in Puerto Rico serves 149,000 students in 882 schools. However, special education services are not often provided within this system. When it is offered, the cost and expenses are high, exceeding the mean annual income of the typical Puerto Rican family.[8]

Despite the legal status, the government of Puerto Rico has financial limitations, even political and administrative barriers, to provide all the individualized services that children need with their special education and in their transition from adolescence to adulthood. The process of requesting services is often slow and difficult, sometimes requiring going through legal channels. This often triggers migration to the United States. Recent natural disasters and the COVID-19 pandemic have worsened these difficulties.

Communication

Working with children means that the clinical approach must be family-oriented. Initial communication tends to be with the child's caregiver, who is usually the mother. Although in our culture the father is considered the head of the traditional family, it is the mother who often assumes the leadership in childcare and the one who often provides more detailed information about the child's development and the family system.

Age and professional levels tend to be respected, although it partially depends on educational and socio-economic factors. Regardless of socio-economic backgrounds, Puerto Ricans tend to be very respectful toward figures of "authority." With time, that relationship might be perceived as a relationship of trust, and therefore, familiarity. It is important to keep a healthy balance between rapport and professional boundaries with families.

Shaking hands is often the preferred method of greetings, at the beginning and at the end of each session, particularly from and between men, but often as part of a professional relationship in any gender. When there is more trust and feelings of familiarity, a kiss on the cheek can be received from, and between, women. Communicative nonverbal gestures tend to be frequent.

Assertiveness can be a challenge sometimes, either from or to families. Some families are not ready to receive direct information of test results or diagnosis without first talking positively and establishing strong rapport. Empathy is required to gain trust. Empowerment is often needed.

Literacy

Puerto Rico is one of the most literate regions in America, with a literacy rate of 92%.[9] This achievement is due to a large investment in education by the federal government. The Puerto Rican labor force has an average education of 12.6 years of study. About 2.5% reached advanced studies, including a doctorate. As for Puerto Rican migrants in the United States, they are the second group among Hispanics with the highest education. It is estimated that 19% have at least a bachelor's degree.[10] Some of the reasons for the remaining 8% on the Island being illiterate include poverty, gender violence, and immigration. Government literacy programs are available to those adults identified when seeking employment so that they can compete in the job market.[11]

Socio-Economic Status

Over the past two decades Puerto Rico has experienced an economic contraction that has affected all government, private and personal sectors, including health and education services. This has been exacerbated by recent natural disasters: a major hurricane that devastated the Island causing thousands of deaths and the temporary collapse of the communication systems, electrical grid, and water supply and earthquakes on the southwestern part of the Island that destroyed properties and commercial activities. The COVID-19 pandemic has also been causing a significant stagnation in the economy. In 2018, the average annual salary of a working-class Puerto Rican family was $24,563.[12] There are estimations that 36 of the 78 municipalities, or towns of Puerto Rico, have more than 50% of their population under poverty levels. These locations also report the lowest educational levels and limited availability of services. US government welfare is usually available for those below the poverty level.

As mentioned before, the Government of Puerto Rico has policies and resources aimed at providing services and supports for children. Although all families can access these services regardless of their social status, most of the working-class families in Puerto Rico require those services to assist in meeting their child's needs. However, because it can be a slow and difficult process, parents with economic resources often pay for private, complementary services. This is a huge challenge, and to some point a disadvantage, because we all know that optimal outcomes of children with disabilities will be determined by early accessibility to health services, educational opportunities, and evidence-based interventions. Again, for many families, those opportunities are found by migrating to the United States, particularly if they have family ties in the mainland.

Values and Customs

We agree with a recent study[13] that found that the most valuable thing for Puerto Ricans is the family (94%), followed by work (70%), free time (66%), and religion (65%). Good manners (90%), respect for others (77.1%), and responsibility (70.9%) were identified as the qualities to be promoted. Other important values reported were health and environmental protection.

Many of our customs are of Christian origin. One of the most important holidays is Christmas. It is celebrated from the end of November up to mid-January. Yes, we have the world record of celebrating the world's longest Christmas season! There are many other Christian-related festivities, such as the Patron Saint Festivals, in almost every town. US holidays are observed, along with the local ones. National sports are also well celebrated. Those are occasions to gather with family and friends.

Gender and Sexuality

In modern Puerto Rican society, much progress has been made in values, attitudes, and stereotypes, although in certain sectors conservative, sexist, and exclusionary attitudes are still maintained. Although women play an important role in the family, our society is primarily patriarchal.[14] **Machismo** and **marianismo** are still part of our culture. This lack of gender equity manifests itself in a high incidence of violence against females and LGBTQIA+ groups. As per our neuropsychological work, this is a topic that requires sensitive exploration as family values might interpose its management.

Spirituality and Religion

Because of our Spanish heritage, the Catholic Church had a great influence on culture and our life in general. Most of the population identifies as Christians, or at least, believers in God. The rest practice other religions or are religiously unaffiliated.[13] Other spiritual movements are identified in our cultural heritage, particularly from African origin mixed with Catholicism. Nuñez Molina's studies[15] have identified several movements: folkloric, evangelical, **espiritismo**, and **santería**. Even though they might function as a religion for some, they have been considered as a healing system, a philosophy, or a science for others.

Health

According to a recent cross-sectional study,[16] there is a high prevalence of medical conditions among Puerto Ricans, including hypertension (39%), obesity (28%), arthritis (26%), hypercholesterolemia (24%), respiratory problems (21%) and diabetes mellitus (21%). The leading causes of death are similar to those observed in the United States: heart disease, cancer, diabetes, Alzheimer's and cerebrovascular diseases.[17] In youth, asthma is the most prevalent health condition.[18] It is considered, however, that there are general health disadvantages when compared to the United States. Due to the high rate of migration and economic constraint, there are currently fewer specialty physicians and other health providers available for the population's needs.

Mental Health Views

The prevalence of mental disorders in Puerto Rico is estimated at 16% in people between the age of 18 and 64, according to data in official documents of the government of Puerto Rico. The most prevalent diagnoses in both youth and adults are affective and anxiety disorders (colloquially defined as **padecer de los nervios**). Substance use and dependencies disorders are also a public health concern. This data makes Puerto Rico the third largest jurisdiction in the United States with the greatest mental health problems.[19] There is still some stigma associated with receiving psychological or psychiatric treatment, as it may be seen as "being crazy." The deterioration of the economy, social inequality, poverty, limitations on access to mental health services, and recent natural disasters seem to have had psychological sequela with increases in cases of depression, anxiety, and suicides. In addition to the above-mentioned disorders, those factors exacerbated pre-existing conditions and sparked a wave of domestic violence.

Approach to Neuropsychology in Puerto Rico

We will present the following content from the perspective of three Puerto Rican neuropsychologists. All of us completed doctoral degrees in Puerto Rico, and two of us circulated to the United States for completion of post-doctoral fellowships in neuropsychology. We are all bilingual (Spanish/English), and currently work in both academic settings and private practice in Puerto Rico.

In Puerto Rico, as in many places in the world, neuropsychology is a new field. A recent study by Rodriguez-Irizarry and colleagues[20] identified about 25 practitioners on the Island who considered themselves neuropsychologists. Here on the Island, neuropsychology follows the North American model of higher education and government licensure process.[21,22] Currently, access to education related to neuropsychology on the Island is largely dependent on course offerings from doctoral training programs. This allows graduate students to receive basic training in harmony with some of the requirements of the Houston Conference Guidelines. However, the options for completing a predoctoral internship or postdoctoral residency in neuropsychology are very limited. According to the study conducted by Rodriguez-Irizarry,[20] less than half of their sample (44%) completed a postdoctoral residency in neuropsychology. Professional training in neuropsychology represents a central controversy for the recognition or certification of this profession on the Island.

As happens in many parts of the world, particularly in Spanish-speaking countries,[23,24] another challenge of our field is the lack of normative data for Puerto Ricans. At the time of writing this chapter, there were only a select group of tests developed or adapted for Puerto Ricans. Recent international efforts have provided some data of Puerto Rican norms for common neuropsychological tests. A common practice is to translate tests (if needed) and use available normative data from other countries. Others might use direct scores and personalized procedures through clinical practice.[20] We try to manage this issue using the "process approach" in our evaluations, focusing on the qualitative data during procedures.

Obtaining local data is complicated, as research and publications are not often fostered outside of the academic setting. This is further complicated by the fact that the few practitioners on the Island are required to perform in many different scenarios and carry out several different duties, which lead them to become overburdened.[20] Buying new tests and protocols can also be a challenge, as shipping and handling costs are higher than mainland United States and reimbursement and revenue from neuropsychological evaluations are significantly lower when compared to the mean average in the United States.

In Puerto Rico, there is little public awareness of neuropsychology and its contributions to the community. In our experience, even some physicians do not have knowledge of what a neuropsychologist does. Some people think we are neurologists. Many of the families we see have a basic understanding that neuropsychologists have additional training. Those of us with the pediatric specialty have often been associated with neurodevelopmental conditions, and many of our referrals come from school personnel. There are many health-related conditions that we do not see as often as we should, such as epileptic syndromes and head traumas.

In general, we have found that, when working with families, the cognitive domains are not often the primary area of concern and discussion. Rather, the focus lies on obtaining a general picture of what they need in terms of intervention and case management and what is required to access the needed services.

Section II: Case Study — "Too High Functioning To Be Autistic"

Note: Possible identifying information and several aspects of history and presentation have been changed to protect patient identity and privacy.

Joel is a young man whom we have seen for services and consultations since he was 5 years old. This gives us the unique perspective of a longitudinal assessment. The family was part of the working class, from an area of Puerto Rico with a high percentage of poverty and, therefore, limited availability of services. We will be presenting background information and the results of Joel's neuropsychological evaluations and follow-up consultations, together with the cultural and biopsychosocial challenges that he and his family have faced throughout their journey.

Referral

Joel is a left-handed Puerto Rican male from a small town located in the Southwestern part of the Island. He was initially referred to us by a family friend, who was a clinical psychologist, for a diagnostic evaluation. At that time, he was five years old. There were concerns regarding possible autism spectrum disorder (ASD) symptomatology. Per his mother's report, the family had been reporting developmental concerns since Joel was 10 months of age and, while his neurologist and other specialists had noted symptoms of ASD, a formal diagnosis had not been established.

Developmental History

Joel was the product of an uncomplicated pregnancy and delivery. Mild delays in some motor milestones (e.g. holding his head and rolling) were reported, and Joel received physical therapy to support his development. Joel was able to walk at 18 months of age. In terms of his language development, he said his first words on time and was able to repeat songs that he heard on the T.V., but his parents were concerned because he rarely responded to his name being called. He was evaluated by a neurologist and an audiologist, who found clinically negative results but referred Joel to a speech-language pathology evaluation, which identified language delays. Joel eventually began receiving speech-language therapy at age four. At the time of the evaluation, he was speaking both Spanish and English but, despite Spanish being the language spoken at home, he spoke and understood English better. Joel was also presenting with stereotyped speech at the time (e.g. referring to himself in the third person).

Academic History

Joel was enrolled in an educational daycare at two years of age. By age three he had learned to read and write on his own. He was enrolled in kindergarten when he was close to five years of age, where behaviors such as frequent tantrums, ignoring instructions, refusing to work in the classroom, not staying seated, and not socializing with peers were reported.

Psychological and Behavioral History

Joel presented with restrictive and repetitive patterns of behavior, such as lining up toys, walking on his toes, avoiding stepping in between tiles, and pulling on his eyelashes; a history of hand flapping at age one was also reported. Joel was also reported to show inflexibility (e.g. insisting on following certain routines at home) and did not tolerate getting dirty. He was evaluated in a psychological clinic, where ASD symptoms were identified using the Gilliam Autism Rating Scale. However, a formal diagnosis of ASD was not made. He was only provided with intervention for toilet training.

Medical History

Joel suffered from dermatitis and nasal allergies throughout most of his life, for which he was treated with several different medications. He was hospitalized when he was one year old due to rotavirus and was later diagnosed with oxidative metabolic disorder and carnitine deficiency, for which he was treated with levocarnitine by his geneticist. His medical history was otherwise unremarkable.

First Evaluation: Five Years of Age

Joel was first evaluated by the authors at age five. General cognitive abilities were assessed using one of the few Spanish batteries available at that time: the Batería III Woodcock Muñoz (WM-III), Pruebas de Habilidades Cognitivas, as well as a nonverbal reasoning measure, the Raven's Coloured Progressive Matrices, a developmental screener translated to Spanish: the DENVER-II, and a visual-motor integration task: The Bender Visual Motor Gestalt Test, Second Edition. Those were commonly selected tests in our clinic due to the Spanish language used for standardization, the amplitude of age ranges available, and the availability of norms that included a few Puerto Ricans among many other Latino communities in the United States.

Test results showed consistently average functioning in all areas assessed, including verbal comprehension, verbal knowledge, nonverbal reasoning, and visual-motor integration. However, throughout this evaluation and subsequent follow-ups Joel was found to demonstrate deficits in social interaction and communication, as well as restrictive/repetitive patterns of behavior, consistent with the DSM-IV-R criteria for High-Functioning ASD (identified at that time as Pervasive Developmental Disorder Not Otherwise Specified). This diagnosis came as a relief to the parents, who had for years been desperately seeking an accurate explanation for their son's behavioral difficulties.

First Evaluation Follow-Up: The Struggle for Services

Following Joel's diagnosis, the next step was for the family to obtain the recommended services for him. The family attempted to register Joel under the SEP of the Department of Education of Puerto Rico in order to receive services. However, he was initially denied services because he appeared to be "too high functioning to be autistic." What came next was a struggle that is all too familiar for many parents with kids on the spectrum in Puerto Rico, and one that would last for many years: trying to obtain adequate services and accommodations for Joel inside and outside the classroom. At the same time, Joel's parents felt that they were losing the support of many of their extended family members, as they did not understand his diagnosis and could not understand why he had tantrums and sensory issues during family gatherings. These types of behaviors are commonly seen by the community as a consequence of "bad parenting" or "lack of discipline" to the child. The family had to stop attending social events and felt isolated from the social support that had been crucial for them in the past.

During this process, the family sought and found support from a relatively new, local advocacy group called the Autism Alliance. There, they met with parents who understood their struggles and were able to begin navigating the complex process of seeking services for Joel. Evidenced-based services for ASD were scarce, so the family found alternate interventions for Joel's difficulties, including Auditory Integration Training, visual therapy, and a gluten- and casein-free diet. Joel's mother learned as much as she could about his diagnosis and his rights under the IDEIA law and quickly became an active participant and a leader in the Autism Alliance, as well as a fierce advocate for Joel's rights. Eventually, Joel was able to begin receiving services and accommodations under the SEP.

Joel remained in a regular education classroom, but behaviors such as tantrums and elopements made it necessary for him to receive the support of a one-to-one aid. With this support, problem behaviors were significantly reduced and, by the second grade, had ceased to be present. During this period, Joel was noted to begin talking with and having lunch with classmates.

Second Evaluation: Psychoeducational Evaluation at Seven Years of Age

At the time of his second evaluation, Joel was enrolled in the second grade. He was motivated and performing well academically, with strengths in classes related to English and Mathematics. His aid helped with redirection and facilitated his comprehension of instructions. Behavioral concerns at school included falling asleep in class, taking off his shoes, and complaining of itching on his body. Testing was carried out in Spanish, and, because of his age and the recent publication of more Spanish instruments, we were able to administer the following tests: Wechsler Intelligence Scale for Children - IV - Spanish (WISC-IV-Spanish), Ravens Coloured Progressive Matrices, WM-III, Bender Visual Motor Gestalt Test, Human Figure Drawing, a School Behavior Checklist, Child Behavior Checklist (CBCL), and the Behavioral Rating Inventory of Executive Functions (BRIEF).

During testing, Joel was cooperative and followed instructions. He would make spontaneous comments about his favorite videogame characters and respond to direct questions with phrases or short sentences. He had difficulties answering verbal test items and often responded by talking about topics not related to the question being asked. Not surprisingly then, verbal tests were found to be more challenging for him than visual and visual-spatial tests. On the WISC-IV-Spanish, his performance fell in the average to above-average range in visual, visual-spatial, and visual-motor tests but fell in the low average to below-average range on verbal reasoning tests. He was found to present with difficulties in executive functions (e.g. initiation, working memory, cognitive organization, and flexibility). Academically, his reading, writing, and math skills, as assessed with the WM-III, were within age- and grade expectations. Consistent with his ASD diagnosis, continued difficulties in social interaction, imaginative play, social communication, as well as restrictive/repetitive patterns of thinking and behavior were documented.

Second Evaluation Follow-Up

Following the evaluation, Joel began to receive psychological intervention to support his socio-emotional functioning, in addition to speech/language therapy (SLT) and occupational therapy (OT). These services were provided as "related services" by the SEP. Because the therapies were frequent throughout the week, were provided outside the school setting, and many of them were provided after school hours, Joel's parents were feeling overburdened and were missing workdays too often. They enlisted the help of their eldest daughter and some close friends in providing transportation for Joel to and from school and therapy centers.

Third Evaluation: Neuropsychological Evaluation at Nine Years of Age

At age nine, Joel continued to receive SLT, OT, and psychological intervention; he also received visual therapies. Medically, he was being treated with cetirizine for allergic dermatitis and with levocarnitine for metabolic deficiency. With regards to schooling, he was in the fifth grade within a regular education classroom (in Spanish), where he had the support of his one-to-one aid. He presented with sleepiness in school and required a ten-minute nap during the afternoons. He showed difficulties understanding and following directions and remembering to hand in assignments, as well as difficulties with writing and low frustration tolerance. Socially, he enjoyed relating to others, although pragmatic difficulties persisted, as well as compulsive patterns of behavior, obsessions, and rituals. He presented with difficulties organizing language and using vocabulary adequately, although he performed better when speaking in his preferred language, English.

He was assessed using the following tests: WISC-IV-Spanish, Wechsler Abbreviated Scale of Intelligence, Vocabulary Subtest (to assess his English expressive language skills); Tower of London; Trail Making Test; Rey Osterrieth Complex Figure; Beery Developmental Test of Visual Motor Integration; Test de Aprendizaje Verbal Infantil; as well as selected subtests from the Test of Everyday Attention for Children; Evaluación Neuropsicológica Infantil; NEPSY-II; Test of Auditory Processing Skills, Third Edition, Spanish-Bilingual (TAPS-3). The following behavior rating scales were also completed by his parents and teachers (when applicable): ADHD Rating Scale; BRIEF, and Behavior Assessment System for Children, Second Edition (BASC-2 PRS-C).

Joel's neuropsychological profile continued to reflect average-level intellectual abilities, as well as average-level functioning in most other areas assessed. Persistent weaknesses were documented in his executive functions (particularly in cognitive organization and flexibility), language, and fine motor skills. Notable progress was documented in his social skills, although weaknesses in pragmatics persisted (e.g. maintaining conversations, understanding sarcasm). What was particularly striking within the results of this evaluation was how different his language performance was in English when compared to Spanish tests. His understanding of instructions in English was age-appropriate, but he struggled with comprehending instructions in Spanish, which meant that he needed most instructions to be translated to English for him. His performance on the English vocabulary test fell in the average range, while his performance in the Spanish vocabulary test fell well below average. Additionally, difficulties with his production and organization of language were noted when he spoke in Spanish but not in English. He was even speaking in Spanish using English syntax and structure. Due to these difficulties, we included in our recommendations a particular emphasis on allowing him to use English to respond to questions while at school and for school personnel to use language that Joel could understand within this setting while providing direct intervention to help him further develop his language competencies.

Third Evaluation Follow-Up: The Language Barrier

Joel was attending a Spanish-language public school, and it was difficult for school personnel to implement language recommendations, as some did not possess the needed proficiency in English to be able to communicate with Joel in this language. Because he appeared to be so high functioning, many also underestimated his language comprehension difficulties. Joel was struggling with academic demands in Spanish. He also encountered frequent social, or pragmatic, misunderstandings. For example, on one occasion, he did not hear the class bell ring because he was in the library (avoiding the sensory overload of the playground noise). When he arrived late to class and explained this to his teacher, his teacher replied saying that it "was no excuse" for arriving late to class. Joel then proceeded to insist on genuinely explaining to the teacher that it was, indeed, an excuse, not understanding what the teacher really meant (that his excuse was unacceptable and that he should not have been late for class). An argument ensued and Joel was sent to the principal's office as a disciplinary consequence, as he "defied" and "spoke back to" an authoritative figure (which is not appropriate behavior for a child in our culture). Meanwhile, his parents continued to struggle to obtain an adequate school placement for him. They persevered in making adjustments and sacrifices to be able to provide him with the support and intervention that he needed.

Fourth Evaluation: Neuropsychological Re-Evaluation at Age 12

At age 12, Joel was seen for a re-evaluation and update on recommendations. Now in sixth grade, he continued to be enrolled in an all-Spanish regular education classroom in public school, with the support of a one-to-one aid. Continued difficulties with attention, executive functions, compulsive behaviors, and hypersensitivity to noise in crowded classrooms and hallways were reported. Additionally, he was reported to pull his eyelashes out when anxious. Medically, he was being treated with antihistamines and topical steroids to treat his persistent dermatitis. Except for visual therapy, he continued with all other therapeutic services as provided through the SEP.

For this evaluation, all the tests (in both Spanish and English) from the neuropsychological battery administered at age nine were repeated. His cognitive profile appeared to be relatively stable; however, his performance on English and Spanish language tests seemed to even out, with improved performance on Spanish-language tests. Because of continued fine motor difficulties affecting his performance on writing-based tasks, an additional diagnosis of dysgraphia was established.

Third Evaluation Follow-Up: The Language Barrier

Despite his improved performance on Spanish cognitive tests, Joel continued to prefer speaking in English, demonstrated greater fluency when using said language, and struggled with school in Spanish. The family had fought in vain to procure for him accommodations that would allow for the translation of school materials to English. Like many adolescents with ASD, Joel's difficulties began to lead to mood and anxiety issues, for which he was seen by a psychiatrist. Meanwhile, his mother had seen her own health deteriorating and had not had the time to seek medical assistance until her condition became aggravated. She was later diagnosed with a neurodegenerative disease that also needed special care.

Fifth Evaluation: Psychoeducational Re-Evaluation at Age 13

Because of his continued struggle in academic subjects, Joel was brought in for a psychoeducational evaluation the following year, at age 13. By this point, he had been diagnosed with anxiety, depression, and obsessive-compulsive disorder and was under treatment with sertraline and dexmethylphenidate hydrochloride, prescribed by his psychiatrist. He continued to pull out his eyelashes during periods of anxiety or frustration, and difficulties maintaining sleep at night were reported by his mother. Treatment with antihistamines for allergies and dermatitis continued. Although he had friends in school, continued difficulties with pragmatics and making new friends were reported. Academically, he benefitted from the assistance of his one-to-one aide but showed difficulties in reading comprehension, particularly in Spanish, as well as in writing, consistent with his diagnosis of dysgraphia.

The following battery of tests was administered: WM-III, select subtests; Woodcock-Johnson III: Tests of Achievement and Tests of Cognitive Abilities (WJ-III), select subtests; Grooved Pegboard; NEPSY-II: Fingertip Tapping subtest; Dean Woodcock Sensory-Motor Battery: Coordination subtest; TAPS-3, select subtests; BRIEF, parent and teacher ratings; BASC-2 SRP; CBCL; and a School Behavior Checklist.

Like before, testing accommodations had to include translation of Spanish instructions to English to aid in comprehension. Select subtests from both the WM-III (in Spanish) as well as the WJ-III (in English) were alternately administered to compare his oral and reading comprehension, as well as expressive vocabulary in each language. Results showed notable strengths in English comprehension (oral and written), as well as English reading and writing fluency when compared to his performance on Spanish measures. Persistent weaknesses in executive functions and fine motor coordination were noted. Based on the results of this evaluation, it was recommended that Joel be placed in a bilingual (English-Spanish) regular education classroom or, at the very least, that translation to English be provided for instructions and academic materials.

Follow-Up

Having vast evidence to support their claim that Joel needed English-based accommodations, his parents hired a lawyer and embarked on a legal claim with the Department of Education. After a struggle to find the appropriate placement for him, his school finally decided to open a small group (10–11 students) bilingual classroom (English and Spanish) for talented students. This was a great benefit, not just for Joel but for other regular and special education students who were academically motivated and interested in being educated in English. Joel continued receiving the assistance of a one-to-one aide to help manage symptoms of anxiety (such as panic attacks), as well as social challenges. Within this setting, Joel thrived and was able to graduate high school.

Beyond High School: A Hurricane, a New Struggle and a Move

After successfully completing high school, Joel had planned to attend college. However, the process of transitioning from the SEP to the Vocational Rehabilitation Program for adults proved to be lengthy and unfruitful. Although Joel had a legal right to receive transition services and supports, including counseling to help him through this process, he did not receive it on time and was left in his home for a full year, having a drastic change in his routine, and without being able to pursue his goals. During this time, a catastrophic hurricane struck Puerto Rico and, not only was Joel stuck at home, but he was also experiencing the stress caused by the aftermath: spending months without reliable electricity and/or water. This led to a regression in symptoms, as described by the family. Joel became increasingly depressed and anxious, his panic attacks increased, and he stopped eating, which led to significant weight loss. Because of this, and like many other families in Puerto Rico at the time, the family decided that it would be best to relocate with their eldest daughter's home in the United States. Once there, they quickly retook the process of enrolling Joel in a Vocational Rehabilitation program. There, Joel received job and interview training and was able to obtain employment in the fast-food industry within the first months after moving. At the time of writing this chapter, we were able to communicate with Joel and his family. Joel is happy, healthy, and thriving. His family seems to be in a healthy acculturation and assimilation process. We are proud of growing old with Joel and having been a part of his journey.

Section III: Lessons Learned

- Puerto Rico is a colonized country, for centuries from Spain, and over the last century from the United States. Culture and traditions come mostly on a mixture of African, European, and, probably less often, Native American descendants, with the Spanish language being one of the most prevalent heritage. The influence of the North American culture is also taking part in our culture.
- Even though Puerto Rico is a territory of the United States and uses the same health system and education model, public services are not necessarily optimal for timely preventive care. Bureaucracy and economic policies seem to affect health care access.
- There are as many Puerto Ricans on the Island as they are outside of the Island, particularly due to migration movements in the 1960s and 2000s. Most of the migration is to the United States, as people from Puerto Rico were granted US citizenship in 1917. This is a relatively accessible option for Puerto Rican families in need of health, education, employment, and economic opportunities. Moreover, most families already have a family member or friend who has already migrated. Despite assimilation and acculturation processes, Puerto Rican culture is usually maintained.
- Families often move to the United States looking for a better quality of life or seeking needed services for one or more of its members. This happened to Joel's family when he grew up: services were not immediately available for him after graduating high school, and the limited services available were scarce after the aftermath of natural disasters. In addition to representing our family-centered culture, this event also highlights the need for professionals to develop research and promote public policy to assist in the services that children with neurodevelopmental disorders might need when they grow up.
- Neuropsychology is a new discipline in Puerto Rico. There are few neuropsychologists on the Island, and the field is often not recognized in the community. There is a limited culture for research in the profession, in part, because of the few researchers and their many work duties. Consequently, as happens with many Latin American countries, there are few tests available for Puerto Ricans.
- Autism Spectrum Disorder recently started to be in public awareness, as has happened in many parts of the world. Because of the extensive research conducted over the last three decades, new definitions and classifications have been updated, but not all health and education professionals are aware of these. In places like Puerto Rico, identifying what at one point can be considered a rare disease can be challenging. With Joel, there was a denial from health professionals and teachers of him having ASD, as he was "too functional to be autistic." This was a common myth even when the DSM-IV definition was commonly used.
- Spanish is the language predominantly used in Puerto Rico. However, a common phenomenon seen within the ASD population is a preference for speaking English.[25,26] There is some limited work regarding that topic. It seems that it is possibly due to frequent exposure to the English language through videos and games on electronic devices (since a very young age) and/or to reduced grammatical demands and rules in English when compared to the Spanish language. Therefore, neuropsychological evaluations in Puerto Rico, particularly in ASD, require taking into consideration the dominant language of the individual. This might impact the selection of language and test use.
- Test selection in general will continue to be a long-term dilemma, given the limited availability of tests specific for the Puerto Rican population and relatively easy access to tests published in

the United States. Decisions must be made on whether to use a test that is normed in another Spanish-speaking country or to use tests that have been translated from the English language but not adapted or standardized to our population. The decision seems to go beyond formal testing, as it also might impact the educational placement.

- A caring attitude and familiarity are positive attitudes often seen in Puerto Rican families. Joel was able to attend school and receive services because the parents were supported by their daughter, friends, and some extended family members. Some teachers were also helpful. Likewise, the family managed to establish a healthy, and somewhat a familiar, professional relationship over time with us.
- Family needs and diagnosis awareness are often prioritized. This might go beyond the classic practice of neuropsychology. Even though Joel was evaluated within the context of a neuropsychological evaluation, the major concerns were the lack of awareness of the condition in the community and family members, the lack of support from the educational system due to lack of knowledge, and the struggle to get the services he needed. This family in particular took the initiative to become active leaders in supporting many other families in the process of managing autism through the health and education system. The process to obtain services in Puerto Rico is very slow. Therefore, the practice of pediatric neuropsychology in Puerto Rico requires the clinician to be knowledgeable of how the education and public system in general work. One of our many duties in the clinical practice includes becoming case managers.

Acknowledgments

We would like to provide special thanks to Joel and his family for their availability and willingness to collaborate with us in narrating Joel's journey, despite being outside the Island.

Glossary

Espiritismo.   Spiritism. It is a movement or a belief that spirits can affect health, luck and other aspects of human life.

Machismo.   It is a sense of masculine pride and dominance, commonly seen in Latino cultures.

Marianismo.   It is the expectation for females to be passive, submissive and dedicated to the home and family. It is very common in Hispanic communities.

Padecer de los nervios.   Suffer from the nerves. It is a common name used by Puerto Ricans to describe ambiguously psychiatric disorders.

Santeria.   The way of the saints. It is a religious practice of African origin, based on the personal relations between deities, or saints.

References

1. Picó F. Historia General de Puerto Rico. San Juan (PR): Ediciones Huracán; 2008.
2. Del Olmo Frese L. La cultura Taína, Programa de Arqueología y etnohistoria. San Juan (PR): Instituto de Cultura Puertorriqueña; 2018.
3. Hernández Cruz J. Corrientes migratorias en Puerto Rico/Migratory trends in Puerto RIco. San Germán (PR): Universidad Interamericana de Puerto Rico; 1994.
4. Rivero-Vergne A, Berrios-Rivera R. Estudio cualitativo sobre el significado de la felicidad de los puertorriqueños: la felicidad en función de otros. Hato Rey (PR): Publicaciones Puertorriqueñas; 2018.
5. Center for Puertor Rican Studies. New estimates of Puerto Rican Migration Post Hurricane María 2018 [Internet]. 2019 Sept [cited 2020 Sept 9]. Available from: HTTP//centropr.hunter.cuny

6. US Census Bureao. Estimados anuales poblacionales [Internet]. 2020. [cited 2020 Sept 8]. Available from: https//:Censo.estadisticas.PR/Estimadospblacionales
7. US Department of Education. Individuals with Disabilities Education Improvement Act of 2004 [Internet]. 2004. [cited 2020, Sept 8]. Available from: https//sites.ed.gov/idea
8. Instituto de Estadísticas de Puerto Rico. Anuario estadístico del sistema educativo de Puerto Rico 2018–2019. Gobierno de Puerto Rico. 2019.
9. Disdier Flores O, Pesante González F, Marazzi Santiango M. Encuesta de Alfabetización de Puerto Rico. San Juan (PR): Instituto de Estadísticas de Puerto Rico; 2012
10. Noe-Bustamante L, Flores A, Shah S. Facts on Hispanics of Puerto Rican origin in the United States [Internet]. Enciclopedia de Puerto Rico. 2019 Sept 16 Available from: https://www.pewresearch.org/hispanic/fact-sheet/u-s-hispanics-facts-on-puerto-rican-origin-latinos/
11. Sanjurjo L. Giro en el perfil del analfabeta boricua. Primera Hora [internet], 2016 Nov 16 [cited 2020 Sept 6]: Available from: https///www.primerahora.com/noticias/puerto-rico/giro-en-perfil
12. Gobierno de Puerto Rico. La economía de Puerto Rico en 2018 y revisiones años fiscales 2016 y 2017. San Juan (PR): Junta de Planificación; 2018.
13. Hernández Acosta J. Encuesta Mundial de Valores para Puerto Rico. Instituto de Estadísticas de Puerto Rico. 2019 Jun 26. Available from: http://esdisticapr.pr
14. Colón González O. Manifestación de los estereotipos de género en un modelo de educación sustentando en la perspectiva de género: UPR; 2017.
15. Nuñez Molina M. El espiritismo en Puerto Rico [Internet]. Sistemas Folclóricos de Ayuda 2007 [cited 2020 Sept 13]. Disponible en: http://vidadigital.net/
16. Mattei J, Tamez M, Ríos-Bedoya CF, Xiao RS, Tucker KL, Rodríguez-Orengo JF. Health conditions and lifestyle risk factors of adults living in Puerto Rico: a cross-sectional study. BMC Public Health [Internet]. 2018;18(491). Available from: https://doi.org/10.1186/s12889-018-5359-z
17. Chronic Disease Prevention and Control Division. Puerto Rico Chronic Disease Action Plan 2014–2020. Departamento de Salud de Puerto Rico, Secretarial for Health Promotion; 2014.
18. Langellier BA, Martin MA, Canino G, R GH, Ortega AN. The health status of youth in Puerto Rico. Clin Pediatr. 2012 Jun;51(6): 569–573.
19. Estado Libre de Puerto Rico Departamento de Salud. Salud Mental de Puerto Rico: Análisis de situación de la salud en Puerto Rico [Internet]. 2014. [citado 2020 sept 13]. Disponible en: www.salud.gov.pr/documents/acreditación%del%20departamento%20de%20
20. Rodríguez-Irizarry W, Oliveras-Rentas, R., Olabarrieta-Landa L, Arango-Lasprilla JC. La práctica de la neuropsicología en Puerto Rico: implicaciones para la certificación de la especialidad. Revista Iberoamericana de Neuropsicología. 2018;1(1):45–62.
21. Albizu Miranda C, Matlin N. La psicología en Puerto Rico: Apuntes sobre el estado de un arte. Revista de Ciencias Sociales de Puerto Rico. 1967;9:71–80.
22. Velázquez J, Millan F, Colton M, Cabiya I, Rodriguez K, Miranda Y, et al. Una nueva Mirada a la Psicología en Puerto Rico: Apuntes sobre el estado de un arte. Glossa Ambilingual Interdiscip. 2006;I(1):1–14.
23. Arango Lasprilla JC, Stevens L, Morlett Paredes A, Ardila A, Rivera D. Profession of neuropsychology in Latin America. Appl Neuropsychol Adult;2016 June 9:9–13.
24. Oliveras-Rentas RE, Romero-García I, Benito-Sánchez I, Ramos-Usuga D, Arango-Lasprilla JC. The practice of child neuropsychology in Spanish-speaking countries: What we've learned and where to go from here. Dev Neuropsychol. 2020;45(4):169–188.
25. Oliveras-Rentas RE. Phenotypic Characterization of Puerto Rican Children with Autism [dissertation] Ponce, PR: Ponce School of Medicine; 2005.
26. Méndez-Rosselló CA, Oliveras RE. Language preference & proficiency in sequential bilingual children with Autism Spectrum Disorders. In Poster session presented at International Society for Autism Research; 2019 May 1–4; Toronto, CA. Available at: https://insar.confex.com/insar/2019/webprogram/Paper29980.html

Venezuela

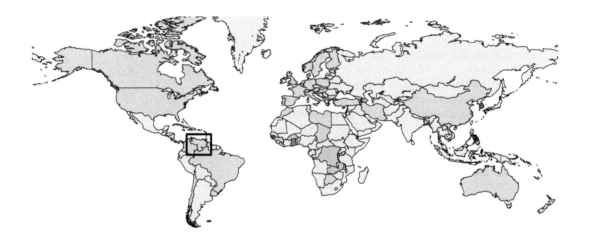

35 Application of the Collaborative Therapeutic Neuropsychological Assessment Approach on a Venezuelan Migrant

Aline Ferreira-Correia

Section I: Background Information

Terminology and Perspective

People from the Bolivarian Republic of Venezuela are referred to as Venezuelans. As part of the Latin American community, we may also be called Latinos, Latinas, or LatinX.

My perspective is that of a cis woman born in Venezuela from European immigrant parents. I graduated as a clinical psychologist from the Central University of Venezuela (Universidad Central de Venezuela/UCV) after the completion of a five-year study program. In the last two years, students choose to specialize and I focused on psychodynamically orientated clinical psychology. In Venezuela, psychologists who wish to become specialized clinicians can do an additional master-equivalent degree over two or three years. My degree had an emphasis on clinical neuropsychology. In 2009, I immigrated to Johannesburg, South Africa, where I obtained my PhD at the University of Witwatersrand. Here, my perspective is that of a white foreign psychologist who is an English second language speaker with dual registration (clinical psychology and neuropsychology). I work as an academic and a clinician in private practice.

Geography

Venezuela is located at the north end of South America. It shares land borders with Colombia on the west and southwest, Brazil to the south, and Guyana to the east. To the north is the Caribbean Sea and the Atlantic Ocean. Venezuela is known for its extraordinary natural beauty. The weather is generally warm and humid, with significant variations in temperature linked to altitude (from the cold-snowy peaks in the Andes to the scorching heat on the coast). We have two seasons: rainy and dry. The total population of Venezuela is approximately 28 million people, with a decreasing birth rate and a large and unprecedented diaspora motivated by the ever-worsening sociopolitical and economic crisis,[1] leading to a population decline.

History

Settlers from North America who arrived during the Paleoindian period (20000 to 5000 BC) first occupied the territory now known as Venezuela. Heterogeneous indigenous groups constituted the original population of Venezuela and several remain in the territory. The arrival of the Spanish colonizers in 1498 also brought white Europeans and black Africans (trafficked as slaves) to the area.[2] Rapid mixing between races and social groups during this period created a complex intersection between class and race, which is reflected in the current social structure in Venezuela. The country

DOI: 10.4324/9781003051862-71

declared independence from Spain on the 5th of July 1810. Toward the middle of the 20th century, Venezuela moved from an agriculture-based economy to one relying exclusively on crude oil. The oil boom brought wealth and a great migration wave from South America and the Caribbean, Europe, Asia, and the Middle East. Our democratic era was established in 1958 but unfortunately has been characterized by consistently corrupt political systems that have depleted a once rich country.[2] Currently, Venezuela is living the worst political, economic and social crisis in its history, creating a humanitarian disaster with horrifyingly high indices of poverty, hyperinflation, and violence.[3]

Immigration and Relocation

Since colonization, Venezuela has received migrants from Europe, South America, and the Middle East. This has played a significant role in its growth and diversity. Until the end of the 21st century, Venezuela offered stability. Now the Venezuelan diaspora represents the largest migration, refugee, and displacement crisis in South America.[4] Motivations for leaving Venezuela have changed in the last decade. Initial migration was to find more opportunities, but is now forced by the need for social security and survival.[5] Approximately five million Venezuelans have left the country to escape political unrest, socio-economic decline, crime, violence, food and medicines shortages, human rights violations, and lack of basic services.[3] A great proportion of those fleeing has incurred great risks by walking to other South American countries.[6] The majority of Venezuelan migrants are living in countries such as Colombia, Peru, Chile, Ecuador, Brazil, and Argentina. Caribbean countries (Trinidad and Tobago and the Dominican Republic), Central (Costa Rica and Panama) and North America (United States of America and Mexico), and Europe (e.g. Spain, Portugal, and Italy) have also received many Venezuelans.[4]

The characteristics of Venezuelan migrants vary by chronological stage.[7] At the end of the nineties and the first decade of 2000, most Venezuelans who emigrated were highly educated, could afford travel, and went through a legal documentation process. This facilitated their adaptation to their receiving countries. In stark contrast, in the past five years, Venezuelans who left on foot have been victims of disaster-induced displacement, tend to be undocumented, poor, and with varying levels of education. They tend to become asylum seekers or refugees and face significant barriers assimilating to their host countries—many of which are now restricting inward-bound movement by Venezuelans. These migrants have left behind loved ones, often carrying only a single bag. Thus, learning about Venezuelan migrants' motivational processes as well as journeys and losses is of paramount importance as a platform for clinical judgment of both their emotional and cognitive functioning.

Language

In Venezuela, Spanish (Castilian) and languages spoken by Indigenous people of the country are the official languages. Accent and lexicon vary by region in Venezuelan Spanish.[8] Most Venezuelans speak Spanish, so the assessment of language proficiency is not common in neuropsychological assessments in the country. Spanish is spoken by 7.5% of the world population,[9] and although there are significant regional differences in terms of lexicon and phonetics, most Spanish-speakers can communicate well with each other.

Communication

Most Venezuelans prefer an informal communication style. The use of titles (e.g. Dr., Ms., Mr.) is quickly abandoned. The use of first names is common in psychologist–client relations. Humor is at the core of everyday life for Venezuelans.[10] It is used to cope and connect with others and also to express dissidence and reflect on reality.[11] Understanding the use of humor is important to consider when working with Venezuelan clients. We tend to make fun of everything, which may cause misunderstandings in multicultural environments. Humor can have great diagnostic and therapeutic power. For example, as a young neuropsychologist working at a large hospital in Caracas, Venezuela, a 63-year-old woman of Portuguese origin was referred to me to explore a memory complaint. She had migrated to Venezuela more than 30 years ago, although she had difficulties speaking Spanish. I attempted the interview in Portuguese, but she made fun of my mistakes and told me to stick to Spanish. Many years later, a South African client (non-Spanish speaker), referred to me for similar reasons, made fun of my accent. From a neuropsychological perspective, both these instances could have been interpreted as a sign of disinhibition, but for my Portuguese-Venezuelan client, it was an acceptable joke—we both laughed and I continued the interview in Spanish. In South Africa, it is considered offensive to make fun of accents of second-language English speakers, so the client's comment was concerning. The neuropsychological assessment and MRI revealed healthy frontal lobes in the first client and executive dysfunction with frontal atrophy in the second.

Venezuelans are prone to minimizing social distance and personal space. We greet others with a hug and one kiss on the cheek. When I first started working in South Africa, one of my colleagues told me that I was a "hugger" which is true. I realized this was culturally influenced a few years later when a Venezuelan client living in South Africa was so happy to have found a Venezuelan psychologist that she asked if she could give me a hug at the end of our first session, because "no one here likes to hug." This was such a powerful way to convey our cultural belonging. It is also worth noting that Venezuelans can be overly familiar with strangers and start spontaneous conversations, which is culturally appropriate. Taking time to discuss confidentiality rules and psychologist-client boundaries is thus very important, particularly when working with family systems and doing collateral interviews.

Education

Since independence, Venezuela's Constitution enshrines the right to education for all its citizens. The government is responsible for providing free and compulsory education to all Venezuelans until high school and for those who wish to continue tertiary studies.[12] The educational system includes six years of primary school and five years of secondary school. Tertiary education may include a technical degree (three years) or a professional degree (five–six years). Masters and doctoral degrees (two–three and five years, respectively) normally include coursework and theses. All levels of education can be completed in government or private institutions. Access to public universities is complex due to limited availability. Inquiring about the history of access to tertiary education is useful, in order to gauge educational opportunities when estimating premorbid level of functioning.

Unfortunately, the current crisis has not spared the educational system. Many educational institutions lack basic services and numerous Venezuelans cannot attend school due to hunger, lack of means to afford school uniforms, materials, or transport. Educators' salaries (approximately $4 a month) is insufficient for basic survival.[13] Obviously, these factors can compromise quality of education, and while the number of years of education is strongly correlated with cognitive performance, there is a need to gather a detailed educational history and use age and education stratified norms when available.[14]

Literacy

The constitution promises compulsory and free education, but despite the social programs designed to eradicate illiteracy, Venezuela's illiteracy rate is 4.9%.[15] Many children of school age are excluded from the educational system and there are significant disparities between Venezuelans in terms of language skills (reading and writing).[12] Venezuela was declared free of illiteracy in 2005,[16] which was far from evident in the neuropsychological unit where I used to work. Many clients arrived describing different reading and writing acquisition processes, which makes evaluating educational history crucial when designing an assessment.

Socio-Economic Status

Venezuela is ranked 127th (out of 140) in economic competitiveness by the World Economic Forum[17] and 179th (out of 180) in the 2020 index of economic freedom.[18] Hyperinflation has been calculated at 10 million percent.[19] At least 80% of the Venezuelan population has reached extreme poverty, which is among the worst in the world. The majority of its citizens are struggling to find food, medicines and have no reliable access to basic services (such as water, sanitation, and energy). Many Venezuelans are now dependent on remittances from family abroad, support from NGOs, and food parcels distributed by the government.[20] This has and will continue to have a negative impact on brain development and mental health.

Values and Customs

Over the past 20 years, Venezuela has rapidly deteriorated, which has impacted the essence of what it means to be Venezuelan.[21] There has been great political polarization and related food, security, healthcare, educational, and judicial inequity that has led to documented human rights violations and crimes against humanity.[3,22] While generalizations about Venezuelans are impossible, it is important to know the people of Venezuela within this context. Notwithstanding the obvious regional and individual differences, there are some values with which Venezuelans commonly identify and are important to keep in mind when offering psychological services.

Strong family ties and friendships (who are considered family)[23] are at the center of a Venezuelan's emotional and social life. They provide significant care and support in times of crisis.[23] Families can be a valuable resource that psychologists have to often rely on due to the unavailability of formal supporting structures (e.g. psychiatric hospitals, halfway houses, safe houses, etc.). At present, nearly all Venezuelans have experienced traumatic separations from family and friends and suffered painful losses, mostly driven by migration, which limits or precludes access to this important source of life support.

Boundaries between family members are therefore often unclear and it is common for people to intervene, participate or give opinions on personal issues that are considered private in other cultures.[23] For example, my client Ana* was concerned about her memory and requested an assessment. A year before our first session, Ana's husband had an affair. Her older sister (a lawyer) organized the divorce papers following the mother's request, which my client quickly signed without reflecting on the issue. Since then, Ana has been feeling sad and resentful because she was rushed into a divorce she did not actively choose and regretted. This exemplifies the importance of family hierarchies where mothers and older or educated members of the family frequently command the highest authority for decision making.

For instance, aggravated by the socio-economic crisis, family and social support are key to survival for Venezuelans. Many Venezuelans work abroad to send money back to family members

---

*I make use of pseudonyms when referring to clients throughout this chapter.

to help them survive.[24] Due to the high levels of criminality and violence, we have internalized a sense of danger and distrust. For example, a Venezuelan would not stop in the road to assist a stranger whose car has broken down, because we fear being robbed or killed by someone pretending to need help.[25] Hence, the neuropsychologist needs to earn the client's trust and identify and manage the client's apprehension.

Due to the economic crisis, it is almost impossible for young Venezuelans to move out of their parents' homes. Many homes thus contain more than one nuclear family and/or extended family members. Similarly, many separated or divorced couples are forced to remain in the same house. Neuropsychologists must be aware of the high levels of interdependency within Venezuelan families when conducting functional or capacity assessments or when evaluating activities of daily living.

The average Venezuelan is kind and likes to express gratitude.[10] Although accepting gifts from clients can elicit undesirable dynamics, when working in certain contexts, it may be considered rude and detrimental to the client to reject a thank you gift at the end of a therapeutic process. Francisco, a five-year-old with severe behavioral issues, was referred to me for psychological assessment in a center that provided free community services. Francisco's grandmother, who brought him to our sessions, was very distressed since the school was threatening to expel him if he did not improve his behavior. Francisco's father was in jail for having killed his mother, so his grandmother was the only caregiver and they were living under extreme poverty. After a full neuropsychological assessment and complex follow-up case management, there was a significant improvement in his behavior and school performance. His granny felt very grateful, and in our last session, she brought me a small bunch of a local fruit (*mamón*), which I accepted as a way to acknowledge her gratitude and her capacity to "give" in a context of so much deprivation.

Gender and Sexuality

Although Venezuela is matricentric (mothers are seen as the backbone of society), structurally the country remains patriarchal and sexist. This is evidenced by the high prevalence of gender-based violence, maternal mortality, teenage pregnancy, over-sexualization of girls and women, and femicide. Women are also the most frequent victims of sexual harassment and xenophobia.[26] High prices and the unavailability of contraceptives have caused staggering increases in unplanned pregnancies and HIV infections.[26] Reports indicate that, although women are allowed to vote and actively participate in the labor market, they are less likely than men to attain positions of political and economic power.[27]

Discrimination in access to education, health services, and employment on any basis, including sexual orientation and gender identity, is illegal. However, instances of exclusions and violations of human rights against the LGBTQI+ community are common and severe.[28] It is upsetting to report that the LGBTQI+ community does not enjoy equal civil and political rights. While not prosecuted, same-sex relationships are not legally recognized, which excludes rights such as marriage, civil unions, and adoption. Additionally, the constitution does not accommodate gender identity changes for transgender people.[8]

Spirituality and Religion

During the colonization process, the Roman Apostolic Catholic Church played a key role in the creation of settlements and consolidation of Spanish rule. Christian missionaries' aggressive proselytization inaugurated a religious society where the majority of Venezuelans today identify as Catholics. Nevertheless, Venezuelan religious and spiritual beliefs and practices are also marked by indigenous animism and African cosmology brought by people trafficked as slaves.

Together, these represent a complex fusion of values, beliefs, and rituals that influences the conscious and unconscious mind of Venezuelans.[29] Venezuelan society is thus religiously syncretic and pluralist,[30] where multiple religious denominations and practices (e.g. Christianism, Judaism, Evangelism, *Santería*, etc.) coexist. Neuropsychologists may encounter clients who ascribe to one religion but engage in cultural practices from different influences.

Acculturation and Systemic Barriers

Venezuelans have seemingly embraced a *"mestizaje"* (mixed-race) culture with abandonment of categorical racial categorizations following independence. However, there is both historical and contemporary evidence of racial discrimination including distribution of wealth along ethnic lines and upholding the European phenotype as the beauty standard.[31] Thus, experiencing and managing race dynamics abroad may be particularly difficult for Venezuelans.

The acculturation process of Venezuelan migrants is diverse and influenced by how Venezuelans are perceived in their receiving countries. For example, despite empirical evidence to the contrary,[32] many countries see Venezuelans as criminals who are stressing their health and educational services. Venezuelans then fall victim to xenophobic attacks of various kinds, particularly in South America.[33] Large cultural, climate, and linguistic distances between the country of origin and receiving countries can exacerbate feelings of alienation, stress, and inadequacy. Many Venezuelans do not have access to passports and other legal documents before they leave Venezuela, which prohibits access to services, employment, and housing abroad. This is an insurmountable barrier in the adaptation process of migrants. Neuropsychologists assessing Venezuelan migrants thus need to explore the individual migration story, which can reveal key contributors to emotional and cognitive symptoms.

Health Status

The socio-economic crisis in Venezuela has impacted the physical and mental health of all citizens in dramatic ways. Difficulties accessing food, medicines, and health services, the exodus of medical practitioners, and the dire working conditions of those who remain in the country have caused an unprecedented health crisis characterized by an increase in preventable infectious diseases (such as malaria, measles, HIV), rampant deterioration of clients with treatable chronic diseases, severe malnutrition and difficulty accessing life-saving treatments.[34] These conditions can have a significant impact on brain function. In an attempt to help, health professionals offer medical and psychological attention to those in need through several civil organizations. For example, Psicodiaspora (psicodiaspora.com) is a network of Venezuelan psychologists and psychiatrists all over the world who offer services to fellow citizens in and out of the country (rates are set by each professional, some offer pro-bono sessions).

Approaches to Neuropsychological Assessment in Venezuela and in My Practice

The development of neuropsychology in Venezuela has been promoted by the efforts of individuals and small teams in different hospitals, universities, and private practices. Its history is fractured and the community remains poorly integrated.[35] One of the founders of neuropsychology in Venezuela, Prof. Otto Lima Gómez, adapted Luria's protocol for the assessment of cortical functions after working with Luria himself. He published the Luria Battery-UCV (Batería Luria-UCV),[36,37] a seminal work for Venezuelan neuropsychologists. Prof Lima Gómez opened an elective course in neuropsychology at the Psychology School in the UCV (Universidad Central de Venezuela), my alma mater. The neuropsychology department in that school was founded shortly thereafter. Members of this department prepared the Manual for Neuropsychological Assessment Luria-UCV and developed norms and published psychometric studies.[38,39]

Two other major contributions to neuropsychological assessment in Venezuela are notable. First, the creation of the Dr. Julio Borges Neuropsychology Section at Hospital Universitario de Caracas UCV (HUC-UCV/University Hospital of Caracas UCV) in 1985. This unit is dedicated to the diagnosis and treatment of clients with cognitive symptoms. It is responsible for providing training in clinical neuropsychology for undergraduate and postgraduate students and has supported the development of several normative studies that have been published in a book edited by Psychologist Ilva Campagna.[14] Second, Prof Magdalena López de Ibañez, from the School of Psychology at UCV, has trained generations of psychologists in neuropsychological assessment and written a seminal book on the topic.[40] I received training in a combination of Russian and North American approaches to neuropsychological assessment and rehabilitation at the aforementioned school and neuropsychology unit.

Neuropsychology in Venezuela is taught within clinical psychology training programs, which influence the scope and style of our work. I have adopted a Collaborative Therapeutic Neuropsychological Assessment (CTNA) approach,[41] which aligns with my training as both a clinical psychologist and neuropsychologist.

The CTNA is a person-centered model where the client is seen as an active and autonomous participant in the neuropsychological assessment process. The client and clinician work together to understand the problems experienced by the client. In this process, the clinician aims to provide an intervention that reduces the client's distress, increases the working alliance, and, ultimately, provides a "transformative experience"[41] (p. 39) because it aims to ease the client's suffering, and facilitate personal development while providing insights into the nature of the cognitive problems. In brief, all encounters with the client in the CTNA approach need to be understood as therapeutic interventions and not processes in which the client is a passive test-taker. This model facilitates the expression and management of culture-dependent dynamics and individual variations because it incorporates the client's constructions of symptoms, therapeutic interventions, and the doctor-client relationship.

During my first session with a client, I aim to establish rapport, understand the problem (reason for consultation) and how the client makes sense of it, and ensure that the client comprehends the neuropsychological assessment process (i.e. why they were referred and what the expected outcome of our relationship will be). I also explore the client's expectations and whether they feel ready to participate in a potentially lengthy and expensive experience moving forward. The process includes an unstructured and client-guided discussion. I also ask clients to complete the Background Questionnaire Adult Version[42] to identify areas that require further exploration and that I might have missed during the interview.

I used the CTNA approach with Veronica, a 64-year-old client with Parkinson's disease. The neurologist considered her an excellent candidate for deep brain stimulation (DBS) and strongly recommended surgery to which she had agreed. My initial impression of Veronica was of a smart, successful, warm woman who was enjoying a fulfilling life. During our first meeting I realized that, unlike with other clients, her experience with Parkinson's disease was not featuring much in our conversation. I reflected this back to her by telling her: "Veronica, I am listening to your life story and I find myself forgetting that you have Parkinson's; this makes me wonder in which ways you imagine DBS will improve your life." Veronica, after a thoughtful silence, replied, "this is probably the most important question to ask myself in this process and I haven't even thought about it; I am working, travelling, doing gardening, taking care of my family ... Parkinson hasn't really impaired my life and perhaps the risk of surgery is not worth it." She left the session having second thoughts about elective surgery, and we agreed that she would think about it until next week's session. Veronica had the opportunity to re-frame the impact of Parkinson's Disease on her quality of life and take an active role in the decision-making process regarding surgery. As a result of this understanding, her trust in the team (and the consideration process) was consolidated.

Clients who understand medical procedures and take active roles therein have better treatment adherence and can better tolerate non-desirable side effects.

If neuropsychological testing is needed when assessing Venezuelan clients, I use tests translated into Spanish and country-specific adaptations and local norms, which should be stratified by age and years of education as these variables have a significant impact on the cognitive performance of Venezuelans (see Appendix). Data on diagnostic validity of neuropsychological tests are limited and affected by the heterogeneity of the population; hence, expert clinical judgment is central in the assessment process, particularly when assessing Venezuelans from rural or indigenous areas. If country-specific norms are not available, the use of stratified norms (by gender and years of education) from Latin American countries should be considered as an alternative option.

Section II: Case Study — "I Lost my Lucidity"

Note: Possible identifying information and several aspects of history and presentation have been changed to protect patient identity and privacy.

Reason for Referral

Miranda was referred to my practice in South Africa by her non-Spanish speaking psychiatrist (Dr. Nkosi), who admitted her to a psychiatric hospital because she was presenting with depression, anxiety, auditory hallucinations, persecutory delusions, attention and concentration difficulties, semantic memory failures, severe difficulties in comprehending and expressing herself in English. In the referral letter, Dr. Nkosi explained that, although this was probably Miranda's first psychiatric admission, Miranda reported experiencing visual hallucinations during childhood and seizures during a recent hospitalization. Given Miranda's history, her presenting symptomatology, and her difficulties communicating in English, Dr. Nkosi requested a neuropsychological assessment by a Spanish-speaking professional in order to further investigate her cognitive symptoms, gather additional history, and assist with the diagnostic process.

I conducted a series of interviews with Miranda to establish rapport, understand her current situation better, gather background information, and guide my selection of tests, if appropriate. Miranda was aware that I was asked to assess her to assist the psychiatrist with the diagnostic process because she was experiencing "*mental confusion*" but did not know she was specifically referred for neuropsychological assessment to explore her cognitive complaints.

Cultural Background

Miranda was a 45-year-old Catholic woman. Her first language was Spanish, and her proficiency in English was low, which limited her ability to communicate with the psychiatrist and treatment team. She was born in Caracas, Venezuela, where she lived until immigrating to Johannesburg with her husband and three children in 2009, at the age of 34. The youngest of three siblings, Miranda never met her father and was raised by her grandmother in a home where she lived with her mother and extended family (including uncles, aunts, and cousins). She experienced significant physical and verbal abuse perpetrated by her family members. At 25, Miranda met Ernesto and they married after a year-long relationship. Ernesto took up a position as an engineer in Johannesburg and the family moved to South Africa during the winter months, which was very difficult for Miranda. Nevertheless, Miranda was excited about moving away from the socio-economic and political stressors of Venezuela and from family conflicts.

Health History

Miranda reported that she was born via vaginal delivery at full term with no complications. She had been generally healthy her entire life. The results from hematological tests and EEG taken during her hospitalization were unremarkable. Miranda's family history included a sibling diagnosed with schizophrenia and two cousins with drug addiction. She described the psychotic episodes of her sibling with ease and was obviously familiar with psychiatric and psychological care. Accessing prolonged psychiatric care in Venezuela is difficult and clients are normally under families' care, who become experts in identifying the onset of symptoms and managing crises. I believe this experience helped Miranda to seek out immediate psychiatric intervention.

I asked Miranda if she ever experienced visions or other types of hallucinations during childhood. She responded that when she and her cousins were little, an uncle used to scare them with "*La Llorona*" and "*La Sayona*," ghost legends that Venezuelans grow up fearing and even "encountering" during childhood. What Dr. Nkosi thought could be a sign of childhood psychosis was in fact a cultural myth to scare children and superstitious people.

Education and Employment History

Miranda has a total of 17 years of formal education (all in Spanish). She completed primary and secondary education in Venezuelan urban public schools. Her performance in school was high-average. Miranda graduated as an economist, with average results from the best public university in Venezuela. Her academic results at university were average. She then worked in the credit card department of a large bank for three years. She resigned when she became a mother.

Clinical Observations

I had three assessment sessions with Miranda and one (jointly) with Ernesto. In our first interview, she was appropriately groomed to her situation (no cosmetics and no jewelry) and wearing EEG electrodes (as she was under 24-hour monitoring). By the third session, Miranda was wearing makeup and had styled her hair. She was polite, friendly, and approachable. Miranda was relieved at being able to express herself in her mother tongue. She addressed me informally (by my first name). I interpreted this as culturally appropriate and responded by addressing her similarly. Her facial expressions were congruent with low mood and she established good eye contact. Rapport was immediately established (facilitated by her sense of relief for having a Venezuelan psychologist) and her interactions were natural and spontaneous.

Miranda was fully oriented and attentive. She answered questions appropriately. She was talkative, had circumstantial speech but was able to come back to the point. Speech rate and volume were normal. Psychomotor functions were preserved. Her mood was generally dysphoric but appropriate and congruent. She was responsive to humor, but tearful, as we addressed painful topics. She reported physical and cognitive fatigue.

At the time of hospitalization, Miranda presented with persecutory delusions, auditory hallucinations (voice in her head), and depersonalization/derealization. Nevertheless, during our meetings she was able to reflect on these symptoms and provided a full logical account of the events that led to their development. Her capacity for insight was excellent as she was able to make good sense of her experience, potential triggers, and contributing factors.

History of Present Illness

Miranda identified the onset of her symptoms two months before seeking help. Her persecutory beliefs had an insidious onset that we traced back to a traumatic episode. While walking home from the supermarket, Miranda was attacked by someone trying to steal her cell phone and was stabbed. During a long hospitalization, she had several seizures, potentially linked to infections, which did not require medication after discharge. After returning home, she felt angry, sad and apprehensive, and resorted to obsessively listening to spiritual and religious videos through earphones all day and night. Sometimes she would stay up all night praying. She believes that the voice in her head was activated by the constant voices coming from the earphones. The voice in her mind was unfamiliar and instructed her to "confess, confess, everyone will find out."

Miranda felt unsupported by her only Venezuelan friend in Johannesburg and became suspicious of those around her. She believed that people in the streets knew she was a foreigner and were planning to attack her again. Consequently, she was reluctant to leave the house and spent more time watching videos. Her crisis peaked when a computer cable was lost, and she believed that her children and husband were hiding it from her. Miranda found the cable a week after it went missing, and realized that she had put it away—a scary thought crossed Miranda's mind: *"Perdí mi lucidez"* (I lost my lucidity). Miranda realized at that moment that there was something wrong with her and called her sibling in Venezuela, who instructed her to consult a doctor. Miranda's sibling had been diagnosed with schizophrenia at 23 and told Miranda that her symptoms sounded like psychotic episodes. Miranda listened to her sibling and was hospitalized immediately. During our interviews, she displayed good insight but was still frequently unsure about the accuracy of some of her interpretations. For example, she was convinced that people did not like her because she was Venezuelan ("Venezuelans have bad reputations all around the world").

Although feeling anxious and sad, Miranda was able to meet her "responsibilities" at home, such as cooking, cleaning, and caring for the children, and maintained her hygiene. She had excellent insight, was able to connect symptoms with specific triggers, and received my feedback and interpretations constructively. For example, she described how she was impacted by South African news on xenophobic attacks on nationals from other African countries where several deaths were reported. She recognized that this may have played a role in her beliefs that she was a potential target which eventually became a reality when she was violently robbed. She would sometimes laugh at herself when describing the ideas she had, which she found "silly."

Application of the CTNA Approach on the Case Study

The CTNA[41] is guided by the assumptions that the client/caregiver/referral source has identified changes in the client's neuropsychological functioning and professional help can ascertain the nature, severity, potential causes, and prognosis of their condition. These functional changes produce distress in the client and their family. Therefore, they are looking to identify ways to reduce the impact that these issues have on different life areas. The model works under the premise that neuropsychological tests provide objective information, which is applicable to the client's life and may provide insight into the current situation and guide the treatment plan. Moreover, CTNA assumes that clients "want to be respected and to be empowered as active and autonomous participants in treatment and decision making process" (p. 41). All sessions, especially the one dedicated to feedback, should be client-centered and empathic, which promotes the client's collaboration in the process, accentuates their active role in the decision-making process, and reduces the resistance to difficult information, therefore strengthening the working alliance between the client and the neuropsychologist.

The first aim in the collaborative information gathering within the CTNA model is to explore the client's understanding of the problem and the emotional experience associated with it. The subjective experience of the issue is as relevant as the objective clinical data. CTNA includes the concept of Central Cognitive-Emotional Complaint (CCEC), which aims to communicate empathic understanding of the client's experience (including the content and associated feelings, and impact on daily life). With this premise in mind, during my first session with Miranda, I used open-ended questions to explore how Miranda was making sense of her current situation (symptoms and hospitalization) and to validate this experience as well as her capacity to make sense of it. Miranda felt relieved for talking in her home language and was open to describing her symptoms and history. Cognitive symptoms were not central features in her narrative around her current and past health history, and she only mentioned experiencing seizures when prompted about her neurological history.

NEUROPSYCHOLOGIST: You mentioned that you had seizures while you were in hospital after the robbery, did you noticed any changes in your cognitive abilities or your capacity to do any activities after you were discharged?

MIRANDA: No. I have felt fine since those seizures. I got those seizures because of the infection I had. I think this is why I have this (EEG) on. When I started feeling like this (referring to the onset of her current episode), I called my sister in Venezuela and she told me that that was exactly how she used to feel before getting hospitalized, so I told my husband to take me to the doctor because I wasn't well.

NEUROPSYCHOLOGIST: What about your concentration? Your memory? You mentioned that you couldn't concentrate well and couldn't remember where you put things, and then thought your kids were taking stuff away from you.

MIRANDA: Honestly, I don't know. I couldn't concentrate well on many things, I was just thinking that everyone was plotting against me. I don't remember putting the cable in where I found it, but what broke me was that I was blaming my poor kids and made them cry (becomes tearful).

NEUROPSYCHOLOGIST: When you saw your kids crying, you worried that something maybe very wrong with you, you felt sad, guilty, and maybe even scared, but it does not sound like the problem was that you 'forgot' where you put the cable, but that you thought your family was hiding the cable from you.

MIRANDA: Exactly! Exactly that. Thank you. My memory is fine. I know Dr. Nkosi is worried about my memory but I don't think that is the problem.

NEUROPSYCHOLOGIST: Miranda, I hear that you are not experiencing major changes in your cognitive abilities, but memory, for example, sometimes can be affected by emotions, like sadness, anxiety. Would it be OK if I ask you a few questions to test your memory now?

Miranda agreed, so I asked her some screening questions that were specific to Venezuelan culture and her life history. For example: In what year was UCV declared a UNESCO world heritage site? Describe the route that can take you from your house to the stadium and describe step-by-step how you would prepare hallacas (a traditional dish of complex preparation). She responded to all questions appropriately and elaborated further on her emotional experience, and accentuated that her neuropsychological performance was not a central aspect of her complaint. I took this opportunity to reflect on her CCEC, as illustrated below.

MIRANDA: I was losing my mind, I was scared, but I did not once forget to fetch my kids from school or to pack them lunch. I was on top of everything in the house ... well, maybe not everything, I wasn't really cleaning much and all I wanted to do was to watch videos, pray, or sleep. You ask me those questions and I know the answer to everything, I can even picture the routes in my head. But I couldn't really understand what the doctor was asking me the other day, she asked me lots of questions that I didn't know the answer to, but you know, I have been here so many years and I can't speak English, my English is really bad (she laughs). My husband helps me but he has to work and now he also has to take care of the kids. I feel ashamed because of my English, people think I'm stupid, so I just shut down. Now that you are here, we speak in Spanish, I can't even tell you, I feel better already, and I feel like I can't stop talking.

NEUROPSYCHOLOGIST: Miranda, I hear that this entire experience has been overwhelming and terrifying for you, not only because of the symptoms you are experiencing but also because your main support structure is not a space that you have been able to trust lately, and they are struggling to understand what is happening to you. Then you come to hospital and cannot communicate with the team caring for you because of the language barrier, so it is also difficult for them to understand what it's happening to you. Talking to me in Spanish now, and being able to make more sense of what you have been feeling is already offering you some relief.

My interventions aimed to investigate the presence of cognitive symptoms using Miranda's report as a starting point and to explore how she constructed these cognitive complaints in relation to her current situation. Miranda was not concerned about her cognitive skills. The next step was to decide with Miranda whether testing was desirable or necessary.

As health practitioners, we have the ethical mandate of informing our clients about the aims, nature, risks, and outcomes of our assessments and interventions. In alignment, CTNA takes this a step forward as it invites the patient to reflect on their fantasies and expectations linked to the assessment process, opening an opportunity for clarification and collaboration. During my meetings with Miranda, we discussed what neuropsychological assessment entails and her thoughts about the potential benefits. Miranda clearly communicated during our sessions that she did not see a significant benefit in getting tested because she did not have neuropsychological concerns. Ernesto agreed as he did not have specific concerns about Miranda's cognitive functioning. Moreover, my clinical assessment did not flag specific cognitive issues that needed immediate exploration. I supported Miranda's decision and, by doing this, reinforced the values of respect, autonomy, empowerment, and collaboration highlighted by the CTNA model. I communicated to Dr. Nkosi that I did not find testing necessary and the need for a full neuropsychological evaluation could be reconsidered in six months. The work done during three sessions with Miranda was sufficient to clarify her diagnosis and provide emotional relief for the client, who recovered well and was soon discharged.

Had we decided to move forward with the assessment, I would have chosen a battery of tests based on those that I have available in Spanish in my South African practice and for which I have Venezuelan norms (e.g. Mini-Mental Status Examination, Rey Auditory Verbal Learning Test, Controlled Oral Association Test, Clock Drawing Test, and Attention Test). If needed, I could have used selected subtests of the Wechsler Intelligence Scale-IV (UK) and the Wechsler Memory Scale-IV (UK) using instructions in Spanish (e.g. Digit Span, Letter-Number Sequencing, Matrix, Block Design, Visual Reproduction, and Symbol Span) taking into consideration interpretation biases due to the use of non-representative norms.

Feedback and Recommendations

For the Psychiatrist

After each of my meetings with Miranda, I discussed my impressions with Dr. Nkosi. My first session with Miranda was used mainly for catharsis, so it was difficult to formulate a hypothesis. Nevertheless, I highlighted that Miranda did not have a childhood history of psychosis and the onset and presentation of symptoms did not support a diagnosis of schizophrenia. Miranda had no history of mania or hypomania. Her depressive symptoms were reactive and did not significantly interfere with her daily functioning. The age of onset was also atypical. The results of the EEG were normal and no major neuropsychological decline was observed. Thus, the diagnoses that had been considered thus far of Schizoaffective Disorder, Bipolar Mood Disorder were excluded. Considering her clinical presentation, Miranda's significant history of trauma, losses, and separations, it is likely that she presented with either a Delusional Disorder (297.1 [F22]) first episode currently in full remission (persecutory type) or a Brief Psychotic Disorder (298.8 [F23]) with marked stressors. The diagnosis of Mild Cognitive Disorder was deferred until the remission of her psychiatric symptoms, which was ruled out after a six-month follow-up.

For the Client

Following her request, I organized a feedback meeting with Ernesto and Miranda. Ernesto hoped to understand Miranda's situation better. During this session, he asked questions about the diagnosis, the risks of recurrent episodes, the medication, and the costs of psychological and psychiatric care. I had a separate feedback session with Miranda, when she was not actively psychotic, with a low mood, but ready for discharge. During this session, I linked Miranda's childhood and recent traumatic history, potential inherited vulnerability to mental health issues on the psychotic spectrum, the alienation experienced by her after immigration, and lack of social support, as potential contributors to her sadness and psychotic episode. "I didn't realise I had so much pain buried in my heart, and that made me disconnect with reality," was her answer. I recommended continuous psychiatric management and psychotherapy. Miranda asked if I could continue to be her psychologist, to which I agreed, and we embarked on a year-long therapeutic process. During this time, Miranda recovered fully.

Section III: Lessons Learned

*   Venezuelans have lived through a catastrophic crisis over the past 20 years, resulting in complicated traumas and bereavement. Clinicians assessing and treating Venezuelan clients need to understand the person within this macro-context and be mindful of their socio-economic and political stressors. Malnutrition, failures in educational systems, poor access to services, unmanageable levels of stress, among other contributors, have a major impact on our mental health, brain development, and neurodegeneration.
*   The practitioner's familiarity with the historical, cultural, and linguistic background of clients influences diagnostic accuracy and treatment effectiveness. Neuropsychologists must not only strive for cultural competence but should aim to improve the diversity of multidisciplinary teams to better cater to an increasingly multicultural society.
*   Providing psychological services in the client's mother tongue can be therapeutic in itself. Clinicians should thus make an effort to provide this option to clients.
*   Traumatic history during childhood has a significant effect on the migration experience in relation to acculturation and the emotional capacity to adapt to the new country. Neuropsychologists must be mindful of the impact of emotional factors on cognitive health when working with migrant communities.
*   Motivations driving migration, subjective experiences in this process, and the legal status of the client in the receiving country should be investigated during the initial interviews in non-threatening ways. This information is key as it provides a route to explore premorbid abilities, current stressors, coping mechanisms, etc.
*   The CTNA approach is ideal for contexts with great cultural variability and for clients experiencing emotional vulnerability.

Recommended Readings

Gorske TT, Smith SR. Collaborative therapeutic neuropsychological assessment. New York (NY): Springer Science & Business Media; 2008.

Acknowledgments

I am grateful to Psychologist Ilva Campagna (Universidad Central de Venezuela), Dr. Victor Sojo (University of Melbourne), and Prof Brett Bowman (University of the Witwatersrand) for their valuable input on the manuscript.

References

1. Cadenas G. The growing Venezuelan diaspora in the United States. In: Arredondo P, editor. Latinx immigrants: Transcending acculturation and xenophobia. Cham: Springer International Publishing; 2018. pp. 211–28.
2. Iturrieta EP. Historia mínima de Venezuela. Ciudad de Mexico, Mexico: El Colegio de México AC; 2018.
3. Venezuela's Humanitarian Emergency. Large-Scale UN Response Needed to Address Health and Food Crises. United States of America Human Rights Watch and The Center for Public Health and Human Rights at Johns Hopkins Bloomberg School of Public Health; 2019.
4. IOM. Venezuelan refugee and migrant crisis [Internet]. 2020. Available from: https://www.iom.int/venezuelan-refugee-and-migrant-crisis
5. Paez T, Vivas Peñalver L. The Venezuelan Diaspora, Another Impending Crisis? Freedom House Report; 2017. https://www.researchgate.net/publication/317099053_The_Venezuelan_Diaspora_Another_Impending_Crisis
6. UNHCR. Venezuela situation [Internet]. 2020 Oct. Available from: https://www.unhcr.org/venezuela-emergency.html
7. Estrada Villaseñor C. ¿Qué perfil tienen los venezolanos que emigran?: The Conversation; 2019 [cited 2020 Oct 13]. Available from: https://theconversation.com/que-perfil-tienen-los-venezolanos-que-emigran-112108
8. Constitución de la República Bolivariana de Venezuela. Gaceta oficial de la República Bolivariana de Venezuela, No 36.860. [Extraordinaria], Marzo 24, 2000; 1999, 30 de Diciembre.
9. Fernández Vítores D. El español: una lengua viva. Informe 2019. Instituto Cervantes, 2019. https://cvc.cervantes.es/lengua/espanol_lengua_viva/pdf/espanol_lengua_viva_2019.pdf
10. Garassini M. La primera fortaleza del venezolano es la gratitud. Revista Debates IESA. 2011;16(2):38–43.
11. Pardo D. El humor es la única forma seria de hablar en Venezuela. BBC News. 2014. https://www.bbc.com/mundo/noticias/2014/06/140624_venezuela_humor_politico_dp
12. Serrón S. De Samuel Robinson a la Misión Robinson: La alfabetización en Venezuela y el proceso de reconceptualización. Sapiens Revista Universitaria de Investigación. 2004;5(99):123–35.
13. Inojosa CV. Los números de la crisis educativa en Venezuela: casi 700.000 estudiantes dejaron la escuela y cerraron 1.275 colegios. INFOBAE; 2020. https://www.infobae.com/america/venezuela/2020/02/20/los-numeros-de-la-crisis-educativa-en-venezuela-casi-700000-estudiantes-dejaron-la-escuela-y-cerraron-1275-colegios/
14. Campagna I. Evaluación neuropsicológica de población venezolana. Caracas: Grafismo Taller Editorial; 2015.
15. Instituto Nacional de Estadística, República Bolivariana de Venezuela. Resultados básicos del censo 2011 [Internet]. 2012 Aug 9. http://www.ine.gov.ve/documentos/Demografia/CensodePoblaciony-Vivienda/pdf/ResultadosBasicosCenso2011.pdf.
16. Freitez A, Correa G. ¿Es realmente Venezuela territorio libre de analfabetismo? Revista temas de coyuntura. 2014;(69):99–107.
17. Forum WE. [Internet] [cited 2020 Oct 20]. Available from: https://reports.weforum.org/global-competitiveness-report-2018/country-economy-profiles/#economy=VEN
18. Miller, T, Kim, AB, Roberts, JM. 2020 Index of Economic Freedom. Washington DC: The Heritage Foundation; 2021 Available from: https://www.heritage.org/index/country/venezuela
19. IMF sees Venezuela inflation at 10 million percent in 2019. OCTOBER 9, 2018. Available from: https://www.reuters.com/article/venezuela-economy-idINKCN1MJ1YX

20. Durán MA. Venezuela al límite de la supervivencia. (20 May, 2021) Available from: https://www.opendemocracy.net/es/venezuela-limite-supervivencia/
21. Acosta Y. Emociones y política: la fuerza de la esperanza. Comunicación. 2016;174:75–89.
22. Independent International Fact-Finding Mission on the Bolivarian Republic of Venezuela. Human Rights Council United Nations, 2020.
23. Guanipa C, Nolte L, Guanipa J. Important considerations in the counseling process of immigrant Venezuelan families. Am J Fam Ther. 2002;30(5):427–38.
24. Degla NA. Understanding the characteristics of remittance recipients in Venezuela: a country in economic crisis. Undergrad Econ Rev. 2019;16(1):3.
25. Cardona L. La violencia enfermó a Venezuela. Debates IESA. 2016;XXI(2):68–71.
26. Collins J. Why you don't want to be a Venezuelan woman right now: The New Humanitarian [Internet]. 2019. Available from: https://www.thenewhumanitarian.org/news-feature/2019/09/17/Venezuela-femicide-maternal-mortality-rates-rising?utm_source=twitter&utm_medium=social&utm_campaign=social
27. Global Gender Gap Report. World Economic Forum, 2020.
28. Human Rights Situation of Lesbian, Gays, Bisexual, Trans and Intersex persons in Venezuela. Red LGBTI Venezuela, 2015.
29. Hidalgo LJR. Lo mágico religioso y el bienestar de los venezolanos. Investigación en Salud. 2006;8(1):31–5.
30. Levine DH. Religion and politics in Latin America: the Catholic Church in Venezuela & Colombia. Princeton (NJ): Princeton University Press; 2014.
31. Gulbas LE. Cosmetic surgery and the politics of race, class, and gender in Caracas. Venezuela: Southern Methodist University; 2008.
32. Bahar D, Dooley M, Selee A. [Internet]. The Brookings Institution; 2020. Available from: https://www.brookings.edu/es/research/inmigrantes-venezolanos-crimen-y-percepciones-falsas-un-analisis-de-los-datos-en-colombia-peru-y-chile/
33. Grattan S. Venezuelan migrants face rising xenophobia in Latin America: The New Humanitarian [Internet]. 2020. Available from: https://www.thenewhumanitarian.org/news-feature/2020/02/13/Venezuelan-migrants-xenophobia-Latin-America
34. Méndez G. Cuál es el panorama de la salud para la Venezuela de 2018: PRODAVINCI [Internet]. 2017 [cited 2020 Oct 21]. Available from: https://prodavinci.com/cual-es-el-panorama-de-la-salud-para-la-venezuela-de-2018/
35. Iribarren Pérez CI. La neuropsicología en Venezuela. Revista Neuropsicología, Neuropsiquiatría y Neurociencias. 2009;9(2):113–20.
36. Lima Gómez O. Protocolo de evaluación neuropsicológica (la batería Luria UCV). Comunicación Preliminar. Gac méd Caracas. 1994;102(2):184–6.
37. Gomez OL, Venezuela UCd. Neuropsicología: Universidad Central de Venezuela; 1996.
38. Lima Gómez O, Roca MJ, Esaá L, Sánchez J, Ruiz M. Confiabilidad y validez del protocolo Luria-UCV. Gaceta Médica de Caracas. 2004;112(4):319–24.
39. Lima Gómez O, Roca M, Esaá L. Evaluación neuropsicológica por grupos de edad. Gac méd Caracas. 1999;107(4):531–6.
40. López de Ibáñez M. Evaluación neuropsicológica. Caracas, Venezuela: CDCH UCV; 1998.
41. Gorske TT, Smith SR. Collaborative therapeutic neuropsychological assessment. New York (NY): Springer Science & Business Media; 2008.
42. Strauss E, Sherman EM, Spreen O. A compendium of neuropsychological tests: administration, norms, and commentary. 3rd ed. Oxford: American Chemical Society; 2006.

G. Persian

Afghan

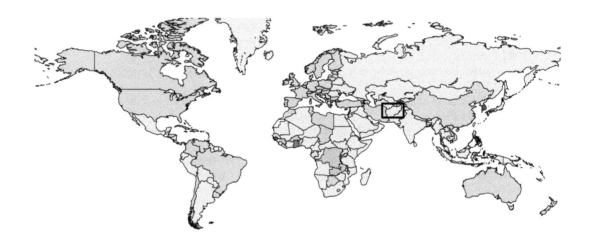

36 Neuropsychological Evaluation of the Afghan, Dari-Persian (Dari-Farsi) Speaking Individual

Clinical and Forensic Considerations

Amir Ramezani, Shushan Tigranyan, Seyed Reza Alvani, Arash Ramezani, and Carlos Oliveira

Section I: Background Information

Terminology and Perspective

Clinicians who work with individuals from Afghanistan or who have an Afghan identity (e.g., here on referred to as Afghan) may enjoy learning about a rich cultural heritage filled with a strong sense of community/friendship, tradition, honor, and resiliency. Specific terms used in the chapter are highlighted in this section. Of note, the term Dari-Persian is the same as Dari-Farsi, and Farsi-Persian is the same as Farsi.

Our perspectives as authors range in training, geographic location, and practice. We all share the same goal, which is to advance cultural awareness. Dr. Amir Ramezani is a bilingual, Farsi-speaking Iranian American neuropsychologist who was trained in the Western portion of the United States and who grew up with Afghans and clinically worked with Afghan Americans. The primary author practices in an academic medical center, integrative health setting, and in private clinical and forensic practice. Dr. Shushan Tigranyan is a bilingual Armenian American psychologist who worked with and did research on ethnic minorities, specifically those of Middle Eastern descent. Dr. Seyed Reza Alvani is a psychologist and an Assistant Professor in Iran and has worked with a diverse Farsi-speaking population clinically. Mr. Arash Ramezani is a bilingual Iranian American, trained in the United States and Sweden, who has studied cognitive science and conducted research in mental health, cognition, and Iranians. Mr. Carlos Oliveira's perspective is a Latino American doctoral candidate trained in the West US region who has worked with Afghan patients with the supervision of the primary author.

Geography

Afghanistan is located in south-central Asia and has over 38 million people. The country lies between Pakistan, Iran, Turkmenistan, Uzbekistan, Tajikistan, and borders China to a much lesser degree. Afghanistan's climate can be characterized as having frigid winters and hot summers.

History

Afghanistan has a rich history. This includes being part of the *Persian Empire* and the city of Herat, where notable intellectual life, art, and poetry thrived. Conflict has also existed in Afghanistan's history since the late 20th century. Generations of people have not experienced peace and have been impacted by war.[1] The country has weathered several invasions, such as from Britain and the Soviet Union. Afghanistan was a peaceful country before the Soviet invasion.[1] Nevertheless,

DOI: 10.4324/9781003051862-73

the people's resistance has been preserved, despite continued insurgency by the Taliban and other groups.[1] This is important contextual information to consider when evaluating patients from Afghanistan since some literature has demonstrated increased risk factors for anxiety and depression of survivors of conflicts in similar geographic regions (e.g., war).[2] War may also lead to potential head trauma, which impacts cognition.

Immigration and Relocation

Afghans began immigrating to the United States in the 1920s, arriving in several waves.[3] Afghanistan stands as one of the few countries that have seen a decline in its population.[4] Since the late 1970s, political unrest has ousted many Afghan citizens to the country's borders and other foreign countries, such as the United States. According to refugee data, from 2001 until approximately 2009, nearly "8,000 Afghan refugees have been resettled in the US ... approximately 2.6 million Afghans continued to seek international protection in Iran and Pakistan" (p. 1248).[5] Based on the US Census Bureau's information, Alemi and colleagues[5] (p. 1248) note that nearly "90,000 people of Afghan ancestry" live in the United States, of which "65,000 are foreign-born." The immigration status of a patient from Afghanistan is critical to help the clinician understand levels of acculturation. Identifying the potential for higher educated and functioning individuals leaving Afghanistan is another important factor to consider during the assessment.

Languages

It is helpful to note that in English, the Farsi language is referred to as the "Persian language." However, native speakers from Afghanistan and Iran refer to the Persian language in their native tongue as the "Farsi language." Afghans refer to the Persian language as Farsi, Dari, or Dari-Farsi. This distinction becomes a bit more complicated when accents or dialects are added. In Afghanistan, it is more common to speak the Dari-Farsi accent or dialect. Since Iranians also speak the Persian or Farsi language, and to avoid confusion, we will be referring to the Afghan Farsi language as the Dari-Farsi language in this chapter. In addition to speaking Dari-Farsi, Afghans also speak Pashto. Please note that some Afghans may also identify as Pashtun, Tajiks, Hazaras, and Uzbeks, which can come with other languages from these ethnic/racial identities.

It may not be uncommon for an Afghan patient to speak more than one language. Research has suggested that bilingualism impacts cognition.[6,7] Bilingualism is common, and switching between dialects is often unnoticeable when working with Afghan individuals. Dari-Farsi and Pashto use the Arabic alphabet, with some adjustments to account for sounds that the Arabic language does not contain. While Dari-Farsi and Pashto are the official languages of Afghanistan, a large portion of Afghans speak Dari-Farsi, and very few speak English. The language structure of Persian and English differ phonetically and phonologically. Individuals who speak one language may struggle with the pronunciation of the others' initial consonant clusters. Consequently, this can lead to omissions of consonants or commissions of vowels to aid with more straightforward pronunciation and simplify challenging consonant clusters and the degree of formality and social closeness can further change the way an individual speaks in Farsi.[8] Therefore, building rapport and having humility are important factors to consider when evaluating spoken language.

Furthermore, there is a need to observe whether switching between languages is purposeful or involuntary as this can be an indication of neuropathology in multilinguals.[9] This can be observed by a Farsi or Pashto-speaking clinician or an interpreter could be made aware of documenting the significance of this switch. Also, in bilinguals, Farsi-speaking individuals who have a neurodegenerative disease may lose their second language first followed by loss of their first language, along with reduction of vowel use in English.[10]

Clinicians may wish to be familiar with the following terms (also found in cultural glossary; "aa" are pronounced like the "a" in the word "tall"):

- *Asaabi:* Feeling nervous or feeling irritable
- *Fekr or Fekr kardan:* Think, to think, or thinking
- *Fishaar:* Literally means pressure, but intended to communicate emotional pressure and a lot of stress
- *Fishaareh Asaaby:* Literally means mental pressure, but implied mental or emotional stress
- *Gham:* Sadness
- *Haafeze:* Memory
- *Jigar Khun:* Means liver blood, but intended to communicate hopelessness, depression, and isolation; Sometimes this can also mean anger and sadness
- *Jinn:* Non-human beings that live among human
- *Tavajo:* Attention
- *Zabaan:* Language
- *Dari-Persian:* Same as Dari-Farsi. Most Afghans will describe their language as Farsi or Dari
- *Farsi-Persian:* Same as Farsi

Communication

Understanding verbal and non-verbal communication is crucial in working with patients from Afghanistan. Typically, individuals from Afghanistan tend to speak both directly and indirectly with others. However, when the person is older or of the opposite gender, communication is more indirect. The language used depends on their age difference, status, and relationship. For example, men of the same age generally refer to each other as "brother," and conversations tend to be informal. On the other hand, the utmost respect is given during a conversation with someone older.[1] When working with older Afghan adults, it is crucial to be mindful of this information since rapport can easily be lost depending on the evaluator's age.

As neuropsychological evaluation includes in-person and at times tele-neuropsychological evaluations, people from Afghanistan consider raising one's voice in public as disrespectful. As such, clinicians need to be mindful about modifications to verbally mediated tests (e.g., list-learning) that may require raising their voice to ensure instructions are heard. At the very least, the clinician should forewarn the individual that the clinician will raise his/her voice during a task.

Non-verbal communication, such as hand use, eye contact, physical contact, and personal space, is also important to consider. Clinicians need to be aware of the Islamic principles that prescribe the left hand for hygiene purposes. As such, the evaluator is encouraged to use the right hand to gesture, touch, or offer items. With left-handed patients, clinicians are advised to verbalize their awareness of handshaking etiquette and ask the patient which hand is preferred for handshaking. Eye contact is another non-verbal gesture to keep in mind. Patients from Afghanistan avoid sustained eye contact with members of the opposite gender. This behavior is considered respectful and observant of differences in gender roles. Similarly, clinicians of various ages are encouraged to consider their age relative to the patient since a clinician of the same age or gender can show direct eye contact without offense.

Generally, it is also acceptable for male friends to show physical affection in public. However, women have more restrictions on the display of physical affection unless they are at home. Understanding this information is vital if evaluating a family system, and it might impact recommendations. Lastly, personal space is crucial during the evaluation. Generally, people of the opposite gender stay within a respectful amount of personal space from one another.[1] This information is essential to consider during screening tasks that require close contact (e.g., sensory-perceptual exam). One approach may be to acknowledge the custom and importance of the test relative to the evaluation and ask for permission in advance.

Education and Literacy

Spink[11] posited that the Afghan education system has experienced a dichotomous divide for decades. On one end, older generations maintained traditional Afghan values of hospitality and respect for others. However, some members of younger male generations had ideology instilled from politicized textbooks since the 1980s that promoted intolerance principles. Spink[11] (p. 204) postulated that "the education system is one of the key contributors to conflicts."

One may consider that this dichotomous divide has important implications for the developing child into an adult. Less emphasis is placed on critical thinking and the acquisition of knowledge. This may change the developmental course of the neuroprotective qualities of cognitive reserve and executive control networks, though this is not fully clear given the limited literature.

The education system consists of six years of primary school from seven to 13 years of age, and three years of middle school (or "Maktabeh Motevaseteh") from 13 to 16 years of age. At the end of ninth grade, students take an exam. Those who pass the exam can go on for higher secondary education ("Doreye Aali") for another three years. Alternatively, students can choose to attend vocational/technical secondary education. In either path, there is a 12th-grade exam that they need to pass in order to receive a 12th-grade graduation certification or diploma. Please note that some vocational/technical education takes two to six years to complete. Clinicians are encouraged to examine the quality of vocation/technical education and the amount of cognitive load/processing it takes in order to closely estimate years of education. To attend post-secondary education or college, students need to take the "Konkor" exam, which is a very difficult exam. While the length of post-secondary education can vary, typically a bachelor's degree takes four years, a master's degree takes two years, and a doctorate degree takes three to four years. A recent article by Shah and colleagues[12] suggested: "an overall literacy rate of 31.74% in Afghanistan"[11] (p. 771). However, poetry is highly valued by the majority of the population and is regarded as one of the most revered art forms.[1] This information has important implications during feedback and rapport. Use of poetry ideas (e.g., Rumi, Ferdowsi, Khushal Khan Khattak, Rahman Baba, Rabia Balkhi, and Nazo Tokhi) can aid in building rapport and creating a stronger alliance.

Values and Customs

Afghanistan is not geographically located in the Middle East, rather in Central Asia.[12] However, culturally, similar values, customs, and traditions are held as individuals from the Middle East. The Afghan government is a Sunni Islamic Republic with its cultural and national identity rooted in Islam. These roots are noticeable through attire, language, dietary restrictions, and prayers. Resilience, loyalty, honor, and hospitality are among the characteristics that are highly valued. There is an emphasis on the family unit, where men and women are ascribed to traditional roles. Women tend to be responsible for household duties, while men perform paid jobs and are financially responsible for the household. The male has additional responsibility for protecting the family's honor and reputation. Men and women do not freely associate with each other unless it is within families. Clinicians are encouraged to consider the gender roles in activities of daily living.

Religion

Afghanistan is considered an Islamic republic, as most of the country's citizens follow Islam. Some estimates suggest that approximately 85% of the population is considered Sunni Muslims, with the remaining percentage constituting Shia Muslims and other minority religions.[1] How people perceive, interpret, and assimilate information can be accounted for by religion. Beliefs about "jinns" are common and are widely held in the Afghan Muslim faith. For instance, Guthrie, Abraham, and Nawaz[13] provide a case report example of a 28-year-old Afghan woman who presented perinatally with possession by jinns. According to Arabian mythology and Islamic theology, jinns are "non-human beings created by Allah from smokeless fire"[13] (p. 1). An important distinction between jinns and other similar belief systems (e.g., spirits in Christianity) is that jinns are not considered spirits but creatures that live among humans and interact with people. Furthermore, jinns are not only malevolent but can also be benevolent and kind and have special powers that include "strength, shapeshifting, and teleportation"[13] (p. 1). Afghan individuals of the Muslim faith may attribute minor ailments or misfortune to jinns. Additionally, psychotic experiences and other psychological phenomena, for some Muslims, could also be attributed to jinns.[13]

Health Status

Hamed's[14] indicated that Afghanistan's health-related conditions, as a developing country, are not well known. However, stroke in the elderly population has been on the rise, and a "rapid increase of neuroimmunological diseases, and diseases resulting from a lack of nutrition are also more frequent in developing regions" (p. 7). This author also noted common neuroinfectious disorders seen in developing countries, such as viral encephalitis, bacterial and tubercular meningitis, and cerebral malaria.[15]

Mental Health Views and Acculturation

There is little data available on the utilization of mental health services, possibly due to Afghanistan's poor mental health infrastructure. Furthermore, like many collectivist groups, support sources tend to come from family, as psychotherapy is typically considered a Western practice.[5] The Afghan culture is collectivistic and emphasizes group interdependence and conformity to group norms. Individuals are representatives of their families, so concealing emotions is praised and encouraged, yet contributes to the stigma around mental health.[16] Seeking mental health services could be viewed as bringing disgrace to their family name and negatively impact the family's reputation.[16] Since seeking psychological services can alert the community that the individual has a mental health illness, this can impact their decision to seek help because of the shame it can bring to their family. It is believed that the individual holds the responsibility to manage their own mental health issues without burdening the family and without seeking external or formal services. An individual is a representation of their family, thus the inability to effectively manage and resolve issues can be perceived as a weakness both individually and as a collective family.[17] If community members become aware of an individual's mental health issues, it can imply that the family is not strong as a unit. This can lead to challenges for family members to enter romantic relationships and get married, something that is highly valued in the Afghan culture. However, support from religious or spiritual figures and trusted, wise, elderly, family members, or friends of the family may act as mental health supports.

When examining Afghans who have immigrated to America, it is important to consider the possible impact of acculturative stress. The need to adjust to an individualistic culture can be challenging with little to no knowledge about the values or customs or language. Immigrants must search for and obtain employment or housing while adjusting to an unfamiliar economic system. This can increase feelings of depression and anxiety. However, these feelings can be left unresolved due to the possible negative attitudes toward seeking mental health services, depending on acculturation levels.[18] Particularly, those with higher levels of association to their heritage culture are more likely to have negative attitudes toward seeking services.[18] In addition, religiosity should be considered, especially since Afghans' religious practices are highly valued. Similar to other Middle Eastern cultures, Afghans who have higher levels of religiosity may be less likely to admit they are struggling with a psychological issue and less open to seeking psychological help.[18] Furthermore, their attitudes toward seeking assistance for psychological issues can be impacted by how strong their faith is and their preference to engaging in rituals and activities privately.[18] Afghans may additionally face challenges speaking about their faith in a mental health setting due to Islamophobia in the United States. Fear of discrimination may hinder the individual's willingness to be forthcoming with information. Withholding crucial information about their faith or religious practices may lead to misdiagnosis or an invalid conceptualization about the presenting problem or other cognitive concerns.

Psychological challenges to consider in the assessment include trauma, loss of family support and erosion of cultural values, feelings of apathy to the culture, a novel sense of identity and independence, and relocation/refugee adjustment.[5,19]

Assessment Needs

There remains very little research on the neuropsychological functioning of Afghans. Some research has been conducted in Iran (e.g., Iranian and Afghan populations living in Iran) with Farsi or Persian validated tests from Iran used to evaluate Afghans. The appendix lists published measures currently available in Farsi or Persian and available for testing in English for bilingual and monolingual Afghans. The appendix can aid clinicians with neuropsychological and psychological assessments with Afghans. Please note that Iranian test norms in Farsi may differ in the level of education, literacy, and quality of education when compared to Afghans. Clinicians should consider these factors when making interpretations. However, clinicians may come across a few challenges when assessing cognitive and emotional functioning. Since many current tests are normed for English speakers, it is not surprising that there is a lack of validated Farsi-language tests for non-English speakers. The lack of normative data and objective interpretative steps of test norms may pose an additional limitation when evaluating Farsi-speaking patients.[10] In addition, cognitive and linguistic confounds such as code-switching can also be impactful. Code-switching occurs when the individual mixes two or more languages during the assessment. This can be a sign of neuropathology, normal or low language proficiency/usage, or problems with organizing or staying in cognitive set.[9] For bilinguals, clinicians may wish to administer tests in one language, then move to another language to avoid this confound.[6]

Understanding the patient's immigration status, in some instances, can provide critical information about the patient's mental health needs, as emotional distress, in the absence of a neurological disorder, is a confound in neuropsychological assessment.[15] A culturally responsive evaluation should account for the possible presence of psychological distress, defined by "mood and anxiety disorders, including depressive and posttraumatic symptomology, respectively"[5] (p. 1248). Additional factors are important to the assessment process. Clinicians must be sensitive to and ask about exposure to war, bomb or missile blast, blast injury, loud noises that impact mental status, chemicals or toxins, and head concussions in Afghanistan.

As Afghan refugees continue to immigrate to the United States, there will likely be variability in "pre-migration traumas (e.g., loss of family members due to death or displacement)" and "post-migration stressors (cultural adjustment and loss of social support)"[5] (p. 1248). This systematic review of Afghanistan refugees' mental health needs suggests a dose-response relationship between trauma and psychological distress levels.[5] Understanding the severity of these experiences of the patient can help a clinician avoid inaccurate inferences during a neuropsychological evaluation. Veliu and Leathem (2016) recommend a balance between assessment integrity and creative approaches due to the lack of research with culturally and linguistically diverse patients.[19]

Section II: Case Study — "The Underpin of an Afghan and a Jinn"

Note: Possible identifying information and several aspects of history and presentation have been changed to protect patient identity and privacy.

Presenting Concerns

Mr. Eshghan (pseudonym) is an Afghan male in his mid-60s, with 12 years of education (high school completed in Afghanistan), who is trilingual in English, Farsi, and Pashto. He is retired and worked as a taxi driver for most of his career. Mr. Eshghan was referred by a neuropsychologist for a bilingual neuropsychological assessment to assist his movement disorder and surgical team in determining his cognitive status and appropriateness for deep brain stimulation (DBS). He has been living with Parkinson's disease for the past six years and has had recent psychiatric and cognitive challenges.

Behavioral Observations

When he arrived at this appointment, Mr. Eshghan and his wife were greeted in Farsi in a humble and inviting way as if they had arrived at a friend's home yet keeping a professional tone of voice. Mr. Eshghan requested that his wife be present for the meeting. Both had many questions about the evaluation. The evaluator took on a relaxed, friendly, and confident attitude in answer their questions. His wife would face this clinician and either nod or shake her head when discussing his cognitive and emotional health. It was clarified that she was communicating, with her nod or shake of her head, that the information Mr. Eshghan was sharing was either true or not true based on her observation. She was observed to be quiet while he was speaking. The evaluating clinician was the first author and a male. Therefore, his wife's freedom of disclosure is worth considering in the context of two males in the room. Taking on a professional and objective attitude while being inquisitive helped to open up dialogue. After Mr. Eshghan left the room to use the bathroom, his wife communicated problems about him believing that someone is present (transient presence hallucinations) and notable jealousy or paranoia about infidelity. This is noteworthy since Afghan women take pride in their loyalty and dedication to family cohesiveness. Also, she communicated that he has periods of hypersexuality and depression. After he returned, permission was requested to discuss family observations, to which Mr. Eshghan agreed. This helped to create respect and maintain his sense of dignity. We discussed his wife's reports of hallucinations openly and Mr. Eshghan acknowledged his own "worries" about his wife and expressed insight into feeling "like someone is there, but I know they are not." During testing, at first glance, he appeared to talk to himself, which could have been concerning for interfering with his performance and scores. However, upon inquiry, he stated that he was praying, a common act he engages in when stressed. This behavior is a common coping skill in Afghans.

Daily Functioning

Mr. Eshghan reported difficulties with problem-solving, following a sequence of actions, and inattention. Yet, functionally, he could perform most daily living tasks except for driving and cooking due to interference from his tremors. Upon inquiry, these limitations had affected his mood and sense of self-worth particularly since he could no longer drive for a living. He was observed to remember when he had to take his medication in our meeting.

Health History

Mr. Eshghan reported reaching developmental milestones appropriately. He was not aware of any medical or substance use problems during his mother's pregnancy with him, including alcohol or drug exposure and high fever. Asymmetric tremors and micrographia were noted 17 years ago. Onset of hallucinations occurred seven years ago. Brain MRI indicated multiple T2 hyperintensities in the bilateral periventricular and subcortical white matter regions five years ago. He denied a family history of Alzheimer's disease, Parkinson's disease, seizure disorders, cancer, or multiple sclerosis. He had good adherence to taking Sinemet 25–100 mg TID (25 mg of carbidopa and 100 mg of levodopa) on schedule. He first noted cognitive changes two years ago.

Educational History

Mr. Eshghan reported severe difficulty staying in his seat while he was in school from the ages of 6 to 12. He stated, "when the teacher went out of class, I was out of my chair and pushing everyone." Mr. Eshghan indicated the reason he would be hyperactive was that he felt bored and restless. He further described multiple inattention and hyperactivity symptoms at home, in school, and with peers. His strong need to get out of his seat distracted him from the content of his classes. His highest level of education was the 12th grade, graduating high school. Yet, the quality of his education was believed to have been poor as the teacher would not correct homework assignments and subject matters were limited. Also, the local political conflict would lead to his school temporarily closing. This may lead to lower performance on cognitive tests, normally.

Language Proficiency

Mr. Eshghan is mainly bilingual in Farsi and Pashto, though he prefers to speak Pashto at home. He expressed being highly fluent in Farsi. He also speaks English but not as proficiently as Farsi. We agreed to test in both Farsi and English to evaluate proficiency in both languages. He was also encouraged to say naming items in any language. Scores in English will likely underrepresent his naming abilities.

Cultural History

Mr. Eshghan was born in Afghanistan and lived in Pakistan for some time before immigrating with his wife when they were in their late 30s, and with their 3 children to the United States. They migrated due to political conflict and war. He has had little integration in the US culture and maintains strong cultural and religious practices in the Afghan community. His overall acculturation level is low.

Emotional Functioning

Mr. Eshghan felt embarrassed to share his emotional health. He wanted his wife to communicate this content to preserve his sense of dignity. In Afghan culture, the male's sense of dignity may be preserved by other family members communicating sensitive topics on their behalf. Past psychiatric diagnoses included psychosis due to a general medical condition/Parkinson's disease, adjustment disorder with depressed and anxious mood, and psychosis due to medication effects. He was ashamed of these diagnoses.

Preliminary Formulation

There are three relevant aspects to Mr. Eshghan's cognitive and psychiatric functioning: mild cognitive changes, mildly depressed mood with periods of hypersexuality, and transient presence hallucinations. Cultural nuances were important to consider in the evaluation, such as acknowledging jinns during feedback to facilitate treatment planning.

Test and Norm Selection

Neuropsychological test results are listed in Table 36.1. When scores from the Repeatable Battery for the Assessment of Neuropsychological Status Update (RBANS) were calculated using age, education, and gender-specific norms from the Duff and Ramezani[20] study, results showed less impairments.[20] See Table 36.2 for details. He had been exposed to the English language for many years. An RBANS was given to understand his global cognition, areas of weakness when tested in English, and the role of demographic-adjusted factors on cognition.

Summary

Mr. Eshghan's premorbid intellectual measure was estimated to be in the low average range. His profile showed poor performance on attention-concentration, working memory, motor speed, executive functioning, and retrieval tasks compared to his premorbid functioning level. Most of his cognitive impairments reflected underlying executive functioning, speed of information processing, and working memory problems. Slow processing speed appeared to lower most of his measures. Mr. Eshghan's best performance was found on language and verbal memory functions in Farsi (see Table 36.1).

Mr. Eshghan's deficits were consistent with a minor neurocognitive disorder when considering his education and level of functioning, particularly when considering the confounding role of processing speed. After adjusting for education, gender, and ethnicity, some of his scores appeared to be within the expected premorbid range with some mild deficits (see Table 36.2, cognitive screen), while other scores were spared. Other considerations include his level of functioning and poor quality of education level. This is worth considering as education-adjusted tests and norms that have 12 years of education are more likely to show him to be more impaired or show more false positives. Etiologically, Mr. Eshghan's impaired ability in processing speed, attention, working memory, executive functioning, and motor speed with spared memory, language, and simple visuospatial functioning coincided with his Parkinson's disease.

His cognitive impairment was also thought to overlap with an attention deficit condition, yet this was not formally tested. He probably has experienced multiple long-standing dysexecutive problems consistent with attention deficit hyperactivity disorder (ADHD), given his early childhood problems with restlessness, hyperactivity, inattention, and disorganization. The cultural context did not have a framework to understand ADHD, which is likely why such neurodevelopmental challenges go undiagnosed and untreated. Family stigma of a "mental health" condition may also be a factor in late diagnoses of cognitive conditions. The current executive functioning, working memory, and attention deficits were considered to have a compounding effect on the accompanying ADHD and Parkinson's disease-related frontal-subcortical cognitive presentations.

Table 36.1 Neuropsychological test results

		Description of performance						
	Impaired	*Borderline impaired*	*Low average*	*Average*	*High average*	*Superior*	*Very superior*	
Percentile	<2	2–8	9–24	25–74	75–90	91–97	>97	

Effort and motivation			
Task	*Test*	*Raw or %ile*	*Clinical classification*
Visual memory effort	Rey 15-Item+ Recognition	23	Valid
Verbal memory effort	Rey Word Recognition	8	Valid
Global cognition effort	RBANS Effort Index	3	Valid
Global cognition effort	RBANS Effort Scale	17	Valid

Global cognitive status			
CNS task	*Test*	*Raw or %ile*	*Clinical classification*
Global functioning	MoCA Farsi Version	20	Below expected

Intellectual functioning			
CNS task	*Test*	*Raw or %ile*	*Clinical classification*
Verbal IQ	Persian Adult Reading Test	24	Low average
Non-verbal IQ	WASI-II Perceptual Organization Index	2	Borderline
	WASI-II Block Design	<1	Impaired
	WASI-II Matrix Reasoning	10	Low average

Attention and working memory			
CNS task	*Test*	*Raw or %ile*	*Clinical classification*
Simple auditory attention	RBANS Digit Span	15	Low average
Visual attention and info. processing	Trail Making Test A (2 norms)	<1 & <10	Below expected
	Errors	0	–

Executive functioning			
CNS task	*Test*	*Raw or %ile*	*Clinical classification*
Flexibility and switching	Trail Making Test B (2 norms)	<1 & <10	Below expected
	Sequencing errors	1	—
	Perseveration errors	0	—
	Set loss errors	1	—
Non-verbal problem solving	WASI-II Matrix Reasoning	10	Low average
Verbal fluency	JFK (phonemic fluency in Farsi)	7	Borderline
	Perseveration errors	1	—
	Set loss errors	0	—
	Fruit + animals (semantic fluency Farsi)	3	Borderline
	Perseveration errors	1	—
	Set loss errors	0	—

(Continued)

Table 36.1 Neuropsychological test results *(Continued)*

	RBANS Semantic Fluency	3	Borderline
	Perseveration errors	0	—
	Set loss errors	0	—
Inhibition	Behavioral Dyscontrol Scale—2	18	Below expected
and	Go-No Go/Red-Green (0–3 rating)	1	—
Impulse	Fist-Edge Palm (0–3 rating)	1	—
Control	Insight (0–3 rating)	3	—
	M-N graphomotor perseveration errors	5+	—

Language functioning

CNS task	Test	Raw or %ile	Clinical classification
Visual confrontational Naming	Persian Naming Test (50 item) in Farsi	49/50	Intact
	Boston Naming Test (60 item)—2 Farsi	<1	Impaired
	Boston Naming Test (60 item)—2 English	<1	Impaired
	RBANS picture naming in English and Farsi	<1	Impaired
Verbal fluency	RBANS semantic fluency (vegetables)	3	Borderline
	JFK (phonemic fluency in Farsi)	7	Borderline
	Fruit + animals (semantic fluency Farsi)	3	Borderline
Speech apraxia	Persian aphasia examination:		
	Response to questions	10/10	Intact
	Speech fluency	10/10	Intact
	Syntax	10/10	Intact
	Repetition	10/10	Intact
	Commands	10/10	Intact
	Naming	20/20	Intact

Visuospatial and sensory perceptual functioning

CNS task	Test	Raw or %ile	Clinical classification
Simple visuospatial	RBANS Figure Copy	1	Impaired
Angle orientation	RBANS Line Orientation	55	Average
Visuospatial problem solving	WASI-II Block Design	<1	Impaired
Spatial neglect	Line Bisection Test Errors (out of 20)	1	Below expected

Learning and memory

CNS task	Test	Raw or %ile	Clinical classification
Verbal memory	RBANS immediate recall in English	—	
	Learning trials	4 3 4 5	—
	List learning	<1	Impaired
	Story memory	57	Average
	RBANS delay memory in English	—	
	List recall	1	Impaired
	List recognition	<1	Impaired
	Story recall	79	High average
	AVLT Trial 1 in Farsi	82	High average
	Trial 2	100	Very superior

(Continued)

Table 36.1 Neuropsychological test results *(Continued)*

	Trial 3	79	High average
	Trial 4	71	Average
	Trial 5	62	Average
	Trial B	2	Borderline
	Trial 6 short delayed recall	97	Superior
	Trial 7 delayed recall	97	Superior
	Recognition (True +)	81	High average
	False Recognition (False +)	1	—
	Total repetitions	2	—
	Total intrusions	2	—
Non-verbal memory	RBANS Figure Copy	1	Impaired
	RBANS Figure Recall	26	Average
	BVMT-R Trials 1	14	Low average
	Trial 2	10	Low average
	Trial 3	3	Borderline
	Total recall	5	Borderline
	Learning	18	Low average
	Delayed recall	7	Borderline
	% Retained	>16	Intact
	Recognition	>16	Intact
	False positives	>16	Intact

Motor functioning

CNS task	Test	Raw or %ile	Clinical classification
Fine motor sequencing	Behavioral Dyscontrol Scale Finger-Thumb Sequencing (0–3 rating)	3	Intact
Visuomotor speed	Trail Making Test A (2 norms)	<1 & <10	Below expected
Echopraxia-mirroring	Behavioral Dyscontrol Scale Head's Test (0–3 rating)	3	Intact

Pain, fatigue, and attention during testing

	Beginning of testing	Middle of testing	End of testing
Pain 0–10	0	0	0
Fatigue 0–10	4	5	9
Attention (5 digits recall)	5	5	5

Table 36.2 Age, education, and gender-corrected RBANS test results

RBANS	Standard norms %ile	Demographic adjusted %ile
List learning	<1	12
Story memory	57	90
Figure copy	1	3
Line orientation	55	80
Picture naming	<1	<1
Semantic fluency	3	21
Digit span	15	12
Coding (n/a)	—	—
List recall	1	20
List recognition	<1	<1
Story recall	79	95
Figure recall	26	45

If the evaluator could go back in time, he would want to recognize the possibility that the patient and the family may have minimized the psychiatric symptoms (e.g., psychosis and hypersexuality) given the stigma, possible family shame, and preserving honor, which would suggest that Parkinson's disease was getting worse. This may place more weight in determining the level of cognitive change. The more moderate to severe cognitive impairments along with psychiatric sequelae of Parkinson's disease do not make for a good DBS candidate. Furthermore, upon reflection, since there were two males and one female in the room, one may hypothesize that his wife may have felt less comfortable talking and showing more deference. This would minimize, again, the clinical presentation. Another consideration is the pattern of his test performance. The results appeared to also overlap with a history of head injury. Though he denied such a history, it would have been worth further examining in the feedback session, particularly since minimization of symptoms could have been an issue.

Feedback Session and Follow-Up

The family was invited for a feedback session. His wife had concerns about her husband's possible possession of jinns (non-human entities that live among humans according to the Muslim faith). We acknowledged jinns as part of their religious beliefs, thus enhancing the alliance, trust-building, and sense of common group belief and problem-solving. Next, education was provided around the role of emotions, depression, anxiety, and panic attacks that might appear in physical ways, along with discussing how psychiatric symptoms can occur with Parkinson's disease (e.g., presence-hallucination), brain function, aging, and cognition. The family felt that there were answers that were more objective and felt less fearful of what was happening with Mr. Eshghan.

His son, who was interested in making more financial decisions, was adamant that he needed to make financial decisions for the family and help with his father's retirement account expenditure. Culturally, the son may assume a leadership role, yet this was not the wishes of his parents. While Mr. Eshghan has cognitive limitations, his capacity for decision-making and functional status did not reach the level where this was in question. Yet concerning psychiatric functioning, his impulse control issues were concerning as an area to examine further. To better address this area, a financial capacity evaluation was needed. Education was provided around his level of functioning, possible attorney consultation, possible forensic assessment needs or financial capacity evaluation, and older adult financial protections (e.g., Adult Protective Service guides to financial misconduct). This helped the family to have a direction with less complications.

Section III: Lessons Learned

The following is a list of tips and suggestions to support clinicians in assessing Afghans. Please note that the following cannot be uniformly applied to all Afghans:

- Afghans have diverse cultural, religious, linguistic, and racial identity backgrounds.
- Providers with the following characteristics are likely to build good rapport: confident, assertive yet friendly, show cultural humility, and humble, be inclusive of family, acknowledge family and gender roles, be respectful, and relationship-oriented (relaxed with time). Knowing a little about the culture and history will strengthen the relationship.
- Asking females if they prefer a handshake or not is a sign of respect for individuals of the Muslim faith. Providing a thorough explanation about the expectations of participation in various tests before the evaluation, especially those involving touching the patient (e.g., Sensory-Perception Exam), can increase trust and build a stronger alliance.

- Literacy, education, work, and functional status in the home country and main country are important factors in determining premorbid functioning.
- Values:
  - Philosophical and religious theories are valued
  - Traditional poetry and music are cherished
  - Relationship and trust between people are important
- Ask clients about or use tools that assess various exposure to emotional, war, and physical trauma.
- Differentiate between culturally appropriate suspiciousness (e.g., a minority is having healthy skepticism toward an authority figure and/or about healthcare providers, and realistically worried about being misunderstood/mislabeled by stigmatizing diagnoses) versus neuropsychiatric symptoms (e.g., presence-hallucinations in Parkinson's disease).
- Make a conscious decision to either refer out to a bilingual or Farsi-speaking provider versus using an interpreter. Select and learn the Farsi tests to use and educate interpreters on reading or administering tests and identifying code-switching. See Ramezani and colleagues (2020) for details. [9]
- Erosion of cultural values or disconnection with either the mainstream or home culture may be a source of acculturation stress and signs of diminished emotional health.
- Naming and verbal memory are often used to determine if there is a presence of neurodegenerative disease. If we were to go back in time, we would have used the Shiraz AVLT as another verbal memory measure. Also, using multiple language/naming tests is recommended to differentiate between language proficiency versus a loss of naming.
- Clinical experience shows that naming scores on the Persian Naming Test are usually near-perfect scores in those without cognitive impairment because there are high-frequency items. The clinician should be suspicious of impairments with scores that are not near perfect scores (e.g., a raw score of less than 45 out of 50 items).
- Knowledge of Dari-Farsi:
  - On some naming and fluency tasks, the patient may not be able to name in English but can name in Dari-Persian. Having a list of translated Dari-Persian items near the examiner may help determine true naming problems. This is particularly important when assessing for neurodegenerative disorders. An interpreter can be helpful in this area.
- Interpreter issues:
  - Ahead of time, clarify with the referring provider (or patient) what language the patient feels comfortable speaking. When requesting an interpreter, request a Dari-Persian-speaking interpreter. Iranians speak Farsi or Persian, while Afghans speak Dari-Persian/Dari-Farsi/Dari, as well as Pashto. Some Afghans may speak other languages as well. An Iranian Farsi-Persian-speaking interpreter can also translate Dari-Persian, but it is worth seeing if this option exists (though this may be rare).
- A patient will likely have various proficiency or literacy levels in Dari-Persian and English. Therefore, evaluating both may yield helpful results.
  - If the monolingual patient has been exposed to the English language for a few years (e.g., working in the United States for five years in a primarily English-speaking environment), it may help gather a quick screen (e.g., RBANS) in English to understand gross cognition. This screening would be in addition to Farsi testing.
- Hallucinations may either be related to trauma, cultural views, or miscommunication.
- You may see some individuals talking to themselves. Clinicians should ask if they are praying to self-soothe. This observation is not to be confused with an individual responding to internal stimuli.

- Multiple recommendations were made for Farsi-speaking patients by Ramezani and colleagues (2019).[10] This article may help manage some of the assessment challenges.
- The Persian Naming Test results will likely show near a perfect score in individuals who do not have temporal lobe involvement, aphasia, Alzheimer's disease, or frontotemporal dementia (FTD) semantic and logopenic (e.g., 50/50 or 47/50). This result is mainly because the stimuli are high-frequency items and commonly used items when speaking, reading, and writing in Farsi. The author of this test suggests a 75% cutoff. It is not clear if this cutoff was meant for inpatient use. However, utilizing multiple naming tests in another language (e.g., RBANS naming and querying on missed items if they had learned and able to know the name in the past in English or Pashto), the consideration of education and functional status, and raising the cutoff to 90% (e.g., PNT <45), would likely increase sensitivity to detect true impairment. This approach is anecdotal and based on clinical experience, discussion with other clinicians, and correspondence with the Persian Naming Test author.
- Clinical judgment:
  - While reliability and validity of tests and results change due to adapting the measure used (e.g., adjusting test instructions to improve understanding, translation, or modification of test administration), the clinician's clinical judgment of results carries more weight. A clinician's years of experience and knowledge base, forming opinions about syndromes and diagnoses should not be discounted simply because a test was adapted to help a patient.[6,10]
  - While demographically adjusted norms are helpful as another data point,[20] clinical judgment should be exercised to ensure false positives or negatives are minimized. Some demographically adjusted norms may overcorrect and shadow true impairments (e.g., regression-based norms may overcorrect a score). Functional status can assist the clinician in determining if scores match up to real-world functioning.[10]

References

1. Evanson J. Afghan culture. 2019 Jan. Available from: https://www.culturalatlas.sbs.com.au/afghan-culture/afghan-culture-communication#afghan-culture-communication
2. Aintablian HK, Melkonian C, Galoustian N, Markarian B, Irmak I, Vardapetyan M, Tigranyan S, Kochkarian Y, Aintablian N. Direct ancestry to a genocide survivor has transgenerational effects on mental health; a case of the Armenian population. J. Hist. Archaeol. Anthropolog. 2018;7(4):233–9. https://doi:10.15406/mojph.2018.07.00235
3. Rabin LA, Spadaccini AT, Brodale DL, Grant KS, Elbulok-Charcape MM, Barr WB. Utilization rates of computerized tests and test batteries among clinical neuropsychologists in the United States and Canada. Prof. Psychol. Res. Pr. 2014 Oct;45(5):368. https://doi.org/10.1037/a0037987
4. Nyrop RF, Seekins DM, editors. Afghanistan: A country study. Washington DC: The Studies; 1986.
5. Alemi Q, James S, Cruz R, Zepeda V, Racadio M. Psychological distress in Afghan refugees: A mixed-method systematic review. J. Immigr. Minor. Health. 2014 Dec 1;16(6):1247–61. https://doi.org/10.1007/s1093-013-9861-1
6. Rivera Mindt M, Byrd D, Saez P, Manly J. Increasing culturally competent neuropsychological services for ethnic minority populations: A call to action. Clin. Neuropsychol. 2010 Apr 1;24(3):429–53. https://doi.org/10.1080/13854040903058960
7. Boone KB, Victor TL, Wen J, Razani J, Pontón M. The association between neuropsychological scores and ethnicity, language, and acculturation variables in a large patient population. Arch. Clin. Neuropsychol. 2007 Mar 1;22(3):355–65. https://doi.org/10.1016/j.acn.2007.01.010
8. Keshavarz MH. The role of social context, intimacy, and distance in the choice of forms of address. Int. J. Sociol. Lang. 2001 May 3;2001(148):5–18. https://doi.org/10.1515/ijsl.2001.015

9. Ramezani A, Alvani SR, Mohajer L, Alameddine LR. Neuropsychology and neuroanatomy of code switching: Test development and application. Psychol. Stud. 2020 Feb 21:1–4. https://doi.org/10.1007/s12646-019-00548-5

10. Ramezani A, Alvani SR, Lashai M, Rad H, Houshiarnejad A, Razani J, Cagigas X. Case study of an Iranian-American neuropsychological assessment in the surgical setting: Role of language and tests. Appl. Neuropsychol. Adult. 2020 Jan 7:1–6. https://doi.org/10.1080/23279095.2019.1706517

11. Spink J. Education and politics in Afghanistan: The importance of an education system in peacebuilding and reconstruction. J. Peace Educ. 2005 Sep 1;2(2):195–207. https://doi.org/10.1080/17400200500185794

12. Shah J, Karimzadeh S, Al-Ahdal TM, Mousavi SH, Zahid SU, Huy NT. COVID-19: The current situation in Afghanistan. Lancet Glob. Health. 2020 Jun 1;8(6):e771–2. https://doi.org/10.1016/S2214-109X(20)30124-8

13. Guthrie E, Abraham S, Nawaz S. Process of determining the value of belief about jinn possession and whether or not they are a result of mental illness. Case Reports. 2016 Feb 2;bcr2015214005.

14. Hamed E. Neurological care in Afghanistan. Pak. J. Neurolog. Sci. 2013;8(3):6–8.

15. Nicholson K, Martelli MF. Confounding effects of pain, psychoemotional problems or psychiatric disorder, premorbid ability structure, and motivational or other factors on neuropsychological test performance. In Young G, Kane AW, Nicholson K, editors. Psychological knowledge in court: PTSD, pain, and TBI. Berlin/Heidelberg, Germany: Springer Science + Business Media; 2006. p. 335–51. https://doi:10.1007/0-387-25610-5_18

16. Abdullah T, Brown TL. Mental illness stigma and ethnocultural beliefs, values, and norms: An integrative review. Clinical Psychol. Rev. 2011 Aug 1;31(6):934–48. https://doi.org/10.1016/j.cpr.2011.05.003

17. Pang KY. Symptoms of depression in elderly Korean immigrants: Narration and the healing process. Cult. Med. Psychiatry. 1998 Mar 1;22(1):93–122. https://doi.org.10.1023/a:1005389321714

18. Tigranyan S. Middle Eastern attitudes toward seeking mental health services [Doctoral dissertation]. Alliant International University; 2020.

19. Veliu B, Leathem J. Neuropsychological assessment of refugees: Methodological and cross-cultural barriers. Appl. Neuropsychol. Adult. 2017 Nov 2;24(6):481–92. https://doi.org/10.1080/23279095.2016.1201483

20. Duff K, Ramezani A. Regression-based normative formulae for the repeatable battery for the assessment of neuropsychological status for older adults. Arch. Clin. Neuropsychol. 2015 Nov 1;30(7):600–4. https://doi.org/10.1093/arclin/acv052

Iranian

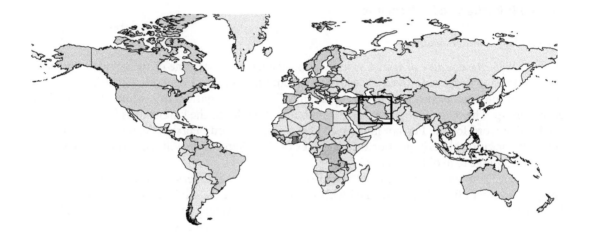

37 Neuropsychological Evaluation of the Iranian American, Persian (Farsi) Speaking Individual

Clinical and Forensic Considerations

Amir Ramezani, Emmanuel A. Zamora, Arash Ramezani, and Maria Soledad Montero

Section I: Background Information

Terminology and Perspective

Prior to 1935, the country of Iran was known as "Persia," and was one of the countries from the Ancient Persian Empire. Individuals who come from the country of Iran often identify as Iranian or Persian interchangeably, but the term "Iranian" describes nationality, while "Persian" is an ethnic group. The official language is Persian, but many refer to the language as "Farsi," which is the Persian word for the Persian language. Therefore, the word "Persian" can refer to language, ethnicity, or cultural heritage. For the purposes of this chapter, we will use Farsi to refer to the Persian language to avoid confusion.

Dr. Amir Ramezani is a bilingual, Farsi-speaking Iranian-American neuropsychologist. His perspective comes from having worked with Iranians in research, clinical, and academic settings. Dr. Emmanuel Zamora is a trilingual Mexican-Portuguese-American neuropsychologist. His perspective comes from having worked with Iranians in psychotherapy and assessment. He is married into an Iranian family, learning Farsi as a fourth language, and finding similarities to his home cultures, primarily the importance of family, respect, affection, and joviality. Mr. Arash Ramezani is a bilingual Iranian American who has studied cognitive science and conducted research in mental health, cognition, and Iranians. His perspective comes from his personal and professional experience working with Iranians in research and health settings. Ms. Maria Montero is a bilingual Mexican American post-doctoral trainee, who has worked with. Farsi-speaking individuals in the neuropsychological setting. Her perspective comes from a multicultural perspective and her clinical experience.

Geography

Iran is in the Western Asia region that encompasses the Iranian plateau. It is the 17th largest and 17th most populous country in the world with 83 million inhabitants. Iran shares its border with Azerbaijan, Armenia, Turkmenistan, Afghanistan, Pakistan, Turkey, and Iraq. It has access to three major bodies of water: the Persian Gulf, the Gulf of Oman, and the Caspian Sea. The country is divided into 5 regions and 31 provinces.

History

Iran has a central location in Eurasia, which historically made it a geopolitical power via numerous imperial dynasties from the 6th century to the 20th century. Iran also has one of the oldest civilizations in the world and reached its territorial height during the Achaemenid Empire (first Persian

DOI: 10.4324/9781003051862-75

Empire) formed by Cyrus the Great. While the politics and government have changed over time, the people of Iran have historically prospered economically and culturally by their location on the Silk Road trade route between the Roman Empire and Asia. Iranians celebrate a rich history of poetry, philosophy, fashion, cuisine, and weaving.

Prior to the 1979 **Islamic Revolution**, Iran had 2,500 years of monarchy. The **Pahlavi dynasty** was last to helm the monarchy. Foreign political involvement, such as the 1953 US/UK led coup d'état, is seen to have had a critical role in leading to the Islamic Revolution, as the monarchy had gained more power after the prime minister was overthrown. The country shifted from a pro-western monarchy to a theocracy, which led to tensions between governments and led many Iranians to seek refuge in countries all over the world.[1]

People

The people of Iran cherish friendships, family, reciprocity, community, and celebration. It may be common for a person to attend 2 or 3 gatherings in a week with friends or family. The people are interconnected, welcoming, and come from a giving culture. At the same time, they have experienced many hardships, including war, separation from their native land, multiple deaths of family and friends, scarcity, economic restrictions, and complex interpersonal and societal trauma. Despite these hardships, the people remain open to worldly ideas and cultures and thrive in cohesive communities. This information may help clinicians to have a framework to better evaluate support systems, coping, strengths, and resiliency in a client.

Ethnicity

Iran's largest ethnic group is Persian, which makes up just over 60% of the population. Other large groups include Azerbaijanis (Azerbaijani Turks), Kurds, and Lurs. In the United States, the majority of Iranian Americans are ethnically Persian.

Immigration and Relocation

The history of Iranian immigration to the United States dates back to the 1950s. The reasons for immigrating to the United States changed with the turn of events between both governments. First, the rapid economic growth in Iran led to a desire to meet the rapid employment demands, which propelled the first wave of Iranian immigrants to the United States. Because of its stable relationship with the United States, the Iranian government supported Iranian students' desire to seek international higher education opportunities.[2] In 1975, the Institute of International Education identified that Iranian students were the largest group of international students (7,797), which more than tripled to 51,310 by 1979 because of the Iranian Revolution.[3]

The second wave of migration from 1972 to 1982, also known as the brain drain [the emigration of highly trained individuals or intelligent people from a country] was precipitated by the Revolution, then the war between Iran and Iraq. The circumstances leading to this second wave were different. This time, many traveled as political refugees or exiles.[4] This time, migrants were middle- to upper-class families, which included individuals with diverse advanced degrees and professions such as artists, journalists, doctors, writers, and musicians. Following the events of the *1980 US and Iran hostage crisis*, the sentiment between both governments changed for the worse. Iranian American immigrants were now facing US government visa scrutiny, which led to significant deportation of Iranians.[5] Even then, the Iran–Iraq war in 1980 led to a third wave of Iranian immigration to the United States. At this time, young Iranians eligible for military service as well as middle-class professionals and unskilled workers sought political asylum in the United States. If asylum was not granted, many still migrated and lived illegally in the United States.

The final wave of Iranian immigration was documented after 2001.[6] Following the September 11 terrorist attacks, enhanced scrutiny targeted individuals from many foreign countries, including Iran. The number of Iranian immigrants in 2003 decreased to just over 7,000, a significant decrease from nearly 14,000 in 2002. Discrimination remained a continued concern as 60% of Iranian Americans report personal discrimination or awareness of discrimination based on ethnicity or country of origin.[7]

Presently, California has the highest concentration of Iranians outside of Iran,[8] with the largest populations in Los Angeles, Orange, and San Diego counties. For most Iranian immigrants, the decision to move to California was based on connecting with an established community. For example, Los Angeles has one of the largest Jewish communities in the world, making it a safe and desirable home for the majority of Iranian Jewish immigrants.[9] California may also remind Iranians of home due to its diverse geography and climate, ranging from snowcapped mountains to arid deserts.

Language

Although the Iranian Constitution recognizes the multi-lingual and multi-ethnic make-up of the country, in 1907, the Farsi language was declared the only official language and script of the country.[10] There are three varieties of Farsi language that clinicians are likely to encounter. Farsi (Iranian Persian) is largely spoken by most Iranians (this can include a wide range of ethnicities: Iranian, Armenian, Kurdish, etc.). Dari-Farsi is largely spoken in Afghanistan and Tajiki-Farsi is spoken by the Tajik people in Afghanistan, Tajikistan, and Uzbekistan.

Contemporary Persian or Farsi is a part of the Indo-European language family. Persian has many loan words from English and French, with a considerable number of Arabic terms that have been Persianized. The Persian alphabet is a modified variant of the Arabic alphabet which includes letters not found in Arabic. Many dialects exist throughout the Persian-speaking world, with the Tehrani accent being the basis for standard Iranian Persian.

Communication

Iranians communicate in a friendly and socially desirable manner. They are not likely to say no as this may reflect disrespect (Note: please see Cultural section for the concept of **Taarof**). They are likely to show disagreements through non-verbal gestures, such as short disapproving glance, as well as pauses in conversations, requests to consult with family or friends prior to approval, or show hesitation in their agreement. This does change with the level of acculturation. Education, social status, and age are prioritized and recognized in communication. For example, a professor, doctor, or engineer will be referred to as such their title (e.g., "hello doctor Reza") in verbal communications. Respecting professional and societal rules may build trust in a clinical relationship. If speaking Farsi with a patient, it is important to use formal pronoun for you, which is **shomâ**, rather than the familiar pronoun for you, which is *to*. It is also important to use proper titles, such as **aaga** for mister and **khaanum** means miss.

Education

Education is a strong Iranian value. According to the 2000 US Census, about 50% of Iranian immigrants attained a bachelor's degree, with 25% holding an advanced degree. In a 2020 survey of Iranian Americans, 86% of respondents earned a college degree.[7] Iranians in America pride themselves in their level of education and are the most highly educated ethnic group in the United States.[11]

Adult immigrants from Iran have varying levels of educational attainment, depending on the socio-economic group they were part of in Iran. Prior to the revolution, students would often pursue education in Europe and the United States, which is why many educated Iranians were multi-lingual prior to immigrating. However, those from lower socio-economic groups were often illiterate or semi-literate if immigration occurred before the 1970s. Literacy was only commonplace for wealthy families until a substantial effort by the government took place called the *literacy corps*.

Currently, primary education in Iran is compulsory and children attend school until about age 15. High school is completed from ages 16 to 18 (this range may vary in rural regions). Students will take a college entrance exam called the *Konkur* to be placed in the desired field of study. Islamic values have been integrated into all aspects of general education since the revolution. Instruction is primarily in Farsi, but Arabic is also taught in order to read the Koran. Students are also required to take an additional foreign language for five years, where English is typically favored. Similar studies are taught in the United States.

Literacy

Iranian Americans are largely literate and often in both English and Farsi. However, immigrants originally from rural or very low socio-economic regions may be illiterate or semi-literate. Usually, this question can be explored when asking about educational attainment. It is important to determine dominance for both spoken and written language to provide the appropriate measures. Farsi script is written and read from right to left, with numerical information embedded from left to right. The script is written in cursive and there is no print version, as in Latin scripts.

Socio-Economic Status

As expected with their high level of education, many Iranian Americans hold top-ranking employment positions, including leadership positions in fortune 500 companies and academic positions at universities. Data from the 2020 National Public Opinion Survey of Iranian Americans[7] indicated that 48% of Iranian Americans made over $100,000 a year, 34% made between $50,000 and $100,000, while 18% made less than $50,000. The number of Iranian Americans making more than $100,000 a year is significantly higher than 90% of other American earners.[12]

Gender and Sexuality

While Iranians typically take a more traditional view of gender roles, it does not appear like other masculine societies. Due to the great importance of family, it is common for men to engage in child-rearing, household activities, and cooking. Iranian women have some traditional expectations but do not hold a meek or diminutive position in the family. Pre-revolution Iranian women had equal rights to education, financial opportunities, and political freedoms. After the revolution, women's financial value, as in compensation for death or inheritance, is half of men. Women are expected to be covered in public and only allowed to show their face and hands. Many Iranian women typically use a headscarf or *rusari* in public.

In the United States, many Iranian families were raised or come from a largely pre-revolution socialized period and tend to have more equitable views of gender. However, sexuality and gender identity are rarely discussed openly.

It is important to ask females if they prefer to handshake or not, as a sign of respect for the Muslim religion. Explaining in detail what you will do and if the testing involves touching the client (e.g., Sensory Perceptual Examination) and asking permission from the client prior to evaluation may help build trust.

Spirituality and Religion

Islam has been the official religion of Iran since the Muslim conquest of Persia in mid-600s. Prior to the conquest, Iranian's were mainly **Zoroastrian**. Iranian's who fled after the revolution largely identify as irreligious or as **Shiite Muslim**. However, there is a sizable population of Iranian Jews, Christians, and Baháís in the United States.[7]

Acculturation and Integration

The acculturation process of Iranian Americans has been met with many challenges due to the relationship between the United States and Iran. Following the events of September 11, 2001, the degree of acculturation was forced to extremes. For example, some fully acculturated by adopting the US culture, including westernizing their names and only speaking English. On the other extreme, some completely refused to adopt the US culture, while others adjusted between both cultures.[13]

Despite historical challenges, Iranian Americans are highly integrated. Socially, Iranians interact with a diverse group of people and have a high level of intermarriage with non-Iranian Americans.[6] Like other immigrant groups, the first generation tends to communicate in their native language, while subsequent groups have full fluency of Farsi and English or English alone.

Culture, Values, and Customs

Iranians are some of the friendliest and welcoming people in the world. It would not be unusual to have an Iranian patient invite you to their home for tea or a meal. Etiquette and respect are key values for Iranians. A term that is important to learn is *Taarof*, which describes a ritualized politeness to promote equality and value of relationship over all else. In terms of hospitality, a host may offer a guest food or drink, while the guest is obliged to refuse it, typically three times. This refusal is the guest's attempt to not inconvenience the host. Taarof can be present in a conversation where an individual may minimize their accomplishments for the sake of humility, especially if there are socio-economic differences in the group. Iranians tend to respect values such as being selfless and dutiful to others.

Respect for elders in the family is paramount. Parents and grandparents are expected to be highly influential in the decisions of their children. When older family members can no longer adequately care for themselves, their child or relative is expected to open up their home and care for them. Placing an older adult in a nursing home is becoming more commonplace in the United States but may be frowned upon in more traditional Iranian communities.

Iranian society is generally more collectivistic than individualistic.[14] Interdependence on a network of family and close friends is considered socially congruent. Children tend to live at home until they marry or leave for school. It is common for large families to live relatively close to one another. In the United States, these cultural values remain consistent to a large degree. The acculturative process may instill more individualism in younger immigrants or children of immigrants.

Mental Health Views

Age, education, family values, and acculturation levels can impact the level of acceptance of behavioral health and neuropsychological services. While Iranian Americans are more accepting of behavioral health service, others may have traditional views whereby such services are looked down upon or stigma may block access to services. Natural/non-medical ways to support emotional and physical health are preferred. It is helpful to educate the client and the family about behavioral health or neuropsychological services as this can greatly enhance rapport, cooperation, and reduce misunderstandings.

Health Conditions

There is a risk of multiple sclerosis, hypertension, cardiovascular disease, and diabetes in Iranians living in Iran, but many of the risks are mitigated when environmental factors are improved.[15] Iranians tend to seek professional treatment if symptoms persist after home remedies.[15]

Approach to Neuropsychological or Psychological Evaluations

Iranian clients may not know why they have been referred to neuropsychology and what will be done in the evaluation. Worries about how the results will be used and impact their work, independence, and family may often be on their mind. Education may be needed to explain the service, process of evaluation, consent form, and communication with healthcare providers and family. Explaining that there will be an interview, testing, and feedback sessions will help clients know what to expect and why the relationship will be terminated after feedback. For clients who are worried about psychiatric factors, the neuropsychological service acts to bridge neurological concerns to behavioral health care. For clients who are worried about neurocognitive factors, such as capacity, decision making, and future planning, the service acts as a way for the client and family to put life in order and have realistic expectations for the future.

When testing, we recommend not testing in Farsi and English at the same time or alternating between languages. Instead, testing in one language and then moving to the next language avoids language interference effects or code switching.[16] Also, consider processing speed in reading tasks as the Farsi language is usually read from right to left. Note that clients may not want to take a break because of *taarof* or being too polite. Therefore, fixed time points for breaks will be helpful. Individuals who show obvious impairments on testing will likely minimize both cognitive and behavioral/emotional factors to "save face" or preserve their dignity.

Currently, it is common to use White norms when scoring due to a lack of Iranian norms or normative adjustments. A list of tests and norms have been provided in the Appendix that can be used for Farsi-speaking populations; however, there remains notable variability. Therefore, caution, clinical judgment, and experience need to be exercised within a cultural context when making interpretations.

Iranian American clients may expect advice or recommendations that are tangible and practical. If clients are referred for behavioral health services, it could be helpful to explain that this is your professional advice. Asking if they wish to have a Farsi-speaking professional and whether they wish for their partner or family to be involved would be considered respectful.

Please note that The Persian Naming Test will likely show perfect score (e.g., 50/50 or 47/50) because the items are high frequency and used commonly in speaking, reading, and writing. Therefore, examiners need to be mindful that slight deviations in scores (<45/50) may suggest difficulties. It is common for Iranians to have exposure or usage of the English language. If a monolingual client has been exposed to the English language for a few years (e.g., working in the United States for five years in a primarily English-speaking environment), it may be helpful to gather a quick screen (e.g., Repeatable Battery for the Assessment of Neuropsychological Status [RBANS]) in English to understand gross cognition. This would be in addition to Farsi testing. Anecdotal clinical experience shows that some clients who use English more than their native language, despite having a short duration in the main country, can show better performance in English. This is rare but worth considering. To evaluate language, using the Persian aphasia tests and simple translated items from the Boston Diagnostic Aphasia Examination (BDAE), in a qualitative manner (e.g., reduced fluency and agrammatic features on the cookie theft writing and speaking section) can yield pathognomonic signs that can assist with diagnosis.

Section II: Case Study — "Primary Persian Aphasia in Translation"

Note: Names and other identifying information have been changed to ensure privacy.

Reason for Referral

Ms. Sohbat was a late 60 year old, right-handed, Iranian female with 18 years of education (master's degree in the United States, worked in nuclear imaging) who spoke English and Farsi. She was referred by a memory clinic to assist with differential diagnoses and to determine her cognitive status.

Cognitive Complaints

Upon arrival, Ms. Sohbat was noted to make paraphrasing errors of the phonemic type in Farsi. She was also noted to have reduced fluency and difficulties with articulating sounds. Ms. Sohbat reported difficulties with concentrating, following conversations, word finding, articulation, and recalling names of familiar people. Although she would have liked to speak English, she switched to Farsi when she could not find words in English. At times, language switching was automatic. Her family was noted to speak for her when she could not find the right words.

Psychiatric Complaints

Ms. Sohbat had trouble with anxiety and uncontrollable worrying since she was an adolescent, though this worsened much more after the Iran-Iraq War, and this continues to be a problem.

Functional Status

Ms. Sohbat reported that her cognitive symptoms did not affect her ability to perform daily activities (e.g., dressing, bathing, feeding, cooking, medications adherence, and grocery shopping). However, she did have notable problems following steps when using a computer. Ms. Sohbat's driving status was reportedly active. When asked about accidents or driving problems, her family reported that she was driving and had not gotten in any accidents, yet her neuropsychological profile suggested otherwise. Such discrepancies may lead one to hypothesize if the family or patient is minimizing symptoms such as medication adherence and driving abilities.

Collateral Information

Ms. Sohbat provided permission to speak with her son, daughter, son-in-law, and husband. When asked what specific cognitive, language, and/or motor problem started first, it appeared that writing fluency, word finding, and reduced verbal fluency were her initial symptoms. Word finding and reduced fluency problems were believed to have started three years prior and preceded cognitive symptoms. Course of cognitive complaints was reportedly slowly worsening over two years.

The family described that one year ago she confused the closet for the bathroom, was found kneeling and had soiled herself. She had two periods of confusion in the preceding year. Ms. Sohbat had a recent history of crying easily in response to emotionally charged experiences. The family described that her second language, English, had slowly reduced and she was speaking more Farsi, a common finding in bilinguals who show neurodegenerative changes.[17] Her family did note functional difficulties and her husband has been taking care of most of her financial activities.

Medical History

Ms. Sohbat reported having high blood pressure. She was taking amlodipine 10 mg, which has helped her manage her blood pressure. She was also currently taking Zoloft 25 mg. She noted anxiety increasing as a result of starting this medication. She last tried Paxil and found it to be helpful with anxiety. Though she wanted to not take medications because "it is not natural," she appeared to be in such a vulnerable space in her life where she had to become open to taking medications. The neurology and memory clinic included possible frontal temporal dementia and primary progressive aphasia as rule-in diagnoses.

Her last EEG was unremarkable one year ago. A brain MRI was also unremarkable around the same time but she did have scattered white matter fluid-attenuated inversion recovery (FLAIR) hyperintensities in both cerebral hemispheres in a non-specific pattern. Lab work was unremarkable.

One year prior, she scored 23/30 on a Mini-Mental State Exam (MMSE) in English. She was unable to do serial 7s past 93, spell her last name backward, or draw in the numbers of a clock (she wrote in the following clock numbers: 12, 1, 2, 6, 45").

Family Medical History

Ms. Sohbat's father had a history of heart disease. She reported that her uncle had a stroke and transient ischemic attack (TIA), as well as high blood pressure. Her aunt was suspected to have Alzheimer's disease. Records note that her father also had dementia, but the patient and her husband denied this.

Other Relevant Medical History

Ms. Sohbat had a prior neuropsychological evaluation. This report was not available for review. It was unclear if she was thinking that her cognitive screen was a neuropsychological evaluation. She denied personal history of seizures, head injury, loss of consciousness, toxic exposure, learning disability, or attention-deficit/hyperactivity disorder.

Development History

Unremarkable.

Language Background

Ms. Sohbat's primary language was English. Ms. Sohbat also spoke Farsi but was more fluent in English, per her and her family. Ms. Sohbat spoke English 80% of the time at home, 100% at her past work, and 50% with friends. She noted that she spoke more English with her children than her husband. Preference for testing and interview was requested to be conducted in English; however, some of the questions were also asked in Farsi when language barriers were present.

Cultural/Ethnic Background

Ms. Sohbat was born in Iran. She lived abroad in Europe most of her life. She came to the United States with her husband. Ms. Sohbat's self-described cultural/ethnic background was Iranian American. Using a 0–100 scale, where 0 is not adopting any cultural practices and 100 is adopting cultural practices, her percentage of acculturation in American culture was reportedly 100% and she felt she was 50% acculturated in the Iranian culture. She was a first-generation immigrant who came to the United States in her early 30s, post-Islamic revolution and present for part of the Iran-Iraq War. She did not affiliate with any specific sociopolitical parties or religious beliefs, though her parent identified as Muslim. She came from an upper socio-economic status background.

Living Situation

Ms. Sohbat was living with her husband.

Test Results and Impression

The test and norm selection was based on the research and test that have been in use in the first author's clinical setting. Selection was also based on experience with the clinical utility and how such uses match clinical impressions over the years.

To estimate premorbid functioning, the following were considered: scores from the Persian Adult Reading Test, master's degree, working in a tech-heavy areas in the United States. States, education in Iran, and literacy in both languages. These factors would suggest a minimum of high average functioning.

In order to arrive at a more accurate depiction of her clinical presentation, a qualitative understanding of the language-based tests (e.g., 100% correct or incorrect, 10/10 raw scores, examining high frequency of naming items) was considered in the context of family reports, cultural background, and Ms. Sohbat's minimization of symptoms. We used both English and Farsi norms to get a gauge of her performance.

Overall, global impairments were found with notable executive functioning, language, and memory problems. Her effort measure was invalid due to having difficulty with impaired visual processing (see visuospatial section), writing fluency/speed (Rey-15 free recall), and getting stuck on repeating items recalled during free recall. This was not due to feigning, rather due to notable impairments. Summary of test data is given in Table 37.1.

Diagnostic Impressions

Major neurocognitive disorder (FTD, PPA).

Summary

There appeared to be three aspects to Ms. Sohbat's cognitive and psychiatric functioning. This included prominent executive dysfunction, language problems, and anxiety.

Regarding cognitive functioning, Ms. Sohbat's premorbid intellectual functioning was estimated to be in the high average range and therefore her current functioning was expected to fall in the same range. Results showed global impairments. Results would point to more severe executive dysfunction and frontal system deficits, as well as language deficits marked by reduced fluency, grammar, writing, comprehension of sentences and paragraphs, phonemic paraphasia, and articulation problems. Qualitative analysis of her cookie theft writing fluency showed grammatical errors and reduced writing fluency. Such qualitative analyses of the data were much more helpful than normed results as language challenges appeared to be prominent and quantitative depictions would minimize impairments. When considering the fluctuating course of her concentration, problem-solving, memory, and language deficits starting three years prior, she

Table 37.1 Neuropsychological testing results from Ms. Shobat's evaluation

Performance validity			
Task	*Test*	*Raw/score*	*Clinical classification*
Visual memory effort	Rey 15-Item + Recognition	12	Invalid

Intellectual functioning				
Central nervous system task	*Test*	*Raw/score*	*%ile*	*Clinical classification*
Verbal IQ	Persian Adult Reading Test (PART)	—	74	Average
Non-verbal IQ	TONI-4	87 IQ	19	Low average

Attention and working memory				
Central nervous system task	*Test*	*Raw/score*	*%ile*	*Clinical classification*
Auditory attention working memory	RBANS Digit Span	7	6	Borderline
Visual attention and info. processing	Color trails 1	7 min	<1	Impaired
	Errors	2	—	—

Executive functioning				
Central nervous system task	*Test*	*Raw/score*	*%ile*	*Clinical classification*
Flexibility, inhibition, and impulse control	Color Trails 2	Could not understand instructions	n/a	Below expected
	Behavioral Dyscontrol Scale-2	—	—	Below expected
	Go-no go/red-green (0–3 rating)	1	—	—
	Fist-edge palm (0–3 rating)	1	—	—
	Insight (0–3 rating)	2	—	—
	M-N graphomotor perseveration errors	Could not do	—	—
Visuospatial problem solving	Clock Drawing Test (20–4)	4/10	—	Below expected
	Hand error	1	—	—
	Organization error	1	—	—
	Stimulus bound error	1	—	—
	Missing numbers error	1	—	—

Language functioning				
Central nervous system task	*Test*	*Raw/score*	*%ile*	*Clinical classification*
Farsi language	Bilingual Aphasia Test—Farsi Syntactic comprehension errors	1	—	Intact
	Bilingual Aphasia Test—Farsi Grammar judgment errors	2	—	Below expected
	Basic reading of Farsi words	10/10	—	Intact

(Continued)

Table 37.1 Neuropsychological testing results from Ms. Shobat's evaluation *(Continued)*

Visual confrontational naming	Persian Naming Test	48/50	—	Intact
	Semantic paraphasias	0	—	—
	Phonemic paraphasias	2	—	—
	RBANS Picture Naming	10	73	Average
Word comprehension	BDAE-III basic word discrimination errors	1	—	Intact
	BDAE-III word comprehension by category errors	2	—	Below expected
	BDAE-III semantic probe errors	1	—	Intact
Comprehension of instructions	BDAE-III commands errors	0	—	Intact
Word discrimination	BDAE-III word identification—lexical decision (real vs. non-sense word) errors	0	—	Intact
Reading comprehension	BDAE-III oral reading basic oral word reading errors	1	—	Intact
	BDAE-III oral word reading special word list errors	3	—	Below expected
	BDAE-III oral reading sentence errors	3	—	Below expected
	BDAE-III reading sentence comprehension errors	0	—	Intact
	BDAE-III reading comprehension—sentence and paragraphs errors	2 Very slow	—	Below expected
Writing	BDAE-III writing errors in cookie theft	Reduced fluency, could not read, misspellings, and agrammatic	—	Below expected
Auditory response naming	BDAE-III responsive naming (out of 20)	10 Due to processing speed being slow	—	Below expected
Verbal fluency	FAS (phonemic fluency) Farsi	8	<1	Impaired
	Animal and fruits (semantic fluency) Farsi	21	44	Average
	BDAE-III cookie theft verbal fluency	Very little verbal production		Below expected

Visuospatial and Sensory Perceptual Functioning

Central nervous system task	Test/task	Raw/score	%ile	Clinical classification
Simple vision	Near vision errors (vision adequate for perception of stimuli)	0	—	Intact
Color vision	Color vision error (color vision adequate for perception of stimuli)	0	—	Intact
Right-left confusion	Right-left orientation errors	0	—	Intact

(Continued)

Table 37.1 Neuropsychological testing results from Ms. Shobat's evaluation *(Continued)*

Gross sensory, auditory, and visual	Reitan–Klove Sensory Perceptual Examination			
	Tactile	L = 0, R = 0, Bil = 0	—	Intact
	Auditory	L = 1, R = 2, Bil = 3	—	Below expected
	Visual field	Up L = 0, Up R = 0, Up Bi = 0, Mid L = 0, Mid R = 0, Mid Bi = 0, Lo L = 0, Lo R = 0, Lo Bi = 0	—	Intact
Simple visuospatial	BVMT-R Copy	9/12	0	Below expected
Angle orientation	RBANS Line Orientation	14	18	Low average
Visuospatial problem solving	Clock drawing test (20–4)	4	—	Below expected
	Number spacing error	1	—	—
	Circle shape error	1	—	—
	Neglect error	unclear	—	—
Spatial neglect	Line bisection test errors (out of 20)	2 missed lines	—	Below expected

Learning and memory

Central nervous system task	Test	Raw/score	%ile	Clinical classification
Verbal memory	Shiraz Verbal Learning Test	—	—	—
Encoding	Learning trials	8, 10, 10, 11, 10	—	—
Retrieval	Total learning trials	49	45	Average
Storage	Short-delay free recall	5	1	Impaired
	Short-delay cued recall	11	30	Average
	Long-delay free recall	8	4	Borderline
	Long-delay cued recall	11	21	Average
	Long-delay yes/no recognition hits	16	>97	Very superior
	Long-delay yes/no recognition false positive	8	—	Below expected
Verbal memory	RBANS	—	—	—
Encoding	Learning trials	2, 5, 6, 9	—	—
Retrieval	List learning	22	9	Low average
Storage	List recall	5	32	Average
	List recognition	19	37	Average
Non-verbal memory	BVMT-R	—	—	—
	Trial 1	1	2	Borderline
	Trial 2	2	<1	Impaired
	Trial 3	3	<1	Impaired
Encoding	Total recall	6	<1	Impaired
Retrieval	Learning	2	18	Low average
Storage	Delayed recall	2	<1	Impaired
	% Retained	67	3–5	Borderline
	Recognition	6	>16	Intact
	False positives	3	<1	Impaired

was likely experiencing a possible neurodegenerative condition marked by frontotemporal lobe dementia (FTD).

Regarding psychiatric functioning, Ms. Sohbat and her family reported anxiety and uncontrollable worry, which were longstanding. They had not made the connection between the impact of the Iran-Iraq War on her level of anxiety. This had been a problem and presented with repeated worrying, fear, involuntary flashes of memories of childhood events, and avoidance of activities due to fear of something going wrong. These symptoms impacted relationships and led to a need for reassurance. It was later discovered, per the family, that she lived during the time of war and had experienced seeing multiple dead bodies. Though she did not meet clear criteria for post-traumatic stress disorder (PTSD), it was clear that trauma played a major etiological role in her general wellbeing.

During the feedback, the family was concerned that Ms. Sohbat was going to make "drastic" decisions with her property in Iran. Recently, she had decided to "cash out" all her retirement and give it to her daughter. Issues of conservatorship and capacity were raised. It was advised that they speak to an attorney to better protect her and manage her foreign and domestic properties and considering there was no durable power of attorney or financial power of attorney on file. Recommendations to meet with a family therapist and individual therapist were provided to better help the family make decisions and protect individuals' wishes.

Section III: Lessons Learned

The following are both lessons learned from this case as well as general lessons learned when working with Iranians. Please note that this may not apply to all Iranians.

- Iranians are proud of their cultural heritage (e.g., Persian dynasty, empire, and worldly historic, philosophical, and artic contributions). Acknowledgment of Persian heritage can assist in building rapport.
- Interviewing multiple people in the family can help with timelines and symptom onset.
- Family members and patient may minimize symptoms and functional impairments.
- Prior to the assessment, clarify with the referring provider what language the client feels comfortable speaking (Farsi).
- Iranian Americans may prefer to test in English because of their high acculturation and high English language usage, but testing in both English and Farsi, and examining qualitative aspects of languages tests (e.g., cookie theft) can assist with a better clinical picture.
- Building good rapport in a non-passive, gentle yet directive manner may help to increase cooperation (e.g., showing humility, including family, acknowledgment of family and gender roles, being respectful).
- Literacy, education, work, and functional status in the home country and main country are important factors in determining premorbid functioning.
- It may be helpful to ask about exposure to wars, bomb or missile blasts, blast injuries, loud noises that impact mental status, chemicals or toxins, and head concussions in Iran.
- If using an interpreter, assess for culturally appropriate over-compliance or agreeableness (e.g., taarof).
- Select and learn the Farsi tests to use and educate the interpreter on how to read or administer the test.
- Consider that naming test stimuli in Farsi or the Persian language can have low difficulty levels:
  - The Persian Naming Test will likely show perfect score (e.g., 47+/50) in individuals who do not have temporal lobe involvement, aphasia, Alzheimer's Disease, or FTD semantic and logopenic type. This is mainly because the items are high frequency and used commonly

in speaking, reading, and writing. The author of this test suggests a 75% cutoff. It is not clear if this cutoff was meant for inpatient use. However, based on outpatient clinical experience, discussion with other clinicians, and correspondence with Persian Naming Test author, it appears that utilizing multiple naming tests (e.g., RBANS naming and querying on missed items if they had learned and able to know the name in the past) in another language (e.g., English and Farsi), considering education and functional status, and raising the cutoff to 90% (e.g., PNT <= 45), would likely increase sensitivity to detect true impairment. This is anecdotal and remains to be researched but may be helpful for a qualitative, clinical understanding.

- Clinicians may wish to consider various norms. Please see norm table in the Appendix.
- Specific recommendations for Farsi-speaking patients can be found in the article by Ramezani et al.[18] This article may help manage some of the assessment challenges.
- Having a list of translated Farsi items near the examiner may help determine true naming problems. This is particularly important when assessing neurodegenerative disorders.
- Asking the patient to rate acculturation and language usage in one or more languages can assist the clinician to broadly estimate the influence of such factors on cognitive and language test results.
- Clinicians have years of experience observing, administering, and interpreting findings on tests. Clinical judgment needs to be exercised when making interpretations of test that have been modified or translated, despite the change in reliability and validity.
- Families may wish to use the neuropsychological evaluation to make legal and financial decisions. Education about the appropriate resources and usage of the evaluation may be needed.

Glossary

Aaga. Mister.

Asabi. Feeling nervous or feeling irritable.

Fishar. Literally means pressure, but intended to communicate emotional pressure and a lot of stress.

Gham. Sadness.

Haafeze. Memory.

Iranian coup d'état. Democratically elected Prime Minister Mohammad Mosaddegh was overthrown by the United States and England efforts due to his promotion of nationalization of the Iranian Oil industry.

Islamic Revolution. In 1979, the Islamic republic/theocratic republic replaced the monarchy of Shah (the king of Iran at the time) with Ayatollah Khomeini, who created the constitution of the Islamic Republic of Iran.

Khaanum. Miss.

Pahlavi dynasty. From 1925 to 1979 (prior to 1930's Iran was Persia), the Pahlavi dynasty (Mohamed Reza Pahlavi, Reza Shah Pahlavi, or Shah) led Iran and political affairs between the United States and England.

Shiite Muslim. A branch of Islam that has blood lines from the Islamic prophet Muhammad designated Ali ibn Abi Talib as his successor.

Shomâ. Formal way to refer to a person.

Taarof. Culturally appropriate offerings or agreeableness to show respect. This is a complex concept and beyond the scope of this chapter.

Tavajo. Attention.

Vasvaas.   Obsessive.

Zabaan.   Language.

Zoroastrian.   One of the oldest religions in Iran, that promote appreciation of natural elements such as fire, and encourage free will and good thought, speech, and action.

References

1. Axworthy M. Revolutionary Iran: a history of the Islamic republic. 2nd ed. Oxford: Penguin; 2019.
2. Ditto S. Red Tape, Iron Nerve: The Iranian Quest for U.S. Education. Policy Focus. Washington, DC; 2014.
3. Bozorgmehr M. From Iranian studies to studies of Iranians in the United States. Iran Stud. 1998;31(1):5–30.
4. Bozorgmehr M, Douglas D. Success(ion): second-generation Iranian Americans. Iran Stud [Internet]. 2011;44(1). Available from: https://www.tandfonline.com/action/journalInformation?journalCode=cist20
5. Hanassab S, Tidwell R. Intramarriage and intermarriage: young Iranians in Los Angeles. Int J Intercult Relations. 1998 Nov 1;22(4):395–408.
6. Public Affairs Alliance of Iranian Americans. Iranian Americans: immigration and assimilation [Internet]. Washington, DC; 2014 Apr [cited 2020 Nov 18]. Available from: https://paaia.org/wp-content/uploads/2017/04/iranian-americans-immigration-and-assimilation.pdf
7. Public Affairs Alliance of Iranian Americans. 2020 National Public Opinion Survey of Iranian Americans [Internet]. Washington, DC; 2020 Oct [cited 2020 Nov 18]. Available from: https://paaia.org/wp-content/uploads/2020/10/PAAIA-2020-survey.pdf
8. Virtual Embassy Tehran. Iranian Americans free to thrive in the U.S. [Internet]. U.S. Embassy. 2018 [cited 2021 May 14]. Available from: https://ir.usembassy.gov/iranian-americans-free-to-thrive-in-the-u-s/
9. Bozorgmehr M, Sabagh G, Der-Martirosian C. Beyond nationality: religio-ethnic diversity. In: Kelley R, Friedlander J, editors. Irangeles. Los Angeles, CA: University of California Press; 1993. p. 57–80.
10. Mirvahedi SH. Nationalism, modernity, and the issue of linguistic diversity in Iran. In: The sociolinguistics of Iran's languages at home and abroad [Internet]. Springer International Publishing; 2019 [cited 2020 Nov 18]. p. 1–21. doi:10.1007/978-3-030-19605-9_1
11. Mostashari A, Khodamhosseini A. An overview of socioeconomic characteristics of the Iranian-American community based on the 2000 Census [Internet]. 2004 [cited 2020 Nov 18]. Available from: http://web.mit.edu/isg/
12. Social Security Administration. Wage statistics for 2019 [Internet]. 2020 [cited 2020 Nov 18]. Available from: https://www.ssa.gov/cgi-bin/netcomp.cgi?year=2019
13. Public Affairs Alliance of Iranian Americans. 2014 National Public Opinion Survey of Iranian Americans [Internet]. Washington, DC; 2014 Mar [cited 2020 Nov 18]. Available from: https://paaia.org/wp-content/uploads/2016/06/2014-paaia-survey-of-iranian-americans.pdf
14. Koutlaki SA. Among the Iranians: a guide to Iran's culture and customs. Boston: Intercultural Press; 2010.
15. Haifizi H, Steis M. People of Iranian heritage. In: Purnell L, Fenkl E, editors. Textbook for transcultural health care: a population approach [Internet]. 5th ed. Cham: Springer International Publishing; 2021 [cited 2020 Nov 18]. p. 529–40. doi:10.1007/978-3-030-51399-3_20
16. Ramezani A, Alvani SR, Mohajer L, Alameddine LR. Neuropsychology and neuroanatomy of code switching: test development and application. Psychol Stud (Mysore) [Internet]. 2020 Jun 21;65(2): 101–14. Available from: http://link.springer.com/10.1007/s12646-019-00548-5
17. McMurtray A, Saito E, Nakamoto B. Language preference and development of dementia among bilingual individuals. Hawaii Med J [Internet]. 2009 Oct;68(9):223–6. Available from: http://www.ncbi.nlm.nih.gov/pubmed/19842364
18. Ramezani A, Alvani SR, Lashai M, Rad H, Houshiarnejad A, Razani J, et al. Case study of an Iranian-American neuropsychological assessment in the surgical setting: role of language and tests. Appl Neuropsychol Adult. 2019 Dec 27. https://doi.org/10.1080/23279095.2019.1706517

H. Russian

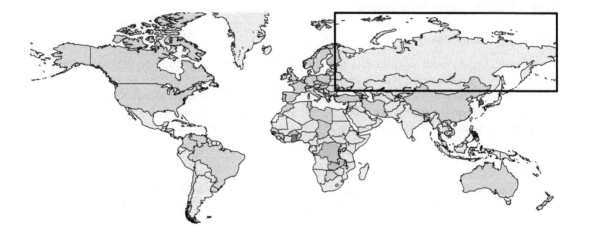

38 Neuropsychological Assessment with Older Russian-Speaking Immigrants
Narrative Matters

Irene Piryatinsky and Dov Gold

Section I: Background Information

Terminology and Perspective

For consistency, Russian immigrants referred to throughout this chapter are first-generation immigrants, who came from Russia to the United States as adults. The perspective provided in this chapter is that of a native Russian speaker brought to the United States as a teenager by a first-generation Russian immigrant (IP). I completed high school and all higher education in the United States, where I currently practice in a private outpatient setting.

Geography

Russia comprises much of central, northern, eastern Europe and northern Asia. It borders Norway, Finland, Estonia, Latvia, Lithuania, Poland, Belarus, Ukraine, Georgia, Azerbaijan, Kazakhstan, Mongolia, China, and North Korea. It is the world's largest country and its climates, vegetation, and soils span vast distances from tundras, coniferous forests, grasslands, and semi-deserts.

History

During the Soviet period, wars, epidemics, famines, and state-sanctioned mass killings claimed millions of lives. During the famine in the 1920s and 1930s, the Great Terror of Joseph V. Stalin in the 1930s, and World War II, an estimated 33.6 million people died. The long-term effects of such disasters lingered and were felt for generations. In the 1990s, the government identified significant reduction in birth rates, increased mortality among males, and declining life expectancy for the population. As the Soviet Union fell apart, immigration to Russia increased in numbers, creating a multicultural state. Representatives from Soviet republics (Ukraine, Georgia, Belarus, Armenia, Azerbaijan, Kazakhstan, Kyrgyzstan, Moldova, Turkmenistan, Tajikistan, and Uzbekistan) announced that they would no longer be part of the Soviet Union. Instead, they declared they would establish a Commonwealth of Independent States. As the iron curtain was lifted, the Soviet Union collapsed, and instead of seeing an influx of mostly Jewish Soviet immigration, waves of refugees of other ethnic groups, such as ethnic Russians, Ukrainians, Belarusians, Armenians, Georgians, and Uzbeks immigrated to the United States from the former Soviet republics.

DOI: 10.4324/9781003051862-77

Education and Literacy

The educational attainment levels and professional status of immigrants from the Former Soviet Union have been relatively high. Universal primary education ensured literacy among the population. The educational system was subdivided into shifts; early morning classes were reserved for younger students whereas older cohorts took courses in the afternoons. The sciences and mathematics were strongly emphasized, though special clubs were freely available and covered a range of other topic areas. Institutes and Universities were a major part of higher education, allowing those outside the Former Soviet Union in the mid-1970s to be exposed to the culture and ideals of the **USSR**. Despite having high levels of education, however, older Russian-speaking immigrants may not be able to fully transfer their skills to the US labor market.[1] Currently, levels of education in Russia are comparable to that of the United States, despite differences in the overarching structure of two systems.

Immigration and Relocation

Per estimates provided by the US Census Bureau in 2019,[2] over two million Russian Americans are living in the United States; though less than a quarter of this number reflects foreign-born citizens. Most immigrants identify Russian as their first language, and are originally from the urban centers of Russia, Ukraine, and Belarus. A smaller subgroup is from other former Soviet republics, such as Kazakhstan and Uzbekistan. They vary widely in terms of years of residence in the United States. A recent survey by Remennick[3] points out that even after over a decade of close co-existence, social and cultural gaps remain between host countries and Russian immigrants.

Language and Communication

Russian is the 7th most common spoken language in the world, with about 260 million people speaking the language globally and about 150 million native Russian speakers.[4] Chiswick[5] states that Russian immigrants in the United States appear to willingly "surrender" to the hegemony of English, consider it superior to Russian and other Slavic languages, and realize its utmost importance for economic success in the United States. Interestingly, but not surprisingly, despite using English in professional domains, Russian-Americans speak primarily Russian at home,[5] though more research is needed to further investigate this.

Russian speakers should be carefully assessed on whether Russian language is their native "mother tongue" to establish their familiarity, prior to making an assumption that Russian is the most preserved language. If a regional dialect exists, it should be documented, and attempts should be made to ensure that the examiner is able to understand the patient and ensure adequate receptive language. If the examiner is not familiar with the dialect enough to conduct an evaluation, it is imperative to ensure that the interpreter is experienced with the particular regional dialect of the patient.

Socio-Economic Status

According to the 2019 US Census Data[2] the average individual income was just below 60,000 dollars for over 2 million self-identified Russian-Americans. 4.9% of families fell below the federal poverty line, and 6.8% of all households qualified for food stamps or federal nutrition assistance program such as Supplemental Nutrition Assistance Program (SNAP) benefits.[2]

Values, Customs, and Risks of Cultural Mismatching

Russian-speaking immigrants tend to appreciate and value economic stability, religious freedom, high-quality education, medical care (e.g., right to choose their providers), and right to choose where to live. Additionally, Granovetter[6] commented that Soviet immigrants had different concepts of friendship in which friends were "confined to a very small circle of personal friends with whom people developed strong family-like personal ties, while a broader circle of people, with whom the individual has contacts, is perceived as consisting of either indifferent or even hostile individuals."

Immigration to the United States is less common among Russian millennials, making it difficult to directly comment on the culture and values of this generation and how it may differ from their predecessors. This younger group is nonetheless present in the current US education system and workforce, however, they appear to be less motivated than older cohorts to make a permanent home in the United States. In our (IP & DG) experience, this group often arrives in the United States with relatively stronger English skills, financial resources, and academic strengths which would (in theory) promote their integration in the mainstream US culture. Despite these advantages however, this younger generation, much like their predecessors, may lack the cultural fluency to seamlessly integrate themselves among their US contemporaries. Consequently, if patients cultural backgrounds and level of acculturation are not appropriately considered, there is a high risk of miscommunication, which may lead to social isolation, suicidality, legal consequences, academic/occupational difficulties, and over-diagnosis or oversimplification of an individual. Further, we (IP & DG) have seen that much like older Russian immigrants, this younger generation may possess attitudes around mental health (described below) that are prohibitive to obtaining treatment prior to their symptoms becoming unbearable.

In attempting to build rapport, evaluators should make efforts to strike a connection with their Russian-speaking patients. There are certain factors to promote rapport building including perceiving the neuropsychologist as educated, experienced, and knowledgeable. Speaking Russian may further promote rapport; however, it is important to be aware that an educated Russian-speaking older adult may correct providers' grammar in the "mother tongue" when an opportunity presents itself. Gender or age of the examiner may influence this as well.

Russian-speaking patients appear to be more receptive to accept recommendations and even make positive changes when recommendations focus on physical health and safety. Motivational interviewing may promote integration of family members in a discussion to ensure patients "stay young" to help with grand- or great-grandchildren. This motivational lens may allow neuropsychologists to collaborate with family further to help reduce impact from pain, sleep disturbance, or mood.

When conducting feedback with families of older adults seen for neuropsychological evaluations, providers should note that dementia diagnoses are often considered "bad news" or a "verdict." Patient's families may be accustomed to being the first to receive the results (even before patients themselves) and making the decision of whether or not to share information with the patient.[7] I (IP) have experienced partners and children spending time in feedback sessions interrupting, rephrasing, paraphrasing, and "sugarcoating," to avoid the words "dementia" or "Alzheimer's disease." This presents an ethical quandary for psychologists practicing in America, whose ethical standards implore them to make feedback available to patients in a comprehensible manner using terms they understand.[8] Thus, it falls to the psychologist to balance respect of cultural norms and fulfillment of the ethical obligation to patients. We strongly encourage readers to use interpreter services during these conversations, rather than relying on family members who may be reasonably motivated to downplay the severity of the results.

Health Status

Research on life expectancy around the time of Soviet Union's collapse shows a decreased life expectancy among both men and women,[9,10] as well as increases in alcohol and tobacco use among Russian adults who lived through this period.[11,12] Compared to a small sample of American citizens, Russian immigrants showed higher rates of vascular disease compared to their same-aged white counterparts.[13,14] Interestingly, a recent study by Mehta and Elo[15] found that disabled Russian immigrants in the United States are more independent in activities of daily living compared to their Russian-residing counterparts. This may reflect relative differences in services available or even the accessibility among the two countries. Regardless of the precise mechanisms at play, successful immigration to the United States may have yielded a net-positive effect for this group, despite the long-term health implications from the conditions surrounding the former Soviet Union's collapse.

While many patients have cardiac problems or other chronic medical conditions, underlying concerns of mistrust of the healthcare system and relatively lower health literacy have been found to impede healthcare utilization among Russian immigrants.[16] In my (IP) practice, common diseases seen in Russian-speaking immigrants include diabetes, hypertension, coronary artery disease, gastrointestinal problems, and alcohol and substance abuse. There is a perception that an illness or disability comes from something the individual has done (e.g., poor diet, not dressing warm enough). I often hear from my older patients, "If I am not in pain, I am in good health." Thus, diabetes, hypertension, and hyperlipidemia, may go unnoticed and untreated.

Mental Health Views

In my (IP) experience, Russian-speaking immigrants are often reluctant to seek help or share their personal issues with people outside of their immediate family. Shame is at times one of the main reasons. Some Russian immigrant patients arrive at the United States with common diagnoses, such as Major Depression and Generalized Anxiety,[17] whereas others with relatively lower levels of acculturation to American culture are less likely to seek mental health treatment.[18] In some cases, it is clear that mood disorders dominate Russian immigrants' presentations. Despite openness and willingness to take medications to manage mental health, there is often reluctance to engage in psychotherapy. This may stem from both a cultural lens of viewing psychotherapists as authority figures, and beliefs that gaining relief from talk therapy is unrealistic. Kohn, Flaherty, and Levav used the term "psychophobia" when describing Soviet Jewish immigrants' tendencies to avoid considering their problems as psychological with preferences for viewing them as biological or physiological.[19] However, even when patients are willing to engage in psychotherapy, there is often a lack of counseling services available in Russian, presenting yet another barrier for these patients. In my (IP) experience, formal diagnosis of mental illness may carry stigma or be perceived as limiting one's employment opportunities and social prospects. I have found rapport and trust building opens opportunities for discussions around identity, trauma, and uncertainty that many immigrants experience in silence.

Neuropsychological Approach

Neuropsychology's history in Russia dates back to the early 20th century with Alexander Luria's and Lev Vygotsky's work of characterizing brain-behavior relationships.[20] At a time when studying outwardly observable phenomena (e.g., behaviors and reflexes) was the dominant dogma of psychological research, Vygotsky presented a novel theoretical framework promoting the measurement of cognitive aspects of psychology. Vygotsky's ideas quickly caught the attention of a young Alexander Luria, who, along with others in their research group, provided the foundation for quantifying and qualifying higher mental processes.[20] Luria's subsequent contributions and methodology to studying and localizing attention, language, memory, and self-regulatory systems in the brain would go on to influence clinical neuropsychology as we know it today.[20,21] Notable among the many outgrowths of his contributions is the clinical-theoretical approach of syndrome analysis to identify disrupted cognitive functions and their relation to patients' behavior.[21]

The ideas seeded by Luria and Vygotsky continue to spread and evolve across the world, influencing contemporary assessment tools and approaches to neuropsychological evaluations.[21,22] Further, Luria's belief in the brain's capacities to reorganize itself and recruit intact cognitive abilities in a compensatory effort remains among his most profound contributions to neuropsychology and neurorehabilitation.[23-25] To say the least, the Vygotsky-Lurian framework is deeply imprinted on modern methods for diagnosing and managing neurocognitive dysfunction, even in the United States.[23,26] We recommend Luria's The Working Brain[27] and Higher Cortical Functions in Man[28] to readers interested in learning more about his principles and contributions.

Luria's approach continues to be prevalent in neuropsychological assessment within the Former Soviet Union. As Glozman[29] puts it, "A psychophysiological orientation for Russian neuropsychology, in contrast to the predominantly neurological orientation in Western contributions, favored the continued development of this field in Russia and assured its predominance in several areas of study: the first descriptions of sensory aphasia and visual agnosia, the first linguo-statistic analysis of aphasia, strong foundations for the systematic approach to investigations of brain damages, and so on (p. 177)."

Research continues to examine clinical validity of tests developed and normed in the United States with Russian-speaking individuals. Presently, assessment tools in Russian are limited.[30,31] Most measures that do exist, do not have validated documented norms and lack publications pertaining to their reliability and validity. This shortage of psychometrically evaluated assessment instruments makes it challenging for clinicians in the United States to draw clear and consistent distinctions between normal aging and potential cognitive impairments, and measure reliable change over time.[32] Available normative data for Russian immigrants is listed in the Appendix.

I (IP) often find that older Russian patients living in mainstream culture may have difficulty communicating their early disease symptoms, which may lead to more difficulty being accurately diagnosed and treated in the early phases of their disease. Furthermore, it is sometimes the case that family members or partners of these immigrant elders do not have the language skills to explain the symptoms, or may be reluctant to share and communicate their symptoms with family members who can assist with translation to avoid overwhelming them.

In my (IP) practice, the most common scenario for evaluating bilingual and bicultural older immigrants with cognitive decline consists of utilizing language interpreters, translating self-report measures, and administering selected subtests with minimal dependency on language and culture. This approach of test selection is often further burdened by the fact that concepts do not always perfectly translate across languages. Further, language abilities may decline in individuals with possible neurodegenerative processes, forcing a qualitative examination of language skills or even greater deviation from standardized administrative protocols. Further, a 2021 study by Melikyan, Puente, and Agranovich[33] suggested that urban-dwelling Russians may underperform on neuropsychological tests compared to their American counterparts due to differing cultural attitudes toward timed performance, multiple-choice format, attention to detail, and short-term memory demands. Disclaimers are therefore included to ensure scores are interpreted with caution due to necessary modifications to accommodate our patients as well as the scarce normative samples representing an individual's cultural and linguistic group.

Section II: Case Study — "From Motherland to the Land of Opportunity"

To help illustrate some of the concepts described in the preceding section, we provide a de-identified case study of a right-handed, married, Russian immigrant gentleman in his mid-80s who was seen for neuropsychological testing in 2018 and again in 2019. He presented with a basic knowledge of conversational English (based on informal observations), however, he preferred to speak in Russian whenever possible.

Referral Question and History of Presenting Illness

The patient was referred by his primary care physician to assess for cognitive impairments and provide treatment recommendations. During his initial evaluation, the patient reported a two-year history of worsening decline in attention, concentration, and recall of information (with some benefit from cuing). He added that he enjoys learning poems but finds it more challenging to learn and retain new material. He has attempted to develop compensatory strategies with inconsistent success. There was no reported decline in the management of his personal or instrumental activities of daily living (ADLs).

Of note, the patient displayed slight word finding difficulties during the 2018 interview. He was unable to state the exact age of his siblings, how many years he had worked in the United States and when he retired. He also could not give names of his grandchildren, which is atypical due to strong familial ties, and the importance of family and of connection to children and grandchildren within the Russian culture. For Russian immigrants, family members may very well be their main social contacts. Many older adults and their children maintain close ties through regular and frequent visitation and phone conversations.[34,35]

The patient described being frustrated with his perceived cognitive declines and lack of improvement with management of his medical conditions. He was previously on a blood pressure medication for two years and discontinued his medication due to perceived ineffectiveness in improving his cognition. He had not reached out to his medical care team due to not wanting to burden others with his concerns. He felt ashamed of "cognitive slippage," worried that his family and friends would notice, leading to increased isolation and depression. He preferred to be seen by his medical doctors without an interpreter to ensure he is viewed as competent and capable of explaining himself, which may have interfered with providers hearing his exact concerns. As his cognitive difficulties persisted, his wife became his spokesperson, and decision-maker, thereby continuing the pattern of limited acknowledgment of his cognitive decline.

Medical History

Medical history was notable for hyperlipidemia, hypothyroidism, chronic kidney disease, and osteoporosis. He denied any history of significant psychiatric illness or mood disturbance; however, he was prescribed nitroglycerin, pravastatin, citalopram, and aspirin at the time of our evaluation. When asked about why he was taking citalopram, he responded that his doctor thought he needed it. This dynamic likely reflects the cultural perceptions surrounding mental illness noted earlier in the chapter; while the patient does not identify as having a mental illness, he is willing to take an antidepressant on recommendation from his physician. This begs the question if this patient was fully aware of the nature of this medication, or if he was instead minimizing his depressive symptoms for fear of stigmatization.

Prior Neurodiagnostic Studies

MRI of the patient's brain in 2011 showed a few tiny foci of T2 hyperintensities suggestive of small vessel disease. He underwent neuropsychological testing at a major medical center in the area in 2016; however, this evaluation was completed entirely in English. The evaluator's impressions were that the patient presented with a mild, non-amnestic cognitive impairment of unclear etiology, with potential contributions from sleep problems and vascular risk factors.

Personal History

The patient was born and raised in Russia and is fluent in Russian. He left Russia at age 65 for economic reasons and to avoid antisemitism for himself but mostly for his children. He "has never looked back" or considered returning to his country of birth. He took English language courses upon arrival and passed the US Citizenship examination without difficulty. He described having a limited number of friends who were all Russian-speaking immigrants. He reported that he did not miss his country of birth, but did miss family and friends, most of whom were Jewish Russian refugees in other parts of the United States and Israel. His parents spoke Yiddish, which he did not learn to speak fluently. His father and mother died around the ages of 81 and 70, respectively, without signs of cognitive decline. He has a brother in his 50s without cognitive problems. The patient held a doctoral degree and worked in Engineering while in Russia. Upon arrival in the United States, he worked as a computer programmer after completing a certification and retired in early 2000s. After his retirement, he volunteered at a local school.

Results and Impressions of Initial Neuropsychological Evaluation

The evaluation was conducted in Russian, including translation of all neuropsychological measures used during the assessment. Tests developed by the Consortium to Establish a Registry for Alzheimer's Disease (CERAD) were utilized as this battery has been already successfully translated into German and French[36,37] and the Russian adaptation was utilized with permission from Dr. Glezerman[30] (personal communication with Dr. Glezerman; http://www.scarletline.com/aglezerman/CERAD.html). Appropriate age and educationally corrected norms were used (see Appendix). Additional measures administered included a standard core battery that is given to most Russian-speaking immigrants referred for baseline evaluation in my practice to rule out a neurodegenerative process (see Table 38.1). WAIS-III Digit Span was utilized because it is easily translatable to Russian.[31] The Clock Drawing Test was used as a screening measure of spatial planning using scoring adapted by Mendez, Ala, and Underwood[38] and normative data from Suhr et al.[39] The Color Trails Test[40] was used, as it has been shown useful in cross-cultural studies and is similar to Trail Making Test A and B, with studies suggesting that even colorblind individuals are able to differentiate the difference between colors on the basis of differing grayscales. Color Trails allows for measurement of speed of processing and set-shifting. Semantic fluency was measured with an Animal category fluency task[41] using normative data from Mitrushina, Boone, and D'Elia.[42] Phonemic fluency was measured by selecting letters previously examined by Dr. Glezerman and her team (personal communication with Dr. Glezerman and http://www.scarletline.com/aglezerman/CERAD.html). The Behavioral Dyscontrol Scale (BDS) was utilized to examine motor planning/sequencing, and simple inhibition.[43] The Beery Visual-Motor Integration Test (VMI) was administered as a measure of construction ability.[44,45] The Line Orientation subtest from the Repeatable Battery for the Assessment of Neuropsychological Status (RBANS) was administered to examine visuospatial abilities.[46]

During testing, more complex instructions had to be repeated and slight perseveration and difficulties with inhibitory control were noted. The patient lost set several times on more challenging tasks. The results of the testing were felt to reflect an accurate estimate of his neurocognitive functioning at that time. He paid close attention to the examiner's pronunciation and use of Russian language, at times correcting the examiner when a more appropriate word could have

Table 38.1 Results of neuropsychological testing

Test name	2018		2019	
	Raw	*Z-score*	*Raw*	*Z-score*
Clock Drawing Test	17	−0.7	7	<−3.0
Cancellation A's	5 omissions	−	10 omissions	−
WAIS-III Longest Span Forward	6	0	6	0.1
WAIS-III Longest Span Backward	4	0	2	−2.2
Trails 1 (secs)	86″	−1.3	145″	<−3.0
Trails 2 (secs)	346″	−3.0	Discontinued	_
Wisconsin Card Sorting Test	Discontinued	_	_	Not administered
Phonemic fluency	42	0.7	30	−0.3
BDS	See text	−	See text	−
RBANS: Line orientation	16	0.2	Not administered	Not administered
Beery VMI	25 (Pic. 3)	0	22 (Pic. 4)	−0.7
CERAD list learning	2/1/3	−1.7/−3.8/−3.1	3/3/3	−1.1/−2.4/−3.1
CERAD delayed recall	0		0	
CERAD Savings	0%		0%	
CERAD recognition True Positives	2	−5.6	7	−1.8
CERAD recognition true negatives	8	−6.0	9	−2.9
BVMT-R total learning	10 (3/4/3)	−1.7	6 (0/3/3)	−1.5
BVMT-R delayed recall	2	−1.9	2	−1.6
BVMT-R % retained	50	−2.2	67	−1.1
BVMT-R recognition	6	0.5	5	−1.2
Boston Naming-15 item	13	0.3	13	−0.3
Semantic fluency (Animals)	1 (lost set)	<−3.0	2	<−3.0
GDS-S	6	−	−	−

Abbreviations: BDS = Behavioral Dyscontrol Scale; Beery VMI = Beery-Buktenica Developmental Test of Visual-Motor Integration; BVMT-R = Brief Visuospatial Memory Test-Revised; CERAD = Consortium to Establish a Registry for Alzheimer's Disease; GDS-S = Geriatric Depression Scale-Short Form; RBANS = Repeatable Battery for the Assessment of Neuropsychological Status; Trails = Color Trail Making Test; WAIS-III = Wechsler Adult Intelligence Scale-Third Edition.

been utilized when explaining a task. Throughout the evaluation, he was acutely aware of when he was being timed, making sure that the examiner was aware that he valued accuracy over speed.

The information below reflects the more salient aspects of his performance in the context of his cultural background. A more comprehensive list of his results is provided in Table 38.1.

He was only partially oriented to time, stating it was "1918" and the date was the 30th (only one day off). He could not name the President of the United States, adding, "I can never remember his name." He incorrectly stated the name of the previous US President; however, he correctly named his immediate two predecessors. He could not tell me the name of other locally elected officials. This was somewhat atypical for this patient given his longstanding interest in national and local politics.

He could not correctly spell "WORLD" backward in Russian. On the BDS, which is generally devoid of cultural and linguistic components, Luria's reciprocal motor programming tasks were performed slowly with multiple perseverative errors (right hand worse than left). On go-no-go tasks, performance was notable for echopraxic errors. He was not able to perform simple or complex motor sequences. Gesture mirroring was performed incorrectly, even after prompting. His ability to copy a clock to command was within expectation (Figure 38.1).

During a task of pattern recognition and cognitive flexibility based on examiner feedback, he failed to enter the task set and the task was discontinued.

Notable observations regarding his language included him requiring repetition of two-step instructions and impaired Semantic fluency; though the latter reflected loss of and failure to regain task set.

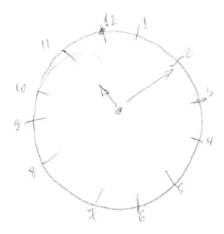

Figure 38.1 Clock drawing 2018 evaluation

Turning to memory, learning of a wordlist in his native language was impaired, without evidence of benefit from repetition of the information. He could not recall any of the words following a brief delay, which may owe to his poor learning. Overall recognition discriminability was in the impaired range, and he identified 2/10 words without any false positive identifications.

On a mood questionnaire translated to Russian, he endorsed mild symptoms of depression, including feeling that his life is empty, experiencing slight hopelessness and helplessness. He did appear to be very concerned about perceived cognitive changes.

Overall, results of his initial evaluation were suggestive of a Mild Neurocognitive Disorder given the level of impairment observed on testing in the context of a man with high educational and occupational attainment. Although there were no declines in his ADLs, the level of impairment on testing raised concerns for an incipient Major Neurocognitive Disorder. Cognitive dysfunction secondary to cerebrovascular disease burden seemed to be the most salient contributor to his presentation. Poor orientation to time raised concerns for contributions from an emergent Alzheimer's disease; however, intact object naming and visual memory storage made this difficult to rule-in or rule-out definitively.

We encouraged him to obtain updated brain imaging and repeat neuropsychological testing in 9–12 months for further monitoring of his cognitive problems and additional etiological clarification.

Follow-Up Evaluation One Year Later

The patient returned for follow-up testing and was accompanied by his wife and his child. His wife stated that she had noticed changes leading up to their move to their new place of residence this year, and that she found it easier to handle the move without his involvement (a considerable change from how they previously handled such situations). She reported observing poor follow-through on tasks, losing items around their home, and more tangentiality in conversation. He also began contacting his wife several times a day at her job for re-assurance and to ask repetitive questions. His wife took over their finances around 12 months prior to this appointment, and he was no longer driving alone because his wife was concerned about his safety.

Additionally, his wife reported that he began referring to her as someone else around two months ago. Specifically, there were times when he talked about his wife as if she was not present. He has also developed visual hallucinations (i.e., seeing children and young adults) within the last three months, which he does not experience as distressing.

Per our previous recommendation, the patient obtained updated neuroimaging. An MRI of his brain from 2018 revealed mild chronic small vessel ischemic changes and moderate prominence of perivascular spaces bilaterally. There were generalized atrophic changes, with notable prominence of the Sylvian fissures, which were more pronounced relative to 2011. Hippocampal atrophy and posterior parietal atrophy were also noted. An old microhemorrhage was noted within the right basal ganglia as well as chronic microhemorrhages in the left inferior frontal lobe.

Results and Impressions of Follow-up Neuropsychological Evaluation

Orientation was limited; he knew the year, but not the month, date, or day of the week. He could not name the current President or the previous President of the United States. He could not identify the city he was living in; however, he could identify his previous town of residence with prompting. During the meeting, he appeared to vaguely recall the examiner. After re-establishing rapport, he no longer eagerly corrected the examiner's grammar or sentence structure. Spontaneous speech was reduced significantly.

On testing, simple and complex motor programming tasks were performed with errors and difficulty. He made impulsive and repetitive errors during simple motor programming and failed to correctly execute a complex motor program. His clock drawing, which he had previously completed without error, was notable for omission of numbers and one of the clock hands (Figure 38.2). In terms of language, confrontation naming was intact. Semantic fluency was impaired. Visuoconstruction was low average, and significantly lower than his performance in 2018. Verbal and visual learning were impaired, as were delayed spontaneous recall. Recall of verbal and visual information were similarly impaired when assessed with a recognition format.

Overall, results were most notable for declines in orientation, processing speed, aspects of executive functioning, and visuoconstruction, as well as ongoing impairments with verbal and visual memory. We felt a Major Neurocognitive Disorder was appropriate given then recent declines in his ADLs. The etiology was likely multi-factorial, with contributions from cerebrovascular disease which likely contributed to the emergence of a Capgras delusion (i.e., thinking his wife is someone else). His pattern of decline and consistently impaired memory alongside evidence of hippocampal atrophy on imaging suggested an emergent Alzheimer's disease process was also contributing.

The discussion of results of assessment for both authors is the most important part of the evaluation process. Subsequently, for this patient, it was prudent to deliver verbal feedback to the

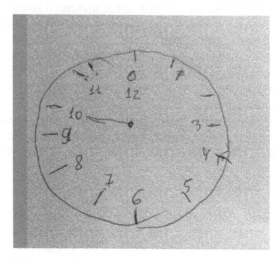

Figure 38.2 Clock drawing 2019 evaluation

patient and his family as well as his referring providers. Recommendations were also provided both verbally and in writing.

We made the following recommendations:

1 Metabolic and blood testing were strongly encouraged to ensure medication compliance and that necessary adjustments can be made.
2 We recommended recruiting this man's existing support system to help support his functioning in daily life. Importantly, his cognitive deficits and neuropsychiatric symptoms were framed in the context of a medical or physical illness to help reduce risks of stigma associated with these problems.
3 Although this patient may have been inclined to withdraw from social situations due to his cognitive problems, we advised him and his family to make opportunities for him to engage with others in a meaningful way to promote higher levels of cognitive engagement and better mood.
4 We offered his wife counseling caregiver support either with the examiner or, if she preferred, another Russian-speaking psychologist at our practice.
5 We advised the patient to identify a trusted advisor or confidant for making financial decisions. We also attempted to facilitate conversations around advanced care planning, power of attorney, and healthcare proxy.

Section III: Lessons Learned

- The health status of patients must be taken into consideration and careful review of medical records is strongly encouraged, including any available neurological and metabolic panels.
- Educational milestones, occupational history in their native country and the country of resettlement, and the degree of bilingual experiences should be considered, as they may impact cognitive performance.
- Mechanisms of translation should also be carefully examined before using adapted measures. Sociocultural factors, the linguistic and cultural gaps relative to the sample population of the test standardization must be considered.
- Although normative data for this population is limited, there is clinical value in obtaining neuropsychological performance at multiple timepoints for purposes of intra-individual comparisons.
- Like many cultures outside the United States, speed when completing tasks or standardized tests is not emphasized in Russian education in the manner it is within the United States.[31,33] Therefore, slow completion times on timed measures may reflect artifacts of this cultural difference rather than a true cognitive deficit.
- Signed consent to allow communication with the patient's treating providers (i.e., primary care, neurologist, psychiatrist) is encouraged to share diagnostic impressions and treatment recommendations, as patients and their families may be reticent to do so spontaneously, as was the case with this gentleman.
- Although this was not a pre-surgical evaluation, we feel it is important to emphasize that Russian-speaking patients referred for pre-surgical workups may need more assistance from trusted family members, which may be encouraged/emphasized at the time of the feedback.

Glossary

Soviet Union/Union of Soviet Socialist Republics (USSR).   A former socialist state lasting from 1922 to 1991 comprising multiple European and Asian republics who came together to topple the provisional government which had taken control following the fall of the Russian Monarchy.

References

1. Remennick L. Russian Jews on three continents: identity, integration, and conflict. New Brunswick (NJ): Transaction Publishers; 2013. p. 427.
2. US Census Bureau. American Community Survey (ACS) [Internet]. The United States Census Bureau; 2019 [cited 2021 May 22]. Available from: https://www.census.gov/programs-surveys/acs
3. Remennick L. Language acquisition, ethnicity and social integration among former Soviet immigrants of the 1990s in Israel. Ethn Racial Stud. 2004 May 1;27(3):431–54.
4. Russian Language. Wikipedia [Internet]. [cited 2021 May 22]. Available from: https://en.wikipedia.org/wiki/Russian_language
5. Chiswick BR. The occupational attainment of American Jewry: 1990 to 2000. Cont Jewry. 2007 Oct 1; 27(1):80–111.
6. Granovetter MS. The strength of weak ties. Am J Sociol. 1973;78(6):1360–80.
7. Althausen L. Journey of separation: elderly Russian immigrants and their adult children in the health care setting. Soc Work Health Care. 1993;19(1):61–75.
8. American Psychological Association. Ethical principles of psychologists and code of conduct (2002, amended effective June 1, 2010, and January 1, 2017) [Internet]. 2017. Available from: https://www.apa.org/ethics/code/
9. Leon DA, Chenet L, Shkolnikov VM, Zakharov S, Shapiro J, Rakhmanova G et al. Huge variation in Russian mortality rates 1984–94: artefact, alcohol, or what? Lancet. 1997 Aug 9;350(9075):383–8.
10. Shkolnikov VM, Cornia GA, Leon DA, Meslé F. Causes of the Russian mortality crisis: evidence and interpretations. World Dev. 1998 Nov 1;26(11):1995–2011.
11. Britton A, McKee M. The relation between alcohol and cardiovascular disease in Eastern Europe: explaining the paradox. J Epidemiol Community Health. 2000 May;54(5):328–32.
12. Gilmore A, Pomerleau J, McKee M, Rose R, Haerpfer CW, Rotman D et al. Prevalence of smoking in 8 countries of the former Soviet Union: results from the living conditions, lifestyles and health study. Am J Public Health. 2004 Dec;94(12):2177–87.
13. Mehler PS, Scott JY, Pines I, Gifford N, Biggerstaff S, Hiatt WR. Russian immigrant cardiovascular risk assessment. J Health Care Poor Underserved. 2001 May;12(2):224–35.
14. Fridman V, Vandalovsky E, Bergmann SR. Cardiac risk factors, medicine usage, and hospital course in immigrants from the former Soviet Union. J Health Care Poor Underserved. 2006 May;17(2):290–301.
15. Mehta NK, Elo IT. Migrant selection and the health of U.S. immigrants from the former Soviet Union. Demography. 2012 May;49(2):425–47.
16. Benisovich SV, King AC. Meaning and knowledge of health among older adult immigrants from Russia: a phenomenological study. Health Educ Res. 2003 Apr;18(2):135–44.
17. Blomstedt Y, Johansson S-E, Sundquist J. Mental health of immigrants from the former Soviet Bloc: a future problem for primary health care in the enlarged European Union? A cross-sectional study. BMC Public Health. 2007 Feb 28;7(1):27.
18. Stepanova Y. Mental health attitudes among Russian-speaking immigrants in the United States [Doctoral dissertation]. Fullerton (CA): California State University; 2019.
19. Kohn R, Flaherty JA, Levav I. Somatic symptoms among older Soviet immigrants: an exploratory study. Int J Soc Psychiatry. 1989;35(4):350–60.
20. Akhutina T, Shereshevsky G. Cultural-historical neuropsychological perspective on learning disability. In: Yasnitsky A, van der Veer R, Ferrari M., editors. The Cambridge handbook of cultural-historical psychology. Cambridge: Cambridge University Press; 2014. p. 350–77.
21. Tupper DE. Introduction: Alexander Luria's continuing influence on worldwide neuropsychology. Neuropsychol Rev. 1999 Mar 1;9(1):1–7.
22. Glozman JM. Russian neuropsychology after Luria. Neuropsychol Rev. 1999 Mar;9(1):33–44.
23. Mikadze YV, Ardila A, Akhutina TV. A.R. Luria's approach to neuropsychological assessment and rehabilitation. Arch Clin Neuropsychol. 2019 Aug 28;34(6):795–802.
24. Tupper DE. Introduction: neuropsychological assessment Après Luria. Neuropsychol Rev. 1999 Jun 1; 9(2):57–61.

25. Akhutina TV, Melikyan ZA, Mikadze YV, Mervis JE, Bisoglio J, Goldberg E. History of neuropsychology in Russia. In: Oxford Handbook of History of Clinical Neuropsychology [Internet]. 2016. doi:10.1093/oxfordhb/9780199765683.013.10

26. Akhutina TV, Pylaeva NM. Overcoming learning disabilities [Internet]. Cambridge: Cambridge University Press; 2012 [cited 2021 May 22]. Available from: https://www.cambridge.org/core/books/overcoming-learning-disabilities/CAE8F6C2EBBEAF26723132DE1B6DB7B3

27. Luria AR. The working brain [Internet]. New York (NY): Basic Books; 1973 [cited 2021 Feb 27]. Available from: https://www.goodreads.com/work/best_book/417216

28. Luria AR. Higher cortical functions in man [Internet]. New York (NY): Basic Books; 1980 [cited 2021 Feb 27]. Available from: https://www.goodreads.com/work/best_book/417216

29. Glozman JM. A.R. Luria and the history of Russian neuropsychology. J Hist Neurosci. 2007 Jun;16(1–2):168–80.

30. Glezerman A, Drexler ML. The Russian adaptation of the CERAD battery (CERAD-RA) [Internet]. San Francisco, CA; 2001. Available from: http://www.scarletline.com/aglezerman/CERAD.html

31. Agranovich AV, Puente AE. Do Russian and American normal adults perform similarly on neuropsychological tests?: preliminary findings on the relationship between culture and test performance. Arch Clin Neuropsychol. 2007 Mar 1;22(3):273–82.

32. Allen MJ, Yen WM. Introduction to measurement theory. IL: Waveland Press; 2001. p. 321.

33. Melikyan ZA, Puente AE, Agranovich AV. Cross-cultural comparison of rural healthy adults: Russian and American groups. Arch Clin Neuropsychol. 2021 Apr 21;36(3):359–70.

34. Gelfand DE. Assistance to the new Russian elderly. Gerontologist. 1986 Aug;26(4):444–8.

35. Day K, Cohen U. The role of culture in designing environments for people with dementia: a study of Russian Jewish immigrants. Environ Behav. 2000 May 1;32(3):361–99.

36. Morris JC, Heyman A, Mohs RC, Hughes JP, van Belle G, Fillenbaum G et al. The Consortium to Establish a Registry for Alzheimer's Disease (CERAD). Part I. Clinical and neuropsychological assessment of Alzheimer's disease. Neurology. 1989 Sep;39(9):1159–65.

37. Beeri MS, Schmeidler J, Sano M, Wang J, Lally R, Grossman H et al. Age, gender, and education norms on the CERAD neuropsychological battery in the oldest old. Neurology. 2006 Sep 26;67(6):1006–10.

38. Mendez MF, Ala T, Underwood KL. Development of scoring criteria for the clock drawing task in Alzheimer's disease. J Am Geriatr Soc. 1992 Nov;40(11):1095–9.

39. Suhr J, Grace J, Allen J, Nadler J, McKenna M. Quantitative and qualitative performance of stroke versus normal elderly on six clock drawing systems. Arch Clin Neuropsychol. 1998 Aug;13(6):495–502.

40. D'Elia LF, Satz P, Uchiyama CL, White T. Color Trails Test: professional manual. Odessa (FL): Psychological Assessment Resources; 1994.

41. Rosen WG. Verbal fluency in aging and dementia. J Clin Neuropsychol. 1980 Oct 1;2(2):135–46.

42. Mitrushina M, Boone KB, Razani J, D'Elia LF. Handbook of normative data for neuropsychological assessment. 2nd Edition. Oxford, New York: Oxford University Press; 2005. p. 1056.

43. Varkovetski M, Pihkanen K, Shanker S, Parris BA, Gurr B. What type of inhibition underpins performance on Luria's Fist-Edge-Palm task? J Clin Exp Neuropsychol. 2020 Aug;42(6):544–55.

44. Beery KE, Beery NA. The Beery-Buktenica Developmental Test of Visual-Motor Integration (Beery VMI): with supplemental developmental tests of visual perception and motor coordination and stepping stones age norms from birth to age six: administration, scoring, and teaching manual. Pearson; 2010.

45. Malloy P, Belanger H, Hall S, Aloia M, Salloway S. Assessing visuoconstructional performance in AD, MCI and normal elderly using the Beery Visual-Motor Integration Test. Clin Neuropsychol. 2003 Dec 1;17:544–50.

46. Randolph C. Repeatable Battery for the Assessment of Neuropsychological Status (RBANS). Psychological Corporation San Antonio (TX); 1998.

I. Sub-Saharan African
Overview

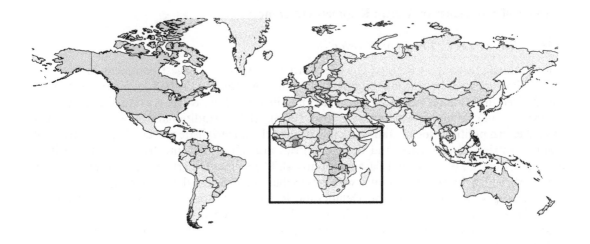

39 The Sub-Saharan African Context and the Birth of Neuropsychology

Jean N Ikanga and Lingani Mbakile-Mahlanza

Division of Sub-Saharan Africa: Regional Differences

Africa's History and Its Impact on Division

The World Bank Annual Report[1] considers Africa the second largest continent in both area (11.7 million square miles) and inhabitants (1.3 billion people) after Asia. Before colonization, Africa was divided into empires (e.g., Kongo, Luba) and kingdoms (e.g., Kush, Aksum, Carthage, Mali, Zimbabwe, etc.). After the conference of Berlin (1885), Africa's traditional frontiers were reshaped to fit Western political, social, and economic needs. The imperialistic powers divided Africa into many countries (53 countries) and these countries are subdivided into five regions (Northern, Southern, Central, Western, and Eastern countries). The Sahara Desert became another historical landmark, which divided Africa into two parts (Saharan and Sub-Saharan Africa).

As neuropsychologists from the Democratic Republic of Congo and Botswana, who were trained in the United States and Australia, we will focus on the Sub-Saharan Africa context in this chapter. This Sub-Saharan region is geographically and ethnoculturally distinct from the Middle East and North African region of primarily Arab League states. We will provide an overview of some relevant aspects of the region as well as the current state of the development of neuropsychology in the Sub-Saharan African context.

From Colonial Divisions to Linguistic Divisions

The conference of Berlin led Western countries to colonize Africa. Africa was divided mostly into French and British colonies (almost twenty-five countries each), Portuguese (six countries), Italian (five countries), German (four countries), Belgian and Spanish (three countries each) colonies. This colonial division led to three main African linguistic divisions involving English-, French-, and Portuguese-speaking countries. The colonization ignored African languages, which imperial powers considered as "poor" and inadequate for science and civilization. After colonization, many African leaders have tried to return to traditional roots and languages.

Linguists have estimated between 1,500 and 2,000 African languages.[2] These languages are subdivided into four groups: (1) Afro-Asiatic (spoken in the Northern Africa); (2) Nilo-Saharian (spoken mostly in Central and Eastern Africa); (3) Niger-Saharian/Niger-Congo (comprising of more than 1000 languages called Bantu and spoken in Central, Southern and Eastern Africa); and (4) Khoisan (mostly spoken in Western parts of Southern Africa[3]). Therefore, an African is apparently a polyglot who speaks the tribal language, national language, and colonial language.[4-6] During neuropsychological evaluations, it becomes important to consider which languages a person speaks and which language they might be most comfortable with for an evaluation.

DOI: 10.4324/9781003051862-79

Impact of Political Division

Colonization has shaped the African political life and antagonized ethnic divisions. As indicated previously, the two main colonial powers were British and French. The British imperial approach was of "assimilation," which wanted to make African countries an extension of the United Kingdom, with British training the next generation of African leaders and scientists. The French (also Belgians) imperial approach was the principle of "paternalism" where colonizers were considered as "fathers" and Africans as "children." Comparing the two approaches, the British approach has been "more conducive to growth" than the one of France or other colonizers, with British former colonies having had better political stability, economic growth, and public goods provision compared to French and other colonies.[7] In the Sub-Saharan Africa, neuropsychology has been taking roots mostly in British colonies. In addition, understanding this context can help appreciate the mindset that African migrants may have toward assimilation or acculturation in host countries.

Education and Its Barriers

The World Bank Annual Report[1] reported an increase in children completing primary school across the continent from 27% to 67% between 1971 and 2015. Yet, the educational system in Africa faces many challenges, including language barriers where children have to be educated either in colonial, national, or mother tongues. In its World Education Report,[8] the United Nations Educational, Scientific and Cultural Organization (UNESCO) pointed concerns about lack of facilities, libraries, manuals, and educators. Due to the low economic status of many Africans, parents may be unable to pay tuition, textbooks, and transportation costs for their children. In French-speaking countries, education is additionally challenged by ongoing conflicts/wars (e.g., Mali, Ivory Coast, Democratic Republic of Congo). Teachers in Africa also earn a very low salary, which can lead to corruption and low motivation. Overall, the educational system in Africa is not set to stimulate academic excellence but to build the intellectual scheme of "minimum" or "at least 5/10 passing grade." As a result, many children may be unable to read a letter, do basic calculations, or write an essay.[9] In its World Education Report,[8] UNESCO estimates rate of adult illiteracy in Africa to be at 39%. Women have the highest illiteracy rates (an estimated 94 million) since many girls tend to be forced to get married very young (between the ages of 12 and 14). Finally, there are differences in educational quality depending on proximity to urban areas as those in the city have greater access to materials.[10] As a result, inquiring about access to education, quality of education, and any barriers is crucial in a neuropsychological evaluation with the African population.

Cultural Considerations

Africa is a large continent with diversity of cultures, beliefs, and traditional systems that predominate it. However, there are some more frequent cultural traditions that are worth being aware of from a psychological perspective, with the understanding that each patient will have their own unique cultural beliefs to share.

Ancestors and Traditions

The ancestral wisdom and legacies in Sub-Saharan African societies have mostly been transmitted through oral tradition. Often, elders utilize evenings around the fire to transmit traditions through metaphors, symbolisms, proverbs, and stories. Through this process, elders build strong family bonds and emphasize the sense of tribe, clan, and family so an individual learns to be "We" rather than "I." This creates importance for tradition, respect for elders, and ancestors. From a neuropsychological perspective, the question remains whether many Africans' experience on auditory acquisition of information provides a benefit to verbal processing approach over visuospatial modalities. This remains an outstanding research question relevant to neuropsychology.

Belief in Supreme Being, Spirits, and Witchcraft

Many Africans believe in the Supreme being and in spirits which can be harmful to human beings.[11] One of the most harmful spirits is the "spirit of witches," which comes from witchcraft. Witchcraft is understood as "belief that the spirit of living human being can be sent out of the body on errands of doing havoc to other persons in body, mind, or estate."[11] John Mbiti[12] has argued that witches can operate in three ways: (1) alone; (2) through other human beings invisibly, or (3) through a lower creature such as an animal or a bird. Therefore, many Africans could generally find the origin of every biological, mental, and spiritual diseases in bad spirits and witchcraft. Any misfortunes in life and death could be viewed as caused by the spirits of witches in the family or clan. From a neuropsychological perspective, for example, epilepsy or seizures and neuropsychological syndromes could be viewed as a possession by evil spirits.

Traditional African Religions

These beliefs in the Supreme Being and spirits are the source of traditional religious activities. Many Africans have a strong sense of what is in the sphere of profane and sacred. They may offer rituals and incantations to God, spirits, and ancestors in every important life event (i.e., conception, marriage, birth, and death). Scholars have argued that "Religion is to the Africans an ontological phenomenon which pertains to the question of existence or being."[13] Many Sub-Saharan Africans tend to be Christians while Northern Africans tend to be Muslims. Therefore, Sub-Saharan Africans will easily discuss their faith during clinical interview or neuropsychological evaluation process.

Concept of Time

It has been argued that Africans do not have notion of time. John Mbiti[12] has articulated that time in Africa is an event rather than being mathematically oriented as it is in the Western cultures. Passed events are what mark the past time. The eventful moments of the present are what constitute the present. However, Mbiti continued in affirming that Africans do have shorter understanding of future. This Sub-Saharan African understanding of time can lead to conclude that Africans do not do longer planification of their life and anticipate life's events.[12] Another consequence of this notion of time is well expressed in the African saying: "There is no hurry in Africa." From a neuropsychological perspective, many Sub-Saharan Africans have difficulty with neuropsychological tests which require mathematical concepts of time or timing (e.g., processing speed, verbal fluency, etc.) and involve planning. Many experts have pointed out influences from the change in traditional agrarian-based African societies due to urbanization and modernization.[10]

Clinical Health Considerations

Many scholars have reported the presence of communicable diseases (CDs), particularly infectious diseases[14–16] and non-communicable diseases (NCDs) in Africa, which have neurological and neurocognitive sequelae.[17–19]

Infectious Diseases

Public health experts have indicated that infectious diseases are the most prominent source of burden and causes of illness in Sub-Saharan Africa.[14–16] The most prevalent CDs in Africa include infectious diseases such as tuberculosis, Human Immunodeficiency Virus/Acquired Immune Deficiency Syndrome (HIV/AIDS), typhoid fever, and parasitic infections such as human African trypanosomiasis ("sleeping sickness") and malaria.[20] Other prevalent infectious diseases in Africa include amoebiasis, neuroschistosimias, cysticercosis, neurocysticercosis, onchocerciasis, and Chagas disease. Tropical infectious diseases which are often neglected include filariases, leprosy, rabies, ascaris suum, and nematodes.[21] Finally, some areas of Sub-Saharan Africa (Democratic Republic of Congo, Guinea, Liberia, etc.) have been the epicenters of Ebola infection. Neuropsychological sequala of these infectious diseases in Africa have been neglected.

Toxic Diseases

Africa is also impacted by toxic diseases which therapeutically need neurocognitive expertise. Conditions which impact the nervous system include abuse of Khat (leaves of shoots of khat trees), konzo (a non-progressive motor neuron disorder associated with cassava toxicity), food preservation issues, snake venom exposure, as well as air and water pollution related toxicities.[21,22]

Psychiatric Disorders

Many Africans are exposed to violence, civil combat, and continual displacement. These traumatic events increase risks for psychiatric disorders such as depressive disorders, anxiety disorders, and trauma and stress-related disorders (post-traumatic stress disorder). As Hill-Jarret, Ikanga, and Stringer[10] have reported the presence of traumatic brain injuries among Africans exposed to wars, along with the presence of unsanitary hygienic practices and diseases of poverty among African refugees who are fleeing conflict conditions and political unrest. Many of these conflict and war-torn areas also struggling with food insecurity and malnutrition which has subsequent psychiatric manifestations.

Non-Communicable Diseases

The aging population in Sub-Saharan Africa is also grappling with NCDs such as cardiovascular disease, cancer, obesity, and neurodegenerative disorders.[17–19] These diseases are often associated with cognitive deficits,[23,24] but may not be adequately assessed, especially if using neuropsychological measures originally developed for non-African populations.

Health Care Barriers

African countries vary significantly in socio-economic status, but many African healthcare systems face difficult issues such as lack of trained healthcare professionals, absence of adequate medical equipment, neuroimaging, or diagnostic technologies.[25] The few healthcare professionals and medical equipment that do exist are often only in big cities and remain inaccessible to people in the rural areas.[10] This creates challenges for early identification and treatment of neuropsychologically relevant health conditions.

Current State of Neuropsychology in Sub-Saharan Africa

Although the last three decades have seen enormous growth in the field of neuropsychology, this growth has been more apparent in North America, Australia, and Europe. The profession in these regions is well established and several training and certification programs are available.[26] In contrast, academic programs for neuropsychology in Sub-Saharan Africa are sparse, mainly due to a shortage of financial and human resources. There is also a paucity of data on the number of neuropsychologists in practice as well as on the academic institutions that offer training in neuropsychology.[27]

Neuropsychology Training and Practice

Given the clinical issues and different disease conditions that face the continent, there is a great need to develop the discipline of neuropsychology in Africa. Yet, due to limited capacity in terms of training facilities, the few neuropsychology service providers that do exist, tend to receive their training outside the continent.

Countries such as South Africa have however made greater strides in training efforts. For example, a Master of Clinical Neuropsychology is offered at the University of Cape Town (UCT) and a Master of Clinical Neuropsychology program has also been established in Zambia. This program in Zambia is an 18-month program with a dissertation that has been running since 2009. To date, the program has produced around 60 Clinical Neuropsychologists. The majority of the people who took the course were already employed as Teachers, Special Education Teachers, Nurses, or doctors, who then went back to their place of work following the training. One joined the Department of Psychiatry as Lecturer and two joined the Department of Psychology of the University of Zambia. They all have strengthened these departments and delivery of services. There are others who have gone into private practice as counselors (personal communication with head of department). In Rwanda, a neuropsychology-training program has also recently been established in conjunction with Emory University.

In tandem with limited training programs in Sub-Saharan Africa, the practice of neuropsychology is also in its infancy. A recent literature review by Kissani and Naji[28] found only 7 published indexed articles related to the state of neuropsychology in Africa, highlighting low levels of focus on neuropsychology on the continent. There is even more varied service delivery and availability of neuropsychology across regions in Africa. For example, relatively speaking, there has been much more significant development of neuropsychology in South Africa, although the services are often only largely available to privileged few. Most other countries in Sub-Saharan Africa have no neuropsychologists or practice of neuropsychology. For example, in the Botswana context, neuropsychological assessment is still very limited due to a lack of neuropsychologists and health care facilities that specialize in the treatment and rehabilitation of cognitive impairment.[29] Countries such as Namibia and Botswana have one neuropsychologist in their respective country. In addition, since the description of what constitutes a neuropsychologist and the scope of practice is vague, other professionals such as psychiatrists, general practitioners, or neurologists are often called upon do neuropsychological work.[27]

Neuropsychological Testing Challenges

Neuropsychological tests are needed to screen for cognitive impairments caused by illnesses, diseases, and brain injuries,[30] as well as for recovery and rehabilitation. Yet, the majority of test batteries that are available and currently being used have been developed, normed, and standardized mainly in Western countries, and are not suitable in various regions of Sub-Saharan Africa, especially given the linguistic diversity on the continent.

While there remains an urgent need for robust cognitive tools that are culturally sensitive with good psychometric properties and consider effects of education and languages, there is currently an absence of focused efforts to develop different types of tools needed. This includes a lack of development of comprehensive neuropsychological batteries that require expertise to administer, as well as briefer cognitive assessments that are accurate at screening for neurocognitive disorders and can be administered by non-specialists, and functional assessments.

This is relevant because in the West, there is awareness that changes in brain function and structure are the earliest signs of progressive neurocognitive disorders, followed by cognitive and functional impairment.[31] High standards of care typically entail dementia diagnosis following comprehensive neurological, cognitive, functional, neuroimaging, and biomarker assessments. Yet, many countries in Africa lack both material and instrumental resources, and neuroimaging technology or biomarker studies are not readily available or too expensive. Along with a lack of culturally appropriate neuropsychological tests and normative data, this hampers good quality brain healthcare and creates barriers to diagnosis, treatment, and care for African patients.

In the Democratic Republic of Congo, Ikanga and Stringer[32] have developed the African Neuropsychological Battery (ANB) and efforts for validation across various countries are underway. The African Neuropsychological Battery consists of tests of visuospatial perception, language, memory, abstract reasoning, and problem solving, as well as sensory and motor screening tests. ANB uses content and stimuli that are based in Sub-Saharan Africa cultures, with versions in French, English, Swahili, Lingala, Tshiluba, and Kikongo. Initial research on the reliability and validity of the ANB has been encouraging. The individual ANB tests have been shown to have generally high internal consistency (0.64–0.93) and test-retest (0.44–0.91) reliability coefficients, comparable to similar tests used in Western countries.[33] Further, our team is examining whether currently available computerized and pen and paper-based tests often used to diagnose dementia can be culturally adapted and validated to improve the diagnosis of dementia for people in Botswana.

Research Developments in Neuropsychology

It is important to consider the clinical utility of the neuropsychological tests used and ensure that they are efficient and practical for various African contexts. The need for local standardization of tests cannot be over emphasized. There is currently limited investment in research infrastructure. Most of the current research in Sub-Saharan Africa focuses on HIV with funding mainly coming from the United States. For example, in Botswana a neurocognitive battery for assessing school-aged children and adolescents with HIV is being developed with a partnership between The University of Pennsylvania and the Botswana-Baylor Children's Center of Excellence in Gaborone.

The Future of Neuropsychology in Africa

Overall, there is a need for the countries in Sub-Saharan Africa to further develop and disseminate neuropsychology services across all levels of health care. One way this can happen is if positions for neuropsychology are created at the primary health care level. This can aid in early diagnosis and treatment and reduce the healthcare burden in their respective countries and de-centralize services in countries that do have services. As previously mentioned, resources are scarce in Sub-Saharan Africa, therefore we need to leverage what is already in existence in terms of resources. While there is a need to develop neuropsychology graduate programs in various countries, to ensure that services can be available more widely, it is also prudent to train non-neuropsychologists including psychometrists and psychology assistants, health auxiliaries, nurses and doctors, teachers, other psychologists as well as patients and their careers. This training could be in the form of professional development or short courses on brain health (assessment, diagnosis, protective factors, etc.). Further training on administering screening tools as well as more comprehensive assessments could be beneficial. There is also clearly a need to develop and utilize cognitive and functional assessment instruments that are culturally appropriate and adapted to common approaches to clinical evaluation across Sub-Saharan African countries. Local normative data collection also needs to be a priority. Capacity building in clinical service delivery and research needs to be a priority in Sub-Saharan Africa to further support the growth of neuropsychology in Africa.

References

1. World Bank 2020. The World Bank Annual Report 2020: supporting countries in unprecedented times. Washington (DC): World Bank Group; 2020.
2. Heine B, Nurse D. African languages: an introduction. Cambridge: Cambridge University Press; 2000. p. 396.
3. Greenberg J. Languages of Africa. Bloomington (IN): Indiana University; 1963. p. 171.
4. Bialystok E, Craik FIM, Luk G. Bilingualism: consequences for mind and brain. Trends Cogn Sci. 2012 Apr;16(4):240–50. Available from: https://www.ncbi.nlm.nih.gov/pmc/articles/PMC3322418/
5. Kave G, Eyal N, Shorek A, Cohen-Mansfield J. Multilingualism and cognitive state in the oldest old. Psychol Aging. 2008 Mar;23:70–8.
6. Schweizer TA, Ware J, Fischer CE, Craik FI, Bialystok E. Bilingualism as a contributor to cognitive reserve: evidence from brain atrophy in Alzheimer's disease. Cortex. 2012 Sep;48(8):991–6.
7. Lee A, Schultz K. Comparing British and French colonial legacies: a discontinuity of Analysis of Cameroon. Quart J Poli Sci. 2012 Feb 21;7:1–46.
8. United Nations Educational, Scientific and Cultural Organization. World education report 2000. Paris: UNESCO; 2000. p. 168.
9. Evans DK, Acosta AM. Education in Africa: what are we learning? J African Econ. 2021 Jan;30:13–54. doi:10.1093/jae/ejaa009
10. Hill-Jarret T, Ikanga J, Stringer AY. Neuropsychology in Africa. In: Kreutzer JS, DeLuca J, Caplan B, editors. Encyclopedia of clinical neuropsychology. 2nd ed. New York (NY): Springer; 2018. p. 3773.
11. Emeka CE, Ekeopara C. God, divinities and spirits in African traditional religious ontology. Amer J Social Man. 2010 Dec;1(2):209–18.
12. Mbiti J. Introduction to the African religion and philosophy. 2nd ed. Johannesburg: Heinemann; 1989. p. 288.
13. Nieder-Heitmann JH. An analysis and evaluation of John S. Mbiti's theological evaluation of African traditional religions [dissertation]. University of Stellenbosch; 1981.
14. Fenollar F, Mediannikov O. Emerging infectious diseases in Africa in the 21st century. New Microbes New Infect. 2018 Nov;26:S10–8.
15. Gouda HN, Charlson F, Sorsdahl K, Ahmadzada S, Ferrari AJ, Erskine H et al. Burden of non-communicable diseases in sub-Saharan Africa, 1990–2017: results from the Global Burden of Disease Study 2017. Lancet Glob Health. 2019 Oct 1;7(10):1375–87.
16. Mudie K, Jin M, Tan, Kendall L, Addo J, Dos-Santos-Silva I et al. Non-communicable diseases in sub-Saharan Africa: a scope review of large cohort studies. J Glob Health. 2019 Dec;9(2):020409.
17. Lekoubou A, Echouffo-Tceugui JB, Kengne AP. Epidemiology of neurodegenerative diseases in Sub-Saharan Africa: a systematic review. BMC Publ Health. 2014 Jun 26;14:653.
18. Lopez AD, Williams TN, Levin A, Tonelli M, Singh JA, Burney PGJ et al. Remembering the forgotten non-communicable diseases. BMC Med. 2014 Oct 22;12:200.
19. Ravindranath V, Dang H-M, Goya R, Mansour H, Nimgaonkar V, Russell V et al. Regional research priorities in brain and nervous system disorders. Nature. 2015 Nov 18;527:S198–206.

20. Karim SSA, Churchyard GJ, Karim QA, Lawn SD. HIV infection and tuberculosis in South Africa: an urgent need to escalate the public health response. Lancet. 2009 Sep 12;374(9693):921–33.

21. Bentivoglio M, Cavalheiro EA, Kristensson K, Pater NB. Neglected tropical diseases and conditions of the nervous system. New York (NY): Springer; 2014. p. 401.

22. Boivin MJ, Giordani B. Neuropsychology of children in Africa: perspectives on risk and resilience. New York (NY): Springer; 2013. p. 347.

23. Mavrodaris A, Powell J, Thorogood M. Prevalence of dementia and cognitive impairment among older people in sub-Saharan Africa: a systematic review. Bull World Health Org. 2013 Oct 1;91(10):773–83.

24. Yiengprugsawan VS, Browning CJ. Non-communicable diseases and cognitive impairment: pathways and shared behavioral risk factors among older Chinese. Frontiers Public Health. 2019 Oct 23;7:296.

25. Mbakile-Mahlanza L, Manderson L, Downing M, Ponsford J. Family caregiving of individuals with traumatic brain injury in Botswana. Disab Rehab. 2017 Mar;39(6):559–67.

26. Ponsford J. International growth of neuropsychology. Neuropsychology. 2017 Nov;31(8):921–33.

27. Truter S, Mazabow M, Morlett Paredes A, Rivera D, Arango-Lasprilla JC. Neuropsychology in South Africa. Applied Neuropsy Adult. 2017 Mar 21;25(4):344–55.

28. Kissani N, Naji Y. Neuropsychology in developing countries: what situation for the African continent. J Neurosci Neuropsy. 2020;3:107.

29. Mbakile-Mahlanza L, Manderson L, Ponsford J. The experience of traumatic brain injury in Botswana. Neuropsy Rehab. 2015 Jan 6;25(6):936–58.

30. Zhang JY, Feinstein A. Screening for cognitive impairments after traumatic brain injury: a comparison of a brief computerized battery with the Montreal Cognitive Assessment. Clin Res Reports. 2016 Jun 3;28(4):328–31.

31. Jack Jr CR, Knopman DS, Jagust WJ, Petersen RC, Weiner MW, Aisen PS et al. Tracking pathophysiological processes in Alzheimer's disease: an updated hypothetical model of dynamic biomarkers. Lancet Neurol. 2013 Feb;12(2):207–16.

32. Ikanga J, Bragg P, Howard C, Stringer A. African enculturation and performance on the African Neuropsychology Battery. Paper Presented at: National Academy of Neuropsychology Conference; 2019 June 5; San Diego.

33. Ikanga J, Basterfield C, Taiwo Z, Bragg P, Bartlett A, Howard C et al. The reliability of the African neuropsychology battery: data from Congo and America. Arch Clin Exper Neuropsych. Forthcoming 2021.

Nigerian

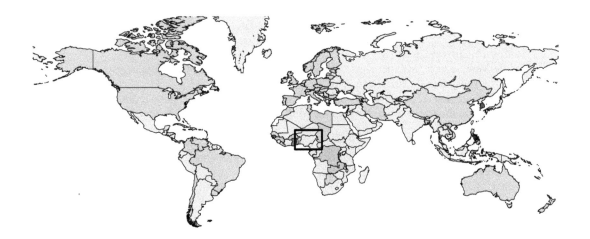

40 The Use of Neuropsychological Assessment in Psychiatric Treatment Formulation in Nigeria

Valentine Afamefuna Ucheagwu
and Bruno Joseph Giordani

Section I: Background Information

Terminology and Perspective

Nigeria is a country located in sub-Saharan Africa with a predominantly Black population of Nigerians. People are known as Nigerians, but by its composition, it is a multi-ethnic country with over 250 indigenous languages and multi-ethnic identification. Nigeria prides herself on the maxim: Unity in Diversity. For ease of communication, the national language is English (British English).

My (VAU) perspective is that of a bilingual, Nigerian trained clinical/counseling psychologist who received additional post-doctoral training at the University of Michigan in Neuropsychology. I teach (undergraduate and post-graduate) and do research at Nnamdi Azikiwe University Awka, which is a public university in southeast (SE) Nigeria. I am engaged in the private practice of clinical psychology and neuropsychological assessment in a suburban town near my university. My practice interest is on assessment and psychotherapy of severe mental disorders and mild cognitive impairment. Due to the nature of the patients that I see, I collaborate with other mental health professionals, particularly psychiatrists and social workers.

BJG is a professor of psychiatry, neurology, psychology, and nursing at the University of Michigan Ann Arbor. He has garnered over four decades of experience in clinical psychology, physiological psychology, and neuropsychology as a researcher, lecturer, and practitioner. He trains and mentors post-doctoral fellows in neuropsychology and was the former head of the Neuropsychology section, Department of Psychiatry, University of Michigan. Presently, Dr. Giordani is the chief psychologist in psychiatry, the associate director of the Michigan Alzheimer's Disease Research Center and senior director of Mary A. Rackham Institute at the University of Michigan. He has done extensive neuropsychology research in Africa and was co-editor of the first book on neuropsychology of children in Africa.[1]

The below information is provided from the authors' perspective and their knowledge of Nigeria and her people.

Geography

The Federal Republic of Nigeria is a West African country on the Gulf of Guinea. It is the largest democracy on the continent with estimated population of over 210 million people by 2020 (www. Worldometer.info). Nigeria is made up of 36 states and 6 geo-political zones, based on similar ethnic groups, and/or common political history. Nigeria shares land borders with the Republic of Niger to the north, Chad to the northeast, Cameroon to the east, and Benin to the west. The coastal region is a low-lying area with sandy beaches and mangrove swamps which merge into an

DOI: 10.4324/9781003051862-81

area of rainforest where palm trees grow to over 30 m (100 ft). From here the landscape changes to savannah and open woodland, rising to the central Jos Plateau at 1800 m (6000 ft). The northern part of the country is desert and semi-desert, marking the southern extent of the Sahara.

History

Nigeria in the pre-colonial years was comprised of independent entities existing and surviving within their regional ethnic spaces. In the eastern part of the country, we have predominantly Igbo people and other ethnic groups. In the west, we have predominantly the Yoruba ethnic group while in the north we find the Hausa and the Fulani with other ethnic minorities. Before colonization, people were governed by kings and traditional rulers including the Ezes (for the Igbos), Obas (for the Yorubas), and Emirs (for the Hausas/Fulanis). In pre-colonial days, Nigeria was governed via protectorates. The colonizers divided the country into northern and southern protectorates with various systems of governance depending on the behavior of the protectorate. In the southern protectorate, the eastern part is governed through indirect rule and the use of warrant chiefs. Because of the political interests of her colonial rulers, Nigeria in 1914 was amalgamated, thereby joining the southern and northern protectorates to become one Nigeria. As some individuals will argue, the amalgamation was not in the interest of the people as they were not consulted before the amalgamation. Some argue that the culture and historical origins of the two protectorates did not warrant amalgamation. To some extent this appears to be true as there are many agitations from various regions in the country for outright break away from Nigeria. The most recent is the agitation from the Indigenous People of Biafra (IPOB) for an independent nation-state.[2]

Nigeria had her independence from British colonial rulers in 1960 followed by post-independence civil war in 1967 (between the then old Eastern region and the rest of the country) that lasted for three years. Many agitators (like the IPOB and other) from different regions of the country are of the opinion that the reasons for the civil war have not been resolved. Post-civil war, the country has been ruled by the military with coups and counter coups that have devastated the country socio-economically and psychologically. Currently, Nigeria is running a democratic system of governance. To some extent Nigeria is more divided across ethnic polarities that negatively affect social behaviors including group to group and person to person interactions across ethnic lines.

People

The case presented in this chapter is that of a male from the *Igbo*-speaking part of Nigeria, specifically SE Nigeria. Aside from the Igbo ethnic group, Nigeria has other ethnic groups including the *Hausa, Yoruba, Ibibio, Itsekiris, Ijaws*, etc. However, there are three major ethnic groups in Nigeria: Igbo, Hausa, and Yoruba. For the purpose of this chapter, the following background information will focus on the Igbo ethnic community.

The SE Nigerians are known by other regions of the country for hard work and diligence. They are predominantly entrepreneurs and can be found all over the country. The nature of their entrepreneurialism begins with apprenticeship after 12 years of education. Apprenticeship in this situation is synonymous to mentoring whereby the apprentice spends five to six years learning a particular trade under a mentor who has been in the business for a given number of years. It is expected that after a period of apprenticeship, the trainee will be given some funds and other social supports by the master and members of the trainee's family to start his own business. This opportunity is not gender specific, although career choice and selection is, to a large extent, gender related. There are businesses that are taken as male related while there are others that are taken as female related.

Immigration and Relocation

The SE people of Nigeria are known for migration and relocation from their ancestral homes for business-related opportunities. One remarkable thing about this group of Nigerians is their inherent capacity to adapt to their new environments and contribute immensely to building their host environment. The SE people have the culture of returning to their ancestral homes once every year, particularly during Christmas time to reunite with their kinsmen.

Language and Communication

The SE people of Nigeria have a traditional language known as the Igbo language. The remarkable thing about the Igbo language is its variants in dialects within the language. This means that among the Igbo-speaking people, there are different forms of dialects with one dialect central among them all. Communication within the region is through the central dialect, although individuals from a given area within the region communicate together in their own form of dialect. Nigeria, because of its multi-ethnic nature, adopted the English language (the language of her colonial rulers) as their formal means of communication. The SE people, like other Nigerians from other regions of the country, have an elementary knowledge of the English language to enable them to communicate with people from other regions of the country. There are times when interpreters may be needed particularly during psychological and neuropsychological assessment. There are some English words that a client with six years of education may not be able to understand if it was not interpreted in the client's local language.

Education

Nigeria runs a 6-6-4 system of education that includes six years of primary education, six years of secondary school education (three years of junior secondary and three years of senior secondary), and four years of tertiary education. The government has a standing mandate that all Nigerian children have at least nine years of education (six years primary and three years junior secondary) and in line with that has made level of education free for all citizens. The SE people are known to attend a minimum of nine years of education before starting apprenticeship. Generally, people from low socio-economic strata strive to finish 9 to 12 years of education before going to learn a trade. Children with behavior problems or low sufficient intellectual endowment may have significant difficulty in education and often complete only the sixth or ninth year of education. The literacy rate in Nigeria is improving due to government insistence on nine years minimum education. There is rise in university education secondary to the increase in private universities, part-time university education, and government subsidies to public universities to help citizens afford university education.

Socio-Economic Status

Compared to other regions of Nigeria, the poverty rate appears lower in SE part of Nigeria (https://zerofy.ng/poorest-tribes/). This is attributed to their love for trade, an entrepreneurial spirit, and independent minds. Although Nigerian society tends to be highly egalitarian and collectivistic, the SE people, considering that trait, have a high level of independence and motivation for success when compared with other regions of the country. Among Nigerians, the people of the SE are more successful, particularly in business.

Values and Customs

The SE Nigerians attach strong values to family, kinship, marriage, morality, and life. They view life as sacred and can only be given and taken by God. They have strong family values and take maintaining family relationships very seriously. They have strong beliefs in a kinship system and practice a patriarchal family system. They value and maintain their lineage and ancestral heritages and practices.

Gender and Sexuality

The SE, and indeed all of Nigeria, are a male-oriented society, although gender equality is recently gaining attention. The male is believed to be and seen as the head of the family and takes significant responsibility for the security and upkeep of the family. Traditionally, it is the males that pay dowry for marriage, and expectations are that the woman in return changes her name to that of the groom's family. People are always expected to dress decently and not to give an impression of promiscuity in dress. Same-sex relationships and marriages are seen as taboo in SE and are not allowed by law in Nigeria. Sexual minorities tend to do so in secret to avoid public stigma, rejection, and punishment. Sexual discussions and sex education were not common during the examinee's childhood. Children and adolescents rarely talk or ask questions about genitals and sexual issues with parents although they may secretly discuss with peers. Although, recently in Nigeria, there are rising efforts to promote sex education.

Spirituality and Religion

The Igbo people of Nigeria are very religious and believe very much in the existence of spirits and life after death. There are various totems and deities that are worshipped and or venerated in the Igbo land, and people believe that such gods determine their survival in life and in the world beyond. The people's religion is tied to their day-to-day lives and reflected in the names they give their children.

With the advent of Christianity, a majority of the people from the SE were converted to Christianity. It has been over a century and half since the Christian religion came into the region. Christianity has flourished in the SE (https://en.wikipedia.org/wiki/Christianity in Nigeria) such that pastors are all indigenous and are also moving out to other parts of the world for evangelism. However, one also observes that in spite of adherence to Christianity, SE people also carry along with them the traces of their traditional religion and always find a way to reconcile it with their Christian beliefs. For example, SE people believe in reincarnation, influence of the dead on the living, and spirit possession. To a significant extent, the Christians of SE region believe that the cause of their problems is spiritual and more or less man-made. A typical SE person is more likely to believe that the cause of his/her child's psychotic reactions is evil eyes cast upon the family by an enemy. In that case, they inadvertently ignore the science behind the sickness. This belief will significantly affect a family's solution for the problem. They are more likely to look for an exorcist in the Christian religion to help cast away the evil spirit or consult a traditional witch doctor or healer to help with the problem.

Mental Health Views

There are misconceptions about mental health in Nigeria, predominately characterized by the notion that mental health issues are the result of evil spirit possession and can be treated with prayers and or by a traditional way of exorcism. Even when a person is taken to the hospital, the family is still in dissonance as to whether orthodox management will help. Particularly in dementia and psychosis, patients are misunderstood and sometimes misdiagnosed. When patients are misunderstood and family perceives their behavior as intentional, they are often treated harshly. There is present awareness and efforts by professional bodies to encourage people to understand that mental illness is another physical illness, and that patients should be understood and loved.

Approaches to Neuropsychological Assessment in Nigeria

Neuropsychological assessment is a nascent area in Nigeria. There is no post-graduate training that has neuropsychology as a separate area of study. Some limited aspects of brain influence on behavior are taught in clinical psychology programs at masters and doctoral levels. Overall, clinical psychologists in Nigeria test for brain dysfunction during their psychological assessment. The main aim of this evaluation is to determine the extent to which presenting psychiatric behaviors or symptoms have an organic origin. Predominantly, the Bender Visual Motor Gestalt Test (BVMGT)[3] and the Mini Mental Status Examination (MMSE)[4] are used as initial tests of organicity during psychiatric assessment in Nigeria. The scope of neuropsychology is otherwise just emerging.

Section II: Case Study — "I Am Ok, It's Just That I Cannot Concentrate or Learn What You Are Teaching"

Note: Possible identifying information and several aspects of history and presentation have been changed to protect patient identity and privacy.

Behavioral Observations

Chidi (male, 41 years old) came to a community rehabilitation center at the insistence of his outpatient psychiatrist who had been seeing him for over 18 months. The referral was for inpatient cognitive and emotional rehabilitation of schizophrenic symptoms, medication management, and neuropsychological evaluation due to treatment resistance.

Chidi was neatly dressed, except that the side beards were not shaved. He came in the company of the elder sister and his brother-in-law. In severe psychiatric cases, patients are accompanied by their relatives who will be able to give a detailed history of the patient and sit in for the patient's psychiatric admission. Upon arrival to the center, he was restless, pacing within the waiting room and was asking his sister what to do and when to see the doctor. On entering the consulting room, he was very quick to greet the doctor (VAU) and try to initiate rapport. Overall, his behavior suggested an anxious disposition and uncertainty. This was understandable, as his psychiatrist had told him and the family that he would be admitted to the center for behavioral rehabilitation. This clinical decision did not go down well with Chidi, and he was hoping that the clinicians at the rehabilitation center would not find him so distressed to be admitted. In Nigeria, the family of a severely psychiatrically impaired patient makes the decision for hospitalization, particularly if the person is judged as incapable of making sound decisions. This was the situation in which Chidi found himself, and he felt he was at the mercy of the clinicians at the rehabilitation center to determine if he would be admitted for treatment or would go back to his home to continue outpatient treatment with his psychiatrist.

The first meeting with Chidi and his family was an initial therapeutic interview. Here I (VAU) discussed with Chidi and his family the presenting concerns, the report from the psychiatrist, as well as the family report. Using motivational interviewing and insight-oriented techniques of interviewing, Chidi became convinced of the need to stay in the rehabilitation center to work on the emotional and behavioral concerns presented by the family and the attending psychiatrist. At the end of the 1-hour interview, Chidi agreed to rehabilitation for one month.

Presenting Concerns

Chidi presented with severe auditory hallucinations and somatic and persecutory delusions. He said he heard voices talking to him from Zimbabwe and that his late mother talked to him at times. He believed that he was an Angel of God and that he had powers to heal. Many times, he replied to the voices that were talking to him, as if they heard him. Chidi always complained that he found it hard to understand complex discussions and alleged that someone removed something from his body and that was the cause of his inattention and inability to understand. Chidi was sent to Onitsha in Anambra state to learn a trade after his secondary school education. Often, he accused the master of removing glomerulus from his body and that the removal of the glomerulus made his penis very small and that no woman would marry him. He also alleged that the removal of the glomerulus was the origin of his mental confusion. Although it was somehow clear to Chidi that his behavior was not normal, he believed firmly in the reality of the voices he heard and his delusions, including the belief that some people were after him and wanted to take his destiny or good luck.

Daily Functioning

Chidi performed fairly well in activities of daily living (ADL), but poorly in instrumental ADL. For example, he could wash his clothes, take his bath, and manage money to buy things from the grocery store for his upkeep. However, he found it very difficult to keep his room clean and attend to daily routines without further prompting and could not manage his bills. He was always occupied with thoughts and voices coming to his mind and could respond to the voices for close to six hours without stopping. Due to this, he was incapacitated for daily events and was not able to hold a job. He was not able to manage his psychiatric medications as prescribed by his psychiatrist, making adherence very poor. He could become very aggressive with his family members, particularly when his delusion and hallucinations were challenged.

Health History

Chidi's family denied any problems with his birth and early development. However, they noted that he was impulsive in behavior while growing up as a teenager. Chidi further reported no physical ailments, even now as an adult other than periodic malaria, which he treated with anti-malarial medicine, as many Nigerians do. He denied ever being diagnosed with cerebral or acute malaria that required hospitalization. His malaria as the patient reported was mild and lasted two to four days. His most recent physical examination and blood work ordered by his psychiatrist were unremarkable. He had no history of smoking, drinking, or other forms of drug abuse.

Chidi was involved in a serious physical fight three years prior to seeing the psychiatrist that left him with some bruises on his body. Chidi has been manifesting symptoms since his secondary school completion. The fight was a result of his brother challenging his delusion. After the fight, they had to send him back to Nigeria from Zimbabwe (because of their inability to manage his delusions). Family medical history was remarkable for two of his elder brothers being diagnosed with schizophrenia and manic disorder, respectively, prior to Chidi developing his symptoms.

Educational History

Chidi completed 12 years of education in Nigeria, meaning that he had completed primary and secondary school education and had passed the senior secondary certificate examination by the West African Examination Council. He was an average student during his primary and secondary school days and had not repeated any class. He attempted entrance examination into university but was not successful because his score did not reach the university entrance point. According to Chidi, he was not able to pass the entrance examination organized by the Joint Admission and Matriculation Board at two sittings, and so decided to go for apprentice to learn shoe trading instead.

Language Proficiency

Chidi is bilingual and speaks Igbo and English languages fluently. He first acquired Igbo language, because that was the mother tongue learned through his family prior to starting formal education. For Nigerians, English is acquired when formal education is started in kindergarten. English was the vehicle of communication in Nigerian schools and so Chidi was also proficient in the English language and sat for his final exam in the secondary school. When asked about his fluency in the language, he said he had better proficiency in speaking and understanding Igbo language, but better proficiency in writing in English. It was clear that Chidi's dominant language was Igbo, followed by English and then Ndebele. His English language proficiency was sufficient to match education and age-based expectations of available English-based neuropsychological test measures to be administered. He expressed a preference for testing in English and further explanation in Igbo language when the need arose. This approach to use a language combination in both English and Igbo languages was the most accurate way to ensure that the testing captured his current cognitive status.

Cultural and Personal History

Chidi came from a monogamous family and was the last of eight children (five boys and three girls) born into a Catholic family in SE Nigeria. Chidi lived with his parents and siblings while growing up in an urban area 20 km from their native village. Consistent with the Igbos of Nigeria, they combined traditional beliefs with Christian doctrine. Prior to the coming of the missionaries, the people had their beliefs and conceptions about God and existence. Even after accepting the Christian religion, they still fall back to their traditional beliefs while explaining the nature and cause of events. His family believed strongly that human parts could be used for rituals to acquire wealth. This may account for why Chidi strongly believed that his glomerulus was removed by his master and that was why he found it difficult to concentrate and believed that he could not get a woman pregnant, even though he never tried.

Chidi's father was an upper-middle-class Nigerian engaged in cloth trading. He was able to build houses in the city and one in the village. His mother was also very industrious and joined in her husband's trade. Chidi reported being happy during childhood and presented no history of abuse, whether physical, emotional, or sexual. He reported that his experience of failure started when he noticed that his penis was very small and did not look like that of his peers. He indicated feeling inferior and self-devalued as he had no one with whom to share his concerns. He said that it will be an abomination to discuss such thoughts with his parents or his elder siblings. Furthermore, all the efforts he made to get a girlfriend were not successful, though his mates were moving forward in heterosexual relationships during the last year of secondary school. At graduation, he managed to interact with a girl, but was totally discouraged by her mother who noticed the relationship. Since then, Chidi started masturbating to gratify his sexual urges because he continued to believe that his penis was small and that he was not capable of having meaningful and lasting relationships. Also, he believed that being in an amorous relationship would put him at crossroad with the God, as his mother had always preached.

After two attempts to enter university, Chidi, at the advice of the parents and siblings, opted for apprenticeship. In apprenticeship, you are asked to live with a person who has mastered the trade. You are to live with the person and learn the trade for at least five to seven years. The essence is to master the skills of the business and be independent to start your own business. Chidi stayed with someone who was in the business of importing and selling shoes. It was one year into the learning of the trade that Chidi started complaining of psychotic symptoms. His first symptom presentation was at the age of 20. In their time, it was the culture that new boys that came to learn trade would be initiated into manhood. This is no other thing than the person's private parts be shaved by the older apprentice in the evening. It was a traumatic experience for Chidi, as he was already ashamed of the smallness of his penis and did not want to expose it to people.

In my analytic interpretation, I saw that as part of the precipitating factor that led to the collapse of ego defense mechanisms and paved the way for anxiety and subsequent psychotic manifestations. It was two weeks after this ritual that Chidi reported gradual onset of anxiety, complaints of voices which at first were taken as simple worries, then as they persisted began to focus on evil spirit possession and later founded the reason to consult the first psychiatrist he met. Since then, Chidi has met with five different psychiatrists and has been on anti-psychotic medications. At one point, he had remission then traveled to Zimbabwe to live with his senior brother and help in trading. He was able to hold on for six months before relapse. Part of the relapse as presented by his elder sister was his inability to manage his medication and total refusal for others to help him. When he could not stay with his brother's family in Zimbabwe, he was brought back to Nigeria.

Emotional Functioning

Chidi was emotionally unstable with high levels of anxiety and insomnia when he presented to the clinic. He was always worried and confused about the thoughts and voices bombarding his head, as well as having to put up with the family challenging the authenticity of his thoughts and voices. He was further worried about his inability to start a trade and his family's unwillingness to sponsor him in another trade because of his emotional instability.

Preliminary Formulation

At the end of the initial therapeutic interview with Chidi and the family (two elder sisters), followed by another two weeks of hospital observation in our center, it was clear that Chidi suffered from schizophrenia. In our center, we follow the DSM-5 diagnostic criteria augmented with clinical objective and projective tests and neuropsychological assessment when need arises. In Nigeria the use of neuropsychological assessment in psychiatric hospitals is not common. Chidi met DSM-5 criteria for schizophrenia. He presented symptoms of delusion, hallucination, disorganized speech and grossly disorganized behavior, particularly silliness and resistance to instructions. He had marked disturbance in the level of functioning in work, social relationship, interpersonal relationship and IADL as compared to prior onset of his disorder. He was diagnosed with this disorder more than ten years before coming to our center. His behavioral disturbance was not attributed to physiological effects of a substance or another medical condition. Since the referral appeal was for inpatient cognitive and emotional rehabilitation, medication management, and neuropsychological evaluation following treatment resistance, Chidi was admitted to the male public ward for psychotherapy and medication management.

One remarkable thing that we observed was that he always complained following individual and group psychotherapy that he could not concentrate or understand the teachings in psychotherapy groups. The group psychotherapy was a didactic form that was based on psychoeducation while the individual therapy was interpersonal process therapy with high level of integration with other therapies. Based on his referral for neuropsychology and informed of neuropsychology literatures on subtypes of schizophrenia with varied neuropsychological presentations, we administered neuropsychological tests to Chidi one month after his admission in the rehabilitation center to better understand brain–behavior relationship in the illness.

Test and Norm Selection

We selected an available test battery that could be administered to Chidi based on his age and educational achievements and also based on history of the test having been used for research in Nigeria. One benefit of neuropsychological testing in Nigeria is that many of the tests can be administered in the English language and language proficiency tends to be relatively good. This is because many Nigerians are exposed to the English language, because that is the lingua franca and is learned in kindergarten. For individuals with 12 years of education, understanding and doing neuropsychological tests in English language is not difficult. Moreover, in our rehabilitation center we have a culture of giving task instructions in both English and local languages to improve task understanding. That said, we also acknowledge that no comprehensive demographically corrected normative neuropsychological test data are available for Nigerians, although some of the tests have been used locally for studies. Where applicable we use test norms derived from local samples. Otherwise, original test norms and clinical judgment were used for test interpretation of this client.

The following tests were available for administration:

1 Montreal Cognitive Assessment (MoCA)[5]
2 Bender Visual Motor Gestalt Test (BVMGT): The Hutt Adaptation as presented by Lack[6] was used for assessment of organic dysfunction in the client.
3 Number Span Test (J Kramer)[7]: Forward and Backward
4 Craft Story 21 Recall (S Craft)[8]: Immediate and Delayed
5 Benson Complex Figure Copy (J Kramer)[9]: Immediate, Delayed and Recognition
6 Trail Making Test: Part A & B
7 Multi-lingual Naming Test (MINT) (TH Gollan)[10]
8 Verbal Fluency: Phonemic Test (F,L) (AE Hillis)[11]
9 Paced Auditory Serial Addition Test (PASAT) (DM Gronwall)[12]

For number span test, Craft Story 21, Benson Complex Figure Copy and Verbal Fluency: Phonemic Test see Uniform Data Set (UDS) of the National Alzheimer's Coordinating Center (NACC).[8,9]

Test Results and Impressions

Chidi performed below the norm on the MoCA which measures global cognition. His score of 23 as against Normal ≥26 (See NACC UDS Version 3.0 form C2) suggested global cognitive impairment. Nigerian data for people between the ages 50 and 70 was >20 for education above 12 years and >15.75 for 12 years education.[13] Using those local norms, Chidi scored above the mean score for his education group although his age of 41 was very much below the age norms. Overall, the impression was that Chidi may be operating within a borderline range for global cognition.

Subtest analysis for MoCA showed that Chidi performed very poorly on delayed verbal recall (0/5) and language fluency (5/11 per 60 seconds). This accounted for his overall poor performance. On BVMGT brain impairment indices, he had four impairment indices on simplification (Bender drawing, figure 3), perseveration (Bender drawing, figure 3), closure difficulty (Bender drawings, figures 7 and 8) and angulation difficulty (Bender drawing, figure 2) and took 25 minutes to draw the figures against a 15-minute benchmark[6] with extreme care and deliberation. The total error score was 5 showing possible organic dysfunction.[6] On Benson Complex Figure test, he performed well above the norm (N) on immediate recall: 16/17 (N > 15) and delayed recall: 15/17 (N > 12.8) as well as recognition where he recognized the original stimulus from the four options. His Trails A & B was without error and within normal time (Trail A: <150 seconds; Trail B: <300 seconds).

His Craft Story 21 immediate recall was 17/44 (Mean(N) > 22.8, SD: 6.8) while delayed recall was 19/44 (N > 21.3, SD: 6.1). Although his scores were below the mean, they did not fall below 1 SD from the mean. His Number Span Test Forward: total correct was 10/14 (N > 8.8, SD:2.7); length of longest correct series: 7/14 (N > 6.8, SD: 1.3) were above the mean score but not up to 1 SD above the mean and the Backward: total correct: 5/14 (N > 8, SD:2.9); length of longest correct series: 4 (N > 5.5, SD: 1.7) were below the mean and 1SD. He appeared to manifest impairment in attention and concentration as well as measure of working memory. His PASAT score was 41/60 (N > 46.7, SD:9.1) was 1SD below the mean.

His MINT total score was 25/32 (N > 29.7, SD: 1.7) which was below the mean and 2 SD below the mean. On phonemic verbal fluency he scored 4/40 (N > 14.8, SD: 3.2) on F and 5/40 (N > 14.4, SD:3.9) on L. Obviously he performed below 4 SD from the mean on F and L, respectively.

Overall, the picture of the neuropsychological test presented some remarkable issues for psychiatric diagnosis and management:

1 There was concern about organicity (brain impairment) following Chidi's BVMGT and MoCA performance.
2 His visual–spatial performance as evidenced from Benson figure test and Trails showed no impairment.
3 There was significant impairment in language naming and verbal phonemic fluency tests signifying serious impairment in language, executive function, and frontal lobe dysfunction.
4 Poor performance on PASAT and number span particularly the backward showed impairment in attention and concentration as well as working memory load.
5 Attention and concentration impairments coupled with his verbal fluency and language impairments likely accounted for his inability to make sense of his psychotherapy sessions. Psychotherapy is a complex exercise that requires reasonable cognitive entry for proper understanding especially with the more verbally dependent forms of psychotherapy that Chidi was receiving.

Feedback Session for Further Treatment

Feedback was presented to the treatment team at hospital conference meeting following assessment. It is the tradition of the rehabilitation center to hold weekly conference meeting of treating professionals to discuss treatment outcomes of their patients as well as review reports of psychological assessments. Chidi's neuropsychological report was presented to the board and below were the consensus decisions following his report:

1 Chidi was switched from talk therapy to behavior therapy in recognition of his language, attentional, and executive functioning limitations. The consensus was that he may benefit more from behavior therapy that involves more performance goals than relying on verbal activities. Particularly, behavior therapy would start by working on his aggression and reactions to his auditory hallucination. The use of operants in the form of reinforcement was recommended along with the use of tokens. Since Chidi wanted to leave the hospital as soon as possible, it was recommended that he should be asked to work toward receiving sufficient tokens that would earn him discharge from the hospital. Particularly, the token economy was designed to improve his performance on ADL and medication adherence.
2 It was recommended that Chidi receive adjunct brief cognitive therapy to work on his irrational thoughts and delusion, with reliance on more visually based strategies rather than

verbal. It was recommended that the therapy be very brief and not more than 30 minutes because of his problems with concentration.

3 The panel further made contacts to enroll Chidi in cognitive training research that was about to be started in a university nearby.

4 The consulting physician further recommended pyritinol hydrochloride as cognitive enhancer. Neuroimaging was not part of the patient's assessment because of the associated costs and the worry that the patient may not be able to stay in the scanner for the period of imaging.

5 The consensus was communicated to the family as part of clinical feedback. Families are given feedback from neuropsychological and personality assessment reports to carry them along to future therapists and doctors to guide their treatment.

Section III: Lessons Learned

- In a multi-ethnic and multi-lingual nation like Nigeria, socio-geopolitical perspectives, linguistic and religious schemas can mitigate the manifestation and perception of behavioral health conditions and their management.

- There are challenges in conducting assessments in settings with limited resources where neuropsychology is nascent, particularly when mental health conditions are viewed with skepticism and patients are stigmatized for their symptoms.

- Conventional psychological assessment of severe psychotic disorders in psychiatric hospitals in Nigeria may not provide all the information required for patients' treatment planning, particularly when treatment is seen as non-effective. While typical diagnostic approaches in Nigeria include interviewing, observation, family report, and administration of objective psychological tests particularly MMPI, BDI, and sparingly intelligence tests; it is sometimes necessary to include measures of cognitive testing to support proper treatment planning.

- The case reviewed reflected the cultural orientation of working with both professionals and families of patients in order to support comprehensive treatment and rehabilitation. It also highlighted the incremental value of using neuropsychological approaches within the Nigerian context, to provide tailored, cognitively informed treatment recommendations.

- In a region where neuropsychology is nascent, being well integrated in a professional community can enhance the ability to educate allied health providers about the scientific underpinning of behavioral symptoms and benefits of neuropsychological evaluations.

References

1. Boivin MJ, Giordani B. Neuropsychology of children in Africa. New York (NY): Springer; 2013. p. 347.
2. The Guardian Newspaper on June 9, 2020. https://guardian.ng/
3. Bender L. Bender motor gestalt test: cards and manual of instructions. New York (NY): American Orthopsychiatric Association; 1946.
4. Folstein MF, Folstein SE, McHugh PR. Mini-Mental State Examination. PAR Test Publishers; 1975.
5. Nasreddine ZS, Phillips NA, Bedirian V, Charbonneeau S, Whitehead V, Collin I et al. The Montreal Cognitive Assessment, MoCA: a brief screening tool for mild cognitive impairment. J Am Geriatr Soc. 2005 Apr;53(4):695–9. doi:10.1111/j.1532-5415.2005.53221.x.
6. Lacks P. Bender Gestalt screening for brain dysfunction. New York (NY): Wiley; 1984. p. 223.
7. Kramer J. Uniform Data Set (UDS) of the National Alzheimer's Coordinating Centre. Number Span Test. 2013. https://naccdata.org/data-collection/forms-documentation/uds-3

8. Craft S. Uniform Data Set (UDS) of the National Alzheimer's Coordinating Centre. Craft Story 21 Recall. 2013.

9. Kramer J. Uniform Data Set (UDS) of the National Alzheimer's Coordinating Centre. Benson Complex Figure Copy. 2013.

10. Gollan TH, Weissberger GH, Runnqvist E, Montoya RI, Cera CM. Self-ratings of spoken language dominance: a Multilingual Naming Test (MINT) and preliminary norms for young and aging Spanish-English bilinguals. Biling Lang Cogn. 2012 Jul;15(3):594–615. doi:10.1017/S1366728911000332.

11. Hillis AE. Uniform Data Set (UDS) of the National Alzheimer's Coordinating Centre. Verbal Fluency: Phonemic Test. 2013.

12. Gronwall DM. Paced auditory serial addition task: a measure of recovery from concussion. Percept Mot Skills. 1977 Apr;44(2):367–73. doi:10.2466/pms.1977.44.2.367.

13. Ucheagwu VA, Ajaelu C, Okoli PC, Ossai J, Ofojebe PC, Ugokwe-Joseph R. Roles of demographics, anthropometric and metabolic syndrome on cognition among mid adults from rural population in Nigeria. Ann Alzheimer's Dement Care. 2019 Aug;3(1): 003–10. doi:10.17352/aadc.000007

Somali

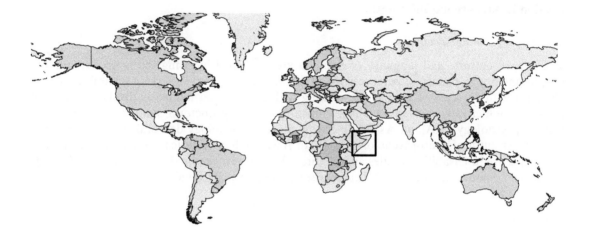

41 Exploring a Social-Ecological Systems Approach to Assessment through a Composite Somali Refugee Case

Jacob A. Bentley, Mohammed Alsubaie, Kimi Hashimoto, Mansha Mirza, and Farhiya Mohamed

Section I: Background Information

Terminology and Perspective

The people, culture, and language of Somalia are described by using the noun Somali. This chapter integrates a range of perspectives: a Caucasian, European-American rehabilitation psychologist with 15 years of experience working with people internationally displaced by socio-political conflict (JB), a Saudi Arabian clinical psychology doctoral student with interest in trauma psychology (MA), an Asian American clinical psychology doctoral student with interest in cross-cultural neuropsychology (KH), an Asian Indian American occupational therapist with expertise in Disability Studies and factors salient to refugees with disabilities (MM), and a US-based Somali community leader and organizer with a background as a social worker (FM).

Geography

Somalia is a long, narrow country located in Eastern Africa that wraps around the Horn of Africa. Somalia has a long coast bordering the Red Sea and the Indian Ocean. It occupies an important geopolitical position for trading zones, with cross-border trade and international import and exports through various ports. Somalia has a harsh, desert climate overall with seasonal monsoons in some parts. Somalia is prone to recurrent droughts, frequent dust storms in the Eastern Plains, and flooding during the rainy seasons. Famine, deforestation, overgrazing, soil erosion, and desertification have become significant issues in recent decades. Following the Civil War of 1991, the country consists of three zones: the northwest (known as Somaliland), the northeast (known as Puntland), and south/central Somalia.

History

Colonial rule of Somalia by France, Britain, Italy, and Ethiopia began in the mid-1800s, dividing the land inhabited by ethnic Somalis into several territories.[1] In July 1960, British Somaliland and Italian Somaliland peacefully obtained their independence and united to form the current borders of Somalia. At the time of independence, a civilian government was established in Somalia.

In 1969, General Mohammed Siad Barre led a coup and created a socialist military government with himself as its President. Initial popular support for his regime waned after increasing oppression and human rights violations. In the late 1970s and early 1980s, clan-based militias developed to oppose and overthrow Barre. Political instability increased in the early 1990s, resulting in a humanitarian crisis and a territorial civil war. The United States supplied military and economic

DOI: 10.4324/9781003051862-83

aid to Somalia but suspended their efforts in 1989 because of the Barre government's human rights record. Civil war erupted from 1988 to 1991, culminating in Barre's exile in January 1991.[2-4]

Since 1991, various clan militias have fought against each other for control of the country.[2-4] Government in Somalia has been unstable since, contributing to cyclical violence and famine.[1,5] The US Army estimated that by the fall of 1992, 40% of the population of Baidoa, a city in the southwestern Bay region of Somalia, and 20% of Somali children under age five had died due to famine. In late 1992, the US and UN forces intervened in Somalia to aid the humanitarian crisis and by March 1994 all foreign troops had withdrawn.

At the present time, inter-clan disputes continue within some regions of Somalia forcing many Somalis to relocate to other countries to escape famine and risk of death. Recent elections have been peaceful and demonstrated signs of progress toward sociopolitical stability, but Somalia remains divided by insurgent groups and rival militaries.

People

Ethnic Somalis are unified by culture, language, Islamic religion, and common ancestry. People of Somali origin account for approximately 85% of the population, with minority ethnic groups accounting for the remaining 15%.[2-4]

Ethnic groups in Somalia are furthered divided into clans.[2-4] Clans hold social and political importance and membership is determined by paternal lineage. Those of Somali origin or "nobles" belong to one of four patrilineal clans: Darod, Hawiye, Dir, and Rahanweyn (which includes the Digil and Mirifle people). These clans dominate modern government and politics, in addition to economy and urban life. Somalia's minority clans are very diverse and are not defined by ethnicity, religion, or linguistic variance but may also be identified by social and historical distinctions. Minority clans live in poverty and have been subject to discrimination and exclusion.

Clans are a very sensitive topic for many Somalis due to enduring tension and ongoing conflict. The US Centers for Disease Control and Prevention recommends that clinicians avoid discussing clans with Somali patients as many may find it disrespectful or offensive.[6]

Immigration and Relocation

Somalis began emigrating in 1991 to escape widespread hunger, rape, and death after years of civil war, famine, unequal distribution of aid, and poor economic prospects. Over a million Somalis fled to neighboring countries such as Ethiopia, Kenya, Djibouti, Yemen, and Burundi. Many stayed in refugee camps established to house them and resettlement programs enabled families to migrate to Europe and the United States. Somalis in the United States have relocated primarily to Minnesota, New York, Southern California (e.g., Los Angeles and San Diego), Washington, DC, and Washington State (Seattle).

Language

Somali is the official language of Somalia and was primarily an unwritten language until a uniform script was adopted in the 1970s based on the Latin alphabet.[1] The second official language is Arabic, mostly spoken in northern Somalia or in coastal towns. It is mainly used to read the Quran. Until the 1970s, education was conducted in the language of colonial rule; therefore, older Somalis from northern Somalia are conversational in English, while Somalis from southern Somalia are conversational in Italian. Somali is the language of instruction in schools, although Arabic, English, and Italian may also be used.

Communication

Somalia is a collectivistic society and communication depends on affinity and trust. For example, talking with a fellow Somali is significantly different from talking to a non-Somali. Communication with elders tends to be softer and indirect and often preceded by a term of respect such as *adeer or abti* (uncle) or *eedo or habaryar* (aunt). Additionally, gender boundaries are commonly known and accepted. Cultural norms are more emphasized in communication with the opposite gender, and physical touch (e.g., handshaking) is generally avoided.

Building rapport is essential with Somali clients. For example, it's helpful to start the evaluation with a cultural greeting like *salam,* ask generally relevant rather than personal questions, and be clear about the purpose of the encounter. Additionally, it is important to ask about and consider gender-match if possible and avoid handshakes with the opposite gender if not offered. These considerations might help build trust and rapport, especially considering the power differential between Western providers and Somali clients.

Education and Literacy

The civil war in Somalia decimated the educational system. Many schools were destroyed, and teaching materials became unavailable. Prior to the war, the government endorsed literacy campaigns in the 1970s–80s and all levels of education including higher education or college were free until 1991. Private schools were only available for those who could afford them. The Civil War rendered both public and private schools inaccessible. Somalia has one of the world's lowest school enrollment rates with only 25% of children enrolled in primary schools and 6% enrolled in secondary schools[3]. School enrollment is substantially higher for boys than girls. Literacy among Somalis is very low. Among those 15 years of age or older, male literacy is approximately 49.7% while literacy among women is at 25.8%[3].

Socio-Economic Status

Social and economic infrastructures in Somalia collapsed after the Civil War. Ongoing conflict and economic shock from increased global food and fuel prices led to the collapse of the Somali currency and unprecedented levels of poverty. An estimated 43% of the population lives in extreme poverty. Somalia's economy is mainly based on agriculture, livestock, and fishery.

Values and Customs

Family structure is organized within a patriarchal framework. The father is the head of the Somali household and is responsible for providing for the family. Most household responsibilities and childcare are maintained by women. Extended family and close family friends additionally help with childcare.

Gender and Sexuality

Gender roles in the Somali culture stem from cultural values. Men are expected to provide for the family and ensure its safety, while women take care of children and elders and the household chores. Such roles, however, have been impacted by different societal, political, and economic changes over the last two decades, and many families are cared for by single mothers or have women who are the main breadwinners.[3,4]

Sexuality is a sensitive topic for Somalis, especially regarding established norms and accepted behaviors of each gender. For example, female behavior is viewed as more reflective of her family's honor and that of her clan at large, so she might be punished or shamed if she behaves in a way that violates established norms.[3] Diverse forms of sexuality such as same-sex attraction are highly stigmatized and individuals who identify as sexual minority may face discrimination and punishment.[3]

Considering such cultural nuances is important for providers. For example, clients may not be comfortable disclosing sexual matters outside the boundaries of accepted norms or may avoid talking about sexual dysfunction. Thus, providers must attend to subtleties in expressions that might warrant a culturally sensitive examination of clients' sexuality and how it associates with their symptoms.

Spirituality and Religion

Majority of Somalis are Sunni Muslims. For those that practice Islam, religion entails a predominant role in life compared to what is typical in the Americas or Europe. Islam is considered a belief system, culture, government structure, and a way of life. The provisional federal constitution of Somalia recognizes Islam as the state religion and requires all laws to comply with the general principles of **sharia**. Attitudes, social customs, and gender roles in Somalia are primarily rooted in Islamic tradition.

Acculturation and Systemic Barriers

After resettlement in a host country, Somalis face various barriers to utilizing mental health services.[7] Common cultural barriers include stigma, concerns about privacy, and the struggle to recognize the need for professional care (e.g., seeking services for physical illness only). Additional systemic barriers include lack of information about services available, scarcity of interpreters, and economic and financial challenges.[2,3] Such barriers breed misinformation and mistrust in the system and overarching goals of available services. For example, some might fear disclosing information about interpersonal or familial discord lest agencies like Child Protective Services get involved. These factors may impact the types of services sought in all aspects of the clinical or neuropsychological evaluation, from the initial introduction to feedback and follow-up.

Somalis' level of acculturation to a host country and its system may impose yet another challenge for mental health utilization. Acculturation has been found to influence mental health symptoms across different cultures. Research shows that Muslims resettled in the United States. who maintained their culture of origin and identified more with their culture endorsed more severe depressive symptoms.[8] Moreover, for Somali adolescents, acculturative stress is associated with post-traumatic stress disorder (PTSD) and depressive symptoms.[9] Acculturative stressors are often rooted in practical considerations that influence functioning and wellbeing in ways that may be invisible to Western providers. For example, like other Muslim communities, Somalis may encounter stressors related to purchasing housing and/or transportation with financial assistance because of the Islamic concept of **riba** that prohibits use of economic interest.

Health Status

Research on health conditions experienced by internationally displaced Somalis is limited. Available data suggests similarities with other communities of refugees and asylum seekers.[10] For example, data collected by the Somali Health Board of Seattle in November 2014 identified most prominent health concerns in a sample of 141 Somalis (age range 18–78, with 94% of the respondents born in Somalia). A subsequent survey about common conditions treated within the community was collected from 21 Seattle-based health providers in March 2015. High blood pressure, diabetes, high cholesterol, heartburn, and arthritis were the top diagnoses, in order of highest to lowest frequency, reported by respondents from the Somali community. Healthcare providers identified diabetes, depression, PTSD, h. pylori and obesity as the top five diagnoses treated.

Mental Health Views

Generally, Somalis think of mental health in two broad categories: sane or insane, with some research suggesting that the concept of mental health and treatment is fairly new among many Somalis.[2] Many psychological difficulties are recognized as part of the individual's personality or as a result of daily stressors.[2,3] Such view is intertwined with the stigma surrounding mental health terminology, diagnoses, and treatment. In understanding mental health symptoms, many Somalis rely on religious and cultural concepts pertaining to the cause and appropriate healing of symptoms.[11,12] Common explanations for mental ailment are predetermined fate, punishment from Allah for lack of faith or poor life decisions, and interference of supernatural forces such as evil spirits and witchcraft. With that said, more Western contributors to mental illness are known in the Somali culture such as life stress, aversive events, and excessive negative emotions.[3,13]

Not all Somalis who seek neuropsychological services refuse conventional ways of treatment or adhere to traditional views. However, the consideration of these cultural views and practices is important for rapport, evaluation approach, case conceptualization, and treatment.

Approaches to Neuropsychological or Psychological Evaluations

Like clinical psychology more broadly, clinical neuropsychology does not exist in Somalia. Moreover, there are currently no neuropsychological instruments normed for use with Somali clients. Considering cultural differences and nuances is important for successful clinical and neuropsychological evaluations.[14] Not many Somalis self-refer due to various cultural differences and barriers mentioned above. Additionally, Somalis may present their difficulties differently or may emphasize somatic symptoms rather than emotional or otherwise psychological concerns.

If interpretation services are utilized, providers are encouraged to ensure the quality of such services.[15] When working with interpreters in small communities, it is important to ensure an agreement and understanding of confidentiality. For example, an evaluator who serves the Somali community might want to ask the client whether they know the interpreter and assess their level of comfort disclosing information in the interpreter's presence.

Traditional approaches to psychological and neuropsychological formulation may need to be adjusted in a way that captures the multi-systemic and inter-related mechanisms behind symptom presentations by Somalis, particularly those who migrated to the United States as refugees or asylum seekers. While the biopsychosocial model[16] presents a more comprehensive framework compared to the biomedical model, it does not capture the cultural factors or multi-systemic barriers that influence the refugee experience. Thus, utilizing a conceptual model that highlights different systemic levels that interact with the individual's subjective experiences may provide a more accurate understanding of their symptoms and help in offering a more acceptable and effective treatment. The case study we present next illustrates the potential utility of an integrated social-ecological framework for evaluating psychosocial and environmental challenges encountered by refugees.[17,18]

Section II: Case Study — "All Pains Are Connected"

Note: The following composite case represents life experiences and themes that have emerged in Somali refugee cases encountered by the authors in clinical and community contexts. Potentially identifying information and personal history have been altered and combined across people to protect patient identity and privacy.

Mr. Yousuf Adam is a 40-year-old Somali man referred by his primary care physician in a local International Medicine Clinic to evaluate symptoms of "confusion" and generalized cognitive difficulties. The referral noted diffuse somatic symptoms for which there was no medical explanation after a thorough medical examination and neuroimaging work-up.

Behavioral Observations

Mr. Adam arrived for his appointment with his wife. He was alert, fully oriented, and cooperative but somewhat guarded. He was conversational in English and requested that the evaluation be conducted in either Somali or Arabic. The clinical interview and testing were conducted by an English-speaking psychologist assisted by a Somali-speaking certified medical interpreter. When conversing through the interpreter, Mr. Adam never bypassed the interpreter, either by responding before what the psychologist had said was interpreted, or by responding in English. This suggests that he was much more comfortable in Somali than in English. The rest of his informed consent process and mental status exam was unremarkable. No difficulties were noted in vision, hearing, movements, speech, language, social or sensory-motor functions. Mr. Adam displayed a mildly restricted range of affect and tended to be subdued. His facial expressions were generally blunted when discussing his history. He appeared anxious at the outset and initially expressed uncertainty about what to expect from the evaluation. He visibly relaxed as the interview progressed and after the assessment procedure was clarified. I (JB) prefaced my questioning by describing my previous professional experience with the Somali community and communicating that my goal was simply to try to understand his experience as best as possible to hopefully be of assistance. Rapport was gradually developed and well-maintained throughout the evaluation. Mr. Adam appeared aware of the quality of his test performance, gave good effort on the tests, tolerated frustration well, but occasionally benefited from encouragement on particularly challenging tasks. The evaluation appeared to provide a generally accurate reflection of factors influencing his functioning; however, test interpretation required significant caution due to the absence of directly applicable norms or validation studies of neuropsychological instruments in Somali (see the Test and Norm Selection section for details).

Presenting Concerns

Mr. Adam reported concerns about "not feeling like [him]self" due to experiences of "confusion," episodes of "thinking too much," headaches, and diffuse body aches. He described forgetfulness in daily activities and somewhat frequent instances of misplacing his personal items (e.g., wallet, car keys). These symptoms had reportedly been present for several years but worsened over the last several months. Consistent with his medical records, he denied any acute medical events or chronic health conditions that could potentially explain these cognitive difficulties. His wife had expressed concern to him about times where he seemed "blank" and interpersonally distant.

Daily Functioning

Mr. Adam was employed as a data entry technician for a longitudinal research project at a local academic institution until grant funding ended approximately six months ago. He had a driver's license and worked as a delivery and rideshare driver since the data entry job ended. He was able to cook some foods, although his wife did most of the cooking in the household. He managed all financial bills in the family. He reported no problems with managing finances and had a bank account and a credit card. He scheduled and managed his own medical appointments through use of a calendar. Mr. Adam was proficient at computer searches, social media, and GPS navigation. He reported recent marital difficulties but mentioned no concerns about sexual function, although this represented a culturally sensitive topic that was not thoroughly assessed. He indicated his family had many family friends from the mosque where they worshiped, but over the past year or so he did not feel connected to them and avoided most social activities.

Health History

Mr. Adam was not aware of any problems with his birth or with his mother's pregnancy. He denied knowledge of any childhood health problems but noted historical, intermittent food insecurity within his family of origin. He denied having any premorbid history of medical or psychiatric conditions. He had no prior history of surgery or hospitalization. There were no known toxic exposures. As an adult, he had experienced occasional headaches treated with over-the-counter medications. His most recent bloodwork was unremarkable, with normal thyroid function and nutrient levels. Recent brain scans were also unremarkable. He had no history of substance use. His family medical history was largely unknown but appeared notable for hyperlipidemia, hypertension, and type II diabetes. His father had a history of stroke with residual lower limb paralysis and expressive language impairment. There was no known family history of dementia or other neurologic conditions.

Educational History

In Somalia, Mr. Adam received approximately 12 years of formal education. He described his educational experience as intermittent and often interrupted due to family responsibilities and occasional concerns for safety resulting from nearby violence in Mogadishu. He denied being held back in classes or any history of academic difficulty in any subject. He reported occasional difficulty with focusing during school due to distractions associated with local violence and, as he got older, the need to help support his family through paid work. He put forth effort in school and thought that he could have performed at a higher academic level if not for worry about safety and economic stability in his family. He later received further education on Islam through a madrassa (religious school) in Kenya, but instruction was curtailed by resource limitations and inconsistent access to teachers. He could read the Quran in Arabic and had participated in occasional classes at the local mosque since his arrival in the United States nine years ago.

Language Proficiency

Mr. Adam spoke Somali and learned to speak Arabic from an early age. At the refugee camp in Kenya, he received some instruction in English. Though he had not otherwise completed any formal English as Second Language classes, Mr. Adam's English language skills were conversational for common interactions in daily life. His degree of English language proficiency meant that age-based norms of available English-based neuropsychological test measures would likely be limited in their applicability. He expressed a preference for testing in either Somali or Arabic, the languages he felt most confident in reading and speaking. An evaluation in his native language was the most accurate way to ensure that the testing approximated his current cognitive status rather than simply obtaining a proxy for his English language proficiency.

Cultural History

Mr. Adam was born in Mogadishu, the capital of Somalia. He attended primary and high school in his hometown. He was the oldest of nine children, with four sisters and four brothers. His extended family lived nearby and often shared housing. His father worked as a cross-country truck driver; his mother worked as a homemaker. Mr. Adam described his family of origin as "loving" and mentioned that his father worked hard to save money for their extended family. As a result of his father's frequent work travel and in response to expectations as the oldest son in a traditionally patriarchal culture, Mr. Adam was often responsible for maintaining household responsibilities. This meant taking time away from school to help with providing food and taking care of the family's home and property. He characterized his childhood as "good" overall, without any early childhood traumatic exposure or abuse, though local famine contributed to periodic food insecurity within his family of origin.

He was 25 years old when he was forced to leave Somalia. A few years prior to leaving Somalia, he had begun working as a field interviewer for a research firm that did work for non-governmental organizations on regulations related to food supply and irrigation. During this time, his work became increasingly dangerous because the projects he was working on angered local political groups who did not want to see the results published. Mr. Adam reported that some local government officials also opposed the work as they wanted to avoid potential financial losses and the appearance of corruption if the data were made public. According to Mr. Adam, he and his colleagues were a visible part of this work as they interviewed local communities and thus were at high risk. Ultimately, they were targeted for their work thus forcing Mr. Adam to flee to neighboring Kenya for safety (see Emotional Functioning section below for more information about secondary impacts of his displacement and migration process). After residing in a Kenyan refugee camp for six years, he was able to seek refugee status in the United States with the assistance of an international non-governmental organization.

Since arriving in the United States, Mr. Adam had been able to connect with local East African and Muslim communities. His parents still lived in Mogadishu, but several of his siblings resided in areas of Canada and Europe. He married a Somali-American woman seven years ago and had three children, ages two to six. At times, he and his wife had difficulty relating to each other. His wife did not see him as reliable at the time of evaluation, stating that he seemed distracted and not present at times. He felt a strong sense of responsibility to support and provide for his family. In addition to efforts to provide financial security for his wife and children, he also regularly sent money to his parents and extended family in Somalia. Financial pressures had been a consistent recent source of stress. Mr. Adam had also experienced racist and Islamophobic encounters that impacted his social integration. For example, he had been called a "terrorist" when overheard speaking in his native language in the community and questioned about whether he knew any "pirates" when disclosing his Somali heritage to members of the majority culture. In response, he tried to ignore these encounters and seek solace through Islam and the local East African community. The mosque he attended had been vandalized multiple times, with broken windows and threatening xenophobic graffiti.

Emotional Functioning

Mr. Adam's emotional status appeared associated with traumatic experiences related to displacement from Somalia as well as stressors encountered since relocating to the United States (e.g., financial instability; Islamophobia; racism).

Regarding pre-migration traumatic exposure, one event clearly troubled Mr. Adam more than others. Several years into his work as a field researcher, Mr. Adam began receiving threatening text messages from private numbers such as, "stop what you are doing" and "if you don't, we're going to come after you." He believed these texts were related to the anti-corruption project he was completing at the time. He indicated that the language of the text messages made it clear that the persons knew where he was and suggested that they were following him. For example, he relocated to remain safe from these threats but then received texts indicating that these people knew where he had moved. He forwarded these texts to his employer, at which point he received a response stating that this was just part of the work and that he needed to persist. Shortly thereafter, Mr. Adam and colleagues were traveling by car down a remote road from a village outside of Mogadishu when a group of men in another vehicle forced them to pull over. He and his colleagues were then forced out of their car. After a brief exchange, the other group of men pulled out firearms and shot at Mr. Adam and his co-workers. A bullet grazed Mr. Adam's head and he reported that he remembered feeling it pass through his hair. He was the first to fall to the ground, quickly followed by his colleagues. Their bodies covered him. He remained still, not fully understanding what had just happened, until the other group of men returned to their vehicle and sped away. He recalled being covered in blood; as he struggled to stand, he began to realize that he was the only survivor and that the blood he felt was not his own. Following this event, he became certain that these individuals would eventually kill him if he did not flee from Somalia.

In the clinical interview, Mr. Adam described often feeling "confused," reported extended periods where he kept to himself and mentioned sometimes "just thinking too much" during those times of isolation. He referred to feeling preoccupied by thoughts of guilt related to surviving the roadside attack while his colleagues perished. He had decreased interest in previously enjoyed activities and relationships, difficulty sleeping, felt fatigued during the day, and described frequent headaches and diffuse body pains. As mentioned above, he was also distressed by noticing situations in which he would walk into a room and realize that he had forgotten why he entered it to begin with and other instances in which he would misplace objects such as his car keys. He denied any active suicidal ideation, citing his faith and familial commitments as protective factors.

Preliminary Formulation

At the end of the interview, it was clear to the psychologist that Mr. Adam was experiencing symptoms of post-traumatic stress and depression but did not recognize it. In addition to pre-migration trauma, post-migration and acculturative stressors were clearly influencing his clinical presentation. Mr. Adam had experienced multiple layers of personal loss related to his safety, security, and professional standing as well as communal losses experienced through separation from family and ongoing sociopolitical strife in Somalia. Additional barriers included poverty, racist and Islamophobic experiences, and an overarching sense of disconnection from dominant culture in the United States.

Test and Norm Selection

Considering the referral question and presenting problems, I selected a test battery that enabled a Process Approach to test the limits of performance across a variety of domains.[19,20] This Process Approach seemed beneficial considering lack of relevant norms, influences of language and use of an interpreter in test administration, cultural impacts on timed tests, and potential lack of familiarity with healthcare evaluations based on paper and pencil tests. Given the lack of documented history of neurologic involvement and clinical hypothesis related to potential PTSD and mood disturbance, the battery was intended to provide impressions about attention, memory, executive, and intellectual functioning through both verbal and visual modalities. I administered the following tests, generally recommended for people with potential trauma-related psychological conditions and potential comorbidities[21]:

- Test of Memory Malingering[22]
- Grooved Pegboard Test[23]
- Montreal Cognitive Assessment (MoCA, Arabic version[24,25])
- The following subtests of the Wechsler Adult Intelligence Scale-Fourth Edition (WAIS-IV[26]):
  - Block Design
  - Matrix Reasoning
  - Visual Puzzles
  - Digit Span
  - Symbol Search
  - Coding
- Hopkins Verbal Learning Test-Revised[27]
- Brief Visuospatial Memory Test-Revised[28]

For emotional functioning, in addition to the clinical interview, I administered brief questionnaires assessing symptoms of PTSD, depression, anxiety, and somatization in Somali with the help of a certified medical interpreter. These questionnaires included the Posttraumatic Stress Disorder Checklist (PCL-5[29]), Patient Health Questionnaire (PHQ-9[30]), Generalized Anxiety Disorder Scale (GAD-7[31]), and the Somatic Symptoms Scale-8 (SSS-8[32]).

Test Results and Impressions

According to age- and education-adjusted norms, Mr. Adam's performance fell in the borderline to low average range across all cognitive domains assessed. Considering the number of cultural-linguistic factors present in the case, these findings likely represented somewhat of an underestimate of his cognitive abilities. For example, time-based visuospatial processing subtests (e.g., Symbol Search; Coding) tended to cluster in the borderline range (2nd percentile) based on norms. When allocating additional time and prompts to the context of the task, his performance appeared more consistent with low average performance (16th percentile). On learning and memory subtests, Mr. Adam demonstrated initial difficulties with encoding information during early trial. Through repetition, he showed a steady learning arc and retention of the acquired information over time. The encoding difficulties seemed consistent with his borderline performance on working memory tasks. Otherwise, language and executive functions provided no notable findings. Overall, his neurocognitive functioning appeared intact but was most likely influenced by emotional and psychosocial factors.

Emotionally, he reported significant symptoms of post-traumatic stress related to the Criterion A traumatic event detailed earlier in the chapter. His symptoms spanned DSM-5 clusters, with prominent loadings on re-experiencing and avoidance domains. Mr. Adam also reported severe symptoms of depression and moderate anxiety. Elevated symptoms of anxiety (GAD-7 score of 10) and depression (PHQ-9 score of 18) included anhedonia and hopelessness, but also appeared partially driven by somatic indicators. This was also reflected in an elevated score on a somatic symptom measure (SSS-8 score of 12). He reported being "bothered a lot" by somatic symptoms of headaches, trouble sleeping, dizziness, and diffuse body aches (e.g., back pain; pain in arms, legs, or joints).

Mr. Adam met full criteria for PTSD with comorbid major depressive disorder, moderate severity. I also acknowledged problems related to his employment status (Z56.7), migration and acculturation difficulties (Z60.3), discrimination (Z60.5), marital distress (Z63.0), and social exclusion and isolation (Z60.4) experienced within the context of previous exposure to war and conflict (Z65.5).

Feedback Session and Follow-Up

For his feedback session, both Mr. Adam and his wife returned to discuss next steps. The same certified medical interpreter participated in the feedback session. Mr. Adam's initial questions related to his somatic symptoms and possible etiologies. I began by briefly summarizing the medical documentation provided by the International Medicine Clinic, which provided no immediate explanation for his concerns. In summarizing the testing results, I shared a conceptualization that "all pains are connected" in an attempt to affirm his experiences while also shifting to a conversation about the range of psychosocial challenges and traumatic stressors described in our initial meeting. This provided a pathway to discuss the interacting and compounding effects of exposure to violence in Somalia, stressors incurred through forced displacement and migration, and ongoing challenges encountered following resettlement in the United States (e.g., poverty; discrimination; under-employment). Through this conversation, we were able to collaborate on a plan to remain engaged with his medical care to further rule out potential physical health explanations and establishing additional supports for addressing other psychosocial contributing factors.

In navigating the conversation, I took care to frame the discussion around efforts to seek healing as opposed to nesting it within a Western biomedical terminology (e.g., psychotherapy) related to mental health and assumptions related to mind-body dualism. Instead, we focused on existing resources within his local community that could be drawn upon. Specifically, with their approval and input, this meant connecting Mr. Adam and his wife to a Somali community-based organization focused on providing family education and resources. The connection was intended to provide a family systems intervention, such that Mr. Adam and/or his wife could gain culturally consistent and community-driven support for psychosocial challenges common within the East African community.

Recognizing that there is no word for "psychological trauma" within the Somali language, I began talking with Mr. Adam about how exposure to war and violence can influence wellbeing in ways that cannot always be seen. I used an analogy to describe how a physical wound can become infected and cause complications throughout the body if left untreated. Similarly, people can experience changes in their thoughts, feelings, and behavior after being exposed to war, violence, and threat to personal safety. If left unattended, over time, these changes can influence additional areas of life just as an infection in one area of the body can affect other seemingly disparate systems. The analogy resonated, and we began talking about compounding effects of losses and stressors they had experienced in their life. Intersections of his faith and a sense of seeking community and reconciliation emerged through the conversation, even if his ability to fully engage had been clouded by the range of challenges he encountered. I tried to validate his experience and normalize the presence of post-traumatic difficulties, while also working to establish a plan to reduce his distress going forward.

To manage his trauma-related symptoms, we talked through a variety of options. With his approval and written permission, I reached out to the International Medicine Clinic to collaborate with the clinic's consulting psychiatrist. Shortly after, Mr. Adam began taking a selective serotonin reuptake inhibitor (SSRI) to assist with his mood symptoms. He also began taking prazosin, an anti-hypertensive medication shown to aid in the management of nightmares experienced by trauma-exposed individuals, including refugees and asylum seekers.[33] In addition, I provided Mr. Adam with information about a faith-based trauma intervention group co-developed by and piloted within the local Somali community. The program, Islamic Trauma Healing,[34,35] integrates evidenced-based trauma treatment principles (e.g., cognitive-restructuring; imaginal exposure) with faith practices (e.g., Quranic readings; prophet stories; prayer). The program is led by trained leaders in the Somali community and groups run through local mosques. Mr. Adam expressed openness to learning more about the program and later attended an informational session.

Section III: Lessons Learned

- Somali culture represents a rich tapestry of clan-based heritage, oral tradition, and communal practices deeply influenced by Islam.
- Mental illness has historically been stigmatized in Somali culture due to a "sane/insane" cultural dichotomy and reinforced through a history in Somalia of chaining people that have been institutionalized for mental illness.[36,37]
- Symptoms of conditions such as depression, anxiety, and post-traumatic stress may present somatically. Somatic symptoms and expressions of "confusion" or "thinking too much" may represent idioms of emotional distress.[38,39] A thorough medical evaluation is critical for ruling out physical health conditions before assuming a psychosomatic presentation given vulnerabilities for refugees to go under-diagnosed due to fragile health systems in their country of origin, healthcare gaps encountered through migration, and barriers to post-resettlement healthcare access.
- Somalis may respond favorably when discussing health within the context of the Islamic worldview. Providing Somalis with the opportunity to share religious and spiritual beliefs can help to reduce stigma, develop an understanding within the practitioner about perceptions of wellness, and increase follow through with recommendations and referrals.
- Refugees experience stressors, challenges, and barriers that extend across multiple systemic levels. Conceptual frameworks grounded in ecological systems theory can provide practitioners with mechanisms for thinking through systemic factors. According to Bronfenbrenner's theory,[40] people are influenced by the various environmental systems with which they interact. Environmental factors are stratified across several nested systems and the interconnections among them. Systems include the (a) microsystem (e.g., an individual and their immediate environments), (b) mesosystem (e.g., interaction between microsystems such as the linkages between the person's family and the health system), (c) exosystem (e.g., systems with which the person is only indirectly associated such as a caregiver's workplace), (d) macrosystem (e.g., sociocultural and political ideologies, practices, values, customs, and laws), and (e) chronosystem (e.g., transitions across the lifespan).
- The Adaptation and Development after Persecution and Trauma model (ADAPT[16]) incorporates features salient to the refugee experience. The ADAPT model provides a broad framework that helps organize a wide range of recursive challenges encountered by refugees at individual, family, and community levels.[17] Table 41.1 summarizes the five core pillars of the model. Several themes from the ADAPT model were apparent in the case of Mr. Adam, including the following: threats to his sense of *Safety and Security* stemming from his history of trauma and early exposure to sociopolitical conflict, fragmentation in his social *Bonds and Networks* through forced displacement, and significant shifts in his *Roles and Identities*

Table 41.1 Five pillars of the ADAPT model[16]

Safety and security	Sense of safety in the environment is important to recovery
Bonds and networks	Ability to form new bonds or grieve the lost bond due to separation from home country
Justice	Clinical experience has shown that ongoing preoccupation with injustice of the past may hinder psychological recovery
Roles and identities	Refugees must overcome possible unemployment and marginalization to find their role in the new country
Existential meaning	Understanding and finding meaning in the experiences refugees have encountered in the past is important to their health

through changes in his employment status that also interact with prescribed gender roles within traditional Somali culture.

- By integrating Bronfenbrenner's bio-ecological theory[40] and Silove's ADAPT model,[17] Wong and Schweitzer[18] proposed a bio-ecological adaptive model (BEAM) that provides a holistic framework to conceptualize the impact of individual, pre-migration, and post-settlement factors. The BEAM framework considers unique characteristics of the refugee experience and accounts for the reciprocal interactions that exist between the individual and various socio-ecological systems. Figure 41.1 provides a graphical depiction of the BEAM model with examples of relevant factors nested within each Bronfenbrenner systemic level.

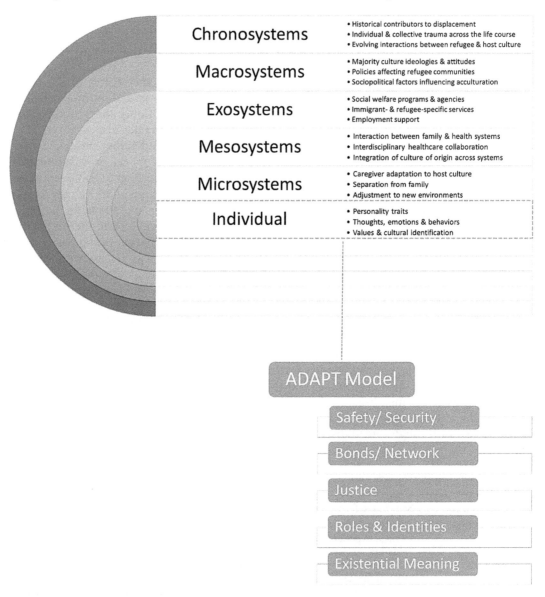

Figure 41.1 The bio-ecological adaptive model (BEAM[17]) applied to multi-systemic psychosocial considerations when assessing refugees

- Qualitative research focused on the service needs and gaps experienced by refugees has identified cross-cultural disconnect with healthcare providers as a primary concern in addition to various barriers to accessing social service and healthcare systems.[41] Table 41.2 provides a list of healthcare utilization challenges commonly experienced by refugees.[41]

Table 41.2 Barriers to healthcare utilization and service provision for refugees

- Separation from family and practical factors (e.g., employment; housing; education) may supersede medical care as immediate priorities
- Exposure to trauma and risk for psychological sequelae (often unrecognized)
- Anti-immigrant and anti-refugee sentiments in the United States
- Public health screening results are often not communicated to chronic care providers
- Refugees with complex medical conditions are often unable to establish care quickly
- Competing demands for services may overwhelm finite resources (e.g., time; finances)
- Unfamiliarity with the biomedical concepts and healthcare bureaucracy
- Mental illness stigma in the culture of origin and/ host community
- Health system limitations in origin country leading to undiagnosed or poorly controlled chronic health conditions
- Language differences

Note: Summarized and adapted from Jackson et al.[41]

- Mr. Adam's case underscored the importance of conceptualizing multiple influences on the clinical presentation of refugee clients by considering pre-migration exposures, migration-related risk factors, and post-migration psychosocial stressors distributed across time and systemic levels. This case also demonstrates the utility of local community partnerships that can inform biopsychosocial-spiritual formulations relevant to the neuropsychological/ psychological assessment process.

Glossary

Sharia.　An Arabic word that means the "pathway to be followed." It consists of a set of principles that are mainly based on Quranic verses and Hadith (Prophet Mohammed's sayings and way of conduct) and are interpreted by scholars to guide Muslims' social, political, and legal matters. For a more detailed discussion.[42]

Riba.　The word Riba in contemporary Islamic banking refers to the monetary interest or increase above the amount owed. Riba is prohibited in Islamic or Sharia law and is sometimes translated to mean usury or unjust practice. Muslim scholars define more than one form of Riba and discuss different interpretations and practices.[43]

References

1. Lewis, T. (2009). *Somali cultural profile*. EthnoMed: Harborview Medical Center's Ethnic Medicine Website. Retrieved from: https://ethnomed.org/culture/somali/
2. Bentley, J. A., & Wilson Owens, C. (2008). *Somali refugee mental health cultural profile*. EthnoMed: Harborview Medical Center's Ethnic Medicine Website. Retrieved from: https://ethnomed.org/resource/somali-refugee-mental-health-cultural-profile/
3. Cavallera V, Reggi M, Abdi S, Jinnah Z, Kivelenge J, Warsame AM, Ventevogel P. Culture, context and mental health of Somali refugees: a primer for staff working in mental health and psychosocial support programmes. Geneva: UNHCR; 2016.

4. Heger Boyle E, Ali, A. Culture, structure, and the refugee experience in Somali immigrant family transformation. Int Migr. 2010;48(1):47–79.

5. Maxwell DG, Majid N. Famine in Somalia. Oxford: Oxford University Press; 2016.

6. Centers for Diseases Control and Prevention. Somali refugee health profile [Internet]. US Department of Health and Human Services; 2018. Available from: https://www.cdc.gov/immigrantrefugeehealth/pdf/Somali-Refugee-Health-Profile.pdf

7. Bentley JA, Thoburn JW, Stewart DG, Boynton LD. Post-migration stress as a moderator between traumatic life events and self-reported mental health symptoms of Somali refugees. J Loss Trauma. 2012;17(5):452–469. doi:10.1080/15325024.2012.665008

8. Abu-Bader SH, Tirmazi MT, Ross-Sheriff F. The impact of acculturation on depression among older Muslim immigrants in the United States. J Gerontol Soc Work. 2011;54(4):425–48.

9. Burgess M, Somali Health Board. Somali health survey and health disparities [Internet]. Harborview Medical Center's Ethnic Medicine Website; 2020. Available from: https://ethnomed.org/resource/somali-health-survey-and-health-disparities/

10. Bentley JA. Cross-cultural assessment of psychological symptoms among Somali refugees. Seattle (WA): Seattle Pacific University; 2011.

11. Bentley JA, Ahmad Z, Thoburn J. Religiosity and posttraumatic stress in a sample of East African refugees. Ment Health Relig Cult. 2014;17(2):185–95. doi:10.1080/13674676.2013.784899

12. Kuittinen S, Mölsä M, Punamäki RL, Tiilikainen M, Honkasalo ML. Causal attributions of mental health problems and depressive symptoms among older Somali refugees in Finland. Transcult Psychiatry. 2017;54(2):211–38.

13. Rivera Mindt M, Byrd D, Saez P, Manly J. Increasing culturally competent neuropsychological services for ethnic minority populations: a call to action. Clin Neuropsychol. 2010;24(3):429–53. doi:10.1080/13854040903058960

14. Mirza M, Harrison E, Bentley JA, Chang H, Birman D. Communication challenges and best practices when working across languages: an exploratory survey of mental health providers and interpreters. Societies. 2020;10(3):66. doi:10.3390/soc10030066

15. Engel GL. The clinical application of the biopsychosocial model. Am J Psychiatry. 1980;137(5):535–44. doi:10.1176/ajp.137.5.535

16. Silove D. The ADAPT model: a conceptual framework for mental health and psychosocial programming in post conflict settings. Intervention. 2013;11(3):237–48. doi:10.1097/WTF.0000000000000005

17. Wong CW, Schweitzer RD. Individual, premigration and postsettlement factors, and academic achievement in adolescents from refugee backgrounds: a systematic review and model. Transcult Psychiatry. 2017;54(5–6):756–82.

18. Casaletto KB, Heaton RK. Neuropsychological assessment: past and future. J Int Neuropsychol Soc. 2017;23(9–10):778.

19. Kaplan E. The process approach to neuropsychological assessment. Aphasiology. 1988;2(3–4):309–11. doi:10.1080/02687038808248930

20. Silveira K, Garcia-Barrera MA, Smart CM. Neuropsychological impact of trauma-related mental illnesses: a systematic review of clinically meaningful results. Neuropsychol Rev. 2020;30:1–35.

21. Tombaugh TN. Test of memory malingering: TOMM. Toronto, Canada: Multi-Health Systems; 1996.

22. Klove H. Grooved Pegboard Test. Lafayette, IN: Lafayette Instrument; 1963.

23. Nasreddine ZS, Phillips NA, Bédirian V, Charbonneau S, Whitehead V, Collin I, et al. The Montreal Cognitive Assessment, MoCA: a brief screening tool for mild cognitive impairment. J Am Geriatr Soc. 2005;53(4):695–99.

24. Saleh AA, Alkholy RSAEHA, Khalaf OO, Sabry NA, Amer H, El-Jaafary S, Khalil MAEF. Validation of Montreal cognitive assessment-basic in a sample of elderly Egyptians with neurocognitive disorders. Aging Ment Health. 2019;23(5):551–7.

25. Wechsler D. Wechsler Adult Intelligence Scale-fourth edition: administration and scoring manual. San Antonio, TX: Pearson; 2008.

26. Benedict RH, Schretlen D, Groninger L, Brandt J. Hopkins Verbal Learning Test–revised: normative data and analysis of inter-form and test-retest reliability. Clin Neuropsychol. 1998;12(1):43–55.

27. Benedict RH, Schretlen D, Groninger L, Dobraski M, Shpritz B. Revision of the Brief Visuospatial Memory Test: studies of normal performance, reliability, and validity. Psychol Assess. 1996;8(2):145.

28. Blevins CA, Weathers FW, Davis MT, Witte TK, Domino JL. The posttraumatic stress disorder checklist for DSM-5 (PCL-5): development and initial psychometric evaluation. J Trauma Stress. 2015;28(6):489–98.

29. Kroenke K, Spitzer RL, Williams JB. The PHQ-9: validity of a brief depression severity measure. J Gen Int Med. 2001;16(9):606–13.

30. Spitzer RL, Kroenke K, Williams JB, Löwe B. A brief measure for assessing generalized anxiety disorder: the GAD-7. Arch Intern Med. 2006;166(10):1092–7.

31. Gierk B, Kohlmann S, Kroenke K, Spangenberg L, Zenger M, Brähler E, Löwe B. The somatic symptom scale–8 (SSS-8): a brief measure of somatic symptom burden. JAMA Intern Med. 2014;174(3):399–407.

32. Boynton L, Bentley JA, Strachan E, Barbato A, Raskind M. Preliminary findings concerning the use of prazosin for the treatment of posttraumatic nightmares in a refugee population. J Psychiatr Pract. 2009;15(6):454–9. doi:10.1097/01.pra.0000364287.63210.92

33. Bentley JA, Feeny NC, Dolezal ML, Klein A, Marks LH, Graham B, et al. Islamic Trauma Healing: integrating faith and empirically-supported principles in a community-based program. Cogn Behav Pract. 2021; 28(2):167–92. doi:10.1016/j.cbpra.2020.10.005

34. Zoellner LA, Graham B, Marks LH, Feeny NC, Bentley JA, Franklin A, Lang D. Islamic Trauma Healing: initial feasibility and pilot data. Societies. 2018;8(3):47. doi:10.3390/soc8030047

35. Boynton L, Bentley JA, Hussein N, Jackson C. Images in psychiatry: Hargeisa Group Hospital Psychiatric Ward. Am J Psychiatry. 2010;167(7):762. doi:10.1176/appi.ajp.2010.10030299

36. Boynton L, Bentley JA, Jackson C, Gibbs TA. The role of state and stigma in the mental health of Somalis. J Psychiatr Pract. 2010;16(4):265–8. doi:10.1097/01.pra.0000386914.85182.78

37. Bentley JA, Thoburn JW, Stewart DG, Boynton LD. The indirect effect of somatic complaints on report of posttraumatic psychological symptomatology among Somali refugees. J Trauma Stress. 2011;24(4):479–82. doi:10.1002/jts.20651

38. Kaiser BN, Haroz EE, Kohrt BA, Bolton PA, Bass JK, Hinton DE. "Thinking too much": a systematic review of a common idiom of distress. Soc Sci Med. 2015;147:170–83.

39. Bronfenbrenner U. The ecology of human development: experiments by nature and design. Cambridge, MA: Harvard University Press; 1979.

40. Mirza M, Heinemann AW. Service needs and service gaps among refugees with disabilities resettled in the United States. Disabil Rehabil. 2012;34(7):542–52.

41. Jackson JC, Haider M, Wilson Owens C, Ahrenholz N, Molnar A, Farmer B, et al. Healthcare recommendations for recently arrived refugees: observations from EthnoMed. Harv Public Health Rev. 2016. Available from: http://harvardpublichealthreview.org/case-based-recommendations-for-the-health-care-of-recently-arrived-refugees-observations-from-ethnomed/

42. Berger MS. Understanding Sharia in the West. J Law Reli State. 2018;6(2–3):236–73. doi:10.1163/22124810-00602005

43. Nomani, F. The interpretative debate of the classical Islamic Jurists on Riba (Usury) [Internet]. n.d. Retrieved March 14, 2021. Available from: http://meea.sites.luc.edu/volume4/NomaniRevised.htm

South African

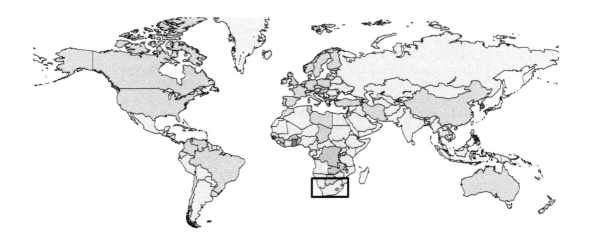

42 Culturally Responsive Neuropsychological Assessment in South Africa

Kate Cockcroft and Sumaya Laher

Section I: Background Information

Terminology and Perspective

South Africa is infamous for apartheid (legislated racial segregation between 1948 and 1884), which led to racial classifications still used by Statistics SA today (for census and employment purposes). These include "**Colored**" for those of mixed-race ancestry, "White" for those of European ancestry, "Black" for indigenous African inhabitants, while those from South Asia (primarily India) are collectively referred to as "Indian." People from East Asia (China and surrounding countries) are termed "Asian," while "Malay" denotes people from Singapore, Malaysia, and countries in Southeast Asia. This blend of people means that South Africa is a nation with a multitude of cultures and traditions.

The first author's perspective is influenced by her ancestry from immigrant parents from Great Britain. She was born in Zimbabwe but has lived in South Africa most of her life and identifies as South African. The second author's perspective spans multiple identities as a mother, wife, daughter, and sister in a communal culture in Johannesburg. She identifies as South African with ancestry stemming from immigrant grandparents from India. Both authors studied at the University of the Witwatersrand, Johannesburg, where they teach psychological assessment and neuropsychology among other subjects.

Geography

South Africa is located at the southernmost tip of Africa with a population of approximately 58 million people.[1] It is described as the Cradle of Humankind evidencing some of the earliest human populations.[2]

Early History

The African cultures that inhabited the region prior to colonization (pre-13th century) relied on an oral tradition to record their history. Thus, there are few written accounts of the early history of the country. The Khoi and San people were the original inhabitants of South Africa, particularly in the Western regions. These were nomadic tribes that operated as collectivist societies with no leadership structures. They lived off the land and their history is inscribed in cave paintings. The Nguni tribes came to the region later and consisted of the Bantu groupings who lived across the Great Lakes region of Africa. Many migrated south in search of better land for their animals and crops. These tribes had a sophisticated social structure with chiefs and leaders, and established settlements to the east of South Africa. As the Nguni tribes migrated south toward the sea, they displaced much of the Khoisan population.[3]

DOI: 10.4324/9781003051862-85

Colonial History

South Africa was colonized by the Dutch (1652–1795; 1803–6) and the British (1795–1803; 1806–1961). During these periods, slaves, workers, and prisoners were brought in from colonies in Malaysia, Singapore, and India. Colonialism laid the ground for apartheid (separate development of different racial groups which privileged White people). During the apartheid era (1948–94), legislation was passed to enforce segregation in all spheres of life (education, employment, residence, health care, and public facilities), with better resources reserved for White South Africans. Apartheid was abolished in 1994, and a democratically elected government was introduced, led by Nelson Mandela. The new South African constitution promotes equality and dignity for all. The country's diversity is evident in the official recognition of eleven languages, with most South Africans speaking at least two of these. Unfortunately, the country is plagued by systemic challenges related to poverty, unemployment, crime and violence, and high rates of HIV infection.[4] Psychological assessment needs to be understood within this broader historical context.

Cultural Factors

African cultures in South Africa are described as collectivist and it is common for extended families to live in the same household. There is a strong sense of community, or **Ubuntu**, among South Africans, which in many indigenous languages is communicated as, "A person is a person through other persons" (with the isiZulu expression of this, "*Umuntu ngumuntu ngabantu*" often cited). Consequently, there is often support from family, friends, and the community, but the close-knit nature of communities means that health concerns are often not private. This can lead to stigma and discrimination associated with neuropsychological difficulties, and families may hide problems. It is often more culturally acceptable to visit traditional healers as this does not carry the same stigma associated with a psychologist or mental illness.[5] Also, traditional healers are more accessible and affordable than university-trained practitioners.[6] The traditional healer is viewed as the most important person in the community after the chief of a village.

isiZulu terms are used here to describe common traditional illnesses, while acknowledging that practices like *Ubuntu* and traditional healing extend to many African cultures.[7] A common ailment is related to ancestral displeasure (**abaphansi basifulathele**). The role of the ancestors (**amadlozi**) in African tradition is to protect the family and in return the ancestors need to be mollified. Failure to do this can result in ancestral displeasure and illness. Traditional healers distinguish between medical and spiritual conditions. Illnesses due to medical conditions (**Ukugula kwashukela**) include head injuries, cerebrovascular accidents, and diseases of old age. Both medical health professionals and traditional healers may be consulted. The former tend to be a resource for providing alleviation of physical symptoms, while the latter are used to discover causes of psychological disturbance. Western psychological models tend to locate the source of psychological difficulties within the individual, with treatment usually taking place on an individual level. In contrast, many African cultures locate both the source of individual psychological distress and responsibility for its treatment within the community.[8]

Language

Twenty-eight languages are spoken in South Africa, of which eleven are officially recognized. Most South Africans are multi-lingual, and not always sufficiently proficient in English to complete tests (English proficiency tends to be linked to urbanization). Literacy rates are lowest among the older population, with a literacy rate of 54.5% in those aged 65 years or older; 79.3% for those between 35 and 64 years; and 87% in those 15 years and older.[9] Few neuropsychological tests exist in the indigenous South African languages, despite the fact that these are spoken by the majority of the population. Consequently, psychologists often resort to ad hoc procedures to adapt tests, such as using family members to translate (if professional translators are unavailable) or giving extended time with practice examples.[10] Although this is changing, most psychologists are White, English speakers, while most South Africans are Black, English second- or third-language speakers, necessitating specific training in cross-cultural sensitivity.[11]

Socio-Economic Status

Although South Africa is classified by the World Bank as a middle-income country, this hides the discrepancies between rich and poor, as reflected in a Gini coefficient of 0.63.[12] Socio-economic status (SES) is an important demographic to consider in neuropsychological assessment because past apartheid policies still persist in the form of socio-economic inequality, and so the majority of South Africans belong to low SES backgrounds.[13] This economic divide results in differing access to resources and education, as well as varying levels of acculturation.

Education

The educational systems (former Model C, ex-DET, and privately funded) offer education that differs vastly in quality. Former Model C government schools were previously reserved for White children under apartheid and were modeled on British public schools. They are comparable to privately funded schools and generally provide a high standard of education. In contrast, schooling provided by the previous Department of Education and Training (DET) for Black children under apartheid remains constrained by limited resources and large classes despite new educational policies that mandate fairer allocation of resources. Although many Black children now attend the former Model C and private schools, most have no option but to attend the ex-DET schools.[14] An advantaged, Western-style schooling teaches problem-solving, as well as test-taking skills, which are drawn on in neuropsychological tests.[15] Consequently, psychologists take both level and quality of education into consideration when evaluating neuropsychological test performance.[16]

Health Status

Despite being a middle-income country, South Africa has poor health outcomes. These include high mortality levels resulting from its quadruple burden of disease (a combination of communicable diseases, such as HIV/AIDS and tuberculosis; maternal and child mortality; non-communicable diseases, such as hypertension and cardiovascular diseases, diabetes, cancer, mental illnesses, and chronic lung diseases like asthma; as well as injury and trauma[17]). Most of the population depends on the public health system to provide for its health care needs, yet these facilities are too few, under-resourced, understaffed, and challenged by management crises.[18] A parallel private healthcare system exists that services only 16% of the population. Black South Africans, the less educated, the unemployed, and the poor are less likely to have adequate access to health care.[19]

Psychological Assessment

Segregationist policies influenced all aspects of South African life, including psychological assessment. Imported, Western psychological tests were used in their original formats with African children and adults to demonstrate "low" native intellect and justify apartheid. Between the 1960s and 1980s, political sanctions limited access to international psychological assessments and several local tests were developed, modeled on Western counterparts. However, these were primarily developed for the White population only.[20] In the 1980s and 1990s, there was a growing awareness of the need for psychological tests that were fair and valid for all South Africans. This led to the development of tests that incorporated differential ability testing, such as the General Scholastic Aptitude Test[21] and the Ability, Processing of Information, and Learning Battery (APIL-B[22]). Tests were also normed on a broader demographic. For example, the Senior South African Scales-Revised (SSAIS-R), a test of intellectual ability in children, was standardized for English- and **Afrikaans**-speaking White, Colored and Indian South African children, but not for African children.[20] In 2000, the Differential Aptitude Tests were developed and the Wechsler Adult Intelligence Scale, Third Edition (WAIS-III) was adapted and standardized for all South Africans. In the same year, the Learning Potential Computerised Adaptive Test (LPCAT), a computer-based test of learning potential, was developed. The LPCAT comprises non-verbal, figural items based on the premise that these are less biased than verbal items for testees from disadvantaged backgrounds.[23]

A challenge facing psychological assessment in South Africa is the fair testing of individuals from very diverse backgrounds. This is exacerbated by the lack of appropriately standardized, culturally relevant tests. Unequal educational opportunities, as well as cultural and linguistic differences in the comprehension of underlying test constructs, often manifest as lowered test performance, which may not reflect the individual's actual ability.[10] Few neuropsychological tests have been standardized and normed for South Africans, although academics are working to address this.[20]

Below, we present a case study that highlights and integrates many of the issues discussed above.

Section II: Case Study — "A Person Is a Person through Other Persons"

Background and Presenting Concerns

When he was five years old, Phumlani* was hit by a car while crossing the road. He sustained injuries to his left temporal lobe. His Glasgow Coma Scale five hours' post-accident was 8/15. Five months later, Phumlani experienced medically uncontrollable seizures resulting in a left temporal lobectomy, hippocampectomy, and amygdalectomy to surgically contain the seizures. He has been seizure free since then, but experienced several difficulties, some of which existed prior to the surgery. These include academic, attention, and verbal difficulties, social anxiety, withdrawal tendencies, and behavioral difficulties, as well as social and emotional vulnerabilities. Phumlani experiences considerable anxiety, especially about his academic performance and social interactions. His mother reported that Phumlani can be loving and affectionate, but also hostile, argumentative, avoidant, and resistant to completing tasks. At school, Phumlani avoids completing tasks that are challenging for him by engaging in alternative behaviors (e.g., changing the conversation topic, distraction, refusal to do the tasks) or opting out (e.g., going to the bathroom). His mother brought Phumlani to the University clinic for an evaluation based on these concerns.

Phumlani has an identical twin, Jabu, and three older sisters. They reside in an informal settlement in Johannesburg. Their father is deceased, and their mother is employed as a domestic worker. The children speak isiZulu at home and are being educated in English. During the interview, their mother indicated that, prior to the accident, the two boys seemed very similar in terms of their intellectual, social, and emotional development, although Phumlani was more introverted and impulsive than his brother.

---

*Names and identifying information have been changed to preserve the anonymity of the client.

Cultural Considerations

On the insistence of her husband's family, Phumlani's mother took him to a traditional healer after the seizures commenced. The healer diagnosed *ukugula kwashukela* and provided herbal medicine which caused Phumlani to have vivid dreams and hallucinations. Phumlani's paternal family initially believed that he was suffering from *abaphansi basifulathele*, meaning that the ancestors were angry that Phumlani was not following the life course they had chosen for him. This is because the paternal family had previously taken him to another traditional healer who said that Phumlani was ignoring a calling to become a traditional healer. During this time, Phumlani was ridiculed and bullied at school and then acted out aggressively.

Health History

Developmental milestones were reportedly achieved age-appropriately. However, following the accident and the surgery, there were indications of developmental regression, with loss of acquired functions, especially in the verbal domain. In his Grade 1 year, ADHD was diagnosed, and autism was ruled out. Medication and therapeutic inputs were recommended, and Phumlani attended speech and occupational therapy at University clinics for one year. Vision and hearing evaluations ruled out any difficulties in these areas.

Phumlani's general health was reported as good. His mother indicated that he experiences enuresis during sleep, as well as nightmares. He was no longer taking any traditional medicines but was taking stimulant medication prescribed by the psychiatrist at the local hospital. He did not consistently take this as the hospital pharmacy sometimes runs low on supplies, and other times his mother is unable to fetch the medication. There was no family history of epilepsy or psychiatric illness.

Educational History

Phumlani did not attend preschool, which is not compulsory in South Africa. He was looked after by his grandmother and sisters until he started formal schooling. Phumlani was 13 years, 3 months at the time of testing, and in Grade 5. He was kept back a year in Grade 1, and again in Grade 4. His brother, Jabu, is in Grade 7 and has not repeated any years. Phumlani's academic performance is varied, and he failed the recent exams. Reports from the school indicate that he needs structure, supervision, and additional time to ensure that he completes tasks.

Test and Norm Selection

In order to obtain a detailed multidomain evaluation of Phumlani's neurocognitive functioning, the NEPSY-II[24] was selected. Although there are no South African norms for this test, the NEPSY-II manual includes scores from special case studies, including ADHD, intellectual disability, and traumatic brain injury. Each case study was compared to a control sample, matched on age, sex, race, and parent-education level, which allowed some comparison between Phumlani's performance and that of a demographically similar case with a similar difficulty. In addition, the examiner was able to test Phumlani's twin brother as a control case[†] against which to compare Phumlani's performance. All tests were administered in English as Phumlani already had seven years of formal education in English.

[†]Marilyn Adan inspired the assessment of Phumlani's twin, after reporting a similar situation in Nell (15 p. 211).

Phumlani experienced difficulties grasping the assessment tasks, particularly the more abstract ones, and so testing was commenced at a lower age level (five years) and was then gradually advanced to the age-appropriate level. In addition, a dynamic assessment approach was used with some tests, which gave Phumlani extended time and/or practice attempts in order to evaluate his best possible performance. This approach evaluates performance both with and without careful mediational assistance from the tester, and the two levels of performance are contrasted to determine Phumlani's learning potential.[25] As there was variation from standardized testing procedures, the results reported below represent an estimate of Phumlani's functioning across the domains assessed, and are contrasted with the scores attained by his brother.

The following were administered:

1 A Developmental Neuropsychological Assessment, Second Edition (NEPSY-II[24])
2 Rey–Osterrieth Complex Figure Test (ROCF[26]).
3 The Draw-a-Person Test (DAP[27]).
4 Kinetic Family Drawing (KFD[28]).

Behavioral Observations

Phumlani appeared withdrawn and lethargic, he seldom made eye contact, and hid his face in his hands, and turned his body away from the examiner. As he became more relaxed, these behaviors lessened although eye contact remained minimal. Many South African cultures regard direct eye contact as disrespectful,[29] and so avoidance of eye contact was not regarded as inherently problematic. Phumlani tended to give monosyllabic responses to questions, but his speech was fluent when talking about topics that interested him, particularly football. He enjoyed looking at toys, but showed little interest in imaginative play or storytelling. Phumlani's attention and concentration fluctuated throughout the assessment and he was easily distracted.

Phumlani is left-handed, with adequate fine-motor control. However, he experienced difficulty planning and executing drawing tasks. His compliance with test instructions and participation in the various tests had to be negotiated (e.g., testing had to be interspersed with games), to enable task completion. Phumlani seemed accustomed to being rewarded for behaving appropriately. As soon as tasks became mildly challenging, he gave up and frequently requested to go to the bathroom. Systematic repetition of test requirements was needed, particularly for multipart instructions. In contrast, his twin, Jabu, was friendly and engaged, and chatted spontaneously. He was able to comprehend tasks at first instruction and to maintain focus until completion. In many instances, Phumlani's grandmother had to translate the instructions for Phumlani, whereas Jabu understood all without translation. While this is not best practice, given that family members tend to want to assist when translating, it speaks to the South African context where psychologists are often not proficient in the languages that clients are comfortable with and there is a shortage of trained professionals who can assist. Ideally a professionally trained translator should be used.

Test Performance

Attention and Executive Functioning

Phumlani's performance in this domain was well below the expected level for his age. In contrast, Jabu's performance was within the Low Average to Average range, with the exception of the Clocks subtest, which was Below Average. Both boys experienced difficulty with the concept of time, which may be due to lack of exposure. Phumlani's performance suggested difficulties with selective auditory attention (he was easily distracted from tasks and instructions had to be frequently repeated); the ability to prevent impulsive or well-learned responses; the ability to adopt, maintain and change set (he struggled to categorize objects into concrete groups); and the ability to plan and organize. This was coupled with slow responding to tasks with time limits. Phumlani struggled to spontaneously self-correct, showing a lack of awareness of his errors, whereas Jabu showed good self-monitoring, noticing, and spontaneously correcting errors.

Language

While the boys speak isiZulu at home, they have attended an English medium school since Grade 1. Phumlani experienced difficulty understanding verbal instructions of increasing complexity. He struggled to read a Grade 2 level story and showed poor comprehension, which corroborates reports from his school. Jabu, in contrast, was able to read and comprehend in English with few errors. Phumlani could name concrete objects reasonably accurately but very slowly, suggesting delayed access to this vocabulary. His mother and teachers reported similar difficulties in isiZulu. Overall, Phumlani's English communication skills are weak, while Jabu's were in the Low Average range.

Social Perception

Phumlani found it difficult to interpret non-verbal cues, to form impressions of others, to recognize emotions in faces and to use contextual information to make inferences about others (all necessary for social functioning). He also struggled to infer other people's beliefs or intentions. In contrast, Jabu fared in the High Average range in these areas.

Memory and Learning

Phumlani's immediate and long-term visuospatial memory for abstract geometric designs was very poor. Memory for faces was somewhat better, but still below expected levels for his age, although retention after a delay was acceptable, suggesting slow processing. Memory for names connected to faces was very weak both at immediate and delayed recall (isiZulu names of similar lengths were also substituted for the English names, yet performance was equally poor), and a similar pattern was found with immediate memory for word pairs. Jabu's performance was slightly better, falling in the Borderline range.

Phumlani found the age-appropriate narrative memory story too complicated, and consequently the story for younger children (five to ten years) was read aloud. He could recall very few details about it. He was then questioned about it to see whether cues assisted his recall, and was asked to choose between a correct and incorrect fact from the story. His immediate free recall was average for a ten-year old, while cued recall and recognition were extremely poor. After Phumlani was taught some strategies for focusing his attention and for recalling key aspects of a story, a second story was read to him (from the Stories subtest of the Children's Memory Scale[30]). His performance on all aspects improved to that of a 12-year old, suggesting good potential for improvement if taught appropriate learning strategies.

Sensorimotor Skills

Phumlani's fine-motor speed and co-ordination, including finger dexterity and motor speed, and fine motor programming were sound (Low Average), and his performance was similar whether he used his non-dominant or dominant hand. His performance was similar to that of his brother's, which was in the Average range.

Visuospatial Processing

This includes interrelated skills, such as judging line orientation, copying figures, reconstructing designs from a model, mentally rotating figures, breaking a figure into parts, and recognizing part-whole relationships. Phumlani's functioning was at age-appropriate levels, although he struggled as the material became more abstract and when time limits were imposed. In comparison, Jabu showed High Average abilities in this domain. Phumlani's visuo-graphic reproduction of complex material on the Rey Complex Figure Test (RCFT) was quick and careless, with many errors and distortions and signs of perseveration. He could not complete the immediate recall task. Delayed visual recall was also poor and he struggled to recognize elements of the drawing when cues were provided.

This performance is contrasted with Phumlani's sound performance on Design Copying of the NEPSY-II, which assesses similar skills. It is possible he was overwhelmed by the complexity of the RCFT and did not apply the same effort as for the NEPSY-II task, where designs were gradually increased in complexity (starting at age five). This does not necessarily indicate difficulty with visual memory, but with organizing visual material in a coherent and meaningful way to encode it in memory. After dynamic mediation, during which the figure was drawn by the examiner while providing a systematic explanation on how to organize the details of the figure into an integrated structure, Phumlani's copying of the figure improved considerably. This indicates good modifiability (ability to learn) when provided with an appropriate strategy.

Emotional Functioning

Projective tests provided tentative indications regarding Phumlani's self-concept, perceptions of his family, interpersonal functioning, and any emotional issues that he may be experiencing. Current research using these measures with culturally diverse South African samples was considered in their interpretation.[31]

For the DAP Test, Phumlani drew a simplified figure of undetermined gender with little attention to detail. A qualitative analysis revealed possible regression tendencies, vulnerable social and emotional adjustment, anxiety, brain injury, dependency, passivity and impulsivity, need for a protective mother figure, and feelings of immobility and constriction.

The KFD is an unstructured projective technique that reveals the child's feelings in relation to those who he regards as most important and whose formative influence is most powerful. As with the DAP, Phumlani drew in a hurried manner (in order): himself, Jabu, his father (on questioning this was revealed to be his paternal uncle, who plays an important part in the children's lives), and mother. It is typical in many African cultures for an uncle to take over the deceased father's role.[32] There was no interaction between any of the figures. The drawing suggests that Phumlani perceives himself as the most important member of the family and identifies closely with his brother, mother, and uncle, but that his sisters are less important in his life.

Test Results and Impressions

Phumlani's performance in all areas, except sensorimotor functioning, was significantly lower than that of his brother, suggesting that the difficulties are related to the brain injury, epilepsy, and/or surgery. His attention, processing speed, and executive functioning difficulties significantly compromised his performance. However, he responded well when tasks were simplified and he was given a structure for how to complete them. Phumlani employs various coping strategies when confronted with tasks that he perceives as too challenging, such as regression, distraction, resistance, or withdrawal. These have been increasing at school and at home, in response to increased academic requirements and social expectations.

Recommendations

Phumlani's mother was receptive to discussing his medications with his psychiatrist to ensure that dosages are effective, given his attention difficulties. She also agreed that individual therapy, with a focus on learning how different emotions are expressed in himself and others, how to connect emotions to the appropriate verbal labels, how to regulate emotions and behaviors, as well as learning how his behavior may impact others, would be helpful. It was recommended that the psychologist meet with the entire family to discuss Phumlani's difficulties and how the family can assist him. It was also necessary to engage with the family's belief systems, since there was a belief in ancestral wrath as a cause of Phumlani's difficulties. Counseling was recommended for Phumlani's mother in order to support and assist with parenting decisions and stresses, and to negotiate the stressors imposed by her in-laws and the community. Phumlani's sister, a university student, agreed to initiate the contact with the psychiatrist and psychologist and to assist her mother with these meetings. Given his difficulties, it was recommended that Phumlani be placed in a remedial school. We also discussed how Phumlani's sisters could assist him with effective study and learning strategies.

Section III: Lessons Learned

- Due to varying levels of literacy, test-wiseness, and acculturation, local psychologists cannot rely solely on a traditional, psychometric testing approach. Instead, a holistic assessment approach is utilized, including a battery of tests, qualitative observations, a detailed and appropriate history, and collateral information, before making decisions and recommendations.[33]
- In heterogeneous societies, such as South Africa, a biopsychosocial-spiritual approach is typically adopted. This allows practitioners to consider both Western systems like the DSM-5 and ICD-10 together with sociocultural and community beliefs about health and illness. The two approaches should not be regarded as mutually exclusive. It is common in African cultures to seek help from a range of sources in recognition that different practitioners can fulfill different needs. Western medicine is often consulted for symptomatic relief, while advice may be sought from traditional healers about explanations for the illness.[34] This means that practitioners need to be culturally sensitive, and that training in neuropsychological assessment should include an understanding of the inter-relationship between beliefs-attitudes, knowledge, and skills.[35]
- In the face of limited resources, it is prudent to research and adapt existing, psychometrically sound measures for use with local populations wherever possible.[36] For example, phonemic fluency tests are established measures of executive functioning. English phonemic fluency is typically tested using the letters FAS (as in the Controlled Oral Word Association Test, COWAT). Different letter sets have been researched for different South African languages, for example, Afrikaans[37] and isiXhosa.[38] The latter study provides a good example of the adaptation of this test with appropriate test items and norms for isiXhosa-speakers in keeping with the International Test Commission's guidelines for culture-fair testing in multi-lingual populations, and recommendations on how to ensure linguistic equivalence of stimuli.[39]
- Since there are few locally normed neuropsychological tests, a flexible approach is essential and psychologists need to be circumspect in their use of normative data. Working in a less structured paradigm allows psychologists to work more flexibly with clients who have linguistic and educational challenges. Non-verbal tests are useful but also rely on test-wiseness and acculturation, and so tests frequently have to be adapted. For example, it may be more appropriate for testees from rural backgrounds to complete Block Design tasks with more familiar objects such as beads, as many African cultures have a tradition of beadwork. Bead

patterns can also be used to evaluate series formation and sequential memory. Arithmetic problems can be represented in terms of counting cattle, fruit, beads, or food quantities.[40] If a child is unfamiliar with paper and pencil work, she can draw a figure with a stick in wet sand or construct a human figure from clay as an adaptation of the DAP Test.[41]

- Given the high levels of socio-economic deprivation and poor schooling in some areas of South Africa, dynamic assessment techniques are useful for tapping learning potential.[42] However, as with other qualitative approaches, this is time and resource intensive and requires specialist skills. Measures of working memory (often included in general intelligence assessments) may be a relatively easy and inexpensive way of tapping a testee's capacity for learning. As indicators of fluid, flexible problem solving, working memory measures tend to be less influenced by SES or access to resources since the stimuli used tend to be equally unfamiliar to all testees, or entail well-learned stimuli, such as letters and numbers.[16,43,44]
- Recommendations commonly include adapted strategies tailored to a testee's SES and cultural background. For example, parents who do not have access to occupational therapy, can encourage their child to use available materials to develop fine motor skills, such as making daisy chains from flowers and grass, threading bottle tops on a string, buttoning shirts after ironing.[10]
- Psychologists need to be aware of the ways in which bilingualism and multi-lingualism can alter typical performance expectations. For example, semantic fluency in either of the bilingual's languages is generally lower than that of monolinguals.[45] Given the varied levels of English proficiency in South Africa, where most tests only exist in English, the testee's English language proficiency should always be considered.
- Psychologists should be sensitive to ethnocentric biases in the interpretation of projective tests. For example, the differing perceptions of fertility in African and Western countries; in many African cultures, children confer social status, offer social security, assist with labor, secure property rights and inheritance, provide continuity through reincarnation and maintenance of the family lineage, satisfy emotional needs and secure conjugal ties.[46] Similarly, tester effects, such as the presence of a person from a different culture, can impact on testee's responding. This is particularly relevant in South Africa, given its history of racial tensions. Further, the power relations between the tester and testee need to be considered, as this can give rise to socially desirable responding.[31]

Glossary

Abaphansi basifulathele.   An ailment related to ancestral displeasure.

Afrikaans.   A West Germanic language that developed from the 1820 Dutch settlers in South Africa, still in use today.

Amadlozi.   An isiZulu term for ancestors (family members who have died).

Colored.   South African term for people of mixed-race ancestry.

Ubuntu.   A sense of community and togetherness which stresses how all of our actions impact on others and on society.

Ukugula kwashukela.   Illnesses due to certain medical conditions.

References

1. Statistics South Africa (2020). Mid-year population estimates [Internet]. [place unknown]: Department Statistics of South Africa; 2020 Jul 9 [cited 2020 Sep 8]. Available from: http://www.statssa.gov.za/?p=13453
2. Oppenheimer S. Out of Africa's Eden. Jeppestown: Jonathan Ball; 2003.

3. Giliomee H, Mbenga B, editors. New history of South Africa. 2nd ed. Cape Town: Tafelberg; 2007. p. 454.
4. Thompson L. A history of South Africa. 3rd ed. London: Yale University Press; 2000. p. 416.
5. Laher S. An overview of illness conceptualizations in African, Hindu, and Islamic traditions: Towards cultural competence. South African J Psych. 2014 Jun;44(2):191–204.
6. Sehoana MJ, Laher S. Pedi psychologists' perceptions of working with mental illness in the Pedi community in Limpopo, South Africa: the need to incorporate indigenous knowledge in diagnosis and treatment. Indilinga. 2015 Dec;14(2):233–47.
7. Sodi T, Mudhovozi P, Mashamba T, Radzalani-Makatu M, Takalani J, Mabunda J. Indigenous healing practices in the Limpopo Province of South Africa: a qualitative study. Int J Heal Prom Ed. 2011;49(3):101–10.
8. Truter I. African traditional healers: cultural and religious beliefs intertwined in a holistic approach. South African Pharm J. 2007;74(8):56–60.
9. Statistics South Africa (2021). Education [Internet]. [place unknown]: Department Statistics of South Africa; 2021 March 3 [cited 2021 Feb 25]. Available from http://www.statssa.gov.za/?page_id=737&id=4=4
10. Laher S, Cockcroft K. Moving from culturally biased to culturally responsive assessment practices in low resource, multicultural settings. Prof Psych. 2017 Apr;48(2):115–21.
11. De Kock JH, Pillay BJ. A situation analysis of clinical psychology services in South Africa's public rural primary care settings. S Afr J Psych. 2016 Oct 6;47(2):260–70.
12. The World Bank. The World Bank in South Africa [Internet]. Pretoria (ZA): [publisher unknown]; [updated 2019 Oct 10; cited 2020 Sep 3]. Available from: https://www.worldbank.org/en/country/southafrica/overview
13. Spaull N. Poverty and privilege: primary school inequality in South Africa. Int J Ed Dev. 2013 Sep;33(5):436–47.
14. Shuttleworth-Edwards AB, Kemp RD, Rust AL, Muirhead JGL, Hartman NP, Radloff SE. Cross-cultural effects on IQ test performance: a review and preliminary normative indications on WAIS-III test performance. J Clin Exp Neuropsych. 2004 Oct;26(7):903–20.
15. Nell V. Cross-cultural neuropsychological assessment: theory and practice. Hove: Psychology Press; 1999. p. 312.
16. Cockcroft K, Alloway T, Copello E, Milligan R. A cross-cultural comparison between South African and British students on the Wechsler Adult Intelligence Scales Third Edition (WAIS-III). Front Psych. 2015 Mar 13;6(297):1–11.
17. Pillay-Van Wyk V, Msemburi W, Laubscher R, Dorrington RE, Groenewald P, Glass T et al. Mortality trends and differentials in South Africa from 1997 to 2012: second national burden of disease study. Lancet Glob Health. 2016 Sept 01;4(1559):E642–53.
18. Maphumulo WT, Bhengu BR. Challenges of quality improvement in the healthcare of South Africa post-apartheid: a critical review. Curationis. 2019 May 29;42(1):a1901.
19. Burger R, Christian C Access to health care in post-apartheid South Africa: availability, affordability, acceptability. Health Econ Policy Law. 2020 Jan 01;15(1):43–55.
20. Laher S, Cockcroft K, editors. Psychological assessment in South Africa: research and applications. Johannesburg: Wits University Press; 2013. p. 592.
21. Claassen NCW, Van Niekerk HA, Kotze MM, De Beer M, Ferndale U, Vosloo HN, Viljoen M. General Scholastic Aptitude Test—Junior, Intermediate and Senior (GSAT). Mindmuzik 2008. p. 490.
22. Taylor T. APIL and TRAM learning potential assessment instruments. In: Laher S, Cockcroft K, editors. Psychological assessment in South Africa: research and applications. Johannesburg: Wits University Press; 2013. p. 158–68.
23. De Beer M. The learning potential computerised adaptive test in South Africa. In: Laher S, Cockcroft K, editors. Psychological assessment in South Africa: research and applications. Johannesburg: Wits University Press; 2013. p. 137–57.
24. Korkman M, Kirk U, Kemp S. NEPSY-II: clinical and interpretive manual. 2nd ed. San Antonio (TX): The Psychological Corporation; 2007. p. 290.

25. Amod Z, Seabi J. Dynamic assessment in South Africa. In: Laher S, Cockcroft K, editors. Psychological assessment in South Africa: research and applications. Johannesburg: Wits University Press; 2013. p. 120–36.

26. Strauss E, Sherman EMS, Spreen O. A compendium of neuropsychological tests: administration, norms, and commentary. 3rd ed. New York (NY): Oxford University Press; 2006. p. 1216.

27. Harris DB. Children's drawings as measures of intellectual maturity. New York (NY): Harcourt, Brace & World; 1963. p. 367.

28. Burns RC, Kaufman SH. Kinetic family drawings (K-F-D): an introduction to understanding children through kinetic drawings. New York (NY): Brunner/Mazel; 1970. p. 160.

29. Carter JH. Psychosocial/cultural issues in medicine and psychiatry: treating African Americans. J Nat Med Ass. 1995 Dec;87(12):857–60.

30. Cohen MJ. Children's Memory Scale: administration manual. San Antonio, Texas: The Psychological Corporation; 1997. p. 170.

31. Bain K, Amod Z, Gericke R. Projective assessment of adults and children in South Africa. In: Laher S, Cockcroft K, editors. Psychological assessment in South Africa: research and applications. Johannesburg: Wits University Press; 2013. p. 336–54.

32. Clowes L, Kopano R, Shefer T. Who needs a father? South African men reflect on being fathered. J Gen Stud. 2013 Jan 25;22(3):255–67.

33. Foxcroft C, Davies C. Historical perspectives on psychometric testing in South Africa. In: van Ommen C, Painter D, editors. Interiors: a history of psychology in South Africa. Pretoria: University of South Africa Press; 2008. pp. 152–82.

34. Crawford TA, Lipsedge M. Seeking help for psychological distress: the interface of Zulu traditional healing and Western biomedicine. Men Heal Rel Cul. 2004;7(2):131–48.

35. Sue DW, Arredondo P, McDavis RJ. Multicultural counselling competencies and standards: a call to the profession. J Multicult Couns Dev. 1992;20(2):64–89.

36. Shuttleworth-Edwards AB. On not re-inventing the wheel: a clinical perspective on culturally relevant test usage in South Africa. South African J Psych. 1996 Jun 1;26:96–102.

37. Kodituwakku PW, Adnams CM, Hay A, Kitching AE, Burger E, Kalberg WO, et al. Letter and category fluency in children with fetal alcohol syndrome from a community in South Africa. J Stud Alc. 2006 Jul;67(4):502–9.

38. Ferrett HL, Carey PD, Baufeldt AL, Cuzen NL, Conradie S, Dowling T, et al. Assessing phonemic fluency in multilingual contexts: letter selection methodology and demographically stratified norms for three South African language groups. Int J Test. 2014 Apr 28;14(2):143–67.

39. Muñiz J, Elosua P, Hambleton RK. International Test Commission Guidelines for test translation and adaptation: second edition. Psicothema. 2013;25(2):151–157.

40. Foxcroft CD. Ethical issues related to psychological testing in Africa: what I have learned (so far). Onl Readings Psych Cult. 2011;2(2):2307–0919.

41. Matafwali B, Serpell R. Design and validation of assessment tests for young children in Zambia. New Dir Child Adolesc Dev. 2014;146:77–96.

42. Sternberg RJ, Grigorenko EL. All testing is dynamic testing. Issues Ed. 2001;7(2):137–170.

43. Cockcroft K. A comparison between verbal working memory and vocabulary in bilingual and monolingual South African school beginners: Implications for bilingual language assessment. Int J Bil Ed Bil. 2016;19:74–88.

44. Cockcroft K, Bloch L, Moolla A. Assessing verbal functioning in South African school beginners from diverse socioeconomic backgrounds: a comparison between verbal working memory and vocabulary measures. Ed Change. 2016 Jan;20:112–28.

45. Bialystok E, Luk G, Peets KF, Yang S. Receptive vocabulary differences in monolingual and bilingual children. Bilingualism. 2010 Oct;13(4):525–31.

46. Dyer SJ. The value of children in African countries: insights from studies on infertility. J Psychos Obs Gyn. 2007 Jun;28(2):69–77.

Appendix
Test and Norm Resources

Editorial Note: The below neuropsychological resources have been provided by some authors to supplement information from their chapters. Please refer to corresponding chapters for further details. These resources include published or unpublished test adaptations/translations, normative data, references and further readings that the authors suggest exploring when evaluating those from a specific community. These resources are based on the authors' knowledge at the time of submission and are not meant to be an exhaustive list. These resources have also not been editorially verified, and readers are encouraged to confirm all sources, search for updated measures, and carefully consider appropriateness for their own clinical use.

Afghan (Authors: Ramezani, Tigranyan, Alvani, Ramezani, and Oliveira)

The following tests have been found useful in clinical practice:

Test	Citation	Available in Farsi or Persian	Available in English (for bilinguals)
Afghan Symptom Checklist (Farsi, Pashto, or English)	Miller et al. (2006)[1]	✓	✓
Afghan War Experience Scale (Farsi or English)	Miller et al. (2006)[1]	✓	✓
Afghan Acculturation and Language Preference (Farsi or English)	Alemi et al. (2015)[2]	✓	✓
Auditory Verbal Learning or Shiraz Auditory Verbal Learning Test (SAVLT)	Rahmani et al. (2017)[3]	✓	
Bilingual Aphasia Test—Persian or Farsi version	Paradis & Libben (1987); Paradis Paribakht, & Nilipour (1987)[4,5]	✓	✓
Persian Aphasia Battery (PAB)	Nilipour (1993)[6]	✓	
Farsi Aphasia Naming Test	Nilipour (2004, 2011)[7,8]	✓	
Boston Diagnostic Aphasia Test-3 (BDAE-3)	Kaplan, Goodglass, & Weintraub (2001)[9]		✓
Boston Naming Test-2	Kaplan, Goodglass, & Weintraub (2001)[9]		✓
Brief Visuospatial Memory Test-Revised	Benedict (1997); Eshaghi et al. (2012)[10,11]	✓	✓
Color Trails Test	D'Elia (1996); Tavakoli, Barekatain, & Emsaki (2015); Avila et al. (2019)[12–14]	✓	✓
Dot Counting Test	Boone, Lu, & Herzberg (2002)[15]		✓

(Continued)

Test	Citation	Available in Farsi or Persian	Available in English (for bilinguals)
Clock Drawing	Roudsari et al. (2018)[16]	✓	✓
Five Point Test or Ruff Figural Fluency Test	Lee et al. (1997); Ruff (1996)[17,18]		✓
Finger Tapping Test	Reitan (1979)[19]		✓
Grip Strength Test	Reitan, Wolfson (1993)[20]		✓
Line Bisection	Schenkenberg, Bradford, & Ajax (1980)[21]		✓
MMSE Farsi	Seyedian et al. (2008); Ansari et al. (2010)[22,23]	✓	✓
MoCA Farsi	Badrkhahan et al. (2020); Sikaroodi, Yadegari, & Miri (2013)[24,25]	✓	✓
Persian Adult Reading Test or National Adult Reading Test	Haghshenas et al. (2001)[26]	✓	✓
Parallel Picture-Naming Tests	Tahanzadeh, Soleymani, & Jalaie (2017)[27]	✓	
Repeatable Battery for the Assessment of Neuropsychological Status (RBANS) (selected scales)	Randolph (2009)[28]		✓
Rey Auditory Verbal Learning Test (RAVLT)	Jafari et al. (2010); Rezvanfard et al. (2011); Aghamollaei et al. (2012)[29–31]	✓	✓
Rey-15 Item Test	Lezak et al. (2012)[32]		✓
Rey Complex Figure Test	Meyers, Meyers (1995)[33]		✓
Rey-Word Recognition Test	Lezak et al. (2012)[32]		✓
Test of Memory Malingering	Tombaugh (1996)[34]		✓
Test of Nonverbal Intelligence	Brown, Sherbenov, Johnsen (2010)[35]		✓
The Stroop Color and Word Test (Golden Stroop in English and Victoria Stroop in Farsi)	Golden, Freshwater (2002); Malek et al. (2013)[36,37]	✓	✓
Symbol Digit Modality	Smith (1973)[38]		✓
Verbal Fluency (Farsi): JFK, PMK, FAS, Animal, Fruits and Vegetables, Grocery	Ebrahimipour et al. (2008); Dadgar, Khatoonabadi, Bakhtiyari (2013); Ghasemian-Shirvan et al. (2018); Soltani et al. (2019)[39–42]	✓	✓
WCST-64	Avila et al. (2019); Kongs (2000)[14,43]	✓	✓
Wechsler Adult Intelligence Scale (WAIS-IV) (selected subscales)	Wechsler (2008)[44]		✓
Wide Range Achievement Test (WRAT-5)	Wilkinson, Robertson (2017)[45]		✓

Afghan symptom checklist means and standard deviations:

ASCL (Miller et al., 2006)	Range	Mean	Standard Deviation
Women	22–110	68.21	16.70
Men	22–110	50.54	12.10

Note: Miller et al. noted the following in their method s section "The ASCL was administered to 324 adults (162 women and 162 men) in 8 of Kabul's 16 districts over the course of 5 days. The mean age of participants was 41.23 years (*SD* 4.83). We attempted to select districts that had experienced varying levels of war-related violence although, in fact, most of Kabul had been subjected to severe shelling during the war" (p. 426)[1].

Norm tables for memory tests (please also see Chapter 37 on Iranians for additional resources):

Author	Date published	Test name	Language test administered	Bilingual	If yes what language	Total numb	Numb females	Age range
Rahmani (recognition trial not stated but I got from author)	2017	Shiraz Verbal Learning Test (SVLT)	Persian	NO	n/a	1275	676	20–89

SVLT norms by age (Rahmani et al., 2017)

Test administered	Gender	20–29 years M	SD	%	30–44 years M	SD	%	45–59 years M	SD	%	60–69 years M	SD	%	70–79 years M	SD	%	80–89 years M	SD	%
Total trails 1–5	Female	61.1	8.77	0	57.2	8.39	0	53.4	7.8	0	50.1	8.19	0	41.8	5.59	0	33.7	3.23	0
	Males	59.5	9.74	68	54.5	8.6	87	53.02	6.68	95	45.5	8.58	98	39.4	6.61	100	35.5	5.67	100
Short-delay free recall	Female	13.9	2.02	0	13.3	2.11	0	12.3	2.24	0	11.4	2.51	0	10.9	2.8	0	6.14	1.74	0
	Males	13.5	2.56	84	12.5	2.58	91	11.9	2.53	95	8.2	3.05	99	8.39	3.23	99	6.47	2.07	100
Short-delay cued recall	Female	14.2	1.78	0	13.4	1.93	0	12.7	2.22	0	12.2	2.27	0	11.6	1.43	0	8.85	1.98	0
	Males	13.9	2.03	85	12.9	2.22	92	12.8	2.23	92	10.6	2.46	99	9.6	2.33	100	8.76	1.23	100
Long-delay free recall	Female	14.5	1.99	0	13.6	1.99	0	12.5	2.28	0	11.9	2.22	0	10.5	2.27	0	6.85	3.12	1
	Males	14.1	2.17	81	13.1	2.26	90	12.4	2.15	95	9.3	2.87	99	8.9	2.81	99	6.82	1.76	100
Long-delay cued recall	Female	14.7	1.77	0	13.8	1.94	0	12.9	2.16	0	12.7	2.09	0	11.5	1.44	0	9.71	1.92	0
	Males	14.5	1.78	80	13.5	2.06	89	13.2	2	92	10.7	2.26	99	10.1	1.98	100	9.29	0.93	100

Norm table of verbally mediated or language-based tests:

	PMK and animal supermarket fruit fluency								
	Ghasemian-Shirvan et al. (2018) norms data								
	P		*M*		*K*		*Total*		
Age	*M*	*SD*	*M*	*SD*	*M*	*SD*	*M*	*SD*
15–24	11.65	4.056	13	3.713	12.4	3.858	37.05	10.41
25–34	11.8	2.648	11.8	3.503	11.6	3.347	35.2	7.777
35–44	12.05	3.236	11.85	3.703	12.1	3.684	36	8.687
45–54	13	4.507	12.65	4.38	13.15	4.545	38.8	12.042
55–65	12.9	3.447	13.4	4.297	13.15	3.066	39.45	8.696

	Animal		*Supermarket*		*Fruit*		*Total*		
Age	*M*	*SD*	*M*	*SD*	*M*	*SD*	*M*	*SD*
15–24	20.9	5.647	19.65	5.174	18.55	3.663	59.1	12.993
25–34	20.35	6.209	20.85	5.687	19.2	5.307	60.4	14.608
35–44	21.75	4.756	20.75	4.723	18.9	3.11	61.4	9.058
45–54	23.3	4.244	22.7	4.293	21.55	5.624	67.55	11.45
55–65	22.05	4.478	22	4.437	19.7	3.729	63.75	9.711

Author	*Date published*	*Test name*	*Language test administered*	*Total numb*	*Numb females*	*Age*	*Age range*	*Education*	*Edu range*	*Mean*	*SD*
Eshaghi et al. (2012)	2012	Persian Adult Reading Test (PART)	Persian	90	57	33.65	n/a Age SD = 9.48	14.27	n/a	41.25	5.74
Hagh-Shenas et al. (2001)	2001	Persian Adult Reading Test (PART)	Persian	75	52	55+	n/a	n/a	n/a		
		Females	Persian							36.9	6.81
		Males	Persian							35	11.6
		Global	Persian							37	6.83

References

1. Miller KE, Omidian P, Quraishy AS, Quraishy N, Nasiry MN, Nasiry S et al. The Afghan symptom checklist: a culturally grounded approach to mental health assessment in a conflict zone. Am J Orthopsychiatry. 2006 Oct;76(4):423–433. doi: 10.1037/0002-9432.76.4.423. PMID: 17209710
2. Alemi Q, James S, Siddiq H, Montgomery S. Correlates and predictors of psychological distress among Afghan refugees in San Diego County. Int J Cult Ment Health. 2015;8(3):274–288. doi:10.1080/17542863.2015.1006647
3. Rahmani F, Haghshenas H, Mehrabanpour A, Mani A, Mahmoodi M. Shiraz Verbal Learning Test (SVLT): normative data for neurologically intact speakers of Persian. Arch Clin Neuropsychol. 2017;32(5):598–609.
4. Paradis M, Libben G. The assessment of bilingual aphasia. Hillsdale, NJ: Lawrence Erlbaum Associates; 1987.
5. Paradis M, Paribakht TS, Nilipour R. The Bilingual Aphasia Test (Farsi version) [Internet]. Hillsdale, NJ: Laurence Erlbaum Associates Inc.; 1987. Available from: http://mcgill.ca/linguistics/research/bat

6. Nilipour R. Persian Aphasia Battery (PAB). Tehran: Iran University of Medical Sciences Publication; 1993.

7. Nilipour R. Farsi Aphasia Naming Test. Tehran: University of Social Welfare and Rehabilitation Sciences Press; 2004.

8. Nilipour R. Aphasia Naming Test (Revised Version). Tehran: University of Social Welfare and Rehabilitation Sciences Press; 2011.

9. Kaplan E, Goodglass H, Weintraub S. The Boston Naming Test. 2nd ed. Austin, TX: Pro-Ed; 2001.

10. Benedict RHB. Brief Visuospatial Memory Test–Revised. Lutz, FL: PAR; 1997.

11. Eshaghi A, Riyahi-Alam S, Roostaei T, Haeri G, Aghsaei A, Aidi MR et al. Validity and Reliability of a Persian Translation of the Minimal Assessment of Cognitive Function in Multiple Sclerosis (MACFIMS). Clin Neuropsychol. 2012 Aug;26(6):975–84.

12. D'Elia LF, Satz P, Uchiyama CL, White T. Color Trails Test. Lutz, FL: PAR; 1996.

13. Tavakoli M, Barekatain M, Emsaki G. An Iranian normative sample of the color trails test. Psychol Neurosci. 2015;8(1):75–81.

14. Avila JF, Verney SP, Kauzor K, Flowers A, Mehradfar M, Razani J. Normative data for Farsi-speaking Iranians in the United States on measures of executive functioning. Appl Neuropsychol Adult [Internet]. 2019 May 4 [cited 2020 Nov 18];26(3):229–35. Available from: https://www.tandfonline.com/doi/full/10.1080/23279095.2017.1392963

15. Boone K, Lu P, Herzberg DS. The Dot Counting Test. Los Angeles, CA: Western Psychological Services; 2002.

16. Roudsari MS, Kamrani AAA, Foroughan M, Shahboulaghi FM, Karimlou M. Psychometric properties of the Persian version of the Clock Drawing Test (CDT) among the aged people in Iran. Iran J Psychiatry Behav Sci. 2018;12(4):e63386.

17. Lee GP, Strauss E, Loring DW, McCloskey L, Haworth JM, Lehman RAW. Sensitivity of figural fluency on the Five-Point test to focal neurological dysfunction. Clin Neuropsychol. 1997;11(1):59–68.

18. Ruff RM. Ruff Figural Fluency Test. Odessa, FL: PAR; 1996.

19. Reitan RM. Manual for administration of neuropsychological test batteries for adults and children. Tucson, AZ: Neuropsychology Laboratory; 1979.

20. Reitan RM, Wolfson D. The Halstead-Reitan Neuropsychological Test Battery: Theory and clinical interpretation. 2nd ed. Tucson, AZ: Neuropsychology Press; 1993. (vol. 31).

21. Schenkenberg T, Bradford DC, Ajax ET. Line bisection and unilateral visual neglect in patients with neurologic impairment. Neurology. 1980 May 1;30(5):509–17.

22. Seyedian M, Falah M, Nourouzian M, Nejat S, Delavar A, Ghasemzadeh HA. Validity of the Farsi version of mini-mental state examination. J Med Counc IRI. 2008;25(4):408–14.

23. Ansari NN, Naghdi S, Hasson S, Valizadeh L, Jalaie S. Validation of a Mini-Mental State Examination (MMSE) for the Persian population: a pilot study. Appl Neuropsychol. 2010;17(3):190–5.

24. Badrkhahan SZ, Sikaroodi H, Sharifi F, Kouti L, Noroozian M. Validity and reliability of the Persian version of the Montreal Cognitive Assessment (MoCA-P) scale among subjects with Parkinson's disease. Appl Neuropsychol Adult. 2020;27(5):431–9.

25. Sikaroodi H, Yadegari S, Miri SR. Cognitive impairments in patients with cerebrovascular risk factors: a comparison of Mini Mental Status Exam and Montreal Cognitive Assessment. Clin Neurol Neurosurg. 2013 Aug 1;115(8):1276–80.

26. Haghshenas H, Farashbandi H, Mani A, Tahmasbi S. Validity of Persian Adult Reading Test for the estimation of premorbid IQ. Iran J Med Sci. 2001 Jan 1;26(1–2):66–70.

27. Tahanzadeh B, Soleymani Z, Jalaie S. Parallel Picture-Naming Tests: development and psychometric properties for Farsi-speaking adults. Appl Neuropsychol Adult. 2017 Mar 4;24(2):100–7.

28. Randolph C. RBANS update: repeatable battery for the assessment of neuropsychological status. Bloomington, MN: Pearson; 2009.

29. Jafari Z, Moritz PS, Zandi T, Kamrani AA, Malyeri S. Psychometric properties of Persian version of the Rey Auditory-Verbal Learning Test (RAVLT) among the elderly. Iran J Psychiatry Clin Psychol. 2010;16(1):56–64.

30. Rezvanfard M, Ekhtiari H, Noroozian M, Rezvanifar A, Nilipour R, Javan GK. The Rey Auditory Verbal Learning Test: alternate forms equivalency and reliability for the Iranian adult population (Persian version). Arch Iran Med. 2011;14(2):104–9.

31. Aghamollaei M, Jafari Z, Toufan R, Esmaili M, Rahimzadeh S. Evaluation of auditory verbal memory and learning performance of 18–30 year old Persian-speaking healthy women. Audiology. 2012;21(3):32–9.

32. Lezak MD, Howieson DB, Bigler ED, Tranel D. Neuropsychological assessment. 5th ed. New York (NY): Oxford University Press; 2012.

33. Meyers JE, Meyers KR. Rey Complex Figure Test and recognition trial. Lutz, FL: PAR; 1995.

34. Tombaugh TN. Test of memory malingering. Toronto, Canada: Multi-Health Systems; 1996.

35. Brown L, Sherbenov RJ, Johnsen SK. Test of nonverbal intelligence. 4th ed. Austin, TX: Pro-Ed; 2010.

36. Golden CJ, Freshwater SM. The Stroop Color and Word Test: a manual for clinical and experimental uses. Chicago, IL: Stoelting; 2002.

37. Malek A, Hekmati I, Amiri S, Pirzadeh J, Gholizadeh H. The standardization of Victoria Stroop Color-Word Test among Iranian bilingual adolescents. Arch Iran Med. 2013;16(7):380–4.

38. Smith A. Symbol Digit Modality. Los Angeles, CA: Western Psychological Services; 1973.

39. Ebrahimipour M, Shahbeigi S, Jenabi M, Amiri Y, Kamali M. Verbal fluency performance in patients with multiple sclerosis. Iran J Neurol. 2008;7(21):138–42.

40. Dadgar H, Khatoonabadi AR, Bakhtiyari J. Verbal fluency performance in patients with nondemented Parkinson's disease. Iran J Psychiatry. 2013;8(1):55–8.

41. Ghasemian-Shirvan E, Shirazi SM, Aminikhoo M, Zareaan M, Ekhtiari H. Preliminary normative data of Persian phonemic and semantic verbal fluency test. Iran J Psychiatry. 2018;13(4):288–95.

42. Soltani M, Moradi N, Rezaei H, Hosseini M, Jasemi E. Comparison of verbal fluency in monolingual and bilingual elderly in Iran. Appl Neuropsychol Adult. 2019;28(1):80–7.

43. Kongs SK, Thompson LL, Iverson GL, Heaton RK. Wisconsin Card Sorting Test—64 Card Version. Lutz, FL: PAR; 2000.

44. Wechsler D. Wechsler Adult Intelligence Scale. 4th ed. Bloomington, MN: PsychCorp; 2008.

45. Wilkinson GS, Robertson GJ. Wide Range Achievement Test. 5th ed. Bloomington, MN: PsychCorp; 2017.

Chinese (Authors: Wong, Chin and Hong)

Neuropsychological Instruments Validated in Chinese-Speaking Populations*

Performance-based tests:

- Boston Naming Test[1,2]
- Consortium to Establish a Registry for Alzheimer's Disease Neuropsychological Assessment Battery[3]
- CERAD Word List Learning Test[3,4]
- Chinese Version Verbal Learning Test[5]
- Clock Drawing Test[2]
- Color Trails Test[6]
- Hong Kong List Learning Test[7]
- Hong Kong Test of Specific Learning Difficulties in Reading and Writing[8]
- Montreal Cognitive Assessment[9–11]
- Modified Wisconsin Card Sorting Test[12,13]
- Neuropsychological Measures—Normative Data for Chinese 2nd Edition[14]
- Repeatable Battery for the Assessment of Neuropsychological Status[15]
- Rey Complex Figure Test[2]

*This list is compiled based on the authors' best knowledge and is not an exhaustive list.

- Stroop Test[2,16]
- Symbol Digit Modalities Test[9,16]
- Test of Everyday Attention[17]
- Trail Making Test[2,16]
- Verbal Fluency Test[2,16]
- Wechsler Adult Intelligence Scale–IV (Hong Kong)[18]
- Wechsler Adult Intelligence Scale–IV (Taiwan)[19]
- Wechsler Intelligence Scale for Children-IV (Hong Kong)[20]
- Wechsler Intelligence Scale for Children-V (Taiwan)[21]
- Wechsler Memory Scale-Third Edition (Taiwan)[22]
- Wechsler Preschool and Primary Scale of Intelligence-IV (Hong Kong)[23]
- Wechsler Preschool and Primary Scale of Intelligence-IV (Taiwan)[24]

Rating scales:

- Autism-Spectrum Quotient[25]
- Beck Anxiety Inventory[26]
- Beck Depression Inventory-II[27]
- Beck Hopelessness Scale[28]
- Beck Scale for Suicide Ideation[29]
- Cross-Cultural (Chinese) Personality Assessment Inventory[30]
- Patient Health Questionnaire[31]
- Geriatric Depression Scale[32]
- Minnesota Multiphasic Personality Inventory®-2[33]
- Structured Interview of Reported Symptoms-2[34]

References

1. Cheung RW, Cheung M-C, Chan AS. Confrontation naming in Chinese patients with left, right or bilateral brain damage. J Int Neuropsychol Soc. 2004 Jan;10(1):46–53.
2. Li H, Lv C, Zhang T, Chen K, Chen C, Gai G et al. Trajectories of age-related cognitive decline and potential associated factors of cognitive function in senior citizens of Beijing. Curr Alzheimer Res. 2014 Sep 11;11(8):806–16.
3. Liu K, Kuo M, Tang K, Chau A, Ho I, Kwok M et al. Effects of age, education and gender in the Consortium to Establish a Registry for the Alzheimer's Disease (CERAD)-Neuropsychological Assessment Battery for Cantonese-speaking Chinese elders. Int Psychogeriatr. 2011 Jul 5;23(10):1575–81.
4. Sosa AL, Albanese E, Prince M, Acosta D, Ferri CP, Guerra M et al. Population normative data for the 10/66 Dementia Research Group cognitive test battery from Latin America, India and China: a cross-sectional survey. BMC Neurol. 2009 Aug 26;9(1):48.
5. Chang C, Kramer J, Lin K, Chang W, Wang Y, Huang C et al. Validating the Chinese version of the Verbal Learning Test for screening Alzheimer's disease. J Int Neuropsychol Soc JINS. 2009 Dec 11;16(2):244–51.
6. Hsieh S, Tori C. Normative data on cross-cultural neuropsychological tests obtained from Mandarin-speaking adults across the life span. Arch Clin Neuropsychol. 2007 Mar;22(3):283–96.
7. Au A, Chan AS, Chiu H. Verbal learning in Alzheimer's dementia. J Int Neuropsychol Soc JINS. 2003 Mar;9(3):363–75.
8. Chung KKH, Ho CSH, Chan DW, Tsang SM, Lee SH & Xiao XM. The Hong Kong test of specific learning difficulties in reading and writing for junior secondary school students (HKT-JS). Hong Kong: Hong Kong Specific Learning Difficulties Research Team; 2012.

9. An Y, Feng L, Zhang X, Wang Y, Wang Y, Tao L et al. Patterns of cognitive function in middle-aged and elderly Chinese adults—findings from the EMCOA study. Alzheimers Res Ther. 2018 Sep 15;10(1):93.

10. Tsai J-C, Chen C-W, Chu H, Yang H-L, Chung M-H, Liao Y-M et al. Comparing the sensitivity, specificity, and predictive values of the Montreal Cognitive Assessment and Mini-Mental State Examination when screening people for mild cognitive impairment and dementia in Chinese population. Arch Psychiatr Nurs. 2016 Jan 21;30(4): 486–91.

11. Chu L-W, Ng KH, Law AC, Lee AM, Kwan F. Validity of the Cantonese Chinese Montreal Cognitive Assessment in Southern Chinese. Geriatr Gerontol Int. 2015;15(1):96–103.

12. Wang Q, Sun J, Ma X, Wang Y, Yao J, Deng W et al. Normative data on a battery of neuropsychological tests in the Han Chinese population. J Neuropsychol. 2011;5(1):126–42.

13. Shan I-K, Chen Y-S, Lee Y-C, Su T-P. Adult normative data of the Wisconsin Card Sorting Test in Taiwan. J Chin Med Assoc JCMA. 2008 Oct;71(10):517–22.

14. Lee T, Wang K. Neuropsychological measures: normative data for Chinese. 2nd revised ed. Hong Kong: Laboratory of Neuropsychology, The University of Hong Kong; 2010.

15. Cheng Y, Wu W, Wang J, Feng W, Wu X, Li C. Reliability and validity of the repeatable battery for the Assessment of Neuropsychological Status in community-dwelling elderly. Arch Med Sci AMS. 2011 Oct;7(5):850–7.

16. Lee T, Yuen K, Chan C. Normative data for neuropsychological measures of fluency, attention, and memory measures for Hong Kong Chinese. J Clin Exp Neuropsychol. 2002 Aug;24(5):615–32.

17. Chan RCK, Wang L, Ye J, Leung WWY, Mok MYK. A psychometric study of the Test of Everyday Attention for Children in the Chinese setting. Arch Clin Neuropsychol Off J Natl Acad Neuropsychol. 2008 Jul;23(4):455–66.

18. Wechsler D. Wechsler Adult Intelligence Scale—Fourth Edition (Hong Kong). Hong Kong: King-May Psychological Assessment Technology Development, Ltd; 2014.

19. Wechsler D. Wechsler Adult Intelligence Scale—Fourth Edition (Taiwan). Taiwan: Chinese Behavioral Science Corporation; 2015.

20. Wechsler D. Wechsler Intelligence Scale for Children-IV. Hong Kong: King-May Psychological Assessment Technology Development, Ltd; 2010.

21. Wechsler D. Wechsler Intelligence Scale for Children-V. Taiwan: Chinese Behavioral Science Corporation; 2018.

22. Wechsler D. Wechsler Memory Scale—Third Edition. Taiwan: Chinese Behavioral Science Corporation; 2005.

23. Wechsler D. Wechsler Preschool and Primary Scale of Intelligence-IV. Hong Kong: King-May Psychological Assessment Technology Development, Ltd; 2018.

24. Wechsler D. Wechsler Preschool and Primary Scale of Intelligence-IV. Taiwan: Chinese Behavioral Science Corporation; 2013.

25. Sun F, Dai M, Lin L, Sun X, Murray AL, Auyeung B et al. Psychometric properties of the Chinese version of autism spectrum quotient-children's version: A sex-specific analysis. Autism Res Off J Int Soc Autism Res. 2019 Feb;12(2):303–15.

26. Beck AT, Steer RA. Beck Anxiety Inventory. Taiwan: Chinese Behavioral Science Corporation; 2000.

27. Beck AT, Steer RA, Brown GK. Beck Depression Inventory-II. Taiwan: Chinese Behavioral Science Corporation; 2000.

28. Beck AT, Steer RA. Beck Hopelessness Scale. Taiwan: Chinese Behavioral Science Corporation; 2000.

29. Beck AT, Steer RA. Beck Scale for Suicide Ideation. Taiwan: Chinese Behavioral Science Corporation; 2000.

30. Cheung F, Cheung SF, Leung F. Clinical utility of the Cross-Cultural (Chinese) Personality Assessment Inventory (CPAI-2) in the assessment of substance use disorders among Chinese men. Psychol Assess. 2008 Jul 1;20:103–13.

31. Spitzer RL, Williams JBW, Kroenke K. Patient Health Questionnaire Screeners [Internet]. Pfizer Inc; Available from: https://www.phqscreeners.com/

32. Mui AC. Geriatric Depression Scale as a Community Screening Instrument for elderly Chinese immigrants. Int Psychogeriatr. 1996 Sep;8(3):445–58.
33. Butcher JN, Grant Dahlstrom W, Graham JR, Tellegen A, Kaemmer B. Minnesota Multiphasic Personality Inventory®-2 Chinese Edition. Hong Kong: The Chinese University of Hong Kong Press; 1989.
34. Liu C, Liu Z, Chiu HF, Carl TW-C, Zhang H, Wang P et al. Detection of malingering: Psychometric evaluation of the Chinese version of the structured interview of reported symptoms-2. BMC Psychiatry. 2013 Oct 9;13(1):254.

Filipino (Authors: Agbayani, Dulay, Romero and Ordoñez)

Tests and questionnaires created/normed in the Philippines:

- De-Westernized Dementia Screening Scale (DDSS)[1]
- Neuropsychological Assessment for Mild Cognitive Impairment (NAMCI)[2]
- Manila Motor-Perceptual Screening Test (MMPS)[*,3]

Western-based tests validated with Filipinos and/or translated to Tagalog:

- Alzheimer's Disease Assessment Scale—Cognitive (ADAS-Cog)[4]
- Behavioral Assessment and Research System[*,5]
- Eyberg Child Behavior Inventory (ECBI)[*,6]
- Filipino Geriatric Depression Scale short-form[7]
- Filipino version of the Mini Mental Status Exam (MMSE-P)[8]
- Neuropsychological Test Battery from the Uniform Dataset of Alzheimer's Disease Center (UDS-ADC)[4]

[*]For use with children.

References

1. Ledesma LK, Diputado BY, Ortega GO, Santillan CE. Development of the de-Westernized Dementia Screening Scale. Philipp J Psychol. 1993;26(2):30–8.
2. Julom, AM. The development and validation of a neuropsychological assessment for mild cognitive impairment of Filipino older adults. Ageing Int. 2013;38:271–327.
3. Javier SB, Luna-Reyes OB, Walter RT, Ledesma LK, Reyes TM. The Manila motor-perceptual screening test: Its development and field investigation. Santo Tomas J Med. 1988;37:126–69.
4. Dominguez JC, Phung TKT, de Guzman MFP, Fowler KC, Reandelar M, Natividad B et al. Determining Filipino normative data for a battery of neuropsychological tests: the Filipino Norming Project (FNP). Dement Geriatr Cogn Disord. 2019;9:260–70.
5. Rohlman DS, Villanueva-Uy E, Ramos EAM, Mateo PC, Bielawski DM, Chiodo LM et al. Adaptation of the Behavioral Assessment and Research System (BARS) for evaluation neurobehavioral performance in Filipino children. Neurotoxicology. 2008;29(1):143–51.
6. Coffey DM, Javier JR, Schrager SM. Preliminary validity of the Eyberg Child Behavior Inventory with Filipino immigrant parents. Child Family Behav Ther. 2015;37(3):208–23.
7. Ty WEG, Davis RD, Melgar MIE, Ramos MA. A Validation Study on the Filipino Geriatric Depression Scale (GDS) using Rasch Analysis. Int J Psychiatr Res. 2019;2(7): 1–6.
8. Ligsay A. validation of the mini mental state examination in the Philippines. Manila: University of the Philippines Manila; 2003

Greek (Author: Staois)

Screening tools:

- Mini Mental State Examination (MMSE)[1]
- Cambridge Cognitive Examination of the Elderly[2]
- Clock Drawing Test[3]
- Ruff 2 & 7 Selective Attention Test[4]

General intelligence:

- Wechsler Adult Intelligence Scale (4th ed.): Adaptation for Greece (WAIS-IV GR)[5]
- Neuropsychological Test Battery. Unpublished Tests & Norms

New learning and memory:

- Rey Auditory Verbal Learning Test[6]
- Greek Verbal Learning Test7
- Selective Reminding Test8
- The Benton Visual Retention Test[9]
- The 5 Objects Test[10]
- The Hellenic Famous Face Screening Test[11]

Executive Functioning:

- Stroop Test[12]
- Trail-Making Test[13]
- Color Trails Test[14]
- Verbal Fluency[15]

Naming and Language:

- Boston Naming Test[16]

Visuospatial Skills:

- Hooper Visual Organization Test[17]
- Rey Complex Figure Test[18]

References

1. Fountoulakis KN, Tsolaki M, Chantzi H et al. Mini mental state examination (MMSE): a validation study in Greece. Am J Alzheimers Dis Other Demen. 2000;15:342–5.
2. Tsolaki M, Fountoulakis K, Chantzi H et al. The Cambridge cognitive examination (CAMCOG): a validation study in outpatients suffering from dementia and nondemented elderly subjects (including age associated cognitive de- cline patients) in Greece. Am J Alzheimers Dis Other Demen. 2000;15:269–76.
3. Bozikas VP, Giazkoulidou A, Hatzigeorgiadou M et al. Do age and education contribute to performance on the clock drawing test? Normative data for the Greek population. J Clin Exp Neuropsychol. 2008;30:199–203.
4. Messinis L, Kosmidis MH, Tsakona I et al. Ruff 2 and 7 selective attention test: normative data, discriminant validity and test-retest reliability in Greek adults. Arch Clin Neuropsych. 2007;22:773–85.
5. Wechsler D. The Wechsler Adult Intelligence Scale, Fourth Edition (4th ed.): Adaptation for Greece (WAIS-IV GR). Athens: Motibo Publishing. 2014.
6. Messinis L, Nasios G, Mougias A, Politis A, Zampakis P, Tsiamaki E, Malefaki S, Gourzis P, Papathanasopoulos P. Age and education adjusted normative data and discriminative validity for Rey's Auditory Verbal Learning Test in the elderly Greek population. J Clin Exp Neuropsychol. 2016;38(1):23–39. doi: 10.1080/13803395.2015.1085496. Epub 2015 Nov 20. PMID: 26588427.

7. Vlahou CH, Kosmidis MH, Dardagani A, Tsotsi S, Giannakou M, Giazkoulidou A et al. Development of the Greek Verbal Learning Test: reliability, construct validity, and normative standards. Arch of Clin Neuropsychol. 2012;28(1):52–64.

8. Zalonis I, Kararizou E, Christidi F et al. Selective reminding test: demographic predictors of performance and normative data for the Greek population. Psychol Rep. 2009; 104:593–607.

9. Messinis L, Lyros E, Georgiou V et al. Benton visual retention test performance in normal adults and acute stroke patients: demographic considerations, discriminant validity, and test-retest reliability. Clin Neuropsychol. 2009;23:962–77.

10. Papageorgiou SG, Economou A, Routsis C. The 5 Objects Test: a novel, minimal-language, memory screening test. J Neurol. 2014 Feb;261(2):422–31. doi: 10.1007/s00415-013-7219-1. Epub 2013 Dec 27. PMID: 24371005.

11. Proios H, Malatra I, Farmakis N. The Hellenic famous face screening test. J Med Speech Lang Pathol. 2007;15:383–94.

12. Zalonis I, Christidi F, Bonakis A et al. The Stroop effect in Greek healthy population: normative data for the Stroop neuropsychological screening test. Arch Clin Neuropsychol. 2009;24:81–88.

13. Zalonis I, Kararizou E, Triantafyllou NI, Kapaki E, Papageorgiou S, Sgouropoulos P, Vassilopoulos D. A normative study of the trail making test A and B in Greek adults. Clin Neuropsychol. 2008 Sep;22(5):842–50. doi: 10.1080/13854040701629301. Epub 2007 Nov 1. PMID: 17934999.

14. Messinis L, Malegiannaki AC, Christodoulou T, Panagiotopoulos V, Papathanasopoulos P. Color Trails Test: normative data and criterion validity for the Greek adult population. Arch Clin Neuropsychol. 2011;26:322–30.

15. Kosmidis MH, Vlahou CH, Panagiotaki P et al. The verbal fluency task in the Greek population: normative data, and clustering and switching strategies. J Int Neuropsychol Soc. 2004;10:164–72.

16. Patricacou A, Psallida E, Pring T et al. The Boston naming test in Greek: normative data and the effects of age and education on naming. Aphasiology. 2007;21:1157–70.

17. Giannakou M, Kosmidis MH. Cultural appropriateness of the Hooper visual organization test? Greek normative data. J Clin Exp Neuropsychol. 2006;28:1023–9.

18. Tsatali M, Emmanouel A, Gialaouzidis, M, Avdikou K., Stefanatos C, Diamantidou, A. et al. Rey Complex Figure Test (RCFT): norms for the Greek older adult population. App Neuropsychol. 2020: 1–9. doi: 10.1080/23279095.2020.1829624

India (Author: Irani)

Translated/Adapted/Validated/Normed Measures for Indian Context:

Please note: This list is not exhaustive. Most of the below measures can be administered in Indian English as well.

Measures	Languages	References
10/66 Dementia Research Group Cognitive Test Battery	Kannada; low literacy	Sosa et al. (2009),[1] Krishna et al. (2016)[2] (https://1066.alzint.org/)
Addenbrooke's Cognitive Examination—III	Tamil, Hindi, Indian English, Kannada, Telugu, Urdu, Marathi	Mathuranath et al. (2000),[3,4] Mekala et al. (2020)[5]
All India Institute of Medical Sciences (AIMS) Comprehensive Neuropsychological Battery	Hindi	Gupta et al. (2000)[6]
Alzheimer's Disease Assessment Scale—Cog	Tamil	Lakshminarayanan et al. (2021),[7] Panikker et al. (2000)[8]
Bilingual Aphasia Test Battery	Hindi, Kannada, Oriya, Tamil, Urdu, Malayalam	Billingual Aphasia Test[9]
Category and Phonemic Fluency	Malayalam, Hindi	Mathuranath et al. (2003),[10] Waldrop-Valverde et al. (2015)[11]
Community Screening Instrument for Dementia		Sosa et al. (2009)[1]

(Continued)

Measures	Languages	References
Consortium to Establish a Registry for Alzheimer's Disease (CERAD) Word List	Hindi	Ganguli et al. (1996)[12]
CNS Vital Signs	Bengali, Gujarati, Hindi, Kannada, Malayalam, Marathi, Punjabi, Tamil, Telugu, Urdu	https://www.cnsvs.com/ WhitePapers/CNSVS-Languages.pdf
Cognistat-Indian Adaptation		Gupta & Kumar (2009)[13]
Dementia Assessment by Rapid Test		Swati et al. (2015)[14]
Everyday Abilities Scale for Indians	Hindi	Fillenbaum et al. (1999)[15]
Frenchay Aphasia Screening Test	Telugu, Kannada	Paplikar et al. (2020)[16]
Geriatric Depression Scale	Hindi	Ganguli et al. (1999)[17]
Generalized Anxiety Disorder 7 item	Hindi, Gujarati, Kannada, Malayalam, Marathi, Punjabi, Tamil, Telugu, Urdu	https://www.phqscreeners.com/
HIV Cognitive Test Battery	Telugu, Tamil, English	Yepthomi et al. (2006)[18]
Hopkins Verbal Learning Test—Revised (adapted)	Hindi	Waldrop-Valverde et al. (2015)[11]
Indian Aphasia Battery	Hindi	Kaur et al. (2017),[19] Nehra, Pershad, & Sreenivas (2013)[20]
Indian Council of Medical Research Neurocognitive Tool Box	Hindi, Bengali, Telugu, Kannada, Malayalam	Menon et al. (2020)[21]
Indo-US Cross National Dementia Epidemiology Study	Hindi	Ganguli et al (1996)[12] (https:// www.dementia-epidemiology. pitt.edu/indous-norms/)
Instrumental Activities of Daily Living Scale for Elderly people		Mathuranath et al. (2005)[22]
Kolkata Cognitive Screening	Bengali	Das et al. (2006)[23]
Longitudinal Aging Study in India	English, Hindi, Kannada, Malayalam, Punjabi	Lee et al. (2019)[24] (https://www. hsph.harvard.edu/pgda/ major-projects/lasi-2/)
Logical Memory (complex passage)	Indian English	Andrade, Madhavan, & Kishore (2001)[25]
Mini Mental State Examination	Hindi, Gujarati, Marathi, Malayalam, Telegu, Bharmouri	Ganguli et al. (1995),[26] Lindesay et al. (1997),[27] Raina et al. (2013)[28] (https://strokengine.ca/ en/assessments/mini-mental-state-examination-mmse/#In whatlanguagesisthemeasureav ailable)
Mattis Dementia Rating Scale	Hindi	Gopaljee, Dwivedi, & Pandey (2011)[29]
Montreal Cognitive Assessment	Bengali, Kannada, Malayalam, Marathi, Tamil, Telugu, Hindi, Urdu	Krishnan et al. (2015),[30] Nasreddine et al. (2005)[31]
Multi-Domain Cognitive Screening Test		Hota et al. (2012)[32]
Naming Test	Malayalam	George & Mathuranath (2007)[33]
NIMHANS Neuropsychological Battery (Adults, Children, Elderly)	Kannada	Rao & Subbakrishna (2004),[34] Kar et al. (2004),[35] Mukundan & Murthy (1979),[36] Tripathi et al. (2013)[37]
Object Naming Test		Ganguli et al (1996)[12]
Patient Health Questionnaire	Assamese, Bengali, Indian English, Gujarati, Hindi, Kannada, Malayalam, Marathi, Oriya, Punjabi, Tamil, Telugu	https://www.phqscreeners.com/ select-screener
PGI Battery of Brain Dysfunction	Hindi	Pershad & Verma (1990)[38]
PGI Memory Scale		Pershad & Wig (1978)[39]

(Continued)

Measures	Languages	References
Picture-Based Memory Impairment Screen for Dementia	Malayalam	Verghese et al. (2012)[40]
Rowland Universal Dementia Assessment Scale	Malayalam	Iype et al. (2006),[41] Komalasari, Chang, & Traynor (2019)[42]
Seven Minute Screen	Malayalam	de Jager et al. (2008)[43]
Trail Making Test	English	Bhatia et al (2007)[44]
Vellore Screening Instrument for Dementia		Stanley et al (2009)[45]
Wechsler products (e.g. Wechsler Intelligence Scale for Children—Fourth Edition, India; Wechsler Adult Intelligence Scale—Fourth Edition, India, Weschler Abbreviated Scale of Intelligence, Second Edition, India, Wechsler Memory Scale—Third Edition, India	Indian English	https://pearsonclinical.in/pearson-clinical-solutions/
Western Aphasia Battery with Indian Norms	Kannada	Chengappa & Kumar (2008)[46]
Wisconsin Card Sorting Test	English, Hindi, Punjab	Kohli & Kaur (2006)[47]
World Health Organization's Study on AGEing and adult health survey		Carroll et al (2012)[48] (https://www.who.int/healthinfo/survey/SAGESurveyManualFinal.pdf)

References

1. Sosa AL, Albanese E, Prince M, Acosta D, Ferri CP, Guerra M et al. Population normative data for the 10/66 Dementia Research Group cognitive test battery from Latin America, India and China: A cross-sectional survey. BMC Neurol [Internet]. 2009 Aug 26;9:48. Available from: https://pubmed.ncbi.nlm.nih.gov/19709405/

2. Krishna, M, Beulah, E, Jones, S, Sundarachari, R, Kumaran, K, Karat, SC et al. Cognitive function and disability in late life: an ecological validation of the 10/66 battery of cognitive tests among community-dwelling older adults in South India. Int J Geriatr Psychiatry. 2016;31(8), 879–91.

3. Mathuranath PS, Nestor PJ, Berrios GE, Rakowicz W, Hodges JR. A brief cognitive test battery to differentiate Alzheimer's disease and frontotemporal dementia. Neurology [Internet]. 2000 Dec 12 [cited 2021 Jun 18];55(11):1613–20. Available from: https://pubmed.ncbi.nlm.nih.gov/11113213/

4. Mathuranath PS, Cherian JP, Mathew R, George A, Alexander A, Sarma SP. Mini mental state examination and the Addenbrooke's cognitive examination: effect of education and norms for a multicultural population. Neurol India [Internet]. 2007 Apr–Jun;55(2):106–10. Available from: https://pubmed.ncbi.nlm.nih.gov/17558112/

5. Mekala S, Paplikar A, Mioshi E, Kaul S, Divyaraj G, Coughlan G et al. Dementia diagnosis in seven languages: the Addenbrooke's Cognitive Examination-III in India. Arch Clin Neuropsychol. 2020;35(5):528–38.

6. Gupta S, Khandelwal SK, Tandon PN, Maheshwari MC, Mehta VS, Sundram KR et al. The development and standardization of a comprehensive neuropsychological battery in Hindi-Adult form. J Pers Clin Stud. 2000;16:75–109.

7. Lakshminarayanan M, Vaitheswaran S, Srinivasan N, Nagarajan G, Ganesh A, Shaji KS et al. Cultural adaptation of Alzheimer's disease assessment scale-cognitive subscale for use in India and validation of the Tamil version for South Indian population. Aging Ment Health [Internet]. 2021 Jan 25:1–8. Available from: https://doi.org/10.1080/13607863.2021.1875192

8. Panikker D, Bhatt A, Dikshit J, Vas C. The Indian adaptation of the Alzheimer's Disease Assessment Scale-cognitive (ADAS-cog): standardisation on a community-resident sample of older persons. Int J Geriatr Psychopharmacol. 2000 Jan;3:142–7.

9. Bilingual Aphasia Test (BAT) [Internet]. Montreal (QB): McGill; [date unknown; cited 2021 Jun 18]. Available from: https://www.mcgill.ca/linguistics/research/bat#ebat

10. Mathuranath PS, George A, Cherian PJ, Alexander AL, Sarma SG, Sarma PS. Effects of age, education and gender on verbal fluency. J Clin Exp Neuropsychol. 2003 Dec 1;25(8):1057–64.

11. Waldrop-Valverde D, Ownby RL, Jones DL, Sharma S, Nehra R, Kumar AM et al. Neuropsychological test performance among healthy persons in northern India: development of normative data. J Neurovirol. 2015;21(4):433–8.

12. Ganguli M, Chandra V, Ratcliff G, Sharma SD, Pandav R, Seaberg EC et al. Cognitive test performance in a community based non demented elderly sample in rural India: the Indo-US Cross-National Dementia Epidemiology Study. Int Psychogeriatr 1996;8:507–24.

13. Gupta A, Kumar NK. Indian adaptation of the Cognistat: psychometric properties of a cognitive screening tool for patients of traumatic brain injury. Indian J Neurotr [Internet]. 2009 Dec 1 [cited 2021 Jun 18];6(2):123–32. Available from: https://www.sciencedirect.com/science/article/abs/pii/S0973050809800063

14. Swati B, Sreenivas V, Manjari T, Ashima N. Dementia Assessment by Rapid Test (DART): an Indian screening tool for dementia. J Alzheimers Dis Parkinsonism [Internet]. 2015 Dec 3;5(198): doi: 10.4172/2161-0460.1000198.

15. Fillenbaum GG, Chandra V, Ganguli M, Pandav R, Gilby JE, Seaberg EC et al. Development of an activities of daily living scale to screen for dementia in an illiterate rural older population in India. Age Ageing. 1999 Mar;28(2):161–8.

16. Paplikar A, Iyer GK, Varghese F, Alladi S, Pauranik A, Mekala S et al. (2020). A screening tool to detect stroke aphasia: adaptation of Frenchay Aphasia Screening Test (FAST) to the Indian context. Ann Indian Acad Neurol. 23(Suppl 2):S143.

17. Ganguli M, Dube S, Johnston M, Pandav R, Chandra V, Dodge H. Depressive symptoms, cognitive impairment and functional impairment in a rural elderly population in India: a Hindi version of the Geriatric Depression Scale (GDS-H). Int J Geriatr Psychiatry. 1999;14:807–20.

18. Yepthomi T, Paul R, Vallabhaneni S, Kumarasamy N, Tate DF, Solomon S et al. Neurocognitive consequences of HIV in Southern India: a preliminary study of clade C virus. J Int Neuropsychol. 12(3):424–30. doi: 10.1017/s1355617706060516

19. Kaur H, Bajpal S, Pershad D, Sreenivas V, Nehra A. Development and standardization of Indian Aphasia Battery. J Ment Health Human Behav [Internet]. 2017 Jul–Dec;22(2):116–22.

20. Nehra A, Pershad D, Sreenivas V. Indian Aphasia battery: tool for specific diagnosis of language disorder post stroke. J Neurol Sci. 2013 Oct 15;333:e165. doi:10.1016/j.jns.2013.07.687

21. Menon RN, Varghese F, Paplikar A, Mekala S, Alladi S, Sharma M et al. Validation of Indian Council of Medical Research Neurocognitive Tool Box in diagnosis of mild cognitive impairment in India: lessons from a harmonization process in a linguistically diverse society. Dement Geriatr Cogn Disord. 2020;49(4):355–64.

22. Mathuranath PS, George A, Cherian PJ, Mathew R, Sarma PS. Instrumental activities of daily living scale for dementia screening in elderly people. Int Psychogeriatr. 2005 Sep;17(3):461–74. doi:10.1017/s1041610205001547.

23. Das SK, Biswas A, Roy T, Banerjee TK, Mukherjee CS, Raut DK, Chaudhuri A. A random sample survey for prevalence of major neurological disorders in Kolkata. Indian J Med Res [Internet]. 2006 Aug;124(2):163–72. Available from: https://pubmed.ncbi.nlm.nih.gov/17015930/

24. Lee J, Banerjee J, Khobragade PY, Angrisani M, Dey, AB. LASI-DAD study: a protocol for a prospective cohort study of late-life cognition and dementia in India. BMJ Open. 2019;9(7):e030300.

25. Andrade C, Madhavan AP, Kishore ML. Testing logical memory using a complex passage: development and standardization of a new test. Indian J Psychiatry. 2001 Jul;43(3):252–6.

26. Ganguli M, Ratcliff G, Chandra V, Sharma S, Gilby J, Pandav R et al. A Hindi version of the MMSE: the development of a cognitive screening instrument for a largely illiterate rural elderly population in India. Int J Geriat Psychiat. 1995 May;10(5):367–77. doi:10.1002/gps.930100505.

27. Lindesay J, Jagger C, Mlynik-Szmid A, Sinorwala A, Peet S, Moledina F. The mini-mental state examination in an elderly immigrant Gujarati population in the United Kingdom. Int J Geriatr Psychiatry. 1997;12:1155–67.

28. Raina SK, Raina S, Chander V, Grover A, Singh S, Bhardwaj A. Development of a cognitive screening instrument for tribal elderly population of Himalayan region in northern India. J Neurosci Rural Pract. 2013;4(2):147.

29. Gopaljee S, Dwivedi CB, Pandey R. Psychometric evaluation of the Hindi adaptation of Mattis Dementia Rating Scale (HMDRS). Indian J Soc Sci Res. 2011 March–Oct;8(1–2):82–90.

30. Krishnan S, Justus S, Meluveettil R, Menon RN, Sarma SP, Kishore A. Validity of Montreal Cognitive Assessment in non-English speaking patients with Parkinson's disease. Neurol India [Internet]. 2015 Mar 4 [cited 2021 Jun 18];63:63–7.

31. Nasreddine ZS, Phillips NA, Bédirian V, Charbonneau S, Whitehead V, Collin I et al. The Montreal Cognitive Assessment, MoCA: a brief screening tool for mild cognitive impairment. J Am Geriatr Soc [Internet]. 2005 Apr [cited 2021 Jun 18];53(4):695–9. Available from: https://pubmed.ncbi.nlm.nih.gov/15817019/

32. Hota SK, Sharma VK, Hota K, Das S, Dhar P, Mahapatra BB et al. Multi-domain cognitive screening test for neuropsychological assessment for cognitive decline in acclimatized lowlanders staying at high altitude. Indian J Med Res [Internet]. 2012 Sep;136(3):411–20. Available from: https://www.ncbi.nlm.nih.gov/pmc/articles/PMC3510887/

33. George A, Mathuranath PS. Community-based naming agreement, familiarity, image agreement and visual complexity ratings among adult Indians. Ann Indian Acad Neurol. 2007;10:92–9.

34. Rao SL, Subbakrishna DK, Gopukumar K. NIMHANS neuropsychological battery manual. Bangalore (IN): National Institute of Mental Health and Neurosciences; 2004. P. 267.

35. Kar BR, Rao SL, Chandramouli BA, Thennarasu K. Neuropsychological battery for children manual. Bangalore: NIMHANS Publications; 2004.

36. Mukundan CR, Murthy VN. Lateralization and localizing cerebral lesions by a battery of neuropsychological tests. Paper presented at: The Joint Conference of Neurology, Psychiatry, Clinical Psychology and Psychiatric Social Work Societies of India; 1979; National Institute of Mental Health and Neurosciences, Bangalore.

37. Tripathi R, Kumar JK, Bharath S, Marimuthu P, Varghese M. Clinical validity of NIMHANS neuropsychological battery for elderly: a preliminary report. Indian J Psychiatry [Internet]. 2013 Jul;55(3):279–82. Available from: https://pubmed.ncbi.nlm.nih.gov/24082250/

38. Pershad D, Verma SK. Handbook of PGI battery of brain dysfunction. Agra (IN): National Psychological Corporation; 1990. P. 172.

39. Pershad D, Wig NN. Reliability and validity of a new battery of memory tests. Indian J Psychiat. 1978;20:76–80.

40. Verghese J, Noone ML, Johnson B, Ambrose AF, Wang C, Buschke H et al. Picture-based memory impairment screen for dementia. J Am Geriatr Soc [Internet]. 2012 Nov;60(11):2116–20. Available from: https://pubmed.ncbi.nlm.nih.gov/23039180/

41. Iype T, Ajitha BK, Antony P, Ajeeth NB, Job S, Shaji KS. Usefulness of the Rowland Universal Dementia Assessment scale in South India. J Neurol Neurosurg Psychiatry [Internet]. 2006 Apr;77(4):513–4. Available from: https://www.ncbi.nlm.nih.gov/pmc/articles/PMC2077504/

42. Komalasari R, Chang HCR, Traynor V. A review of the Rowland Universal Dementia Assessment Scale. Dementia [Internet]. 2019 Oct–Nov;18(7–8):3143–58. Available from: https://pubmed.ncbi.nlm.nih.gov/30606042/

43. de Jager CA, Thambisetty M, Praveen KV, Sheeba PD, Ajini KN, Sajeev A et al. Utility of the Malayalam translation of the 7-minute screen for Alzheimer's disease risk in an Indian community. Neurol India [Internet]. 2008 Apr–Jun;56(2):161–6. Available from: https://pubmed.ncbi.nlm.nih.gov/18688141/

44. Bhatia T, Shriharsh V, Adlakha S, Bisht V, Garg K, Deshpande SN. The trail making test in India. Indian J Psychiatry. 2007 Apr;49(2):113–6.

45. Stanley R, Kuruvilla A, Kumar S, Gayatrhi K, Mathews P, Abraham V et al. The Vellore screening instruments and strategies for the diagnosis of dementia in the community. Int Psychogeriatr. 2009;21:539–47.

46. Chengappa SK, Kumar R. Normative & Clinical Data on the Kannada Version of Western Aphasia Battery (WAB-K). Lang India. 2008 Jun 1;8(6):5.

47. Kohli A, Kaur M. Wisconsin Card Sorting Test: normative data and experience. Indian J Psychiat. 2006 Jul;48(3):181–4. Available from: https://pubmed.ncbi.nlm.nih.gov/20844649/

48. Carroll BA, Kowal P, Naidoo N, Chatterji S, Kowal P. Measuring cognitive status in older age in lower income countries: results from a pilot of the Study on global AGEing and Adult Health (SAGE). SAGE Working Paper No. 3. 2012 Nov. Available from: http://www.who.int/entity/healthinfo/sage/SAGEWorkingPaper3_Pilot_cognition_Nov12.pdf

Indigenous Canadian (Authors: O'Connell, Panyavin, Bourke-Bearskin, Walker and Bourassa)

Typically employed neuropsychological instruments at the RRMC that **might or might not** be used with Indigenous Peoples who present to the RRMC depending on educational background and cultural context with caveats for interpretation.

Domain	Instrument
Premorbid cognitive status	Advanced Clinical Solutions (ACS)[1]-Word Reading
Suboptimal effort	For all: California Verbal Learning Test-II (CVLT-II)[2] Forced Choice; for those under age 65: ACS[1]-Word Choice
Language	Short Form Boston Naming Test (BNT)[3], Token Test[4]
Visuospatial processing	WMS-IV[5] Block Design, Brief Visuospatial Memory Test-Revised (BVMT-R)[6]; if needed Repeatable Battery for the Assessment of Neuropsychological Status (RBANS)[7]-Line Orientation
Attention and speed of mental processing	WAIS-IV[8] Span and Coding, Delis Kaplan Executive Function System (DKEFS)[9] Trails Visual Scanning, Letter & Number Sequencing, Motor Sequencing; DKEFS[9] Interference Colour & Word Naming
Episodic memory	BVMT-R[6]; CVLT-II[2] short form; WMS-IV[5] Logical Memory
Semantic memory	Short Form BNT[3]; CVLT-II[2] Semantic Clustering; if needed Point & Repeat Test, DKEFS[9] Category Fluency
Executive function	DKEFS[9] Letter Fluency, Category Fluency, Switching; DKEFS[9] Interference, Inhibition, & Inhibition/Switching; DKEFS[9] Trails Number/Letter Switching
Social cognition	Social Norms Questionnaire[10]

If the above tests do not appear appropriate because they do not have normative data for Indigenous Peoples with few years of education or do not appear at all culturally appropriate based on a client's background and context some or all of the following might be given:

Global cognition	Canadian Indigenous Cognitive Assessment[11,12]
Memory	Brief Visuospatial Memory Test-Revised (BVMT-R)[6] only if use of pencil is overlearned
Executive function	Behavioural Assessment of Dysexecutive Syndrome (BADS)[13]—Rule Shift and Problem-Solving Subtasks—qualitative observation vs scoring due to lack of appropriate norms
Language	Boston Diagnostic Aphasia Evaluation (BDAE)[14] qualitatively scored due to lack of appropriate norms
Visuospatial processing	Repeatable Battery for the Assessment of Neuropsychological Status (RBANS)[7]-Line Orientation; if appropriate the color trail making test could also be used

References

1. Wechsler D. Advanced clinical solutions for WAIS®-IV and WMS®-IV: Clinical and interpretive manual. Pearson; 2009.
2. Delis DC, Kramer, J. H., Kaplan, E., Ober, B. A. The California Verbal Learning Test-Second Edition. Psychological Corporation; 2000.
3. Kaplan E, Goodglass H, Weintraub S. Boston naming test. Second edition, Pro-Ed, Austin, Texas: 2001.
4. De Renzi A, Vignolo LA. Token test: a sensitive test to detect receptive disturbances in aphasics. Brain. 1962. 85: p. 665–78.
5. Wechsler D. WMS-IV: Wechsler memory scale-fourth edition. San Antonio, Texas: Pearson; 2009.
6. Benedict RHB. Brief Visuospatial Memory Test - Revised: Professional manual: Psychological Assessment Resources, Inc.; 1997.
7. Randolph C, Tierney MC, Mohr E, Chase TN. The Repeatable Battery for the Assessment of Neuropsychological Status (RBANS): Preliminary Clinical Validity. Journal of Clinical and Experimental Neuropsychology. 1998;20(3):310-9.
8. Drozdick LW, Raiford SE, Wahlstrom D, Weiss LG. The Wechsler Adult Intelligence Scale—Fourth Edition and the Wechsler Memory Scale—Fourth Edition. Contemporary intellectual assessment: Theories, tests, and issues. 4th ed. New York (NY): The Guilford Press; 2018. p. 486–511.
9. Delis DC, Kaplan E, Kramer JH. Delis-Kaplan Executive Function System®(D-KEFS®): Examiner's Manual: flexibility of thinking, concept formation, problem solving, planning, creativity, impluse control, inhibition. Pearson; 2001.
10. Rankin K. Social norms questionnaire. In: Center NAsC, editor. University of Washington; 2013.
11. Jacklin K, Pitawanakwat K, Blind M., O'Connell ME, Walker J, Lemieux AM et al. Developing the Canadian Indigenous Cognitive Assessment for use with Indigenous Older Anishinaabe Adults in Ontario, Canada. Innovation Aging. 2020;4(4):igaa038.
12. Walker J, O'Connell ME, Crowshoe L, Jacklin K, Boeheme G, Hogan D, et al. Adaptation of the Canadian Indigenous Cognitive Assessment in three provinces and evidence for validity. AAIC 2020 Conference Featured Research; 2020.
13. Wilson BA, Alderman N, Burgess P, Emslie H, Evans JJ. Behavioural assessment of the dysexecutive syndrome (BADS). Bury St. Edmunds, England: Thames Valley Test Company; 1996.
14. Roth C. Boston diagnostic aphasia examination. In: Kreutzer JS, DeLuca J, Caplan B, editors. Encyclopedia of clinical neuropsychology. New York (NY): Springer New York; 2011. p. 428–30.

Iranian (Authors: Ramezani, Zamora, Ramezani, and Montero)

The following Persian tests have been found useful in clinical practice:

Test	Citation	Available in Farsi or Persian	Available in English (for bilinguals)
Auditory Verbal Learning or Shiraz Auditory Verbal Learning Test (SAVLT)	Rahmani et al. (2017)[1]	✓	
Bilingual Aphasia Test—Persian or Farsi version	Paradis & Libben (1987); Paradis Paribakht, & Nilipour (1987)[2,3]	✓	✓
Persian Aphasia Battery (PAB)	Nilipour (1993)[4]	✓	
Farsi Aphasia Naming Test	Nilipour (2004, 2011)[5,6]	✓	
Boston Diagnostic Aphasia Test-3 (BDAE-3)	Kaplan, Goodglass, & Weintraub (2001)[7]		✓
Boston Naming Test-2	Kaplan, Goodglass, & Weintraub (2001)[7]		✓
Brief Visuospatial Memory Test-Revised	Benedict (1997); Eshaghi et al. (2012)[8,9]	✓	✓

(Continued)

Test	Citation	Available in Farsi or Persian	Available in English (for bilinguals)
Color Trails Test	D'Elia (1996); Tavakoli, Barekatain, & Emsaki (2015); Avila et al. (2019)[10–12]	✓	✓
Dot Counting Test	Boone, Lu, & Herzberg (2002)[13]		✓
Clock Drawing	Roudsari et al. (2018)[14]	✓	✓
Five Point Test or Ruff Figural Fluency Test	Lee et al. (1997); Ruff (1996)[15,16]		✓
Finger Tapping Test	Reitan (1969)[17]		✓
Grip Strength Test	Reitan, Wolfson (1993)[18]		✓
Line Bisection	Schenkenberg, Bradford, & Ajax (1980)[19]		✓
MMSE Farsi	Seyedian et al. (2008); Ansari et al. (2010)[20,21]	✓	✓
MoCA Farsi	Badrkhahan et al. (2020); Sikaroodi, Yadegari, & Miri (2013)[22,23]	✓	✓
Persian Adult Reading Test or National Adult Reading Test	Haghshenas et al. (2001)[24]	✓	✓
Parallel Picture-Naming Tests	Tahanzadeh, Soleymani, & Jalaie (2017)[25]	✓	
Repeatable Battery for the Assessment of Neuropsychological Status (RBANS) (selected scales)	Randolph (2009)[26]		✓
Rey Auditory Verbal Learning Test (RAVLT)	Jafari et al. (2010); Rezvanfard et al. (2011); Aghamollaei et al. (2012)[27–29]	✓	✓
Rey-15 Item Test	Lezak et al. (2012)[30]		✓
Rey Complex Figure Test	Meyers, Meyers (1995)[31]		✓
Rey-Word Recognition Test	Lezak et al. (2012)[30]		✓
Test of Memory Malingering	Tombaugh (1996)[32]		✓
Test of Nonverbal Intelligence	Brown, Sherbenov, Johnsen (2010)[33]		✓
The Stroop Color and Word Test (Golden Stroop in English and Victoria Stroop in Farsi)	Golden, Freshwater (2002); Malek et al. (2013)[34,35]	✓	✓
Symbol Digit Modality	Smith (1973)[36]		✓
Verbal Fluency (Farsi): JFK, PMK, FAS, Animal, Fruits and Vegetables, Grocery	Ebrahimipour et al. (2008); Dadgar, Khatoonabadi, Bakhtiyari (2013); Ghasemian-Shirvan et al. (2018); Soltani et al. (2019)[37–40]	✓	✓
WCST-64	Avila et al. (2019); Kongs (2000)[12,41]	✓	✓
Wechsler Adult Intelligence Scale (WAIS-IV) (selected subscales)	Wechsler (2008)[42]		✓
Wide Range Achievement Test (WRAT-5)	Wilkinson, Robertson (2017)[43]		✓

Norm tables for memory tests:

Author	Date	Test name	Language	Bilingual	If yes what language	Total sample	Females	Age range
Rahmani	2017	Shiraz Verbal Learning Test (SVLT)	Farsi	No	n/a	1275	676	20–89

SVLT Norms by Age

Test	Gender	20–29			30–44			45–59			60–69			70–79			80–89		
		M	SD	%	M	SD	%	M	SD	%	M	SD	%	M	SD	%	M	SD	%
Total Trails 1–5	Female	61.1	8.77	0	57.2	8.39	0	53.4	7.8	0	50.1	8.19	0	41.8	5.59	0	33.7	3.23	0
	Male	59.5	9.74	68	54.5	8.6	68	53.02	6.68	95	45.5	8.58	98	39.4	6.61	100	35.5	5.67	100
Short-Delay Free Recall	Male	13.5	2.56	84	12.5	2.58	91	11.9	2.53	95	8.2	3.05	99	8.39	3.23	99	6.47	2.07	100
	Female	14.2	1.78	0	13.4	1.93	0	12.7	2.22	0	12.2	2.27	0	11.6	1.43	0	6.14	1.74	0
Short-Delay Cued Recall	Male	13.9	2.03	85	12.9	2.22	92	12.8	2.23	92	10.6	2.46	99	9.6	2.33	100	8.76	1.23	100
	Female	14.5	1.99	0	13.6	1.99	0	12.5	2.28	0	11.9	2.22	0	10.5	2.27	0	8.85	1.98	0
Long-Delay Free Recall	Male	14.1	2.17	81	13.1	2.26	90	12.4	2.15	95	9.3	2.87	99	8.9	2.81	99	6.82	1.76	100
	Female	14.7	1.77	0	13.8	1.94	0	12.9	2.16	0	12.7	2.09	0	11.5	1.44	0	6.85	3.12	1
Long-Delay Cued Recall	Male	14.5	1.78	80	13.5	2.06	89	13.2	2	92	10.7	2.26	99	10.1	1.98	100	9.29	0.93	100

Author	Date	Test name	Language	Bilingual	If yes what language	Total sample	Age range	Education range
Jafari	2010	Rey Auditory-Verbal Learning Test (RAVLT)	Farsi	No	n/a	250	60–80	3–12

Trial	M	SD
RAVLT Trial I	4.8	1.3
RAVLT Trial II	6.31	1.23
RAVLT Trial III	7.71	1.6
RAVLT Trial IV	9.14	1.53
RAVLT Trial V	10.54	1.57
RAVLT Trial B	4	0.95
RAVLT Trial VI (Immediate Recall)	8	1.56
RAVLT Delayed Recall	7.2	1.48
RAVLT Recognition	12.5	1.72

Author	Date	Test name	Language	Bilingual	If yes what language	Total sample	Female	Age range	Education range
Aghamollaei	2012	Rey Auditory-Verbal Learning Test (RAVLT)	Farsi	No	n/a	70	70	60–80	3–12

Trial	M	SD
RAVLT Trial I	8.94	1.91
RAVLT Trial II	11.52	1.72
RAVLT Trial III	13.07	1.41
RAVLT Trial IV	13.67	1.29
RAVLT Trial V	13.7	1.18
RAVLT Trial B	7.64	1.99
RAVLT Trial VI (Immediate Recall)	13.24	1.37
RAVLT Delayed Recall	13.47	1.27
RAVLT Recognition	14.27	0.53

Author	Date	Test name	Language	Bilingual	If yes what language	Total sample	Female	Age range	Education range
Rezvanfard	2011	Rey Auditory-Verbal Learning Test (RAVLT)	Farsi	No	n/a	30	15	31.63 (8.48)	10.50 (6.21)

Trial	M	SD
RAVLT Trial I	7.03	2.43
RAVLT Trial II	9.83	2.32
RAVLT Trial III	11.23	2.3
RAVLT Trial IV	12.23	2.24
RAVLT Trial V	12.57	1.98
RAVLT Trial B	6.07	2.38
RAVLT Trial VI (Immediate Recall)	11.73	2.27
RAVLT Delayed Recall	11.27	2.57
RAVLT Recognition	14.3	1.22

Norm table of verbally mediated or language-based tests

	PMK and animal supermarket fruit fluency								
	Ghasemian-Shirvan et al. (2018) norms data								
	P		*M*		*K*		*Total*		
Age	*M*	*SD*	*M*	*SD*	*M*	*SD*	*M*	*SD*	
15–24	11.65	4.056	13	3.713	12.4	3.858	37.05	10.41	
25–34	11.8	2.648	11.8	3.503	11.6	3.347	35.2	7.777	
35–44	12.05	3.236	11.85	3.703	12.1	3.684	36	8.687	
45–54	13	4.507	12.65	4.38	13.15	4.545	38.8	12.042	
55–65	12.9	3.447	13.4	4.297	13.15	3.066	39.45	8.696	

	Animal		*Supermarket*		*Fruit*		*Total*		
Age	*M*	*SD*	*M*	*SD*	*M*	*SD*	*M*	*SD*	
15–24	20.9	5.647	19.65	5.174	18.55	3.663	59.1	12.993	
25–34	20.35	6.209	20.85	5.687	19.2	5.307	60.4	14.608	
35–44	21.75	4.756	20.75	4.723	18.9	3.11	61.4	9.058	
45–54	23.3	4.244	22.7	4.293	21.55	5.624	67.55	11.45	
55–65	22.05	4.478	22	4.437	19.7	3.729	63.75	9.711	

Author	*Date published*	*Test name*	*Language test administered*	*Total numb*	*Numb females*	*Age*	*Age range*	*Education*	*Edu range*	*Mean*	*SD*
Nejati	2009	Verbal Fluency Test, Fruits and Animals	Persian	124	n/a	41.81	20–69	4.58	n/a	27.53	3.4
		JFK	Persian	124	n/a	41.81	20–69	4.58	n/a	26.24	4.2
Ebrahimpour	2008	Verbal Fluency Test, Animals + Fruit Semantic Verbal Fluency Test	Persian	30	24	31.36	20–45	10	8–12	22.76	4.78
		FAS-Phonemic Verbal Fluency Test	Persian	30	24	31.36	20–45	10	8–12	10.95	3.13
		Verbal Fluency	Persian	30	24	31.36	20–45	10	8–12	16.59	3.66
Eshaghi	2012	Controlled Oral Word Association Test (COWAT)	Persian	90	57	33.65	n/a	14.27	n/a	34.68	12.87

(Continued)

Author	Date published	Test name	Language test administered	Total numb	Numb females	Age	Age range	Education	Edu range	Mean	SD
Eshaghi	2012	Controlled Oral Word Association Test COWAT	Persian	90	57	33.65	n/a	14.27	n/a	34.68	12.87
Dadgar	2013	Verbal Fluency Test, Animals + Fruit Semantic Verbal Fluency	Persian	n/a	n/a	27–70	n/a	n/a	n/a	34.96	6.45
		FAS-Phonemic Verbal Fluency Test	Persian	n/a	n/a	27–70	n/a	n/a	n/a	22.24	7.65
Soltani	2019	Fruit Semantic Verbal Fluency Test	Persian	12	n/a	n/a	65–82	n/a	n/a	10.83	3.48
		Animals Semantic Verbal Fluency Test	Persian	12	n/a	n/a	65–82	n/a	n/a	16.25	4.67
		FAS Total	Persian	12	n/a	n/a	65–82	n/a	n/a	9.75	4.49
		Verbal Fluency, Fruits Semantic Verbal Fluency Test	Persian	12	n/a	n/a	65–82	n/a	n/a	10.83	3.48
		Animals Semantic Verbal Fluency Test	Persian	12	n/a	n/a	65–82	n/a	n/a	16.25	4.67
		FAS Total	Persian	12	n/a	n/a	65–82	n/a	n/a	26.91	11.99

Author	Date published	Test name	Language test administered	Total numb	Numb females	Age	Age range	Education	Edu range	Mean	SD
Nilipour R. [Persian Aphasia Battery (PAB) (Persian)]. Tehran: Iran University of Medical Sciences	1993	Persian Naming Test	Persian	n/a	n/a	n/a	n/a	n/a	n/a	50/50 Raw score	n/a

(Continued)

Author	Date published	Test name	Language test administered	Total numb	Numb females	Age	Age range	Education	Edu range	Mean	SD
Yadeghari	2008	Persian Naming Test	Persian	n/a	n/a	n/a	60–82	9	n/a	50	n/a
Nilipour R. [Persian Aphasia Battery (PAB) (Persian)]. Tehran: Iran University of Medical Sciences	1993	Persian Aphasia Batter (PAB)	Persian								
		PAB Response to Questions								10/10 Raw score	
		PAB Speech Fluency								10/10 Raw score	
		PAB Syntax								10/10 Raw score	
		PAB Repetition								10/10 Raw score	
		PAB Commands								10/10 Raw score	

Author	Date published	Test name	Language test administered	Total numb	Numb females	Age	Age range	Education	Edu range	Mean	SD
Eshaghi	2012	Persian Adult Reading Test (PART)	Persian	90	57	33.65	n/a Age SD = 9.48	14.27	n/a	41.25	5.74
Hagh-Shenas et al. (2001)	2001	Persian Adult Reading Test (PART)	Persian	75	52	55+	n/a	n/a	n/a		
		Females	Persian							36.9	6.81
		Males	Persian							35	11.6
		Global	Persian							37	6.83

References

1. Rahmani F, Haghshenas H, Mehrabanpour A, Mani A, Mahmoodi M. Shiraz Verbal Learning Test (SVLT): normative data for neurologically intact speakers of Persian. Arch Clin Neuropsychol. 2017;32(5):598–609.
2. Paradis M, Libben G. The assessment of bilingual aphasia. Hillsdale, NJ: Lawrence Erlbaum Associates; 1987.
3. Paradis M, Paribakht TS, Nilipour R. The Bilingual Aphasia Test (Farsi version) [Internet]. Hillsdale, NJ: Laurence Erlbaum Associates Inc.; 1987. Available from: http://mcgill.ca/linguistics/research/bat

4. Nilipour R. Persian Aphasia Battery (PAB). Tehran: Iran University of Medical Sciences Publication; 1993.

5. Nilipour R. Farsi Aphasia Naming Test. Tehran: University of Social Welfare and Rehabilitation Sciences Press; 2004.

6. Nilipour R. Aphasia Naming Test (Revised Version). Tehran: University of Social Welfare and Rehabilitation Sciences Press; 2011.

7. Kaplan E, Goodglass H, Weintraub S. The Boston Naming Test. 2nd ed. Austin, TX: Pro-Ed; 2001.

8. Benedict RHB. Brief Visuospatial Memory Test–Revised. Lutz, FL: PAR; 1997.

9. Eshaghi A, Riyahi-Alam S, Roostaei T, Haeri G, Aghsaei A, Aidi MR et al. Validity and Reliability of a Persian Translation of the Minimal Assessment of Cognitive Function in Multiple Sclerosis (MACFIMS). Clin Neuropsychol. 2012 Aug;26(6):975–84.

10. D'Elia LF, Satz P, Uchiyama CL, White T. Color Trails Test. Lutz, FL: PAR; 1996.

11. Tavakoli M, Barekatain M, Emsaki G. An Iranian normative sample of the color trails test. Psychol Neurosci. 2015;8(1):75–81.

12. Avila JF, Verney SP, Kauzor K, Flowers A, Mehradfar M, Razani J. Normative data for Farsi-speaking Iranians in the United States on measures of executive functioning. Appl Neuropsychol Adult [Internet]. 2019 May 4 [cited 2020 Nov 18];26(3):229–35. Available from: https://www.tandfonline.com/doi/full/10.1080/23279095.2017.1392963

13. Boone K, Lu P, Herzberg DS. The Dot Counting Test. Los Angeles, CA: Western Psychological Services; 2002.

14. Roudsari MS, Kamrani AAA, Foroughan M, Shahboulaghi FM, Karimlou M. Psychometric properties of the Persian version of the Clock Drawing Test (CDT) among the aged people in Iran. Iran J Psychiatry Behav Sci. 2018;12(4):e63386.

15. Lee GP, Strauss E, Loring DW, McCloskey L, Haworth JM, Lehman RAW. Sensitivity of figural fluency on the Five-Point test to focal neurological dysfunction. Clin Neuropsychol. 1997;11(1):59–68.

16. Ruff RM. Ruff Figural Fluency Test. Odessa, FL: PAR; 1996.

17. Reitan RM. Manual for administration of neuropsychological test batteries for adults and children. Tucson, AZ: Neuropsychology Laboratory; 1979.

18. Reitan RM, Wolfson D. The Halstead-Reitan Neuropsychological Test Battery: Theory and clinical interpretation. 2nd ed. Tucson, AZ: Neuropsychology Press; 1993. (vol. 31).

19. Schenkenberg T, Bradford DC, Ajax ET. Line bisection and unilateral visual neglect in patients with neurologic impairment. Neurology. 1980 May 1;30(5):509–17.

20. Seyedian M, Falah M, Nourouzian M, Nejat S, Delavar A, Ghasemzadeh HA. Validity of the Farsi version of mini-mental state examination. J Med Counc IRI. 2008;25(4):408–14.

21. Ansari NN, Naghdi S, Hasson S, Valizadeh L, Jalaie S. Validation of a Mini-Mental State Examination (MMSE) for the Persian population: a pilot study. Appl Neuropsychol. 2010;17(3):190–5.

22. Badrkhahan SZ, Sikaroodi H, Sharifi F, Kouti L, Noroozian M. Validity and reliability of the Persian version of the Montreal Cognitive Assessment (MoCA-P) scale among subjects with Parkinson's disease. Appl Neuropsychol Adult. 2020;27(5):431–9.

23. Sikaroodi H, Yadegari S, Miri SR. Cognitive impairments in patients with cerebrovascular risk factors: a comparison of Mini Mental Status Exam and Montreal Cognitive Assessment. Clin Neurol Neurosurg. 2013 Aug 1;115(8):1276–80.

24. Haghshenas H, Farashbandi H, Mani A, Tahmasbi S. Validity of Persian Adult Reading Test for the estimation of premorbid IQ. Iran J Med Sci. 2001 Jan 1;26(1–2):66–70.

25. Tahanzadeh B, Soleymani Z, Jalaie S. Parallel Picture-Naming Tests: development and psychometric properties for Farsi-speaking adults. Appl Neuropsychol Adult. 2017 Mar 4;24(2):100–7.

26. Randolph C. RBANS update: repeatable battery for the assessment of neuropsychological status. Bloomington, MN: Pearson; 2009.

27. Jafari Z, Moritz PS, Zandi T, Kamrani AA, Malyeri S. Psychometric properties of Persian version of the Rey Auditory-Verbal Learning Test (RAVLT) among the elderly. Iran J Psychiatry Clin Psychol. 2010;16(1):56–64.

28. Rezvanfard M, Ekhtiari H, Noroozian M, Rezvanifar A, Nilipour R, Javan GK. The Rey Auditory Verbal Learning Test: alternate forms equivalency and reliability for the Iranian adult population (Persian version). Arch Iran Med. 2011;14(2):104–9.

29. Aghamollaei M, Jafari Z, Toufan R, Esmaili M, Rahimzadeh S. Evaluation of auditory verbal memory and learning performance of 18–30 year old Persian-speaking healthy women. Audiology. 2012;21(3):32–9.

30. Lezak MD, Howieson DB, Bigler ED, Tranel D. Neuropsychological assessment. 5th ed. New York (NY): Oxford University Press; 2012.

31. Meyers JE, Meyers KR. Rey Complex Figure Test and recognition trial. Lutz, FL: PAR; 1995.

32. Tombaugh TN. Test of memory malingering. Toronto, Canada: Multi-Health Systems; 1996.

33. Brown L, Sherbenov RJ, Johnsen SK. Test of nonverbal intelligence. 4th ed. Austin, TX: Pro-Ed; 2010.

34. Golden CJ, Freshwater SM. The Stroop Color and Word Test: a manual for clinical and experimental uses. Chicago, IL: Stoelting; 2002.

35. Malek A, Hekmati I, Amiri S, Pirzadeh J, Gholizadeh H. The standardization of Victoria Stroop Color-Word Test among Iranian bilingual adolescents. Arch Iran Med. 2013;16(7):380–4.

36. Smith A. Symbol Digit Modality. Los Angeles, CA: Western Psychological Services; 1973.

37. Ebrahimipour M, Shahbeigi S, Jenabi M, Amiri Y, Kamali M. Verbal fluency performance in patients with multiple sclerosis. Iran J Neurol. 2008;7(21):138–42.

38. Dadgar H, Khatoonabadi AR, Bakhtiyari J. Verbal fluency performance in patients with nonde-mented Parkinson's disease. Iran J Psychiatry. 2013;8(1):55–8.

39. Ghasemian-Shirvan E, Shirazi SM, Aminikhoo M, Zareaan M, Ekhtiari H. Preliminary normative data of Persian phonemic and semantic verbal fluency test. Iran J Psychiatry. 2018;13(4):288–95.

40. Soltani M, Moradi N, Rezaei H, Hosseini M, Jasemi E. Comparison of verbal fluency in monolingual and bilingual elderly in Iran. Appl Neuropsychol Adult. 2019;28(1):80–7.

41. Kongs SK, Thompson LL, Iverson GL, Heaton RK. Wisconsin Card Sorting Test—64 Card Version. Lutz, FL: PAR; 2000.

42. Wechsler D. Wechsler Adult Intelligence Scale. 4th ed. Bloomington, MN: PsychCorp; 2008.

43. Wilkinson GS, Robertson GJ. Wide Range Achievement Test. 5th ed. Bloomington, MN: PsychCorp; 2017.

Israeli (Authors: Hoofien and Vakil)

Neuropsychological tests validated in Hebrew:

- Rey Auditory Verbal Learning Test[1]
- Children's Test of Attention[2]
- Verbal Fluency Test[3]
- The Word Memory Test[4]
- Delis-Kaplan Executive Function System Sorting Test[5]
- Patient's Perceived Competency Scale[6]
- Temporal Memory Sequence Test[7]
- The Tactual Span Test[8]

References

1. Vakil E, Blachstein H. Rey AVLT: developmental norms for adults and the sensitivity of different memory measures to age. Clin Neuropsychol. 1997;11:356–69.

2. Vakil E, Greenstein Y, Sheinman M, Blachstein H. Developmental changes in attention tests norms: implications for the structure of attention. Child Neuropsychol. 2009;15:21–39.

3. Kavé G. Phonemic fluency, semantic fluency, and difference scores: normative data for adult Hebrew speakers. J Clin Exp Neuropsychol. 2005;27:690–9.

4. Hegedish O, Hoofien D. Detection of malingered neurocognitive dysfunction among patients with acquired brain injuries: a "Word Memory Test" study. Eur J Psychol Assess. 2012:29(4). doi:10.1027/1015-5759/a000154.

5. Heled E, Hoofien D, Margalit D, Natovich R, Agranov E. The Delis-Kaplan Executive Function System Sorting Test as an evaluative tool for executive functions after severe traumatic brain injury: a comparative study. J Clin Exp Neuropsychol. 2012;34:151–9.

6. Hoofien D, Sharoni L. Reliability and validity of the Hebrew version of the PCRS (Patient Competency Rating Scale) as a measurement of self-awareness after traumatic brain injury. Isr J Psychiatry and Allied Sci. 2006;43:296–305.

7. Hegedish O, Kibilis N, Hoofien D. Preliminary validation of a new measure of negative response bias: the Temporal Memory Sequence Test. Appl Neuropsychol. 2014;22(5):348–54.

8. Heled E, Rotberg S, Yavich R, Hoofien D. Introducing the Tactual Span—a new task for assessing working memory in the tactile modality. Assessment[Internet]. 2020. Available from: https://doi.org/10.1177/1073191120949929

Latin American and Caribbean (Authors: Perez-Delgadillo, Ramos-Usuga, Olabarrieta-Landa, Morel-Valdés, and Arango-Lasprilla)

First author	Year	Title	Country	Population	N	Neuropsychological measures	Normative data
Roselli et al.[1]	1990	Normative Data on The Boston Diagnostic Aphasia Examination in a Spanish speaking population	Colombia	Adults	180	Boston Diagnostic Aphasia Examination	Mean and standard deviation
Allegri et al.[2]	1997	Spanish Boston Naming Test norms	Argentina	Adults	200	Boston Naming Test	Mean and standard deviation
Ostrosky-Solís et al.[3]	1998	Neuropsychological Test Performance in illiterate subjects	Mexico	Adults and adolescents	64	NEUROPSI neuropsychological test battery	Mean and standard deviation
La Rue et al.[4]	1999	Neuropsychological performance of Hispanic and non-Hispanic older adults: an epidemiologic survey	Mexico	Adults	797	WAIS-R Digits Forward, Fuld Object Memory Evaluation, Clock Drawing, the Color Trail Making Test	Mean and standard deviation
Ostrosky-Solís et al.[5]	1999	NEUROPSI: a brief neuropsychological test battery in Spanish with norms by age and educational level	Mexico	Adults and adolescents	800	NEUROPSI neuropsychological test battery	Mean and standard deviation
Ostrosky-Solís et al.[6]	1999	Determination of Normative Criteria and Validation of the SKT for use in Spanish-speaking populations	Mexico	Adults	335	Short Cognitive Performance Test	Mean and standard deviation

(Continued)

First author	*Year*	*Title*	*Country*	*Population*	*N*	*Neuropsychological measures*	*Normative data*
Butman et al.[7]	2000	Fluencia verbal en español, datos normativos en Argentina	Argentina	Adults and adolescents	266	Verbal fluency	Mean and standard deviation
Gómez-Pérez et al.[8]	2006	Attention and Memory Evaluation Across the Life Span: Heterogeneous Effects of Age and Education	Mexico	Adults and children	521	NEUROPSI neuropsychological test battery: attention and memory	Mean and standard deviation
Ostrosky-Solis et al.[9]	2007	Same or different? Semantic verbal fluency across Spanish-speakers from different countries	Mexico	Adults and adolescents	2011	Verbal fluency	Mean and standard deviation
Cherner et al.[10]	2007	Demographically corrected norms for the Brief Visuospatial Memory Test-revised and Hopkins Verbal Learning Test-revised in monolingual Spanish speakers from the US–Mexico border region	Border Mexico–US	Adults	127	Brief Visuospatial Memory Test-revised and the Hopkins Verbal Learning Test-revised	Regression
Fernández et al.[11]	2008	A comparison of normative data for the Trail Making Test from several countries: equivalence of norms and considerations for interpretation	Argentina	Adults	251	Trail Making Test	Mean and standard deviation
Marquez de la Plata et al.[12]	2009	Item analysis of three Spanish naming tests: a cross-cultural investigation	US, Spain, and Colombia	Adults	252	The Texas Spanish Naming Test, Modified Boston Naming Test-Spanish, and the naming subtest from the CERAD	Mean and standard deviation
Rosselli et al.[13]	1993	Developmental norms for the Wisconsin Card Sorting Test in 5- to 12-year-old children	Colombia	Children	233	Wisconsin Card Sorting Test	Mean and standard deviation
Rosselli et al.[14]	2001	Neuropsychological test scores, academic performance, and developmental disorders in Spanish-speaking children	Colombia	Children	290	Handedness questionnaire, Seashore rhythm test, FTT, CVLT–C, BVRT, Picture Vocabulary	Mean and standard deviation

(Continued)

First author	Year	Title	Country	Population	N	Neuropsychological measures	Normative data
Armengol, C.[15]	2002	Stroop test in Spanish Children's Norms	Mexico	Children	349	Stroop Test in Spanish of the Camalli-Kaplan version	Mean and standard deviation
Rosselli et al.[16]	2004	Evaluación Neuropsicológica Infantil (ENI): batería para la educación de niños entre 5 y 16 años de edad. Estudio normativo colombiano	Colombia	Children	252	Evaluación Neuropsicológica Infantil (ENI)	Mean and standard deviation
Gutierrez et al.[17]	2006	Effect of age and level of education on semantic fluency: normative data for Spanish-speaking population	Mexico	Children	2221	Verbal fluency	Mean and standard deviation
Ostroski-Solís et al.[18]	2007	NEUROPSI attention and memory: a neuropsychological Test Battery in Spanish with norms by age and educational level	Mexico	Children	521	NEUROPSI attention and memory	Mean and standard deviation
Galindo et al.[19]	2010	Estandarización de la Figura de Taylor en Población Mexicana	Mexico	Children	2100	Figura de Taylor en Población Mexicana	Mean and standard deviation
Rosselli et al.[20]	2010	Performance of Spanish/English bilingual children on a Spanish-language neuropsychological battery: preliminary normative data	USA (Miami-Denver)	Children	180	Evaluación neuropsicológica infantil (ENI)	Mean and standard deviation
Ardila et al.[21]	2011	Gender differences in cognitive development	Mexico and Colombia	Children	788	Evaluación neuropsicológica en adolescentes: Normas para población de Bucaramanga	Mean and standard deviation
Beltrán Dulcey et al.[22]	2012	Evaluación neuropsicológica en adolescentes: Normas para población de Bucaramanga	Colombia	Children	141	Benton visual retention test, Boston Naming Test, Benton Judgment of Line Orientation, Rey Auditory Verbal Learning Test, Trail Making Test, Verbal fluency, Stroop, Rey Complex Figure Test	Mean and standard deviation

References

1. Rosselli M, Ardila A, Florez A, Castro C. Normative data on the Boston diagnostic Aphasia examination in a Spanish-speaking population. J Clin Exp Neuropsychol. 1990 Mar;12(2):313–22.
2. Allegri RF, Villavicencio AF, Taragano FE, Rymberg S, Mangone CA, Baumann D. Spanish Boston naming test norms. Clin Neuropsychol. 1997 Nov;11(4):416–20.
3. Ostrosky-Solis F, Ardila A, Rosselli M, Lopez-Arango G, Uriel-Mendoza V. Neuropsychological test performance in illiterate subjects. Arch Clin Neuropsychol. 1998 Oct 1;13(7):645–60.
4. LaRue A, Romero LJ, Ortiz IE, Chi Lang H, Lindeman RD. Neuropsychological performance of Hispanic and non-Hispanic older adults: an epidemiologic survey. Clin Neuropsychol. 1999;13(4):474–86.
5. Ostrosky-Solís F, Ardila A, Rosselli M. NEUROPSI: a brief neuropsychological test battery in Spanish with norms by age and educational level. J Int Neuropsychol Soc. 1999 Jul;5(5):413–33.
6. Ostrosky-Solís F, Dávila G, Ortiz X, Vega F, Ramos GG, de Celis M et al. Determination of normative criteria and validation of the SKT for use in Spanish-speaking populations. Int Psychogeriatr. 1999 Jun;11(2):171–80.
7. Butman J, Allegri RF, Harris P, Drake M. Fluencia verbal en español. Datos normativos en Argentina. Medicina (Mex). 2000;60(5 Pt 1):561–4.
8. Gómez-Pérez E, Ostrosky-Solís F. Attention and memory evaluation across the life span: heterogeneous effects of age and education. J Clin Exp Neuropsychol. 2006 May;28(4):477–94.
9. Ostrosky-Solis F, Gutierrez A, Flores M, Ardila A. Same or different? Semantic verbal fluency across Spanish-speakers from different countries. Arch Clin Neuropsychol. 2007 Mar;22(3):367–77.
10. Cherner M, Suarez P, Lazzaretto D, Fortuny L, Mindt M, Dawes S et al. Demographically corrected norms for the Brief Visuospatial Memory Test-revised and Hopkins Verbal Learning Test-revised in monolingual Spanish speakers from the U.S.–Mexico border region. Arch Clin Neuropsychol. 2007 Mar;22(3):343–53.
11. Fernández AL, Marcopulos BA. A comparison of normative data for the Trail Making Test from several countries: equivalence of norms and considerations for interpretation. Scand J Psychol. 2008 Jun;49(3):239–46.
12. Marquez de la Plata C, Arango-Lasprilla JC, Alegret M, Moreno A, Tárraga L, Lara M et al. Item analysis of three Spanish naming tests: a cross-cultural investigation. Arango-Lasprilla JC, editor. NeuroRehabilitation. 2009 Feb 9;24(1):75–85.
13. Rosselli M, Ardila A. Developmental norms for the Wisconsin card sorting test in 5- to 12-year-old children. Clin Neuropsychol. 1993 Apr;7(2):145–54.
14. Rosselli M, Ardila A, Bateman JR, Guzman M. Neuropsychological test scores, academic performance, and developmental disorders in Spanish-speaking children. Dev Neuropsychol. 2001 Aug;20(1):355–73.
15. Armengol CG. Stroop Test in Spanish: children's norms. Clin Neuropsychol. 2002 Feb;16(1):67–80.
16. Rosselli M, Matute Villaseñor E, Ardila A, Botero Gómez VE, Tangarife Salazar GA, Echevarría Pulido SE et al. Evaluación Neuropsicológica Infantil (ENI): batería para la evaluación de niños entre 5 y 16 años de edad. Estudio normativo colombiano. Rev Neurol. 2004;38(08):720.
17. Gutierrez A, Ostrosky-Solis F. Effect of age and level of education on semantic fluency: normative data for Spanish-speaking population. Rev Mex Psicol. 2006;23(1):37–44.
18. Ostrosky-Solís F, Esther Gómez-Pérez Ma, Matute E, Rosselli M, Ardila A, Pineda D. Neuropsi Attention and Memory: a neuropsychological test battery in Spanish with norms by age and educational level. Appl Neuropsychol. 2007 Aug 17;14(3):156–70.
19. Galindo G, Molina V, Cruz MEB, Cruz JS, Zamorano ER. Estandarización de la Figura de Taylor en población mexicana. Salud Ment. 2010;33(4):341–5.
20. Rosselli M, Ardila A, Navarrete MG, Matute E. Performance of Spanish/English bilingual children on a Spanish-language neuropsychological battery: preliminary normative data. Arch Clin Neuropsychol. 2010 May 1;25(3):218–35.
21. Ardila A, Rosselli M, Matute E, Inozemtseva O. Gender differences in cognitive development. Dev Psychol. 2011;47(4):984–90.
22. Beltran Dulcey C, Solis-Uribe G. Evaluación neuropsicológica en adolescentes: Normas para población de Bucaramanga. Rev Neuropsicol Neuropsiquiatría Neurocienc. 2012;12(2):77–93.

Mexico (Authors: Strutt, Diaz Santos, Puente Calzada and Sanchez)

Below are some measures and normative data that were selected for the Chapter 33 case study:

Table 33.2: Measures Administered

Domain	Test	Normative data
Informant Questionnaires	Activities of Daily Living Questionnaire-Spanish Version (ADLQ-SV)	Gleichgerrcht et al., 2009[1]
	Neuropsychiatric Inventory Questionnaire (NPI-Q)	Boada et al., 2002[2]
Patient Questionnaires	Generalized Anxiety Disorder 7-Item Scale (GAD-7)	Garcia-Campayo, et al., 2010[3]
	Patient Health Questionnaire-9 (PHQ-9)	Kroenke, Spitzer, & Williams, 2001[4]
Screener	Mini Mental Status Exam-Spanish Version (MMSE)	Folstein, et al., 1975[5]
Premorbid	WAIS-IV* Information	Wechsler et al., 2014[6]
	Word Accentuation Test-Chicago (WAT-C)	Krueger, Lam, & Wilson, 2006[7]
Attention/Concentration	Verbal Series Attention Test (VSAT)	Strutt, et al. (in review)[8]
	WAIS-IV* Coding	Wechsler et al., 2014[6]
	Stroop (Reading and Color naming)	Rivera et al., 2015[10]
Executive Functioning	WAIS-IV* Similarities	Wechsler et al., 2014[6]
	Color Trails 2	D'Elia et al., 1994[11]
	Stroop (Color-Word)	Rivera et al., 2015[10]
Language	Boston Naming Test (BNT)^	Olabarrieta-Landa et al, 2015[12]
	Ponton Satz BNT	Ponton et al., 1996[13]
	Batería Neuropsicológica en Espanol (BNE) – PMR	Artiola i Fortuny et al., 1999[14]
	Animales & Frutas	Olabarrieta-Landa et al, 2015[15] Benito-Cuadrado et al., 2002[16] Rivera, et al., 2019[17]
Memory	Escala de Memoria de Wechsler, Cuarta edición (WMS-IV)^ Memoria Lógica I, II y Reconocimiento; Reproducción Visual I, II y Reconocimiento	Wechsler D., 2008[18]
	Hopkins Verbal Learning Test-Revised (HVLT-R)	Arango-Lasprilla et al., 2015[19]
Visuospatial	Clock Command & Copy	NA
	WAIS-IV* Visual Puzzles	Wechsler et al., 2014[6]
	Rey Complex Figure Test (RCFT) Copy Trial	Rivera et al., 2015[19]

*Mexican version

^Spaniard version

References

1. Gleichgerrcht, E., Camino, J., Roca, M., Torralva, T., & Manes, F. (2009). Assessment of functional impairment in dementia with the Spanish version of the Activities of Daily Living Questionnaire. Dementia and Geriatric Cognitive Disorders, 28(4), 380–388.

2. Boada, M., Cejudo, J. C., Tarraga, L., Lopez, O. L., & Kaufer, D. (2002). Neuropsychiatric inventory questionnaire (NPI-Q): Spanish validation of an abridged form of the Neuropsychiatric Inventory (NPI). Neurologia (Barcelona, Spain), 17(6), 317–323.
3. García-Campayo, J., Zamorano, E., Ruiz, M. A., Pardo, A., Pérez-Páramo, M., López-Gómez, V., ... & Rejas, J. (2010). Cultural adaptation into Spanish of the generalized anxiety disorder-7 (GAD-7) scale as a screening tool. Health and quality of life outcomes, 8(1), 1–11.
4. Kroenke, K., Spitzer, R. L., & Williams, J. B. W. (2001). The Patient Health Questionnaire (PHQ-9)–overview. J. Gen. Intern. Med, 16, 606–616.
5. Folstein, M. F., Folstein, S. E., & McHugh, P. R. (1975). "Mini-mental state": a practical method for grading the cognitive state of patients for the clinician. Journal of psychiatric research, 12(3), 189–198.
6. Wechsler, D. (2009). Wechsler Adult Intelligence Scale–Fourth Edition (WAIS-IV) Mexican version administration and scoring manual. Monterrey, Mexico, Manual Moderno.
7. Krueger, K. R., Lam, C. S., & Wilson, R. S. (2006). The Word Accentuation Test–Chicago. Journal of Clinical and Experimental Neuropsychology, 28(7), 1201–1207.
8. Strutt, A.M., Scott, B., Fogel, T. (under review). The Verbal Series Attention Test: Performance of Spanish-speaking older adults and the effects of education on a brief attentional screening measure.
9. Williams, J., Rickert, V., Hogan, J., Zolten, A. J., Satz, P., D'Elia, L. F., ... & Light, R. (1995). Children's color trails. Archives of Clinical Neuropsychology, 10(3), 211–223.
10. Rivera, D., Perrin, P. B., Stevens, L. F., Garza, M. T., Weil, C., Saracho, C. P., ... & Arango-Lasprilla, J. C. (2015). Stroop color-word interference test: normative data for the Latin American Spanish speaking adult population. NeuroRehabilitation, 37(4), 591–624.
11. Olabarrieta-Landa, L., Rivera, D., Morlett-Paredes, A., Jaimes-Bautista, A., Garza, M. T., Galarza-del-Angel, J., ... & Arango-Lasprilla, J. C. (2015). Standard form of the Boston Naming Test: Normative data for the Latin American Spanish speaking adult population. NeuroRehabilitation, 37(4), 501–513.
12. Pontón, M. O., Satz, P., Herrera, L., Ortiz, F., Urrutia, C. P., Young, R., ... & Namerow, N. (1996). Normative data stratified by age and education for the Neuropsychological Screening Battery for Hispanics (NeSBHIS): Initial report. Journal of the International Neuropsychological Society, 2(2), 96–104.
13. Artiola-i-Fortuny, L., Hermosillo, D., Heaton, R. K., & Pardee, R. E. (1999). Manual de normas y procedimientos para la bateria neuropsicologia en español. Tuscon. AZ: mPress.
14. Olabarrieta-Landa, L., Rivera, D., Galarza-Del-Angel, J., Garza, M. T., Saracho, C. P., Rodríguez, W., ... & Arango-Lasprilla, J. C. (2015). Verbal fluency tests: Normative data for the Latin American Spanish speaking adult population. NeuroRehabilitation, 37(4), 515–561.
15. Benito-Cuadrado, M. M., Esteba-Castillo, S., Böhm, P., Cejudo-Bolivar, J., & Peña-Casanova, J. (2002). Semantic verbal fluency of animals: a normative and predictive study in a Spanish population. Journal of Clinical and Experimental Neuropsychology, 24(8), 1117–1122.
16. Rivera, D., Olabarrieta-Landa, L., Van der Elst, W., Gonzalez, I., Rodríguez-Agudelo, Y., Aguayo Arelis, A., ... & Arango-Lasprilla, J. C. (2019). Normative data for verbal fluency in healthy Latin American adults: Letter M, and fruits and occupations categories. Neuropsychology, 33(3), 287.
17. Wechsler D. Escala de Memoria de Wechler-IV. Manual de corrección y aplicación. Pearson, 2008.
18. Arango-Lasprilla, J. C., Rivera, D., Garza, M. T., Saracho, C. P., Rodríguez, W., Rodríguez-Agudelo, Y., ... & Perrin, P. B. (2015). Hopkins verbal learning test–revised: Normative data for the Latin American Spanish speaking adult population. NeuroRehabilitation, 37(4), 699–718.
19. Rivera, D., Perrin, P. B., Morlett-Paredes, A., Galarza-del-angel, J., Martinez, C., Garza, M. T., ... & Arango-Lasprilla, J. C. (2015). Rey–Osterrieth Complex Figure–copy and immediate recall: Normative data for the Latin American Spanish speaking adult population. NeuroRehabilitation, 37(4), 677–698.

Moroccan (Dutch) (Authors: Uysal-Bozkir, Franzen, and Goudsmit)

Recommended tests to use with older migrants with low education:

Cognitive domain	Test name	Abbreviation
Screening	Rowland Universal Dementia Assessment Test	RUDAS[a,1]
	Cross-Cultural Dementia Screening Test	CCD[a,2]
Attention/executive functioning	Five Digit Test	FDT[3]
	Corsi block tapping[4]	
	Animal fluency	Norms CNTB[a,5]
	Frontal Assessment Battery	FAB
Memory	Modified Visual Association Test	VAT[a,6]
	Enhanced Cued Recall	ECR[7]
	Recall of Pictures Test	RPT[8]
Language	Picture naming	From CNTB
	Supermarket fluency	CNTB
Visuo-spatial/visuoconstruction	Clock reading test	CRT[9]
	Stick Design Test	SDT[10]
Performance validity	Coin-in-the-hand Test[11]	
Informant questionnaire	Informant Questionnaire for Cognitive Impairment in the elderly	IQCODE[a,12]
GDS	Geriatrics Depression Scale	GDS[a,13,14]

[a]Specifically applicable for the Moroccan context.

References

1. Nielsen TR, Jørgensen K. Cross-cultural dementia screening using the Rowland Universal Dementia Assessment Scale: a systematic review and meta-analysis. Int Psychogeriatr. 2020 Mar 9:1–14.
2. Goudsmit M, Uysal-Bozkir Ö, Parlevliet JL, van Campen JPCM, de Rooij SE, Schmand B. The Cross-Cultural Dementia Screening (CCD): a new neuropsychological screening instrument for dementia in elderly immigrants. J Clin Exp Neuropsychol. 2017 Mar;39(2):163–72.
3. Sedó M. The "Five Digit Test": a color-free, non-reading alternative to the Stroop. Int Neuropsychol Soc Liaison Committee Newsletter. 2004;13:6–7.
4. Corsi PM. Human memory and the medial temporal region of the brain. Dis. Abstr. Intl. 1972;34:891B.
5. Nielsen TR, Segers K, Vanderaspoilden V, Beinhoff U, Minthon L, Pissiota A et al. Validation of a European Cross-Cultural Neuropsychological Test Battery (CNTB) for evaluation of dementia. Int J Geriatr Psychiatry. 2019 January 01;34(1):144–52.
6. Franzen S, van den Berg E, Kalkisim Y, van de Wiel L, Harkes M, van Bruchem-Visser RL et al. Assessment of visual association memory in low-educated, non-Western immigrants with the modified Visual Association Test. Demen Geriatr Cogn Disord. 2019;47(4–6):345–54. doi:10.1159/000501151.
7. Solomon PR, Hirschoff A, Kelly B, Relin M, Brush M, DeVeaux RD et al. A 7 minute neurocognitive screening battery highly sensitive to Alzheimer's disease. Arch Neurol. 1998;55(3):349–55.
8. Nielsen TR, Vogel A, Waldemar G. Comparison of performance on three neuropsychological tests in healthy Turkish immigrants and Danish elderly. Int. Psychogeriatr. 2012;24(9):1515–21. doi:S1041610212000440.
9. Schmidtke K, Olbrich S. (2007). The Clock Reading Test: validation of an instrument for the diagnosis of dementia and disorders of visuo-spatial cognition. Int. Psychogeriatr;19(2):307–21.
10. Baiyewu O, Unverzagt FW, Lane KA, Gureje O, Ogunniyi A, Musick B et al. The Stick Design Test: a new measure of visuoconstructional ability. J Int Neuropsychol Soc. 2005;11(5):598–605.
11. Kapur N. The coin-in-the-hand test: a new "bedside" test for the detection of malingering in patients with suspected memory disorder. J Neurol Neurosur Psychiatry. 1994;57(3):385–6.
12. Goudsmit M, Van Campen J, Franzen S, Van den Berg E, Schilt T, Schmand B. Dementia detection with a combination of informant-based and performance-based measures in low-educated and illiterate elderly migrants. Clin Neuropsychol. 2020 Jan;17:1–19.

13. Uysal-Bozkir Ö, Hoopman R, Rooij SE. Translation and validation of the short Geriatric Depression Scale (GDS-15) among Turkish, Moroccan and Surinamese older migrants in the Netherlands. Submitted. Part of dissertation Uysal, Ö. (2016). Health status of older migrants in the Netherlands: Cross-cultural validation of health scales. University of Amsterdam, The Netherlands. https://dare.uva.nl/search?identifier=5cbc8621-c343-4dae-a9b3-5392b5256af0
14. Uysal-Bozkir Ö. (2016). Health status of older migrants in the Netherlands: cross-cultural validation ofhealthscales.UniversityofAmsterdam,TheNetherlands.https://dare.uva.nl/search?identifier=5cbc8621-c343-4dae-a9b3-5392b5256af0

Additional Readings

Cross-Cultural Neuropsychological Battery (CNTB):

Nielsen TR, Segers K, Vanderaspoilden V, Beinhoff U, Minthon L, Pissiota A, Bekkhus-Wetterberg P, Bjørkløf GH, Tsolaki M, Gkioka M, Waldemar G. Validation of a European Cross-Cultural Neuropsychological Test Battery (CNTB) for evaluation of dementia. Int J Geriatr Psychiatry. 2019 Jan;34(1):144–52.

TULIPA Study: Neuropsychological Assessment:

Franzen S, van den Berg E, Goudsmit M, Jurgens CK, van de Wiel L, Kalkisim Y et al. A systematic review of neuropsychological tests for the assessment of dementia in non-Western, low-educated or illiterate populations. J Int Neuropsychol Soc. 2020 Mar;26(3):331–51.

Effects of Illiteracy on Test Results:

Ardila A, Bertolucci PH, Braga LW, Castro-Caldas A, Judd T, Kosmidis MH et al. Illiteracy: the neuropsychology of cognition without reading. Arch Clin Neuropsychol. 2010 Dec;25(8):689–712. doi:10.1093/arclin/acq079. PMID: 21075867.

Portuguese (Authors: Dores, Geraldo and Guerreiro)

The majority of the instruments for assessing neuropsychological functioning developed in Portugal are commercialized by Hogrefe Editora, Lda. To have access to the instruments available and sold by this publisher, you may consult its website: https://www.hogrefe.com/pt/. You can also find some other instruments at Edipsico, Edições e investigações em Psicologia, Lda (https://www.edipsico.pt/testes.html).

A greater effort on the translation, cultural adaptation, and validation of further neuropsychological tests has been registered in the past few years, namely by members of this team. Here we list some examples of the scientific results of this effort, where some normative data for Portuguese population can be found:

Cavaco S, Gonçalves A, Pinto C, Almeida E, Gomes F, Moreira I et al. Auditory verbal learning test in a large nonclinical Portuguese population. Appl Neuropsychol Adult [Internet]. 2015;22(5):321–31. Available from: https://doi.org/10.1080/23279095.2014.927767
Dias E, Pinto J, Lopes J, Rocha R, Carnero-Pardo C, Peixoto B. Phototest: normative data for the Portuguese population. J Clin Gerontol Geriatr [Internet]. 2015;6(2):59–62. Available from: https://doi.org/10.1016/j.jcgg.2014.09.004
Dores AR, Barbosa F, Carvalho IP, Almeida I, Guerreiro S, Martins da Rocha B et al. An fMRI paradigm based on Williams Inhibition Test to study the neural substrates of attention and inhibitory control. Neurol Sci [Internet]. 2017;38(12):2145–52. Available from: https://doi.org/10.1007/s10072-017-3104-5
Lima M, Duro D, Freitas S, Simões M, Santana I. Validation study of the Toulouse-Piéron cancellation test for Portuguese patients with mild cognitive impairment and Alzheimer's disease. Sinapse. 2019;9(1–2):26–23.
Peixoto B, Machado M, Rocha P, Macedo C, Machado A, Baeta É et al. Validation of the Portuguese version of Addenbrooke's Cognitive Examination III in mild cognitive impairment and dementia. Adv Clin Exp Med [Internet]. 2018;27(6):781–6. Available from: https://doi.org/10.17219/acem/68975

Vicente SG, Ramos-Usuga D, Barbosa F, Gaspar N, Dores AR, Rivera D et al. Regression-based norms for the Hopkins Verbal Learning Test-revised and the Rey-Osterrieth Complex Figure in a sample of Portuguese adult population. Arch Clin Neuropsychol [Internet]. 2020:acaa087. Available from: https://doi.org/10.1093/arclin/acaa087

Vicente SG, Rivera D, Barbosa F, Gaspar N, Dores AR, Macialino, G et al. Normative data for tests of attention and executive functions in a sample of European Portuguese adult population. Aging Neuropsychol Cogn [Internet]. 2020. Available from: https://doi.org/10.1080/13825585.2020.1781768

Vicente SG, Benito-Sánchez I, Barbosa F, Gaspar N, Dores AR, Rivera D et al. Normative data for verbal fluency and object naming tests in a sample of European Portuguese adult population, Appl Neuropsychol Adult [Internet]. 2021. Available from: https://doi.org/10.1080/23279095.2020.1868472

In addition, an effort is being made toward a deeper analysis of the existent tools and programs for neurocognitive rehabilitation, as well as the development of new ones, which you can consult in the below-mentioned scientific papers:

Geraldo A, Dores AR, Coelho B, Ramião E, Castro-Caldas A, Barbosa F. Efficacy of ICT-based neurocognitive rehabilitation programs for Acquired Brain Injury: a systematic review on its assessment methods. Eur Psychol [Internet]. 2018;23:250–64. Available from: https://doi.org/10.1027/1016-9040/a000319

Geraldo A, Azeredo A, Pasion R, Dores AR, Barbosa F. Fostering advances in neuropsychological assessment based on the Research Domain Criteria. Clin Neuropsychol [Internet]. 2019;33(2):327–56. Available from: https://doi.org/10.1080/13854046.2018.1523467

Pinto J, Dores AR, Peixoto B, Geraldo A, Barbosa F. Systematic review of sensory stimulation programs in the rehabilitation of acquired brain injury. Eur Psychol [Internet]. 2020. Available from: https://doi.org/10.1027/1016-9040/a000421

Pinto JO, Dores AR, Geraldo A, Peixoto B, Barbosa F. Sensory Stimulation Programs in Dementia: a systematic review of methods and effectiveness. Expert Rev Neurother [Internet]. 2020;20(12):1229–47. Available from: https://doi.org/10.1080/14737175.2020.1825942

Dores AR, Geraldo A, Carvalho IP, Barbosa F. (). The use of new digital information and communication technologies in psychological counseling during the COVID-19 pandemic. Int J Environ Res Public Health [Internet]. 2020;17(20):7663. Available from: https://doi.org/10.3390/ijerph17207663

Puerto Rican (Authors: Oliveras-Rentas, Vega-Carrero, and Rodríguez-Irizarry)

List of tests used in neuropsychology with norms for the Puerto Rican population living in Puerto Rico:

Test and/or batteries of general cognitive abilities:

- Escala de Inteligencia Wechsler para Adultos, Tercera Edición (Puerto Rico) (EIWA-III PR)[1]
- Escala Wechsler de Inteligencia para Niños, Revisada para Puerto Rico (EIWN-R-PR)[2]
- Raven's Coloured Progressive Matrix (RCPM)[3]

Academic achievement:

- Boehm Test of Basic Concepts[4]

Language:

- Boston Naming Test[5]
- Verbal Fluency test[5,6]
- Token Test[5]
- Peabody Picture Vocabulary Test III[6]

Attention:

- Brief Test of Attention[5]
- Digit-Symbol Modalities Test[5,6]
- Trail Making Test A[5,6]
- Stroop Color-Word Interference Test[5,6]
- Concentration Endurance Test (d2)[6]

Working memory/executive function:[5,6]

- Trail Making Test B[5,6]
- Modified Wisconsin Card Sorting Test[5,6]

Visuospatial:

- Rey Complex Figure Test-Copy[5,6]
- Bender Gestalt Test, Second Edition[7]

Learning/memory:

- Rey Complex Figure Test-Delay[5,6]
- Hopkins Verbal Learning Test[5]
- Child-Learning and Verbal Memory Test[6]

Response effort:

- Test of Memory Malingering[5]

Personality/affect:[4]

- Goodenough draw-a-Person test
- Beck Depression Inventories
- Minnesota Multiphasic Personality Assessment for Adolescents

Behavioral rating:

- Inventario de Comportamiento Escolar Bauermeister[8]
- Child Behavior Checklist[4]

References

1. Wechsler D. Escala de Inteligencia Wechsler para Adultos, Tercera Edición: Manual de Administración y Puntuación. Pearson. New York, NY: 2008.
2. Wechsler D. Escala de Inteligencia Wechsler para Niños, Revisada de Puerto Rico: Manual. Pearson; New York, NY: 1992.
3. Ross-Casiano J. Normalización de la Prueba de Matrices Progresivas Raven – Escala Coloreada para Niños Puertorriqueños de 8 a 11 años de edad. 2013. [Unpublished doctoral dissertation, Ponce School of Medicine and Health Sciences].
4. Roca de Torres I. Perspectiva Histórica sobre la Medición Psicológica en Puerto Rico. Revista Puertorriqueña de Psicología. 2008;19(1):11–48.

5. Arango-Lasprilla JC. Commonly used neuropsychological tests for Spanish speakers: normative data from Latin America. NeuroRehabilitation. 2015;37(42); 489–91.
6. Arango-Lasprilla JC, Rivera D. Normative data for Spanish-language neuropsychological tests A step forward in the assessment of pediatric populations. NeuroRehabilitation. 2017; 41(3): 577–80.
7. Vega M. Bender Visual-Motor Gestalt Test, Second Edition: Norms for Puerto Rican Children Ages Eight to Eleven Years. 2012. [Unpublished doctoral dissertation, Ponce School of Medicine and Health Sciences].
8. Bauermeister JJ, Vargas I, Colberg C, González LE, Carroll J. Development of the Inventario de Comportamiento Escolar (IDCE) for Puerto Rican Children. Hispanic J Behav Sci. 1987;9(1):49–67. doi:10.1177/073998638703090104

Russian (Authors: Piryatinsky and Gold)

Neuropsychological tests available in Russian:

- Validity[1]
- Mini-Mental Status Examination[2]
- CERAD[3]
- Verbal Fluency[4]
- Geriatric Depression Scale (https://web.stanford.edu/~yesavage/ACRC.html)

References

1. Green P. (2003). Word Memory Test. Order information paulgreen@shaw.ca. (Malingering test translated into Spanish, French, German, Dutch, Turkish, Italian, Russian, Hebrew, Portuguese, and Mandarin).
2. Folstein MF, Folstein SE, McHugh PR. Mini-Mental Status Examination. Florida: Psychological Assessment Resources; 1975.
3. Glezerman A, Drexler ML. The Russian Adaptation of the CERAD Battery (CERAD-RA). Arch Clin Neuropsychol. 2001;16:826.
4. Munoz-Sandoval AF, Cummins J, Alvarado CG, Ruef ML. Bilingual verbal ability tests. Illinois: Riverside Publishing; 1998.

South African (Authors: Cockcroft and Laher)

Further Reading

The African Journal of Psychological Assessment is an open access journal that publishes research related to psychological assessment in Africa (https://ajopa.org/index.php/ajopa).
Laher S, Cockcroft K, editors. Psychological assessment in South Africa: research and applications [Internet]. Johannesburg: Wits University Press; 2013. Available from: https://library.oapen.org/handle/20.500.12657/25725
Nell V. Cross-cultural neuropsychological assessment: theory and practice. Hove: Psychology Press; 1999.
Suzuki LA, Ponterotto JG, Meller PJ, editors. Handbook of multicultural assessment: clinical, psychological, and educational applications. 2nd ed. San Fransicso (CA): Jossey-Bass/Wiley; 2001.
Foxcroft C. & Roodt G. An introduction to psychological assessment in the South African context (5th ed.). Oxford University Press; 2019.
Laher S. International Histories of Psychological Assessment. Cambridge University Press; 2021.
The South African Journal of Psychology also publishes research using psychological tests in South Africa (https://us.sagepub.com/en-us/nam/journal/south-african-journal-psychology).

South Korean (Authors: Lee and Jo)

Further Reading

Korean Mini-Mental Status Exam (MMSE-KC): This version of the MMSE is accessible through the Korea Citation Index website (https://www.kci.go.kr/kciportal/main.kci?locale=en) by searching for the phrase "A normative study of the Mini-Mental State Examination in the Korean elderly." Select the article by the full title and the authors Jonginn Woo, Jung Hie Lee, and Woo Sung-IL.

Korean version of the Montreal Cognitive Assessment (K-MoCA): Available for free at: https://www.mocatest.org/pdf_files/test/MoCA-Test-Korean.pdf

Korean version of the Rey Auditory Verbal Learning Test (RAVLT) [10]: The test and norms are in the public domain (Cheong et al., 1999) and available at: http://journal.kisep.com/pdf/002/1999/0021999095.pdf

Korean version of the CERAD (K-CERAD: Consortium to Establish a Registry for Alzheimer's Disease): This can be purchased through Duke University at a modest cost: https://sites.duke.edu/centerforaging/cerad/

Clinical Dementia Rating Scale (CDR): The CDR can be useful in situations where it may be helpful to obtain separate information from informants and patients. The CDR is available in Korean for free at the following site: https://knightadrc.wustl.edu/cdr/cdr.htm

Verbal Fluency Norms: Older patient Korean norms for phonemic fluency and semantic fluency can be found at https://doi.org/10.12963/csd.15272. Korean category fluency norms have also been published [21] as have letter fluency norms [22].

A Korean translation of the Patient Health Questionnaire-9 (PHQ-9) as well as the Generalized Anxiety Disorder-7 (GAD-7) can be found at https://www.phqscreeners.com

Spaniard (Authors: Olabarrieta, López, Wongvalle, Rivera, and Lasprilla)

List of community-specific Spanish norms available:

Year	Authors	Test	Population	Age	Education	Methodology
2004	Campo & Morales (2004)[1]	Verbal Selective Reminding Test	Healthy	18–59 years	6–8 years, 9–12 years, and 13 or more years	Mean and standard deviation
2004	Ser Quijano et al.[2]	Short Portable Mental Status Questionnaire Mini Mental State Examination Benton Orientation Test Bell Test Verbal fluency Clock Drawing Test Trail Making Test Free and Cued Figures Recall Logic Memory Naming, Incidental Recall Delayed Recall Similarities IQCODE Questionnaire of Jorm	Home dwelling elderly	71–99 years	Illiterate No study Incomplete primary education At least primary education	Mean and standard deviation

(Continued)

Year	Authors	Test	Population	Age	Education	Methodology
2007	Periáñez et al.[3]	Trail Making Test	Traumatic brain injury, schizophrenia, and normal ageing	15–80 years	2–19 years	Mean and standard deviation Percentile
2008	Nieto et al.[4]	Phonemic (F, A, M) and semantic (animals)	Healthy	6–11 years		Mean and standard deviation
2009	Choca et al.[5]	Spanish WAIS-III	Healthy	16–94 years	did not complete primary school or <8 years of education, primary school, secondary school, and a university degree	Regression Models
2009	Peña-Casanova et al.[6]	Rey–Osterrieth Complex Figure (Copy and Memory), and Free and Cued Selective Reminding Test	Healthy	50–94 years	0–20 years	Regression Models
2009	Peña-Casanova et al.[7]	Visual Object and Space Perception Battery-Abbreviated, and Judgment of Line Orientation	Healthy	50–94 years	0–20 years	Regression Models
2009	Peña-Casanova et al.[8]	Boston Naming Test and Token Test	Healthy	50–94 years	0–20 years	Regression Models
2009	Peña-Casanova et al.[9]	Stroop Color-Word Interference Test and the Tower of London-Drexel	Healthy	50–94 years	0–20 years	Regression Models
2009	Peña-Casanova et al.[10]	Verbal fluency tests: animals, fruits, vegetables, and kitchen tools categories. Letters P, M, and R. ELF tasks	Healthy	50–94 years	0–20 years	Regression Models
2009	Peña-Casanova et al.[11]	Verbal span, visuospatial span, letter and number sequencing, trail making test, and symbol digit modalities test	Healthy	50–94 years	0–20 years	Regression Models
2010	Morales et al.[12]	Spanish Version of the Verbal Selective Reminding Test	Healthy	15–93 years	Low, average, and high education	Regression Models
2011	Quintana et al.[13]	Abbreviated Barcelona Test	Healthy	50–94 years	0–20 years	Regression Models
2012	Aranciva et al.[14]	Norms for the Boston Naming Test and the Token Test	Healthy	18–49 years	8–20 years	Regression Models

(Continued)

Year	Authors	Test	Population	Age	Education	Methodology
2012	Cancela et al.[15]	Symbol Digit Modalities Test	Home care residents	>55 years	Primary, secondary, university	Regression Models
2012	Tamayo et al.[16]	Span verbal, span Visuospatial, letter-number sequencing, trail making test and symbol digit modalities test	Healthy	18–49 years	8–20 years	Regression Models
2013	Calvo et al.[17]	Visual Object and Space Perception Battery and Judgment of Line Orientation Tests	Healthy	18–49 years	8–20 years	Regression Models
2013	Casals-Coll et al.[18]	Verbal fluency tests: animals, fruits, vegetables, and kitchen tools categories. Letters P, M, and R. ELF tasks	Healthy	18–49 years	8–20 years	Regression Models
2013	Llinàs-Reglà et al.[19]	Stroop Color and Word Test	Healthy	35–74 years	Low (up to 8 years); average (8–12 years); high (>12 years of education)	Regression Models
2013	Ortiz Marqués et al.[20]	Spanish Version of the Rey Auditory-Verbal Learning Test	Healthy	61–95 years	≤4 to ≥12 years	Percentile, Scale Score
2013	Palomo et al.[21]	Rey-Osterrieth Complex Figure (copy and memory) and Free and Cued Selective Reminding Test	Healthy	18–49 years	8–20 years	Regression Models
2013	Rognoni et al.[22]	Stroop Color-Word Interference and Tower of London-Drexel University Tests	Healthy	18–49 years	8–20 years	Regression Models
2014	Casals-Coll[23]	BNT Short-Form	Healthy	50–94 years	0–20 years	Regression Models
2015	Aizpurua & Lizaso[24]	Semantic verbal fluency: 20 semantic categories	Healthy	Younger 17–29 Older adults 55–81	Younger: Mean = 12.0 (SD = 1.0) years Older: Mean = 12.2 (SD = 3.0)	Mean and standard deviation
2015	Alegret et al.[25]	Spanish Version of the Face Name Associative Memory Exam (S-FNAME)	Cognitively normal	50–84 years	Elementary, high school, and Bachelor's degree	Mean and standard deviation
2015	Del Pino et al.[26]	Taylor Complex Figure Test	Healthy	18–90	0–20 years	Regression Models
2016	Contador et al.[27]	37 item Version of the Mini-Mental State Examination	Healthy	67–98 years	Illiterate, read & write, primary school, secondary, or higher	Mean and standard deviation Percentiles

(Continued)

Year	Authors	Test	Population	Age	Education	Methodology
2016	Contador et al.[28]	Semantic verbal fluency: animals and fruits categories	Healthy	67–98 years	Illiterate, read & write, primary school, secondary, or higher	Mean and standard deviation Percentiles
2016	Del Pino et al.[29]	Modified Wisconsin Card Sorting Test	Healthy	18–90	0–20 years	Regression Models
2016	Nieto et al.[30]	Addenbrooke's Cognitive Examination-Revised	Healthy	48–89 years	≤3 to ≥13 years	Regression Models
2016	Ojeda et al.[31]	Montreal Cognitive Assessment Test	Healthy	18–90	0–20 years	Regression Models
2016	Peña[32]	The Salthouse Perceptual Comparison Test	Healthy	18–90	0–20 years	Regression Models
2016	Pérez-Pérez et al.[33]	The Hayling Test	Healthy	19–99 years	0–18 years	Regression Models
2017	Arango-Lasprilla et al.[34]	Rey–Osterrieth Complex Figure— copy and immediate recall (3 minutes)	Healthy	6–17 years	Mean Parents Education 0–26 years	Regression Models
2017	Arango-Lasprilla et al.[35]	Modified Wisconsin Card Sorting Test (M-WCST)	Healthy	6–17 years	Mean Parents Education 0–26 years	Regression Models
2017	Arango-Lasprilla et al.[36]	Trail Making Test	Healthy	6–17 years	Mean Parents Education 0–26 years	Regression Models
2017	Arango-Lasprilla et al.[37]	Symbol Digit Modalities Test	Healthy	6–17 years	Mean Parents Education 0–26 years	Regression Models
2017	Olabarrieta-Landa et al.[38]	Peabody Picture Vocabulary Test-III	Healthy	6–17 years	Mean Parents Education 0–26 years	Regression Models
2017	Olabarrieta-Landa et al.[39]	Verbal fluency tests: animals and fruits, categories. Letters F, A, and S	Healthy	6–17 years	Mean Parents Education 0–26 years	Regression Models
2017	Olabarrieta-Landa et al.[40]	Shortened Version of the Token Test	Healthy	6–17 years	Mean Parents Education 0–26 years	Regression Models
2017	Rivera et al.[41]	Stroop Color-Word Interference Test	Healthy	6–17 years	Mean Parents Education 0–26 years	Regression Models
2017	Rivera et al.[42]	Learning and Verbal Memory Test (TAMV-I)	Healthy	6–17 years	Mean Parents Education 0–26 years	Regression Models
2017	Rivera et al.[43]	Concentration Endurance Test (d2)	Healthy	6–17 years	Mean Parents Education 0–26 years	Regression Models
2017	Contador et al.[44]	Story and Six-Object Memory Recall Tests	Healthy	67–98 years	Educational level: illiterate, read & write primary school, secondary, or higher	Mean and standard deviation Percentiles

(Continued)

Year	Authors	Test	Population	Age	Education	Methodology
2017	Duque et al.[45]	Selective Reminding Test Symbol Digit Modalities Test Verbal fluency (letter P; no letter E) Paced Auditory Serial Attention Test	Healthy	16–60 years	Educational level: basic, average, and advanced studies	Regression Models
2018	Grau-Guinea et al.[46]	B of the Spanish-language Free and Cued Selective Reminding Test	Healthy	18–90	0–20 years	Regression Models
2019	Ladera et al.[47]	The 5 Objects Test	Healthy	15–95	2–17	Mean and standard deviation Percentiles
2019	Muñoz-Machicao et al.[48]	Visual Memory Test based on Snodgrass Pictures (VMT-SP)	Healthy Learning disabilities	7–14 years		Mean and standard deviation
2020	Bonete López et al.[49]	Abbreviated-revised Barcelona	Healthy	55–83 years	0–16	Regression Models
2020	Lara et al.[50]	Episodic Memory and Verbal Fluency Tasks	Non-institutionalized adults	Mean = 66.3 (SD = 10.4)	Mean = 9.9 (SD = 6.1)	Regression Models
2020	Muntal et al.[51]	Repeatable Battery for the Assessment of Neuropsychological Status (RBANS)	Healthy	20–89 years	≤5 to ≥16 years	Regression Models

References

1. Campo P, Morales M. Normative data and reliability for a Spanish version of the verbal Selective Reminding Test. Archives of Clinical Neuropsychology. 2004 Jan 1;19(3):421–35.
2. Ser Quijano T del, García de Yébenes MJ, Sánchez Sánchez F, Frades Payo B, Rodríguez Laso Á, Bartolomé Martínez MP et al. Evaluación cognitiva del anciano. Datos normativos de una muestra poblacional española de más de 70 años. Medicina Clinica. 2004 Jan 1;122(19):727–40.
3. Periáñez JA, Ríos-Lago M, Rodríguez-Sánchez JM, Adrover-Roig D, Sánchez-Cubillo I, Crespo-Facorro B et al. Trail Making Test in traumatic brain injury, schizophrenia, and normal ageing: sample comparisons and normative data. Arch Clin Neuropsychol. 2007 Jan 1;22(4):433–47.
4. Nieto A, Galtier I, Barroso J, Espinosa G. Verbal fluency in school-aged Spanish children: normative data and analysis of clustering and switching strategies. Revista de neurologia. 2008 Jan;46(1):2–6.
5. Choca JP, Krueger KR, De la Torre GG, Corral S, Garside D. Demographic Adjustments for the Spanish Version of the WAIS-III. Arch Clin Neuropsychol. 2009 Sep;24(6):619–29.
6. Peña-Casanova J, Gramunt-Fombuena N, Quiñones-Úbeda S, Sánchez-Benavides G, Aguilar M, Badenes D et al. Spanish Multicenter Normative Studies (NEURONORMA Project): norms for the Rey–Osterrieth Complex Figure (Copy and Memory), and Free and Cued Selective Reminding Test. Arch Clin Neuropsychol. 2009 Jun;24(4):371–93.
7. Peña-Casanova J, Quintana-Aparicio M, Quiñones-Úbeda S, Aguilar M, Molinuevo JL, Serradell M et al. Spanish Multicenter Normative Studies (NEURONORMA project): norms for the visual object and space perception battery-abbreviated, and judgment of line orientation. Arch Clin Neuropsychol. 2009 Jun;24(4):355–70.

8. Peña-Casanova J, Quiñones-Úbeda S, Gramunt-Fombuena N, Aguilar M, Casas L, Molinuevo JL et al. Spanish Multicenter Normative Studies (NEURONORMA project): norms for Boston naming test and Token test. Arch Clin Neuropsychol. 2009 Jun;24(4):343–54.

9. Peña-Casanova J, Quiñones-Úbeda S, Gramunt-Fombuena N, Quintana M, Aguilar M, Molinuevo JL et al. Spanish Multicenter Normative Studies (NEURONORMA project): norms for the Stroop Color-Word Interference Test and the Tower of London-Drexel. Arch Clin Neuropsychol. 2009 Jun;24(4):413–29.

10. Peña-Casanova J, Quiñones-Úbeda S, Gramunt-Fombuena N, Quintana-Aparicio M, Aguilar M, Badenes D et al. Spanish Multicenter Normative Studies (NEURONORMA Project): norms for Verbal Fluency Tests. Arch Clin Neuropsychol. 2009 Jun;24(4):395–411.

11. Peña-Casanova J, Quiñones-Úbeda S, Quintana-Aparicio M, Aguilar M, Badenes D, Molinuevo JL et al. Spanish Multicenter Normative Studies (NEURONORMA project): norms for verbal span, visuospatial span, letter and number sequencing, trail making test, and symbol digit modalities test. Arch Clin Neuropsychol. 2009 Jun;24(4):321–41.

12. Morales M, Campo P, Fernández A, Moreno D, Yáñez J, Sañudo I. Normative data for a six-trial administration of a Spanish version of the Verbal Selective Reminding Test. Arch Clin Neuropsychol. 2010 Dec;25(8):745–61.

13. Quintana M, Peña-Casanova J, Sánchez-Benavides G, Langohr K, Manero RM, Aguilar M et al. Spanish Multicenter Normative Studies (Neuronorma Project): norms for the Abbreviated Barcelona Test. Arch Clin Neuropsychol. 2011 Mar;26(2):144–57.

14. Aranciva F, Casals-Coll M, Sánchez-Benavides G, Quintana M, Manero RM, Rognoni T et al. Estudios normativos españoles en población adulta joven (Proyecto NEURONORMA jóvenes): normas para el Boston Naming Test y el Token Test. Neurología. 2012 Sep 1;27(7):394–9.

15. Cancela JM, Ayán C, Varela S. Valores normativos del "Symbol Digit Modalities Test" de aplicación en poblaciones españolas residentes en geriátricos: un estudio piloto. Actas Espanolas de Psiquiatria. 2012 Dec 11;40(6):299–303.

16. Tamayo F, Casals-Coll M, Sánchez-Benavides G, Quintana M, Manero RM, Rognoni T et al. Estudios normativos españoles en población adulta joven (Proyecto NEURONORMA jóvenes): normas para las pruebas span verbal, span visuoespacial, Letter-Number Sequencing, Trail Making Test y Symbol Digit Modalities Test. Neurología. 2012 Jul 1;27(6):319–29.

17. Calvo L, Casals-Coll M, Sánchez-Benavides G, Quintana M, Manero RM, Rognoni T et al. Estudios normativos españoles en población adulta joven (proyecto NEURONORMA jóvenes): normas para las pruebas Visual Object and Space Perception Battery y Judgment of Line Orientation. Neurología. 2013 Apr 1;28(3):153–9.

18. Casals-Coll M, Sánchez-Benavides G, Quintana M, Manero RM, Rognoni T, Calvo L et al. Estudios normativos españoles en población adulta joven (proyecto NEURONORMA jóvenes): normas para los test de fluencia verbal. Neurología. 2013 Jan 1;28(1):33–40.

19. Llinàs-Reglà J, Vilalta-Franch J, López-Pousa S, Calvó-Perxas L, Garre-Olmo J. Demographically adjusted norms for Catalan older adults on the Stroop Color and Word Test. Arch Clin Neuropsychol. 2013 May;28(3):282–96.

20. Marqués NO, Caro IA, Valiente JMU, Rodríguez SM. Normative data for a Spanish version of the Rey Auditory-Verbal Learning Test in older people. Span J Psychol. 2013 Jul 19;16.

21. Palomo R, Casals-Coll M, Sánchez-Benavides G, Quintana M, Manero RM, Rognoni T et al. Estudios normativos españoles en población adulta joven (proyecto NEURONORMA jóvenes): normas para las pruebas Rey-Osterrieth Complex Figure (copia y memoria) y Free and Cued Selective Reminding Test. Neurología. 2013 May 1;28(4):226–35.

22. Rognoni T, Casals-Coll M, Sánchez-Benavides G, Quintana M, Manero RM, Calvo L et al. Estudios normativos españoles en población adulta joven (proyecto NEURONORMA jóvenes): normas para las pruebas Stroop Color-Word Interference Test y Tower of London-Drexel University. Neurología. 2013 Mar 1;28(2):73–80.

23. Casals-Coll M, Sánchez-Benavides G, Meza-Cavazos S, Manero RM, Aguilar M, Badenes D et al. Spanish Multicenter Normative Studies (NEURONORMA Project): normative data and equivalence of four bnt short-form versions. Arch Clin Neuropsychol. 2014 Feb;29(1):60–74.

24. Aizpurua A, Lizaso I. Datos normativos para respuestas a categorías semánticas en castellano en adultos jóvenes y mayores. Psicológica. 2015;36(2):205–63.

25. Alegret M, Valero S, Ortega G, Espinosa A, Sanabria A, Hernández I et al. Validation of the Spanish Version of the Face Name Associative Memory Exam (S-FNAME) in cognitively normal older individuals. Arch Clin Neuropsychol. 2015 Nov;30(7):712–20.

26. del Pino R, Peña J, Ibarretxe-Bilbao N, Schretlen DJ, Ojeda N. Taylor Complex Figure test: administration and correction according to a normalization and standardization process in Spanish population. Revista de neurologia. 2015 Nov 1;61(9):395–404.

27. Contador I, Bermejo-Pareja F, Fernández-Calvo B, Boycheva E, Tapias E, Llamas S et al. The 37 item Version of the Mini-Mental State Examination: normative data in a population-based cohort of older spanish adults (NEDICES). Arch Clin Neuropsychol. 2016 May;31(3):263–72.

28. Contador I, Almondes K, Fernández-Calvo B, Boycheva E, Puertas-Martín V, Benito-León J et al. Semantic Verbal Fluency: normative data in older Spanish adults from NEDICES population-based cohort. Arch Clin Neuropsychol. 2016 Dec;31(8):954–62.

29. del Pino R, Peña J, Ibarretxe-Bilbao N, Schretlen DJ, Ojeda N. Modified Wisconsin Card Sorting Test: standardization and norms of the test for a population sample in Spain. Revista de neurologia. 2016 Mar 1;62(5):193–202.

30. Nieto A, Galtier I, Hernández E, Velasco P, Barroso J. Addenbrooke's Cognitive Examination-revised: effects of education and age. Normative data for the Spanish speaking population. Arch Clin Neuropsychol. 2016 Nov;31(7):811–8.

31. Ojeda N, Del Pino R, Ibarretxe-Bilbao N, Schretlen DJ, Pena J. Montreal Cognitive Assessment Test: normalization and standardization for Spanish population. Revista de neurologia. 2016 Dec 1;63(11):488–96.

32. Peña J, del Pino R, Ibarretxe-Bilbao N, Schretlen DJ, Ojeda N. The Salthouse Perceptual Comparison Test: normalization and standardization for Spanish population. Revista de neurologia. 2016 Jan 1;62(1):13–22.

33. Pérez-Pérez A, Matias-Guiu JA, Cáceres-Guillén I, Rognoni T, Valles-Salgado M, Fernández-Matarrubia M et al. The Hayling Test: development and normalization of the Spanish version. Arch Clin Neuropsychol. 2016 Aug;31(5):411–9.

34. Arango-Lasprilla JC, Rivera D, Ertl MM, Muñoz Mancilla JM, García-Guerrero CE, Rodríguez-Irizarry W et al. Rey–Osterrieth Complex Figure—copy and immediate recall (3 minutes): normative data for Spanish-speaking pediatric populations. NeuroRehabilitation. 2017;41(3): 593–603.

35. Arango-Lasprilla JC, Rivera D, Nicholls E, Aguayo Arelis A, García de la Cadena C, Peñalver Guia AI et al. Modified Wisconsin Card Sorting Test (M-WCST): normative data for Spanish-speaking pediatric population. NeuroRehabilitation. 2017;41(3):617–26.

36. Arango-Lasprilla JC, Rivera D, Ramos-Usuga D, Vergara-Moragues E, Montero-López E, Adana Díaz LA et al. Trail Making Test: normative data for the Latin American Spanish-speaking pediatric population. NeuroRehabilitation. 2017;41(3):627–37.

37. Arango-Lasprilla JC, Rivera D, Trapp S, Jiménez-Pérez C, Hernández Carrillo CL, Pohlenz Amador S et al. Symbol Digit Modalities Test: normative data for Spanish-speaking pediatric population. NeuroRehabilitation. 2017;41(3):639–47.

38. Olabarrieta-Landa L, Rivera D, Ibáñez-Alfonso JA, Albaladejo-Blázquez N, Martín-Lobo P, Delgado-Mejía ID et al. Peabody Picture Vocabulary Test-III: normative data for Spanish-speaking pediatric population. NeuroRehabilitation. 2017;41(3):687–94.

39. Olabarrieta-Landa L, Rivera D, Lara L, Rute-Pérez S, Rodríguez-Lorenzana A, Galarza-del-Angel J et al. Verbal fluency tests: normative data for Spanish-speaking pediatric population. NeuroRehabilitation. 2017;41(3):673–86.

40. Olabarrieta-Landa L, Rivera D, Rodríguez-Lorenzana A, Pohlenz Amador S, García-Guerrero CE, Padilla-López A et al. Shortened Version of the Token Test: normative data for Spanish-speaking pediatric population. NeuroRehabilitation. 2017;41(3):649–59.
41. Rivera D, Morlett-Paredes A, Peñalver Guia AI, Irías Escher MJ, Soto-Añari M, Aguayo Arelis A et al. Stroop Color-Word Interference Test: normative data for Spanish-speaking pediatric population. NeuroRehabilitation. 2017;41(3):605–16.
42. Rivera D, Olabarrieta-Landa L, Rabago Barajas BV, Irías Escher MJ, Saracostti Schwartzman M, Ferrer-Cascales R et al. Newly developed Learning and Verbal Memory Test (TAMV-I): normative data for Spanish-speaking pediatric population. NeuroRehabilitation. 2017;41(3):695–706.
43. Rivera D, Salinas C, Ramos-Usuga D, Delgado-Mejía ID, Vasallo Key Y, Hernández Agurcia GP et al. Concentration Endurance Test (d2): normative data for Spanish-speaking pediatric population. NeuroRehabilitation. 2017;41(3):661–71.
44. Contador I, Fernández-Calvo B, Boycheva E, Rueda L, Bermejo-Pareja F. Normative data of the Story and Six-Object Memory Recall Tests in older Spanish adults: NEDICES population-based cohort. Arch Clin Neuropsychol. 2017 Dec;32(8):992–1000.
45. Duque P, Oltra-Cucarella J, Fernandez O, Sepulcre J, Grupo de Estudio de la Bateria Neuropsicologica Breve En la Esclerosis Multiple G de E de la BNBE la EM. Brief neuropsychological battery for multiple sclerosis. normative data stratified by age and educational level. Revista de neurologia. 2017 Feb 1;64(3):97–104.
46. Grau-Guinea L, Pérez-Enríquez C, García-Escobar G, Arrondo-Elizarán C, Pereira-Cutiño B, Florido-Santiago M et al. Desarrollo, estudio de equivalencia y datos normativos de la versión española B del Free and Cued Selective Reminding Test. Neurología [Internet]. 2018 Jan 1. https://doi.org/10.1016/j.nrl.2018.02.002
47. Ladera V, Perea MV, García R, Prieto G, Delgado AR. The 5 Objects Test: normative data from a Spanish community sample. NeuroRehabilitation. 2019;44(3):451–6.
48. Muñoz-Machicao JA, Fernández-Alcántara M, Correa-Delgado C, González-Ramírez AR, Pérez García M, Laynez-Rubio C. Visual Memory Test based on Snodgrass Pictures (VMT-SP): a New Neuropsychological Measure of Visual Memory on Children with Learning Disabilities. Universitas Psychologica. 2019 Mar;18(2):1–15.
49. Bonete López B, Oltra-Cucarella J, Lorente Martínez R, Sitges Maciá E. Datos normativos del test Barcelona revisado-abreviado para personas mayores cognitivamente activas. Revista Espanola de Geriatria y Gerontologia. 2020 May 1;55(3):137–46.
50. Lara E, Miret M, Sanchez-Niubo A, Haro JM, Koskinen S, Leonardi M et al. Episodic Memory and Verbal Fluency Tasks: normative data from nine nationally representative samples. J Int Neuropsychol Soc. 2020 Aug 7;1–10.
51. Muntal S, Doval E, Badenes D, Casas-Hernanz L, Cerulla N, Calzado N et al. Nuevos datos normativos de la versión española de la Repeatable Battery for the Assessment of Neuropsychological Status (RBANS) forma A. Neurología. 2020 Jun 1;35(5):303–10.

Taiwanese (Author: Paltzer)

Neuropsychological Tests Appropriate for Use with the Taiwanese-Chinese Speaking Population:

- Boston Naming Test, 30 item, modified for the Chinese population[1]
- Chinese Wechsler Adult Intelligence Scale—Fourth Edition (WAIS-IV)[1,2]
- Color Trails Test[3]
- Finger Tapping Test[5]
- Geriatric Depression Scale (Australian Chinese GDS-15)[6]
- Grooved Pegboard Test[7]

- Hong Kong List Learning Test—Second Edition[8]
- Minnesota Multiphasic Personality Inventory-2-RF (MMPI-2-RF)[9]
- Montreal Cognitive Assessment (MoCA) Chinese Version 7.1 (selections)[10]
- Performance validity tests
- Rey-Osterrieth Complex Figure Test[11]
- Taiwan Frontal Assessment Battery (TFAB)[12]
- Verbal Fluency Test[13]
- Wide Range Achievement Test—Fifth Edition (WRAT-5)[14]
- Wisconsin Card Sorting Test (WCST)[15]

References

1. Cheung RW, Cheung MC, Chan AS. Confrontation naming in Chinese patients with left, right or bilateral brain damage. J Int Neuropsychol Soc. 2004;10:46–53.
2. Wechsler D. Wechsler Adult Intelligence Scale Fourth Edition. NCS Pearson, Inc; 2008.
3. Wechsler D, Chen HY, Chen RH, Hua MC. Chinese Wechsler Adult Intelligence Scale Fourth Edition 魏氏成人智力量表. NCS Pearson Inc: 2015.
4. D'Elia LE, Satz P, Uchiyama CL, White T. Color Trails Test. Odessa: Psychological Assessment Resources;1996.
5. Reitan RM. Manual for administration of neuropsychological test batteries for adults and children (unpublished manuscript). Indianapolis University Medical Center; 1969.
6. Rule BG, Harvey HZ, Dobbs HR. Geriatric Depression Scale for younger adults. Clin Gerontol. 1989;9:37–43.
7. Mathews CG, Klove K. Instruction manual for the adult neuropsychological test battery. Madison: University of Wisconsin Medical School; 1964.
8. Chan AS. Hong Kong List Learning Test, 2nd Edition 香港文字記憶學習測驗第二版. The Chinese University of Hong Kong; 2006.
9. Ben-Porath YS, Tellegen A. Minnesota multiphasic personality inventory-2-restrictired form. University of Minnesota Press; 2011.
10. Nasreddine ZS, Charbonneau S, Whitehead V, Collin I, Cummings JL, Chertkow H. The Montreal cognitive assessment, MoCA: a brief screening tool for mild cognitive impairment. J Am Geriatric Soc. 2005;53:695–9.
11. Meyers JE, Meyers KR. Rey Complex figure test and recognition trial. Odessa: Psychological Assessment Resources; 1995.
12. Budois B, Wong ZL, Hong YS, Yang, CC. Frontal Assessment Battery Taiwan Edition 台灣版額葉評估量表. Chinese Behavioral Science Corporation; 2015.
13. Tombaugh TN, Kozak J, Rees L. Normative data stratified by age and education for two measures of verbal fluency: FAS and animal naming. Arch Clin Neuropsychol. 1999;14:167–77.
14. Wilkinson GS, Robertson GJ. WRAT5. Bloomington: Wide Range Inc./Pearson; 2017.
15. Heaton RK, Chelune GJ, Talley JL, Kay GC, Curtiss G. Wisconsin Cart Sorting Test manual: revised and expanded. Odessa: Psychological Assessment Resources; 1993.

Turkish (Author: Nielsen)

Tests with greater ecological relevance for people who are illiterate:

- Brief Cognitive Screening Battery[1]
- Clock Reading Test[2]
- Cross-Linguistic Naming Test[3]
- Five Digit Test[4]

- Fuld Object Memory Evaluation[5]
- Recall of Pictures Test[6]
- Rowland Universal Dementia Assessment Scale[7]
- Stick Design Test[8]
- Supermarket fluency[9]

References

1. Nitrini R, Caramelli P, Herrera JE, Porto CS, Charchat-Fichman H, Carthery MT et al. Performance of illiterate and literate nondemented elderly subjects in two tests of long-term memory. J Int Neuropsychol Soc. 2004;10(4):634–8.
2. Schmidtke K, Olbrich S. The Clock Reading Test: validation of an instrument for the diagnosis of dementia and disorders of visuo-spatial cognition. Int Psychogeriatr. 2007;19(2):307–21.
3. Ardila A. Toward the development of a cross-linguistic naming test. Arch Clin Neuropsychol. 2007;22(3):297–307.
4. Sedó MA. Five digit Test: Manual. Madrid, Spain: TEA Ediciones; 2007.
5. Fuld P. Fuld Object Memory Evaluation Instruction Manual. Wood Dale (IL): Stoelting; 1981.
6. Nielsen TR, Vogel A, Waldemar G. Comparison of performance on three neuropsychological tests in healthy Turkish immigrants and Danish elderly. Int Psychogeriatr. 2012;24(9):1515–21.
7. Storey JE, Rowland JT, Basic D, Conforti DA, Dickson HG. The Rowland Universal Dementia Assessment Scale (RUDAS): a multicultural cognitive assessment scale. Int Psychogeriatr. 2004;16(1):13–31.
8. Baiyewu O, Unverzagt FW, Lane KA, Gureje O, Ogunniyi A, Musick B et al. The Stick Design Test: a new measure of visuoconstructional ability. J Int Neuropsychol Soc. 2005;11(5):598–605.
9. Strauss E, Sherman EMS, Spreen O. A compendium of neuropsychological tests. Administration, norms, and commentary. 3rd ed. New York (NY): Oxford University Press; 2006.

Venezuelan (Author: Ferreira-Correia)

The book edited by Campagna's (2015) includes normative data for Venezuelan adults from 20 to 79 years of age, from 0 to 17 years of education, on the following tools:

- Mini-Mental Status Examination
- Rey Auditory Verbal Learning Test
- Controlled Oral Association Test
- Benton Temporal Orientation Test
- Clock Drawing Test
- Attention Test
- Trail Making Test
- Set Test

Other publications relevant for the neuropsychological assessment of the Venezuelan population are listed under "Further Reading" section.

Further Reading

Campagna I. Ferreira-Correia A. Hooper Visual Organization Test: psychometric properties and regression-based norms for the Venezuelan population. Appl Neuropsychol Adult. 2021. doi:10.1080/23279095.2 021.1882461
Campagna I, Crespo S. Funcionamiento cognitivo de población venezolana sana. Rev Argent Neuropsicol. 2015;27:1–24.

Campagna I, Ferreira-Correia A, Sojo V, Borges J, Crespo S, León A et al. Atención y Memoria en una Muestra de Pacientes con Quejas de Memoria. Rev Argent Neuropsicol. 2014;24:1–15.

Ferreira Correia A, Campagna I. The Rey Auditory Verbal Learning Test: normative data developed for the Venezuelan population. Arch Clin Neuropsychol. 2014;29(2):206–15. doi:10.1093/arclin/act070

Ramírez CI, Moncada Rodríguez CEA, Baptista T. Validez y confiabilidad del Minimental State Examination (MMSE) y del MMSE modificado (3MS) para el diagnóstico de demencia en Mérida, Venezuela. MedULA. 2011;20(1):128–35.

Campagna Osorio I, Castro A, Gamez M, Rasquin M, Vergara K. Validación del cuestionario de comportamiento multitarea IMMAK. Vitae. 2015;(62):4. http://saber.ucv.ve/ojs/index.php/rev_vit/article/view/9124/8954

Vietnamese (Authors: Tran, Nguyen, Ba and Nguyen)

Lists of available tests with Vietnamese translations and/or normative data:

Measures	Translation	Norm
Cognitive Screener		
Mini Mental State Examination[1]	✓	
Montreal Cognitive Assessment[2]	✓	
Visuospatial/Construction		
CERAD Figure Drawing[3]	✓	✓
WAIS-R Block Design[3,4]	✓	✓
Processing Speed/Attention/Working Memory		
Trail Making Test Part A[3,4]	✓	✓
WAIS-R Digit Span[3,4]	✓	✓
Speech and Language		
Animal Naming[5]	✓	
Bilingual Aphasia Test[6]	✓	
Bilingual Verbal Abilities Test[7]	✓	✓
CCNB Confrontation Naming[3]	✓	✓
CCNB Auditory Comprehension[3]	✓	✓
Learning and Memory		
Common Objects Memory Test[8]	✓	
RAVLT-WHO/UCLA version[9,10]	✓	
Executive Functioning		
Trail Making Test Part B[3,4]	✓	✓
Vietnamese Stroop Test[11]	✓	
WAIS-R Picture Completion[3,4]	✓	✓
Mood Functioning		
Phan Vietnamese Psychiatric Scale[12]	✓	
Vietnamese Depression Scale[13]	✓	
Hopkins Symptom Checklist[14]	✓	
Collateral Measure		
Informant Questionnaire of Cognitive Decline in the Elderly[15]	✓	

References

1. Folstein MF, Folstein SE, McHugh PR. Mini-mental state. A practical method for grading the cognitive state of patients for the clinician. J Psychiatr Res; 1975;12(3):189–98.
2. Nasreddine ZS, Phillips NA, Bedirian V, Charbonneau S, Whitehead V, Collin I, et al. The Montreal Cognitive Assessment, MoCA: A brief screening tool for mild cognitive impairment. J Am Geriatr Soc. 2005;53:695–9.
3. Dick MB, Teng EL, Kempler D, Davis DS, Taussig IM. (2002). The Cross-Cultural Neuropsychological Test Battery (CCNB): Effects of age, education, ethnicity, and cognitive status on performance. In Ferraro FR, editor. Minority and cross-cultural aspects of neuropsychological assessment. Lisse, the Netherlands: Swets & Zeitlinger Publishers; 2002. pp. 17–41.
4. Lezak MD, Howieson DB, Bigler ED, Tranel D. Neuropsychological assessment, 5th edn. New York, NY: Oxford University Press; 2012.
5. Kempler D, Teng EL, Dick M, Taussig IM, Davis DS. The effects of age, education and ethnicity on verbal fluency. J Int Neuropsychol Soc; 1998;4(6):531–8.
6. Paradis M, Libben G. The assessment of bilingual aphasia. Hillsdale, NJ: Erlbaum; 1987.
7. Munoz-Sandoval AF, Cummins, J, Alvarado, CG, Ruef ML. Bilingual verbal ability tests. Itasca, IL: Riverside Publishing; 1998.
8. Kempler D, Teng EL, Taussig M, Dick MB. The common objects memory test (COMT): A simple test with cross-cultural applicability. J Int Neuropsychol Soc; 2010;16:537–45.
9. Maj M, Satz P, Janssen R, Zaudig M, Starace F, D'Elia L, Sughondhabirom B, et al. WHO neuropsychiatric AIDS study, cross-sectional phase II: Neuropsychological and neurological findings. Arch Gen Psychiat; 1994;51:51–61.
10. Mitrushina M, Boone K, Razani J, D'Elia L. Handbook of normative data for neuropsychological assessment, 2nd edn. New York, NY: Oxford University Press; 2005.
11. Doan QT, Swerdlow NR. Preliminary findings with a new Vietnamese Stroop Test. Percept Mot Skills; 1999;89:173–82.
12. Phan T, Steel Z, Silove D. An ethnographically derived measure of anxiety, depression and somatization: The Phan Vietnamese Psychiatric Scale. Transcult Psychiatry; 2004;41(2):200–32.
13. Kinzie JD, Manson SM, Vinh DT, Tolan NT, Anh B, Pho TN. Development and validation of a Vietnamese-language depression rating scale. Am J Psychiatry; 1982;139:1276–81.
14. Mollica RF, Wyshak G, de Marneffe D, Khuon F, Lavelle J. Indochinese versions of the Hopkins Symptom Checklist-25: A screening instrument for the psychiatric care of refugees. Am J Psychiatry; 1987;144(4):497–500.
15. The Informant Questionnaire on Cognitive Decline in the Elderly (IQCODE): A review. Int Psychogeriatr; 2004;16:275–93.

Index

Note: *Italicized* page numbers indicate figures and **bold** indicate tables in the text

For Product Safety Concerns and Information please contact our EU
representative GPSR@taylorandfrancis.com
Taylor & Francis Verlag GmbH, Kaufingerstraße 24, 80331 München, Germany

www.ingramcontent.com/pod-product-compliance
Ingram Content Group UK Ltd.
Pitfield, Milton Keynes, MK11 3LW, UK
UKHW030829080625
459435UK00014B/583